W M McDonnell.

Elements of Medical Genetics

Alan E.H. Emery.

A TEXTBOOK
FOR MIDWIVES

A TEXTBOOK FOR MIDWIVES

BY

MARGARET F. MYLES

S.R.N., S.C.M., H.V.CERT., SISTER TUTOR CERT., M.T.D.

FORMERLY EXAMINER TO CENTRAL MIDWIVES BOARD, SCOTLAND:
PRINCIPAL MIDWIFE TUTOR, SIMPSON MEMORIAL MATERNITY
PAVILION, EDINBURGH: DIRECTOR OF EDUCATION, WOMAN'S
HOSPITAL, DETROIT, U.S.A.: EXAMINER TO CENTRAL MIDWIVES
BOARD, NORTHERN IRELAND: TUTOR, MIDWIFE TEACHERS
DIPLOMA (SCOT.) COURSE

FOREWORD BY

MISS JEAN P. FERLIE

O.B.E., R.G.N., S.C.M.

FORMERLY
MATRON IN CHARGE OF THE SIMPSON
MEMORIAL MATERNITY PAVILION
EDINBURGH

SEVENTH EDITION
REPRINT

CHURCHILL LIVINGSTONE
EDINBURGH AND LONDON
1972

First Edition . . .	1953
Reprinted	1955
Second Edition . . .	1956
Reprinted	1956
Third Edition . . .	1958
Reprinted	1959
Fourth Edition . . .	1961
Reprinted	1962
Fifth Edition . . .	1964
Reprinted	1966
Sixth Edition . . .	1968
Reprinted	1969
Seventh Edition . . .	1971
Reprinted	1972

E.L.B.S. Sixth Edition first published	1968
E.L.B.S. Edition reprinted .	1968
E.L.B.S. Edition reprinted .	1969
Seventh Edition E.L.B.S. .	1971
E.L.B.S. Edition reprinted .	1972

ISBN 0 443 00787 X

PRINTED IN GREAT BRITAIN

FOREWORD

The depth of knowledge and accuracy of statement required in writing a textbook such as this can only be achieved after long and intensive study. Mrs Myles has been a serious student of obstetrics for many years and the soundness of her knowledge has been demonstrated in her teaching of pupil midwives and in the articles on midwifery she has contributed to nursing journals.

That she is an experienced teacher is manifest by the arrangement of the book, the lucidity of the explanations given and the way in which theory and practice are co-related. The excellent illustrations, many of which are reminiscent of her blackboard, have eminent teaching value. Mrs Myles was the first Midwife Tutor appointed to the Simpson Memorial Maternity Pavilion, Edinburgh, and during a period of almost fourteen years prepared 3,000 pupil midwives for the Central Midwives Board Examinations.

This is probably the first textbook for midwives in which practical procedures and obstetrical nursing have been described in such detail. It is commendable that many of the techniques perfected by midwives throughout the years are now recorded.

Great care has been exercised in producing a textbook embracing the practical as well as the theoretical aspects of midwifery and designed to meet the needs of pupil midwives. Tutors may find that, with guidance in the use of the book, individual study by their pupils will be facilitated.

Practising midwives will find a wealth of up-to-date information within the pages of this book and those in domiciliary practice will appreciate that " home treatment " of grave emergencies has been given special consideration. Mrs Myles has always shown great interest in Mothercraft and those who are not accustomed to speaking and demonstrating in public will glean much from her practical advice on the teaching of this important subject.

It is with confidence that I cordially recommend this textbook and wish it every success.

JEAN P. FERLIE.

PREFACE TO THE SEVENTH EDITION

Bringing this edition in line with the modern concepts that are inexorably changing the pattern of obstetric practice has been a challenging and formidable task: both obstetrics and neonatal pædiatrics having advanced rapidly and triumphantly in recent years.

The study of genetics, feto-placental physiology and neonatal biochemistry has added a new dimension to the role of obstetrician and pædiatrician which indirectly involves the midwife in saving and improving the quality of fetal life.

Gleaning new material has necessitated diligent perusal of current obstetric and medical literature including the 5 weekly, 7 monthly journals subscribed to. Selecting subject matter of interest, concern, or use, to midwives, sifting it in the light of one's knowledge and experience demands the constant making of decisions. No new matter or procedure is accepted for publication until it has been exposed to the critical appraisal of an authority in the particular branch of obstetrics, pædiatrics or medical speciality.

It is inevitable in this mechanized age that the seventh edition has a technological bias. The introduction of diagnostic devices such as the diasonograph, cardiotocograph, vital signs and apnoea electronic monitors, have altered but not diminished the need for providing personal patient-centred care, as was predicted by some: in fact this has been enhanced. Midwives must comprehend the basic principles underlying the modern techniques they are required to carry out as members of the obstetric team.

Fifty of the 135 new photographs depict some aspect in which mechanical aids are being employed: phototherapy, umbilical arterial catheterization, vacuum aspiration of uterine contents, intermittent positive pressure ventilation, bronchial suction and lavage. The eight photographs illustrating the mechanics of delivery in face presentation and in face to pubes have been much improved.

The fact that 60 per cent of the copies of this book are sold overseas demands consideration for the needs of midwives in hospitals with few modern facilities, and others working alone 300-600 miles from a doctor. Having to cope with grave obstetrical emergencies may entail resorting to methods no longer practised in the more highly developed centres. Increased awareness of such problems has strengthened my desire to retain the chapter on mechanism of labour. That the subject is often taught by rote does not justify its condemnation. It is my deep conviction that midwives should understand " mechanism " and apply this knowledge to management. Fear in coping with malpresentation in a remote area is reduced when manual dexterity is based on mechanism.

Shoulder dystocia occurs more frequently in the practice of midwives whose knowledge of mechanisms is deficient. Further stress has been laid on prevention and five photographs introduced to illustrate coping with this difficulty.

In dealing with obstetrical emergencies greater emphasis has been laid on prophylaxis: (*a*) education of the expectant mother, (*b*) vigilant prenatal care, (*c*) early recognition and prompt action. Modern management of prolapse of cord is described in greater detail. The timing of Syntometrine combined with controlled cord traction, and the inadvisability of waiting for signs of placental descent have been explained more fully.

New matter includes extracts on endotoxic shock, vasectomy, the non-D.D.A. drug pentazocine (Fortral) that midwives may administer, methoxyflurane (Penthrane) given via the Cardiff inhaler.

Subjects that have been expanded are " light for dates " babies, epidural anæsthesia including the midwives duties, nasogastric and bottle feeding, induction and accelera-tion of labour, genetic counselling. Many outdated words have been deleted from the Glossary to admit terms in current use, e.g. autosomes, trisomy, acid base, metabolic acidosis, cytology, prostaglandins, venography. The conversion of weights and measures used throughout the text are those of the British Standards Institution.

Additional objective and structured questions for revision have been incorporated at the end of each chapter; the practical aspect being dominant. Multiple-choice type were excluded (*a*) for lack of space, (*b*) the author's objection to printing an incorrect statement, which the student may subsequently recall.

Every sentence in the book has been scrutinized with meticulous care; amendments having been made on practically every page. Outmoded matter has been discarded where possible, but inevitably the book is enlarged by over 40 pages because of so much new knowledge, the additional photographs and more detailed questions for revision.

The future social and community service commitments of the midwife are fluid at the moment so any attempt to enlarge on this, in the text, has been deferred until a decision is taken regarding (*a*) reorganization of the medical services, (*b*) unification of the maternity service, (*c*) the deliberations of the Committee on Nursing (Briggs).

MARGARET F. MYLES.

14 ASHLEY PARK SOUTH,
ABERDEEN, 1971.

PREFACE TO THE FIRST EDITION

This book has been written with the aim of presenting the subject of obstetrics from the midwife's point of view and in a form suitable for the pupil midwife. An up-to-date textbook is needed, for recent advances in the practice of obstetrics have created many new methods and a multiplicity of treatments which demand from the midwife some knowledge of the various procedures, as well as familiarity with the necessary equipment. It is the midwife's duty to keep abreast of changing trends.

Whilst the needs of the pupil midwife have been kept constantly in mind (and her mental capacity should not be underestimated), the text contains more than the minimum requirements for the Central Midwives Board examination. It is intended that the book will also provide a reference manual for those actively engaged in the practice of midwifery. The lists of equipment and photographs of the " set up " for various procedures will, it is hoped, be of service in an emergency to those unaccustomed to carrying out such measures.

The author has attempted to present her own mode of teaching in textbook form. Maximum attention has been given to basic principles so that practical skill may be built on a sound foundation. This enables the midwife to apply her methods in different environments and to modify them if necessary when complications arise. Much space has been taken up with explanatory matter in order to give the pupil a real understanding of obstetrics, for unless her knowledge is deep enough to arouse interest and give her confidence she is unlikely to become a practising midwife. Important points are stressed by presenting them from different angles throughout the book, a method of subtle repetition which has proved its value in the classroom. Test questions set at the end of each chapter give the pupil an opportunity of consolidating her ideas and assessing her knowledge as her reading of the subject continues.

No bibliographical references have been given because of the vast number of sources which have been tapped in compiling the text and because pupil midwives become confused when they study from more than one or two textbooks. Few pupils would find time to read widely; for those who desire to broaden their field of study the midwife teacher will recommend suitable books.

Although the midwife is concerned mainly with the normal, she must be competent to recognize and report deviations from it and to deal with the abnormal in an emergency. Due consideration has been given to obstetrical complications and also to disorders of the newborn, for it is realized that prompt recognition of these conditions by the midwife will help to reduce both maternal and fetal mortality.

Mothercraft cannot be dissociated from midwifery, and so great is the contribution of the midwife in this field that a separate chapter has been devoted to the subject. The well-being of both the pregnant woman and the fetus *in utero* is to a great extent dependent on the observance of the laws of health. It is certain that better physical and emotional development of the infant, with a higher survival rate during the first year of life, will result from a combination of antenatal instruction in the care of babies and supervision of the baby at an infant welfare centre.

Psychological aspects of pregnancy, labour, the puerperium, the newborn baby, infertility and the menopause all come within the scope of the practising midwife and therefore have received attention in the appropriate chapters.

The wider implications of childbearing have also been considered, for although the birth of a baby is a very personal matter to the mother, at the same time the ultimate health and well-being of the nation depend upon an efficient obstetric service. It is the duty of the midwife to co-operate with those members of the various branches of medicine and the social services who have as their aim the promotion of health and the prevention of disease.

MARGARET F. MYLES.

14 ASHLEY PARK SOUTH,
ABERDEEN, 1953.

ACKNOWLEDGEMENTS

My indebtedness to Scottish obstetricians, neonatal pædiatricians and medical specialists increases every year. The amount of available new knowledge is colossal and without benefit of their mature judgment in evaluating ideas, procedures, equipment and drugs it would be impossible to present a balanced and accurate account of current trends. For their willingness to share their highly specialized knowledge and to elucidate, to one no longer in practice, the more abstruse subjects such as ultrasonography, neonatal biochemistry, chromosomal and blood coagulation disorders my gratitude is profound. Without having had some verbal explanation by experts it would be extremely difficult to present such subjects in a form acceptable to midwives.

I acknowledge with pleasure the opportunity provided when visiting over 150 maternity hospitals in 16 countries during 1969-1970 to observe their obstetric practice and problems. To the consultants, matrons and tutors who expressed their views regarding the needs of the midwife in training and in practice I tender my thanks. The experience will enable me to write with greater understanding, for those in remote areas when prescribing treatment.

To the matrons and tutors of 18 English hospitals visited I express appreciation of their cordial willingness to discuss all aspects of midwife education and to demonstrate new equipment and procedures. Such contacts are essential in writing a textbook.

Simpson Memorial Maternity Pavilion

My indebtedness to the Simpson Memorial Maternity Pavilion Edinburgh exceeds all others. As in former editions the traditions, teaching and practice of that school permeate the text. Professor R. J. Kellar, C.B.E., continues to afford me the courtesy of using the facilities of " The Simpson ", including the department of photography. The consultants are a constant source of erudite information and competent clinical advice.

Dr John G. Robertson, F.R.C.O.G., with his highly expert knowledge of Rhesus incompatibility is my advisor-in-chief on that subject. His counsel on various aspects of practical obstetrics is always sound and has been invaluable.

Dr M. M. Lees, M.R.C.O.G., clarified some problems regarding the physiology of pregnancy. For his discerning appraisal of some of the newer concepts in diagnosis and treatment I am deeply grateful.

Dr R. K. Galloway, M.R.C.O.G. (now consultant at Bellshill Maternity Hospital), assisted with proficiency, attention to detail and infinite patience in " setting up " for photographs involving cardiotocography, Salings procedure and the use of the Sonicaid to diagnose deep vein thrombosis. For his reading of the script concerning these subjects and suggested alterations I record my thanks.

Dr B. H. Hobson, Director Hormone Laboratory, Department of Obstetrics, Edinburgh University, with exceeding courtesy rewrote the section on immunological pregnancy tests. For the help of a world authority on this subject I express my thanks.

Dr S. H. Davies, Director Department of Hæmatology, endeavoured by discussion to simplify the complex topic of blood coagulation disorders, and responded generously to various other questions on his speciality.

Dr L. S. P. Duncan, Physician-in-charge Diabetic Department, read and amended the section on his subject. Expert advice given in practical terms is invaluable to midwives who assist in the care of diabetic women.

Dr Forrester Cockburn's attainments in research, and experience as a clinical pædiatrician gives him competence to be in charge of the neonatal intensive care unit. His ability to explain difficult scientific investigations and findings in practical terms was invaluable during my many requests for enlightenment. His advice on feeding the baby under 1588 G was gratefully accepted. With dexterity and calm assurance demonstrations were set up for photographic purposes involving electronic vital signs and apnœa monitors, the phototherapy unit, and other equipment. My gratefulness to him is immense.

Dr Nancy Loudon, Medical Officer, Family Planning Clinic, read the script on contraception, suggested radical changes and generously imparted some of her vast knowledge of this topical subject.

Dr N. W. Horne, Chest Physician, scanned the subject-matter on pulmonary tuberculosis and brought some of the statements up to date. The improvements he recommended with his usual perception and consideration were gladly accepted.

Dr D. H. H. Robertson, Physician-in-charge, Venereal Disease Department read with exceeding care the chapter on venereal disease in pregnancy. Because of his very thorough revision in addition to a period of discussion, the subject-matter now reflects modern trends in treatment.

Dr D. W. Lindsay, Radiologist, with his usual courtesy discussed many controversial problems in radiology and with Miss I. R. West, radiographer, provided 6 excellent films of the fetus *in utero* to replace the outworn ones. **Dr Bruce Young, Department** of Radiology, arranged the photographic " set up " of the diasonograph in use and the polaroid diasonogram and X-ray film of the anencephalic fetus. His generous co-operation is much appreciated.

Dr T. Durie, Department of Bacteriology, gave much helpful advice on various aspects of his speciality.

Dr Haldane P. Tait, Principal Child Medical Officer, has kept me accurately informed regarding vital statistics and State benefits to which mother and child are entitled.

To Miss M. Auld, Matron of the Simpson Maternity Pavilion, I am deeply grateful for the cordial way she has welcomed me during repeated visits to " The Simpson ". On each occasion, I have received every consideration in visiting departments, meeting consultants and observing procedures. Over a period of 10 days more than 50 photographs were arranged for by Miss Auld and I was most impressed by the proficiency in her organization of procedures and staff who were concerned directly or indirectly. To her my gratitude is sincerely recorded.

Miss A. S. Grant, Principal Tutor, gave advice and assistance regarding setting up procedures for photography. She has read the proofs of this edition with her usual care and exactitude and made a number of valuable amendments and suggestions on various aspects of obstetric practice. For her continued help and co-operation in assessing new ideas and gleaning corroborative evidence I am greatly indebted.

Miss M. Staples, Labour Ward Superintendent, has on numerous occasions answered my questions on matters of technique and assisted with photography. From her vast experience based on substantial knowledge she has generously expressed her opinion and given advice for which I thank her.

Miss M. Taylor, supervisor of the neonatal intensive care unit, permitted me the benefit of her experience in caring for sick neonates.

Miss M. E. Herbertson, Sister in charge, renal dialysis unit, Edinburgh Royal Infirmary, read and amended the section on acute renal failure. For her excellent advice based on knowledge and clinical experience I gratefully express my thanks.

Aberdeen Maternity Hospital

To **Professor Ian Macgillivray** I record my appreciation of his courtesy in permitting me to visit the hospital and discuss ideas, procedures and problems with members of the medical staff. Professor Macgillivray has given me much wise counsel and the benefit of his research and experience regarding pre-eclampsia and other subjects.

Professor Ross Mitchell has on several occasions given helpful suggestions regarding current trends in neonatal care and in the feeding regimen for low birth weight infants. The privilege extended in allowing me to photograph, in the neonatal intensive care unit, procedures involving electronic and other mechanical equipment is gratefully acknowledged.

Dr Arnold Klopper, F.R.C.O.G., is a scholarly source of information on the endocrinology of reproduction. By brilliant exposition he has clarified obscure facts on the feto-placental unit, endocrine aspects of fertility and hormonal treatment of anovulatory infertility. It is a pleasure to record my gratitude to this world authority.

Dr K. J. Dennis, M.R.C.O.G., has an encyclopædic fund of theoretical knowledge, some of it gleaned from participation in research projects such as on the physiology of pregnancy, labour and the puerperium. Because of considerable clinical acumen his advice is always apt and competent. An innate enthusiasm for communicating renders him the logical person to approach with the many problems that arise in writing a practical text-book for midwives. For his generous help I thank him.

Dr M. E. Tunstall, Obstetric Anæsthetist, has had unique experience in his speciality and I consider myself fortunate in having the opportunity to share the fruits of his knowledge of obstetric analgesia. For his assistance in setting up, with utmost patience and infinite attention to detail, the photographs of epidural anæsthesia as well as reading and improving the script I gratefully record my thanks.

Dr G. Russell, Consultant Pædiatrician, has been most patient in response to many requests for explanation of scientific terms and elaboration of complex subjects, *i.e.* blood gas analyses and the metabolism of abnormal respiratory function. His ability to translate and communicate difficult subject matter in non-technical language has been of tremendous assistance in presenting neonatal intensive nursing care to midwives.

Miss M. Turner, Matron, has been most courteous in allowing me to visit the hospital and observe procedures and discuss new techniques with the nursing staff. For her co-operation and competence in arranging for the setting up of numerous photographs she deserves high praise.

Miss M. Mackay, Principal Tutor, carefully checked the page proofs and made some excellent recommendations. She also participated in the presentation of many photographs depicting classroom technique in the delivery of abnormal presentations. Her willingness to consult the appropriate specialist in obtaining new knowledge has been of tremendous help for which I am duly appreciative.

Miss R. Archibald, Superintendent of labour ward, has contributed her opinions on many practical aspects of labour including induction and kept me informed regarding procedures and drugs in current use. She has carried out a number of minor fact-finding projects and is an invaluable adjuvant when assessing new techniques, instruments and equipment for use in normal and abnormal labour.

Miss Ruth Allan, Sister, intensive care nursery, with her extensive experience in nursing sick newborn babies has always been co-operative in sharing her practical knowledge.

Royal Maternity Hospital, Rottenrow, Glasgow

Dr John C. Maclaurin, Consultant in Charge of the neonatal intensive care unit, gave expert advice on the management of "small for dates" babies and respiratory distress syndrome. He also co-operated generously in setting up for photography, complicated resuscitative procedures including intubation, bronchial suction and lavage. His timely suggestions and amendments to the script were of inestimable worth, for which I gratefully express my thanks.

Miss A. McLellan, Matron, with gracious competence gave every facility and opportunity to study the excellent practice and procedures in the pædiatric unit and arranged for staff and equipment to be available for participation in photographic demonstrations.

Miss J. Steele, Midwife Tutor organized a series of features depicting the latest fashions in baby clothes and equipment for the Mothercraft section.

Mrs M. Mackenzie, Supervisor neonatal intensive care unit, had much to contribute from her extensive and successful experience in the nursing of ill and small babies. It was a privilege to be shown up-to-date electronic equipment and other mechanical devices in use and to be informed regarding the modern drugs and treatment employed. Her contribution to writing suitable captions for the many pictures taken in her Department was considerable and I am most indebted to her.

County Maternity Hospital, Bellshill, Lanarkshire

Miss S. P. O. Bramley, Matron, with her usual efficiency and generosity made excellent arrangements for 14 photographic representations of current obstetric practice involving some of their up-to-date equipment. **Miss I. Strachan, Assistant Matron,** supervised the assembly of the various demonstrations concerned with clinical teaching, and the Tutors **Miss E. C. Caldwell** and **Miss M. L. Brown** showed great originality in setting up practical wall displays. It gives me great pleasure to acknowledge their assistance in enhancing the pictorial educational function of the book.

The 135 new photographs were taken by hospital photographers, **Mr H. C. Gray, Glasgow, Mr T. McFetters, Edinburgh,** and **Mr W. Topp, Aberdeen,** to whom I express thanks for their excellent technical skill.

To the publishers I record my appreciation of their continued efforts in maintaining the high standards of production for which they are renowned. **Mr W. G. Henderson, Managing Director,** generously sanctioned the improvement of many existing illustrations and the introduction of over 130 new ones. I express my gratitude for the freedom of ideas and expression accorded to me in the organization and illustration of subject-matter.

Mr A. D. Lewis, Production Director, deserves the highest praise for his forbearance in coping with the colossal number and complexity of the alterations and for his technical advice and unfailing courtesy throughout what was a prolonged and demanding pursuit.

M. F. M.

ACKNOWLEDGEMENTS OF ILLUSTRATIONS

The author gratefully acknowledges her indebtedness for the use of:

Illustrations

The Nursing Mirror, for permission to use Figs. 463, 464, from articles by the author which have appeared in this journal.

Longmans, Green & Co. Ltd. for permission to use Fig. 39 from Gray's *Anatomy*.

Clinical Photographs

Professor R. J. Kellar (Fig. 476).

Professor A. Duncan (Fig. 321).

Professor W. I. C. Morris (Fig. 115).

Dr G. Douglas Matthew (Figs. 236, 363, 364, 475).

Dr D. W. Lindsay, Radiologist, The Simpson Memorial Maternity Pavilion, kindly reproduced the photographs from X-ray films in Figs. 135, 146, 236, 239, 255, 262, 281, 458, 459, 460, 461, 462, 464.

Dr P. C. Steptoe (Fig. 113).

Dr G. P. Hopkin (Fig. 404).

Messrs E. & S. Livingstone have granted permission to use illustrations from the following works published by them:

Baird: *Combined Textbook of Obstetrics and Gynæcology*.

Batchelor and Murrell: *A Short Manual of Venereal Diseases and Treponematosis*.

Behn: *Exercises after Childbirth*.

Bell, Davidson and Scarborough: *Textbook of Physiology and Biochemistry*.

Craig: *Care of the Newly Born Infant*.

Ellis and Mitchell: *Disease in Infancy and Childhood*.

Heardman: *A Way to Natural Childbirth*.

Johnstone: *William Smellie*.

M. F. M.

CONTENTS

xvii

PART V—ABNORMAL LABOUI

PART VI—THE PUERPERIUM

PART VII—THE NEWBORN BABY

PART VIII—MISCELLANEOUS

CONTENTS

1

The Female Pelvis : The Genital Organs

THE BONY PELVIS

The pelvis forms a bony canal through which the fetus must pass during the process of birth, and if the canal is of average shape and dimensions the baby of normal size will negotiate it without difficulty. But pelves vary in size and shape, even within normal limits, so it is essential that the midwife should be competent to recognize

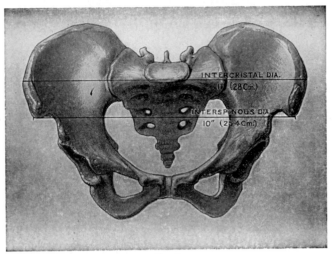

FIG. 1
Normal female pelvis. Pubic arch 90°.

a normal pelvis in the pregnant woman ; she must also be able to detect deviations from normal and the physical characteristics which usually accompany them.

Gross deformities due to maldevelopment or disease are fortunately rare : their diagnosis presents little difficulty and the appropriate treatment, which in such cases is in the hands of the doctor, is usually Cæsarean section.

Knowledge of pelvic anatomy is also needed in the conduct of labour, for the progress made is estimated by the relationship of the fetus to certain pelvic landmarks.

PELVIC BONES

The pelvis is composed of four bones ; two *innominate* or hip bones at the sides and in front, the *sacrum* and *coccyx* behind. The innominate bone consists of three parts the **ilium, ischium** and **os pubis,** which although united by cartilage during childhood, become firmly fused before the 25th year.

2

The ilium is the large flared-out part, and the concave anterior surface of the ala or wing is known as the iliac fossa. The upper curved border is called the iliac crest, the terminal points of which are known as the anterior superior and the posterior superior iliac spines.

The ischium is the lowest part of the innominate bone, and upon the large prominences, known as the *tuberosities* of the ischium, the body rests when in a

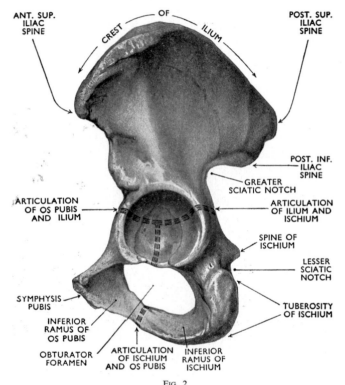

FIG. 2

Left innominate bone, showing important landmarks.

sitting position. Posterior and superior to the tuberosity is a projection, the *spine* of the ischium, which separates the greater and lesser sciatic notches and is an important landmark.

The os pubis consists of a body, a superior and an inferior ramus. Each superior ramus joins the ilium at a slightly roughened point on the brim, the ilio-pectineal eminence. The two inferior rami form the pubic arch, and join the ischium in the lower third of the obturator foramen, an opening in the front of the pelvis covered with membrane. The two pubic bones meet at the symphysis pubis.

The sacrum is a wedge-shaped bone composed of five sacral vertebræ, the first of which is large and projects forwards: the centre of the upper surface of the first sacral vertebra is known as the **promontory of the sacrum.** It is said to be the most important landmark of the pelvis because it encroaches on the antero-posterior diameter of the pelvic inlet and in some cases may prevent the fetal head from entering the brim. The ala or wing of the sacrum articulates with the ilium at the sacro-iliac joint, and the apex or tip articulates with the coccyx at the sacro-coccygeal joint. The anterior surface of the sacrum is concave and is referred to as the *hollow of the sacrum.*

The coccyx is a small bone consisting of four coccygeal vertebræ, tiny nodules of bone, fused together.

PELVIC JOINTS

There are four pelvic joints ; two sacro-iliac, the symphysis pubis and the sacro-coccygeal. In the non-pregnant state there is very little movement in these joints, but during pregnancy a certain amount of softening and stretching of the ligaments takes place, probably due to endocrine activity, which results in slight separation of the joints. In cases where there is a minor degree of disproportion between the fetal head and maternal pelvis, the additional space provided by the " give " of the joints may permit passage of the fetal head.

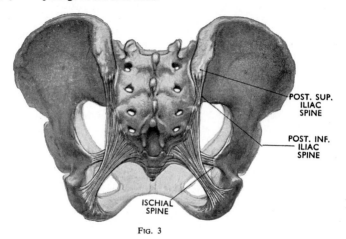

POST. SUP. ILIAC SPINE

POST. INF. ILIAC SPINE

ISCHIAL SPINE

Fig. 3

Posterior view of the pelvis.

The sacro-iliac joint is formed at the articulation of the ala of the sacrum with the ilium, and allows for a limited backward and forward movement of the tip and promontory of the sacrum. During pregnancy there is a good deal of strain on these joints, and multigravid women frequently complain of backache at this time and in the weeks following childbirth.

The symphysis pubis is formed at the junction of the two pubic bones which are united by a pad of cartilage. This joint widens appreciably during the later months of pregnancy, and the degree of movement permitted may give rise to pain on walking.

The sacro-coccygeal joint is formed where the base of the coccyx articulates with the tip of the sacrum, and allows the coccyx to bend backwards during the actual birth of the head.

PELVIC LIGAMENTS

The function of ligaments is to bind bones together, and the ligaments binding the sacrum and ilium at the sacro-iliac joint are the strongest in the whole body. The interpubic ligaments strengthen the symphysis pubis. **The sacro-tuberous ligament** forms an attachment between the sacrum and the tuberosity of the ischium, **the sacro-spinous ligament** connects the sacrum with the spine of the ischium and both ligaments form the posterior wall of the pelvic outlet.

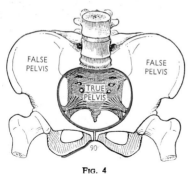

FIG. 4

True and false pelvis.

THE FALSE PELVIS

The bony pelvis is divided into two parts, the false and the true. The false pelvis is that part above the brim and consists mainly of the flared-out iliac bones. It has little obstetrical importance.

THE TRUE PELVIS

The true pelvis is the curved bony canal through which the fetus must pass during birth. It consists of a brim, cavity and outlet.

THE PELVIC BRIM

The pelvic brim is bounded posteriorly by the promontory and alæ of the sacrum, laterally by the ilio-pectineal lines and eminences, and in front by the symphysis pubis. In the gynæcoid or female pelvis the brim is round, except where the promontory of the sacrum projects into it.

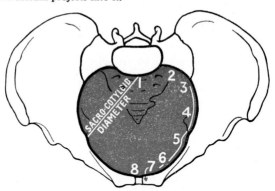

FIG. 5

Brim or inlet of the female pelvis.

1. Promontory of sacrum.	5. Ilio-pectineal eminence.
2. Ala of sacrum.	6. Ramus of os pubis.
3. Sacro-iliac joint.	7. Pubic spine (summit of symphysis).
4. Ilio-pectineal line.	8. Symphysis pubis.

Its size is important, and four diameters are measured :—

1. The antero-posterior.
2. The oblique (right and left).
3. The sacro-cotyloid (right and left).
4. The transverse.

1. **The antero-posterior diameter** is measured from the sacral promontory to a point 1·25 cm. (half an inch) down, on the posterior surface of the symphysis pubis, and measures 10·8 to 11·4 cm. (4¼ to 4½ inches). This measurement is known as the **obstetrical conjugate,** and differs from the true or anatomical conjugate, 12·1 cm. (4¾ inches), which is measured to the summit of the symphysis pubis. As the pubic bone is thick, the obstetrical conjugate *is available* for the passage of the fetal head; not the wider anatomical conjugate.

The diagonal conjugate, the distance from the lower border of the symphysis pubis to the promontory of the sacrum 12·1 to 13·3 cm. (4¾ to 5¼ inches), is measured

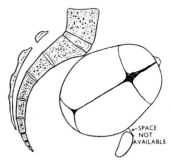

FIG. 6

Note the narrow obstetrical conjugate through which the head must pass. Because of the thickness of the pubic bone, the extra space provided by the anatomical or true conjugate is not available for the passage of the fetal head.

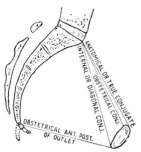

FIG. 7

Median section of the pelvis showing antero-posterior diameters.

per vaginam to assess the length of the antero-posterior diameter of the pelvic brim (see p. 104).

2. **The oblique diameters of the brim** are measured from the sacro-iliac joints to the ilio-pectineal eminences on the opposite sides, and are named right and left, according to the sacro-iliac joint from which they are measured. Both are 11·4 to 12·1 cm. (4½ to 5 inches) in length, but the descending colon encroaches on the left oblique diameter and diminishes the available space. The fetal head sometimes enters in the right oblique diameter of the pelvic brim.

3. **The sacro-cotyloid diameters** measure 8·9 cm. (3½ inches), and lie between the promontory of the sacrum and the ilio-pectineal eminences.

4. **The transverse diameter is the widest part of the brim,** and extends from side to side, immediately behind the ilio-pectineal eminences. It measures 12·7 to 14 cm. (5 to 5½ inches), but is encroached on by the psoas muscles.

THE PELVIC CAVITY

The cavity is the curved canal between the inlet and outlet. The anterior wall is 4·4 cm. (1¾ inches)—the length of the pubic bone. The posterior wall is 12·1 cm. (4¾ inches)—the length of the sacrum and coccyx. The cavity is circular in shape and curves forwards. Its diameters cannot be accurately measured as the cavity is not entirely surrounded by bone, but all the diameters are considered to be 11·4 to 12·7 cm. (4½ to 5 inches).

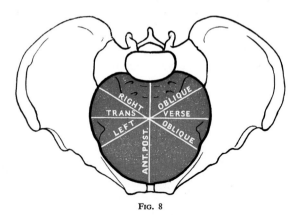

FIG. 8

View of pelvic inlet, showing diameters.

THE PELVIC OUTLET

The upper border of the pelvic outlet is at the level of the ischial spines; the distance between these being known as the **bi-spinous diameter 10·2 cm.** (4 inches). This diameter has great obstetrical importance because it is the transverse measurement of the " narrow pelvic plane."

The lower border of the pelvic outlet is diamond-shaped, and is bounded anteriorly by the pubic arch which, in the gynæcoid pelvis, forms an angle of 90°. Laterally it is bounded by the ischial tuberosities, and posteriorly by the coccyx and sacro-tuberous ligaments.

The antero-posterior diameter is measured from the apex of the pubic arch to the tip of the coccyx, but as the coccyx bends backwards during the birth of the head the diameter is increased by 1·25 cm. (half an inch). This larger diameter is known as the obstetrical antero-posterior diameter, and measures 12·7 cm. (5 inches).

The oblique diameters of the outlet would be measured from the sacro-tuberous ligaments which are not fixed points ; they are therefore not taken.

THE TWO TRANSVERSE DIAMETERS OF THE OUTLET

1. **Bi-spinous** 10·2 cm. (4 inches) at upper boundary of outlet.

2. **Intertuberischial** 10·2 to 10·8 cm. (4 to 4¼ inches) at lower border of outlet extends from the inner borders of the ischial tuberosities.

PELVIC INCLINATION

When a woman is standing in the upright position, her pelvis is not at right angles to her spine, as one might think : the inlet slopes at an angle of 60° with the floor; the tip of the sacrum will be on a level with the summit of the symphysis pubis. The inclination of the cavity is 30°, and at the outlet the inclination is only 11°, being nearly horizontal.

MEASUREMENTS OF THE PELVIC CANAL

	Antero-posterior	Oblique	Transverse
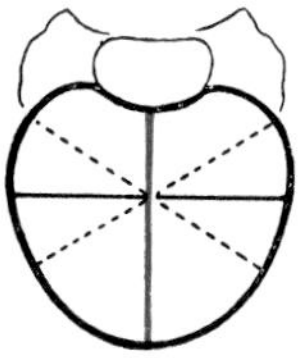 Brim	10·8 to 11·4 cm. 4¼ to 4½ inches	11·4 to 12·7 cm. 4½ to 5 inches	12·7 to 14 cm. 5 to 5½ inches
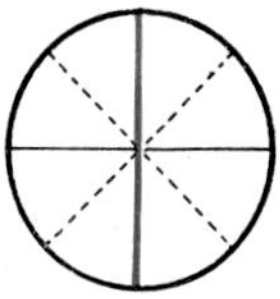 Cavity	11·4 to 12·7 cm. 4½ to 5 inches	11·4 to 12·7 cm. 4½ to 5 inches	11·4 to 12·7 cm. 4½ to 5 inches
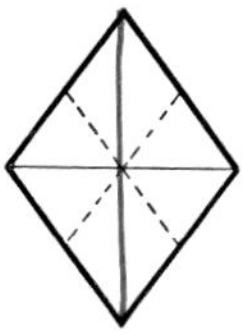 Outlet	12·7 to 14 cm. 5 to 5½ inches	11·4 to 12·7 cm. 4½ to 5 inches	10·2 to 10·8 cm. 4 to 4½ inches

PELVIC PLANES

These are imaginary flat surfaces at various levels of the pelvic canal. The three commonly described are on a level with the brim, cavity and outlet.

The fetus will enter at right angles to the plane of the brim, and the inclination of that plane, as already stated, is 60°. When trying to determine whether the fetal head is small enough to enter the pelvic inlet, the inclination of the plane of the brim should be kept in mind. This will be better understood if Figure 9 is turned sideways to give the impression of a patient in the recumbent position.

Because the plane of the outlet is at an inclination of 11°, it will be necessary for the fetus to turn at an acute angle to enter it. This plane extends from the lower border of the symphysis pubis to the ischial spines and tip of the sacrum.

AXIS OF THE PELVIC CANAL

A line drawn at right angles to the planes of the inlet, cavity and outlet would represent the anatomical axis of the pelvic canal, sometimes known as the curve of

Carus. During the actual birth the midwife facilitates the natural upward curving movement of the baby's head and body.

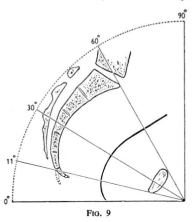

FIG. 9

Median section of true pelvis, showing the inclination of the planes and the axis of the pelvic canal.

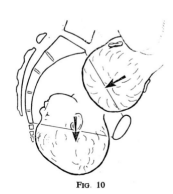

FIG. 10

Fetal head entering plane of pelvic brim and leaving plane of pelvic outlet.

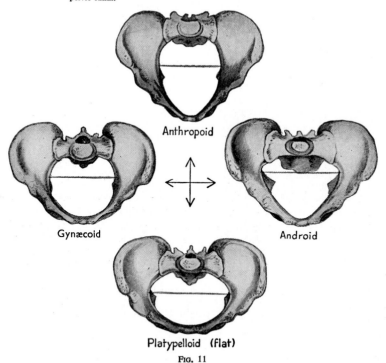

Anthropoid

Gynæcoid

Android

Platypelloid (flat)

FIG. 11

Characteristic inlet of the four types of pelvis. (*Caldwell and Moloy.*)

THE FOUR BASIC TYPES OF PELVIS

Pelves vary in size and shape as much as faces and feet, and women's shoes range from size 2 to 10, with nine widths in each of the average sizes.

Female pelves have been classified by Caldwell and Moloy into four parent groups, according to the shape of the brim.

1. **The gynæcoid,** or true female pelvis, has a round brim.
2. **The android** has a heart-shaped brim.
3. **The anthropoid** has an oval brim, narrow in the transverse.
4. **The platypelloid,** or simple flat pelvis, has a kidney-shaped brim, narrow in the antero-posterior diameter.

The gynæcoid pelvis, is eminently suited for child-bearing. The *brim is round,* except where it is encroached upon by the promontory of the sacrum. *The cavity is shallow* with a broad well-curved sacrum. The greater sciatic notch is wide, the pubic arch forms a right angle, the iliac crest is broad and well curved.

This pelvis would be found in a woman of average build whose hips are broader than her shoulders—**height over 1·6 metres** (5 feet 3 inches), with **shoes size 4 or larger,** and in whom no deformity is evident.

THE PELVIC FLOOR

Although it is desirable that the midwife should be acquainted with the general formation and functions of the pelvic floor, she need not have a detailed knowledge of its anatomy.

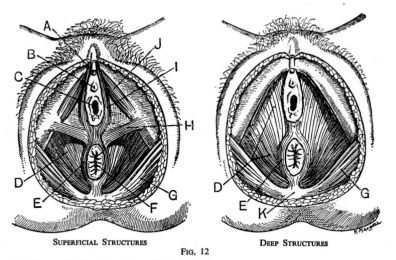

SUPERFICIAL STRUCTURES DEEP STRUCTURES

FIG. 12

(A) Clitoris. (B) Urethral orifice. (C) Vaginal orifice. (D) Levator ani and coccygeus muscles. (E) Sphincter ani externus. (F) Anus. (G) Gluteus maximus. (H) Transverse perinei. (I) Bulbo-cavernosus. (J) Ischio-cavernosus. (K) Coccyx.

It is made up mainly of muscular tissue, but skin, fat, fascia and connective tissue go to form this structure which fills in the irregular-shaped pelvic outlet.

The levatores ani are the most substantial of the six pairs of muscles included in its construction, and by their mode of attachment to the pelvis they act like a sling or hammock. In front they are attached to the lateral part of the os pubis; behind, to the ischial spines and coccyx, and laterally, to the obturator fascia.

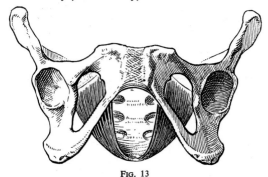

FIG. 13

Diagrammatic representation of the gutter shape of the pelvic floor.

The two levator ani muscles meet to form a gutter which slopes forwards and is perforated by three canals, the *urethra, vagina* and *rectum*. These canals are embraced by fascia which serves to augment the area where they pass through the pelvic floor.

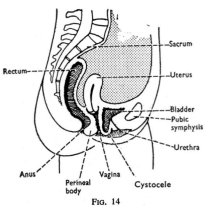

FIG. 14

Note upright backwardly displaced uterus; also cystocele.

The external aspect of the pelvic floor is mainly muscular; the transverse perinei which stretches from the perineum to the ischial tuberosity being the most superficial. The ischio-cavernosus runs from the ischial tuberosity to the region of the clitoris. The bulbo-cavernosus surrounds and strengthens the vaginal orifice and the sphincter ani externus guards the anal canal.

Internally the pelvic floor constitutes the base of the abdominal cavity; it is lined with peritoneum; and the cervix, upper vagina, bladder and rectum are securely anchored in it. These organs are surrounded by connective tissue and sustained by muscle and strong fascial attachments. The connective tissue surrounding the uterus is known as parametrium and it merges with the fascia of the *transverse cervical ligaments* and with the fibres of the levator ani muscles.

INJURY TO PELVIC FLOOR DURING LABOUR

During the last weeks of pregnancy the pelvic floor softens in preparation for labour. If, during the first stage of labour, the patient " bears down "—when she will, of course, be advised to desist—the paracervical tissue and transverse cervical ligaments will be subjected to excessive strain. The uterus may then sag downwards and become retroverted.

When, during the second stage, the fetal head distends the pelvic floor, the perineal body is flattened out until it is quite thin. The stress to which the pelvic floor is subjected may be very great, and an effort should be made to preserve its integrity.

Should the second stage be unduly prolonged, the fascia supporting the bladder may become overstretched; subsequently the anterior vaginal wall prolapses and forms a sac containing bladder, known as a cystocele. When the head is on the perineum too long, the excessive strain to which this structure is subjected will give rise to a lax, sagging pelvic floor that will afford inadequate support to the pelvic organs.

THE VULVA

The term " vulva " is applied to the external genital organs, extending from the mons veneris to the perineum.

The labia majora, or greater lips, are two elongated masses of areolar tissue and fat, covered with skin on their outer surfaces. They arise anteriorly in the mons veneris—a pad of fat lying over the symphysis pubis; posteriorly they merge into

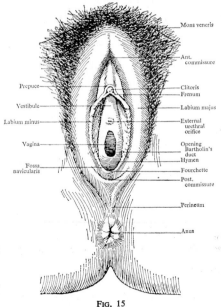

Fig. 15

Female external genital organs.

the perineum; the round ligaments of the uterus are inserted into their anterior portion.

The labia minora are two thin folds of skin, lying between the inner surfaces of the labia majora. Posteriorly they fuse and form a thin fold of skin known as the *fourchette*, or anterior edge of the perineum. In front, the labia minora unite and enclose the clitoris, one fold passing under that structure, the other passing over it like a hood to form the prepuce of the clitoris.

The clitoris, a rudimentary organ analogous to the penis in the male, is a sensitive, highly vascular structure, situated about 2·5 cm. (1 inch) above the external urethral orifice. It serves as a useful landmark in locating this orifice for catheterization when, following childbirth, extensive vulval bruising and laceration are present.

The external urethral orifice is situated in the vestibule, a triangular-shaped area, bounded anteriorly by the clitoris, laterally by the labia minora and posteriorly by the fourchette. Skene's ducts which open on the posterior wall of the urethra just within the orifice are sometimes inflamed, due to infection which may be gonococcal.

The introitus, or orifice of the vagina, is partially closed by the hymen, a thin membrane which tears during the birth of the first child, if it has not previously been torn during coitus. The remaining tags of hymen are known as *carunculæ myrtiformes*.

Bartholin's glands lie embedded in the posterior region of the labia majora, and their ducts open on either side of the vaginal orifice. They secrete a lubricating fluid. If infected, abscess formation may result, and this is frequently, but not invariably, due to the gonococcus. Repeated attacks of infection result in a cystic condition of the gland, which can be recognized on palpating it.

THE PERINEUM

The perineum is the area extending from the fourchette to the anus, and forms the base of the perineal body—a triangular mass of connective tissue, muscle and fat, measuring 3·8 cm. × 3·8 cm. (1½ × 1½ inches). The perineal body fills the wedge-shaped area between the lower ends of the rectum and vagina, and forms a central attachment for the muscles and fascia of the pelvic floor.

INJURY TO PERINEUM

When, during the second stage of labour, the perineal body is flattened out by the descending fetal head, the perineum elongates and becomes so thin that it is liable to tear.

First degree tear. The fourchette only is torn.

Second degree tear. Beyond the fourchette and not involving rectum or anus

Third degree tear. Rectum or anal sphincter is torn.

THE VAGINA

The vagina is a canal extending from the vestibule to the cervix. The posterior wall is 7·6 to 10·2 cm. (3 to 4 inches) long and the anterior wall is 5·1 to 7·6 cm. (2 to 3 inches) being 2·5 cm. (1 inch) shorter because the cervix enters its upper third; the uterus therefore lies almost at right angles to the vagina. The upper end of the vagina is known as the vault and is divided into four arches or fornices by the cervix protruding down into it. The largest arch, known as the posterior fornix, is behind the cervix, the one in front is the anterior fornix, and on the right and left sides are the two lateral fornices.

STRUCTURE

The vagina has four coats and is lined with stratified epithelium which is similar to skin, without the horny layer. This epithelium is thrown into ridges or rugæ which tend to be obliterated with repeated childbearing. The outer connective tissue coat is richly supplied with blood vessels, mainly from the vaginal arteries and branches of the uterine arteries. The muscular layer is not well developed and the vagina is capable of great distension. There are no glands in the vagina; its secretion is a transudation of lymph and cast-off epithelial cells. During pregnancy the vaginal secretion is increased, but if it is profuse, red, purulent, frothy or irritating, this should be investigated.

The acid medium of the vagina tends to inhibit the growth of organisms, and this acidity is maintained by the action of Doderlein's bacillus—a normal inhabitant of the vagina. Certain organisms are found fairly constantly in the vagina, *e.g.* aerobic and anaerobic streptococci, but *not hæmolytic streptococci which are always introduced from without.* Gram-positive cocci and diphtheroids are also found.

ANATOMICAL RELATIONS OF THE VAGINA

The lower half of the anterior wall of the vagina is in close contact with the urethra which runs parallel to it; the upper half is in contact with the *bladder.* (When obtain-

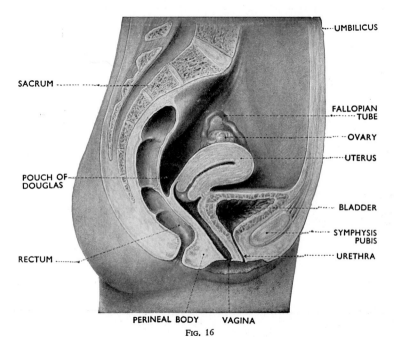

FIG. 16

A median section through the female pelvis, showing bladder, uterus, rectum, vagina and their anatomical relations.

ing a urethral smear for gonococci the gloved finger is inserted into the vagina, and by stroking its anterior wall, secretion can be " milked " from the urethra.) During labour, if difficulty is encountered in inserting a catheter, the gloved finger placed against the anterior wall of the vagina can be used as a guide to direct the catheter into the bladder and thus avoid injury to the urethra.

The lower third of the posterior vaginal wall adjoins the perineal body; the middle part is in apposition with the *rectum,* and it is because of this close proximity of rectum and vagina that rectal examinations may be employed in place of vaginal examinations during labour. **The upper part** is in contact with the peritoneum at the base of the pouch of Douglas. Laterally, the vagina is in relation to the levator ani muscles of the pelvic floor.

THE UTERUS

The uterus, a hollow muscular organ shaped like a flattened pear, is situated in the cavity of the true pelvis, behind the bladder and in front of the rectum. In it the fertilized ovum embeds, is nourished and protected for 40 weeks until, during labour, the fetus is expelled by the powerful contractions of the uterine muscle.

SIZE OF THE UTERUS

The non-pregnant uterus weighs about 57 G. (two ounces) and measures 7·6 × 5·1 × 2·5 cm. (3 × 2 × 1 inches). The corpus or body is 5·1 cm. (2 inches) long, the cervix 2·5 cm. (1 inch) long: the upper part of the corpus is 5·1 cm. (2 inches) broad, the lower part and cervix are 2·5 cm. (1 inch) broad.

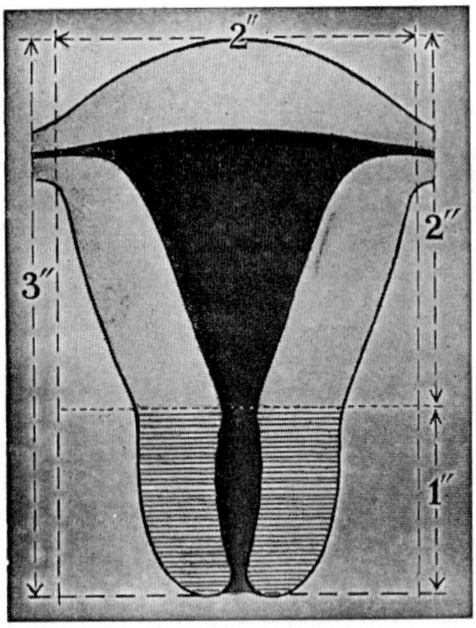

The walls of the uterus are 1·25 cm. (½ inch) thick, and as the anterior and posterior walls are in apposition the thickness of the uterus is 2·5 cm. (1 inch). The cavity is a flat triangular space 6·4 cm. (2½ inches) long, extending from the external cervical os to the fundus.

FIG. 17

Measurements of uterus.

THE CORPUS

The corpus or body forms the greater part of the uterus, and the rounded upper part of the corpus above the insertion of the Fallopian tubes is known as the fundus. The angle where the Fallopian tube is inserted is known as the *cornu* or horn (plural cornua). The body gradually tapers downwards and the constricted area immediately above the cervix is known as the isthmus which distends during pregnancy to form the lower uterine segment.

Endometrium lines the body of the uterus and consists of columnar epithelium, glands, which produce an alkaline secretion, and stroma or connective tissue cells capable of the rapid regeneration necessary following menstruation. The endometrium is richly supplied with blood and is about 1·5 mm. (1/16 inch) thick. When pregnancy occurs the endometrium is known as the decidua, because after labour it will be shed.

The myometrium, or muscle coat, forms seven-eighths of the thickness of the uterine wall and consists of three layers, an inner layer of circular fibres, a middle criss-cross layer and an outer longitudinal layer. These layers are not well defined in the non-pregnant state but develop tremendously in pregnancy. During labour the muscle coat is concerned with the expulsion of the fetus and the control of bleeding.

The perimetrium is a layer of peritoneum, which covers the uterus except at the sides, beyond which it extends to form the broad ligaments. The perimetrium is firmly attached to the uterine wall except at the lower anterior part where, at the level of the isthmus, the peritoneum is reflected on to the bladder.

THE CERVIX

The cervix or neck is the lowest part of the uterus and the vaginal portion projects into the vault of the vagina. The cervical canal is 2·5 cm. (1 inch) long, and the constricted area where the cervix and isthmus meet forms what is known as the **internal os** (mouth): the **external os** is a small round opening at the lowest point of the uterus, but after childbirth it is a transverse slit. In structure the cervix differs from the body of the uterus, containing less muscular and more elastic tissue. Lining the canal is mucous membrane, with glands of the deep racemose type which secrete glairy alkaline mucus. The mucosa covering the outer surface of the cervix is similar to the stratified epithelium of the vagina.

Position of Uterus

The uterus lies in a position which is almost horizontal when the woman stands erect. It leans forwards, and this position is known as *anteversion*; it bends forwards on itself, producing *anteflexion*, with the fundus resting on the bladder. When this position of anteflexion and anteversion is maintained, prolapse is less likely to occur. When the uterus is backwardly displaced or retroverted, it lies in the same axis as the vagina and is more liable to prolapse.

The uterus is maintained in position by four pairs of ligaments and indirectly by the **pelvic floor.** It is capable of a wide range of movement: a full bladder alters its position from horizontal to vertical: a distended colon pushes it downwards and forwards.

LIGAMENTS

2 broad ; 2 round ; 2 transverse cervical ; 2 utero-sacral.

The broad ligament is a double fold of peritoneum continuous with the perimetrium, extending outwards from the uterus and attached to the side wall of the pelvis. The lower border of the broad ligament is thickened and strengthened with fascia, fibrous tissue and muscle to form the most important uterine support, the **transverse cervical ligament,** which, if overstretched or damaged during labour, will cause the uterus to sag downwards.

The round ligament arises at the cornu of the uterus, in front of and below the insertion of the Fallopian tube, and runs between the folds of the broad ligament, passes through the inguinal canal and is inserted into the labium majus. It has little value as a support, but tends to hold the uterus forwards in the position of anteversion.

The utero-sacral ligament consists of folds of peritoneum containing muscular and fibrous tissue, extending backwards from the sides of the isthmus and attached to the sacrum. It forms the lateral border of the base of the pouch of Douglas, and by pulling the cervix backwards helps to maintain uterine anteversion.

BLOOD SUPPLY

The vessels supplying blood to the uterus are the two uterine and the two ovarian arteries. The **uterine artery,** a branch of the internal iliac, is ensheathed in the paracervical tissue forming the transverse cervical ligament, and joins the uterus at the level of the isthmus. It sends a branch to the upper part of the vagina, but the larger branch runs in a convoluted fashion up alongside the uterus between the folds of the broad ligament, giving off branches to the body of the uterus and eventually anastomosing with the ovarian artery. Uterine veins accompany the arteries.

The ovarian artery is a branch of the abdominal aorta and arises just below the renal artery. It enters the pelvis, passes between the folds of the broad ligament, supplies ovary and Fallopian tube, and enters the uterus at the fundus. The veins that drain the upper part of the uterus unite between the folds of the broad ligament to form the pampiniform plexus and from it on either side arise the two ovarian veins which fuse to form one vein: the left joining the left renal vein, the right joining the inferior vena cava. The uterine blood supply is increased during pregnancy and decreased during the puerperium.

The lymphatic drainage from the uterus is abundant and accounts for the successful outcome of many uterine infections. Under the perimetrium there is a lymphatic

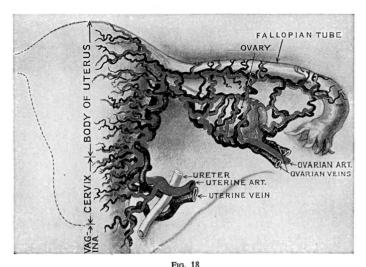

FIG. 18

Blood supply of the uterus and its appendages.

plexus. Some of the lymph vessels pass to the inguinal glands; others go to the internal and external common iliac glands.

THE NERVE SUPPLY

The main nerve supply to the uterus is now considered to be from the sympathetic nervous system, and doubt exists as to whether parasympathetic nerves supply the uterus. It is suggested that impulses transmitted by the sympathetic nerves may be stimulative or inhibitive to the uterus depending on whether they are influenced by chemical agents in the uterus or placenta, or by hormonal factors.

Sympathetic nerve fibres from the hypogastric plexus pass to the pelvic (Frankenhauser's) plexus, in the base of the utero-sacral ligaments, from which are supplied the uterus, vagina, bladder and rectum. This may explain why uterine action is intensified when the bowel is stimulated as by enemata or conversely why in cases of hypotonic uterine action bladder tone is also poor.

Sympathetic nerves from the pelvic plexus pass to the paracervical ganglia, which are sheaths of sympathetic nerve fibres situated close behind and on either side of the cervix. The contact or pressure on the cervix of a well-fitting presenting part results in the transmission of a stimulus through the paracervical ganglia from the nerve endings in the cervix. These stimulative impulses result in stronger contractions of the muscle fibres in the upper uterine segment.

THE FALLOPIAN TUBES

The Fallopian tubes are two muscular canals, extending from the cornua of the uterus and opening into the peritoneal cavity near the ovaries. Each tube measures about 11·4 cm. (4½ inches) in length and is enveloped in the upper fold of the broad ligament. The ciliated mucous membrane, lining the tube, produces a current of

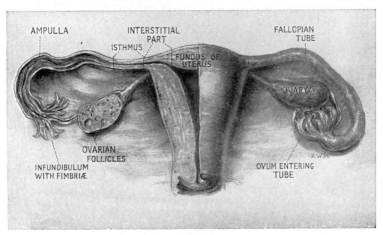

FIG. 19

Diagrammatic representation of Fallopian tube in section, demonstrating the narrow interstitial and isthmic portions. Note ovum entering the fimbriated end of the tube.

lymph which, in conjunction with the rhythmic peristaltic action of the muscle coat furthers the passage of the ovum from the ovary along the tube to the uterus.

Four parts of the tube are described, as follows:

The interstitial passes through the 1·25 cm. (½-inch) thickness of the uterine wall. Its lumen is about 1 mm. in diameter (the size of a common pin).

The isthmus is the narrow part, immediately adjoining the uterus.

The ampulla is the wider portion in which fertilization of the ovum usually takes place.

The infundibulum is the funnel-shaped extremity, the terminal margins of which are fimbriated (fringed); one of the longer fimbria being in contact with the ovary, the fimbria ovarica.

THE OVARIES

The ovaries are two small organs (about the size of an unshelled almond), 3·8 cm. (1½ inches) long, 1·9 cm. (¾ inch) broad. and 1·25 cm. (½ inch) thick. They are situated

3

on the posterior surface of the broad ligaments to which they are attached by the mesovarium.

Blood vessels and nerves enter the ovary at the hilum, a stalk-like structure, on its anterior edge. One end of the ovary is attached to the cornu of the uterus by the ovarian ligament which is about 2·5 cm. (1 inch) long; the other end is connected to the pelvic wall by the suspensory or infundibulo-pelvic ligament. The ovary is brought into contact with the Fallopian tube by one of its longer fimbria, the fimbria ovarica.

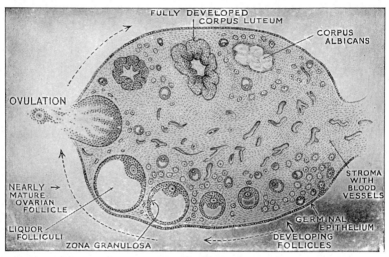

FIG. 20

LIFE CYCLE OF THE GRAAFIAN FOLLICLE.

Schematic representation of the ovary, showing primordial follicles; development of the mature Graafian follicle; ovulation; formation and degeneration of the corpus luteum, resulting in the corpus albicans. The processes occur in the sequence indicated by the arrows.

The ovary consists of a medulla and a cortex. The medulla is a supporting framework of connective tissue, blood vessels and nerves, but the cortex (covering or bark) is the important functioning part and is composed of germinal epithelium, stroma cells and Graafian follicles. The **germinal epithelium** is the membrane from which the ova are derived: it lies under the tunica albuginea which forms the surface of the ovary.

During fetal life the cells of the germinal epithelium form primordial ova which are encased in small sacs of fluid, and at birth about 100,000 of these are present in the ovary. During the years preceding puberty some of the primordial follicles begin to mature, but not until puberty do they ripen, come to the surface and rupture to liberate an ovum.

The mature Graafian follicle is about 8 mm. (⅓ of an inch) in diameter and consists of an outer layer (or theca externa) which is lined with theca interna. Inside the theca interna is a layer known as the membrana granulosa which contains a clear fluid, the liquor folliculi. At one end of the follicle the cells of the membrana granulosa are heaped up to surround the ovum and are called the discus proligerus.

FUNCTIONS OF THE OVARY

1. OVULATION.   2. ENDOCRINE ACTION.

1. **Ovulation,** which consists of the rupture of the ripened Graafian follicle and the expulsion of the ovum, takes place once every month in a normal healthy woman from puberty to the menopause approximately 14 days previous to the first day of the next menstrual period (between the 12th and 16th days after the beginning of the last menstrual period). One follicle comes to the surface of the ovary, ruptures and allows the ovum to escape into the fimbriated end of the tube, cupped underneath it at this time.

The corpus luteum or yellow body is formed in the ruptured Graafian follicle. If the ovum is not fertilized, it dies; the corpus luteum degenerates and is gradually replaced by hyaline tissue (the corpus albicans), which allows the ovary to heal where rupture has taken place, without the formation of scar tissue.

2. **Endocrine action.**—The ovary produces the hormones progesterone and œstrogens. Œstriol, œstradiol and œstrone are ovarian hormones but œstriol is excreted in larger quantities than the other œstrogens.

THE EFFECTS OF ŒSTROGENS AND PROGESTERONE
1. DURING THE MENSTRUAL CYCLE

The œstrogens, under the influence of the follicle stimulating hormone (FSH) of the anterior pituitary gland are produced by the joint action of corpus luteum cells

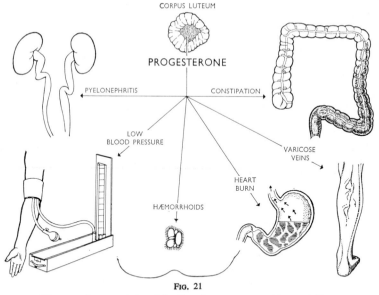

FIG. 21

Diagrammatic representation of the effect of progesterone on plain muscle fibres during pregnancy.

and interstitial cells. Œstrogens have widespread metabolic effects; they are also concerned with the proliferative changes in the endometrium, the activity of the breasts, vaginal epithelium, and cervical glands.

3 A

Progesterone, the hormone produced by the corpus luteum, under the influence of the luteinizing hormone (LH) of the anterior pituitary gland is responsible for the secretory phase—the second two weeks—of the menstrual cycle. Progesterone can only affect tissues that have previously been acted on by œstrogens.

DURING PREGNANCY
ŒSTROGENS

The feto-placental unit is intimately associated in the production of œstrogens but this process is not yet completely understood. In the fetal adrenals a steroid is metabolised and carried to the placenta where it acts as a precursor in the elaboration of œstriol which is the main œstrogenic hormone of pregnancy. Œstriol is essentially a growth hormone concerned with the growth of the fetus, decidua, myometrium and breasts. This hormone is excreted in the urine of pregnant women, and the amount excreted gives some indication of fetal well-being.

When conditions exist that could impair fetal growth the termination of pregnancy would be considered after the 34th week in order to promote fetal survival, so assays of urinary œstriol are made and if low, this signifies that the feto-placental unit is not functioning properly: when below a critical level fetal death may be imminent (see p. 655).

PROGESTERONE

This hormone is thought to be metabolised by the feto-placental unit and is excreted in the urine as pregnanediol.

In early pregnancy progesterone is produced by corpus luteal and interstitial cells under the stimulation of chorionic gonadotrophin. Later the placenta produces increasing quantities; the adrenal cortex may also be involved.

Progesterone causes proliferation of the decidua to meet the nutritional needs of the growing embryo and is also concerned with the secretory function of the breasts. It may play some part in maintaining fluid and electrolyte balance. The surmised sedative action of progesterone on pregnant uterine muscle is not yet fully understood.

Urinary pregnanediol assays reflect functioning of the corpus luteum and are employed in cases of infertility to determine whether ovulation has occurred. They are not of value in later pregnancy.

One of the pregnancy hormones, probably progesterone, is believed to relax plain muscle fibres throughout the body and the result of this action on the various tissues may predispose to the following conditions in pregnant women—

Progesterone

Action	Effect
By relaxing the ureters	pyelonephritis
„ „ „ veins	varicose veins
„ „ „ arteries	lowered blood pressure
„ „ „ intestine	constipation
„ „ „ cardiac sphincter of stomach	heartburn

3. DURING LABOUR

Œstrogens and progesterone are considered to be necessary in the production of powerful rhythmic uterine contractions during labour. Although the level of œstrogens and progesterone is very high at term neither hormone is believed to play any part in the initiation of labour.

After labour œstrogens and progesterone fall rapidly when the placenta, which is a rich source of progesterone and œstrogens, is expelled. Luteotrophin (*prolactin*) the lactogenic hormone, now comes into play and stimulates the production of milk

PITUITARY GONADOTROPHINS

The anterior pituitary gland secretes two hormones that influence ovarian function: (1) the follicle stimulating hormone (FSH) is believed to stimulate the development of the Graafian follicles; (2) the luteinizing hormone (LH) brings about the development of the corpus luteum. Anterior pituitary hormones and ovarian hormones interact on each other, stimulating or inhibiting, as required and so maintaining a correct hormonal balance.

The pituitary growth hormone promotes growth and development of the breasts as well as stimulating lactation.

Chorionic Gonadotrophin

Gonadotrophin produced by trophoblastic tissue (placenta) appears in the urine a few days after implantation of the ovum: Its main function, prolonging the life of the corpus luteum during pregnancy, inhibits menstruation. A peak level is reached at about 60 days from the last menstrual period.

Finding chorionic gonadotrophin in the urine of a woman is accepted as a sign of pregnancy; in fact this is the basis of the immunological and other pregnancy tests. An excessive amount is present in cases of hydatidiform mole.

Human chorionic somatomammotrophin (H.C.S.), formerly known as placental lactogen, is mainly concerned with mobilisation of fat stores in pregnancy. In the metabolism of carbohydrates it counteracts the hypoglycaemic action of insulin.

LUTEOTROPHIN

Luteotrophin produced by the anterior pituitary gland is considered to be identical with and was formerly known as prolactin. It is a mammogenic hormone, essential for the initiation of lactation. **It is not gonadotrophic.**

QUESTIONS FOR REVISION

THE BONY PELVIS

Why is the promontory of the sacrum the most important landmark of the pelvis ?
The true female pelvis is known as...
Differentiate between the gynæcoid, android, and platypelloid pelvis. Write 5 lines on each of the following: the diagonal conjugate; pelvic outlet; false pelvis; pelvic joints.

Practical Application

From inspection of the pregnant woman what would make you suspect a small or deformed pelvis ?
In what way is knowledge of the following facts of value in the practice of midwifery ? (1) The pelvic joints " give " during labour. (2) the inclination of the plane of the brim is 60°. (3) The antero-posterior is the largest diameter of the outlet.
C.M.B.(Eng.) paper.—Describe the brim of the pelvis. What bones form it ? What are its measurements ?

C.M.B.(Eng.) paper.—Describe the female bony pelvis. Give reasons for the importance of knowing its structure.

C.M.B.(Scot.) paper—Describe the female pelvis. Give a list of the diameters and their measurements (inches or centimetres).

C.M.B.(Eng.)—50 word question on the diagonal conjugate of the pelvis.

THE PELVIC FLOOR

The main muscle is the................................. Name the three canals which perforate it.

Practical Application

(1) **The pelvic floor softens and sags at the end of pregnancy.** Relate this to (*a*) lightening ; (*b*) taking the diagonal conjugate. (2) What part does the pelvic floor play in the mechanism of labour ? : how may it be injured during labour ? What damage would be incurred by making a lateral rather than a medio-lateral episiotomy ?

C.M.B.(Eng.) paper.—Describe the anatomy of the pelvic floor. What physiological changes occur and what pathological changes may take place as a result of delivery ? What can you do in an endeavour to prevent such pathological changes ?

C.M.B.(Eng.) paper.—Describe the perineal body. How may this be damaged in labour and what steps can be taken to minimize this damage ?

C.M.B.(Scot.) paper.—Describe the anatomy of the pelvic floor. What changes may take place as the result of child bearing?

THE VULVA

REARRANGE CORRECTLY:

Structure	location		
(1) Clitoris	pad of fat on symphysis pubis	(	)
(2) Fourchette	above urethral orifice	(	)
(3) Vestibule	where labia minora meet posteriorly	(	)
(4) Mons veneris	posterior wall of urethral orifice	(	)
(5) Introitus	posterior area of vestibule	(	)
(6) Skene's ducts	between clitoris and fourchette	(	)

A first degree perineal tear involves the...

A third degree tear involves the...

Practical Application

Describe the vulva of a woman who has previously given birth to a child. How would you locate the urethra when much bruising is present ?

THE VAGINA

The anterior wall, lower half, is in contact with...

The anterior wall, upper half, is in contact with...

The posterior wall, lower third, is in contact with...

The posterior wall, middle third, is in contact with...

Practical Application

(*a*) If difficulty is encountered in passing a catheter during the second stage of labour, what would you do ? (*b*) What is the advantage of the acid medium of the vagina ? (*c*) What types of vaginal discharge should be reported to the doctor ? What is a cystocele ? What conditions predispose to its formation ?

C.M.B.(Eng.) paper.—Describe the anatomy of the cervix. What changes take place in pregnancy and in labour ?

C.M.B.(Eng.) paper.—Describe the vagina and perineum. Explain how injuries to these structures can be minimized during labour.

C.M.B.(Eng.) paper.—Describe the anatomical relations of the bladder in the female. In what ways may the bladder be affected by pregnancy and labour ?

C.M.B.(N. Ireland) paper.—Describe the structure, functions and anatomical relations of the vagina.

C.M.B.(Eng.) paper, 1969.—Describe the anatomy of the vagina. Give its relations.

C.M.B.(Eng.) paper, 1969.—Describe the anatomy of the female bladder and its relations. Why is this knowledge important in midwifery ?

THE UTERUS

Name.—The lining of the pregnant uterus... .... the part where the corpus and cervix meet............................... the nervous system supplying the uterus .... the collection of nerves behind the cervix............... the ligament which is a fibro-muscular fold at the base of the broad ligament............... What does the isthmus form ?............................... The non-pregnant uterus measures............... weighs............... The uterus at term measures............... weighs .... The uterus lies in a position of............... The uterine artery is a branch of............................... The ovarian artery is a branch of...............................

Practical Application

In what way might the woman overstretch the transverse cervical ligaments during labour ? What causes the uterus to increase in size during pregnancy and to decrease during the puerperium ? Why does a retroverted uterus tend to prolapse ?

C.M.B.(Eng.) paper.—What is the normal position of the non-pregnant uterus and how is it maintained ? What may be the consequences of a malposition of the uterus ?

C.M.B.(Eng.) paper.—Describe the supports of the uterus. How may they be damaged in labour ? How can the risk of such damage be reduced ?

C.M.B.(Eng.) paper.—Describe the anatomy of the cervix uteri. What changes occur in it during pregnancy and labour ?

C.M.B.(N. Ireland) paper.—Describe the normal non-pregnant uterus, its position and blood supply.

C.M.B.(Eng.) paper.—Outline the anatomy of the body of the uterus. Describe the behaviour of its musculature in the three stages of labour.

FALLOPIAN TUBES AND OVARIES

Name the following parts of the Fallopian tubes : The part (a) which passes through the uterine wall............................... (b) in which fertilization usually takes place .... (c) immediately adjoining the uterus............................... (d) the widened ends...............................

Name the following structures in the ovary : The functioning part............................... .... The covering membrane............................... The sac containing the ovum...............................

Practical Application

In what way might the Fallopian tubes or the ovaries be responsible for sterility, or infertility ?

If the tubes are narrowed, what may be the result ?............... If they are blocked ? ....

C.M.B.(Eng.) paper.—Describe the pathway through which the fertilized egg passes in order to reach the uterus. What may happen if anything obstructs the passage of the fertilized egg into the uterus ?

C.M.B.(Scot.) paper, 1970.—Describe the hormonal changes which occur in pregnancy. How can a knowledge of these contribute to diagnosis and management ?

2

The Menstrual Cycle : the Ovum—the Placenta

The menstrual cycle is a series of four phases, mainly affecting the tissue structure of the endometrium.

1. REGENERATIVE.	3. SECRETORY.
2. PROLIFERATIVE.	4. MENSTRUAL.

The menstrual cycle is governed indirectly by the anterior pituitary gonadotrophic hormones and directly by the ovarian hormones, œstrogens and progesterone.

1. REGENERATIVE

This phase begins as soon as menstruation ceases and lasts for two days. The remaining glands and stroma cells multiply and the effused blood is absorbed as in the healing of a wound. The endometrium is reformed.

2. PROLIFERATIVE

This phase commences about two days after the cessation of menstruation and lasts until ovulation takes place (14 days previous to menstruation). Œstrogens are responsible for the growth of the endometrium which takes place at this time.

3. SECRETORY

The pre-menstrual phase commences after ovulation, when progesterone causes the endometrium, which has already been growing under the influence of œstrogens, to hypertrophy still further. The endometrial glands increase in size and have a high glycogen content: the capillaries are distended with blood, and small hæmatomata form under the epithelium, producing a red congested surface. This thick soft vascular membrane is admirably prepared for the reception of the fertilized ovum. Should fertilization not take place, the ovum dies, the corpus luteum disintegrates, the secretion of œstrogens and progesterone falls and the endometrium shows degenerative changes which are followed by desquamation and bleeding.

4. MENSTRUAL

The discharge of blood, lasting for three or four days, which occurs every 28 to 30 days from puberty to the menopause in the normal woman, is the terminal phase of the menstrual cycle. If the preparations made during the three preceding phases for the reception of a fertilized ovum are not required, they are discarded. The superficial layer of endometrium is shed, along with blood from the capillaries; the unfertilized ovum being discarded as well.

Although physiologically the menstrual cycle ends with bleeding, it is customary when prescribing contraceptive pills, starting on the 5th day of the cycle, to consider the first day of bleeding to be the first day of the menstrual cycle. This simplifies calculation of the day of starting administration of the pills for the woman concerned.

THE MENOPAUSE

The menopause, change of life or climacteric, is the end of the reproductive period: the ovarian œstrogenic hormones are gradually withdrawn and other complex endocrine changes occur: ovulation ceases. About 50 per cent of women cease menstruating between the age of 45 and 50, but the menopause does rarely occur as early as 35 and as late as 55. The periods may be scanty and irregular for some months and within one year they usually cease, but the menopause is generally considered to extend over a period of two years.

Symptoms commonly attributed to the menopause may arise before menstrual irregularities occur and after they have ceased, and œstrogen withdrawal is not the sole cause of menopausal symptoms.

The midwife should appreciate the grave responsibility she incurs when her advice is sought regarding vaginal bleeding which is profuse, prolonged or irregular, and without exception the woman should be urged to consult her doctor. The possibility and danger of **malignant disease** of the uterus at this time of life should always be kept in mind, for early diagnosis means early treatment and greater hope of recovery.

Throughout this period systems of the body other than the reproductive may be disturbed. The effect on the circulatory system may be evident as palpitation. **Vaso-motor instability** is responsible for one of the most common disturbances, hot flushes. The tendency to obesity is fairly general. The blood pressure may be slightly raised and headaches and noises in the ears may be troublesome. Pains in the joints and the sensation of " pins and needles " in the hands and feet are often complained of. Manifestations of a disturbed nervous system may occur, but they should not arise in a well-adjusted personality: reassurance, sympathetic understanding and much patience are needed in these cases.

Depression, anxiety, insomnia, irritability and tension may be present in slight or severe degrees, and patients with these symptoms usually benefit from the use of sedatives which are, of course, prescribed by the doctor. When menopausal symptoms are distressing to the patient, the doctor may, if there is no vaginal bleeding, order one of the synthetic œstrogenic substances to be taken: the dose given is the least possible and for the shortest possible time. Good food, fresh air and adequate sleep are very necessary.

There is a psychological aspect to this period of life, and women should not be encouraged to expect ill-health. They should lead an active life and maintain an interest in pursuits outside home or employment. Such women should be persuaded to anticipate a long period of happy useful life with greater tranquillity of mind than experienced previously.

THE OVUM

EARLY DEVELOPMENT

When ovulation takes place, the ovum, which is about 0·16 mm. ($\frac{1}{150}$ inch) in diameter (about the size of the point of a fine needle), escapes into the peritoneal cavity and finds its way into the Fallopian tube. How this is accomplished is a matter of conjecture. It is possible that under the influence of œstrogens at the time of ovulation the Fallopian tube becomes arched so that its fimbriated end is cupped underneath and around the ovary to receive the ovum from the ruptured Graafian follicle. The ovum, having no power of locomotion, is wafted along by the cilia, and by the peristaltic muscular contractions of the tube.

CHROMOSOMES

Every cell in the human body has 46 chromosomes. The ovum and spermatozoon each have 46 chromosomes, two of which are sex chromosomes, and the genes contained in the chromosomes transmit to the offspring certain hereditary characteristics of the two parents and their ancestors. Only 46 chromosomes are required by the fertilized ovum so, during a process of maturation, which occurs prior to fertilization, the number in ovum and spermatozoon is reduced by half in order that each parent will contribute 22 chromosomes plus one sex chromosome. This may explain why children of the same parents inherit different characteristics.

The sex chromosome in the spermatozoon determines whether the child will be of the male or the female sex. The two sex chromosomes of the ovum being identical have been designated XX, and can only produce a female child. The two sex chromosomes of the spermatozoon being different have been designated XY and can produce either a female or a male child. If the spermatozoon X chromosome fuses with the ovum X chromosome the sex of the child will be female. If the spermatozoon Y chromosome fuses with the ovum X chromosome the sex of the child will be male.

Father	X	Y
Mother	X	X

Baby girl XX	XY Baby boy

(Statistics show that the sex ratio remains fairly constant—about 106 boys are born to every 100 girls.)

It is now possible to determine the sex of the fetus by examining the sex-chromatin pattern of the desquamated embryonic cells found in amniotic fluid obtained by abdominal amniocentesis.

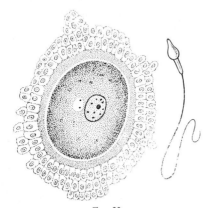

FIG. 22

Showing comparative size of ovum and spermatozoon.

CONCEPTION

The fusion of the ovum and spermatozoon is called conception, fertilization, or impregnation, and initiates the beginning of a new life. The ovary only produces one ovum per month, but as many as 200,000,000 spermatozoa each 0·05 mm. ($\frac{1}{500}$ inch) are deposited in the vagina when coitus takes place. At this time the cervix secretes a flow of alkaline mucus that attracts the spermatozoa and in which they are propelled by the rotary movement of their tails. A limited number of spermatozoa reach the Fallopian tube; a few may penetrate the zona pellucida but only one fuses with the nucleus of the ovum.

Almost without exception fertilization takes place in the Fallopian tube, usually in the ampulla. By means of the sharp point on its head the spermatozoon penetrates the ovum.

The most likely period for conception to take place is immediately following ovulation which occurs 14 days previous to the next menstrual period. **The majority of women conceive between the 10th and 18th day of the menstrual cycle;** but it is believed that conception can take place earlier or later. Neither ovum nor spermatozoon are thought to be capable of fertilization for longer than 48 hours.

DEVELOPMENT OF THE FERTILIZED OVUM

While being propelled along the tube, segmentation or cell division takes place and the fertilized cell or zygote divides into 2–4–8–16 and so on until it consists of a ball of cells like a mulberry, known as the **morula.** (Three to four days are required for the journey along the tube to the uterus, and as the interstitial part of the Fallopian tube through which it must pass has a diameter of 1 mm., the ovum must be very small to pass through it.) A cavity or blastocele forms in the morula which now becomes known as the **blastocyst**. At one point the cells clump together, forming the inner cell mass; the remainder of the cells are pushed to the periphery.

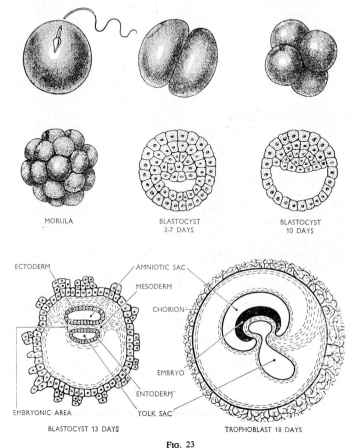

MORULA

BLASTOCYST
3-7 DAYS

BLASTOCYST
10 DAYS

ECTODERM

AMNIOTIC SAC

MESODERM

CHORION

EMBRYO

ENTODERM

EMBRYONIC AREA

YOLK SAC

BLASTOCYST 13 DAYS

TROPHOBLAST 18 DAYS

FIG. 23

Diagrammatic representation of the development of the fertilized ovum.
There is a very slight increase in the size of the ovum until the blastocyst stage.

EMBEDDING OF THE OVUM

Six to seven days may elapse before the fertilized ovum, now at the blastocyst stage is ready for embedding. It comes to rest on the endometrium, and at the area of contact tiny projections or buds appear which could be likened to the sprouting roots of a germinating seed. The outer trophoblastic cells, known as the syncytiotrophoblast, have the power of breaking down tissue, eroding the endometrium and allowing the blastocyst to become embedded.

When the ovum burrows into the implantation cavity, slight bleeding may occur which might be mistaken for a scanty menstrual period. The endometrial cells heal the opening, and the embedding of the ovum is complete,

THE TROPHOBLAST

By the 13th day trophoblastic cells surround the whole blastocyst and form rudimentary chorionic villi which contain no blood vessels; they absorb nutriment from the disintegrated cells in the implantation cavity. **The trophoblast is concerned with the nutrition of the ovum.**

DEVELOPMENT OF THE EMBRYO

Three primitive layers in the ovum can now be differentiated, and from each layer particular parts of the fetus develop.

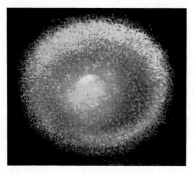

FIG. 24

Ovum in early pregnancy covered with chorionic villi.

The ectoderm forms the nervous system, skin and certain lining mucosa.

The mesoderm forms bone, muscle, the circulatory system, and certain internal organs.

The entoderm forms the mucosa of the alimentary tract, the epithelium of the liver, pancreas, lungs and bladder.

In the inner cell mass two cavities appear:

(1) **The amniotic sac,** which is filled with fluid, and (2) immediately below it the **yolk sac.** The area between these two sacs is comprised of ectoderm, mesoderm, entoderm, and is known as the embryonic area, from which the embryo develops.

The amniotic sac contains and protects the embryo, and as the cavity increases in size the amnion comes in contact with the chorion to which it becomes adherent (about the fourth week).

The yolk sac provides nourishment for the embryo, until the trophoblast develops sufficiently to absorb nutriment from the maternal tissues, and later from the mother's blood.

The embryo is attached to the placenta by a broad band of mesoderm, the body stalk, which envelops part of the yolk sac and other structures. By a complicated process of " folding off " the amniotic sac surrounds the embryo; the yolk sac is constricted and eventually atrophies. Primitive blood vessels appear in the embryo and chorionic villi: blood cells develop, and by the 6th week a primitive form of circulation is established, which at the 12th week is functioning completely.

FORMATION OF THE DECIDUA

Every month, from puberty to the menopause, the uterus prepares for a fertilized ovum. If conception takes place this preparation is intensified, and the endometrium becomes known as the **decidua** (*deciduous means shedding: a baby's first teeth are called deciduous because they are shed*). The increased activity of the decidua is brought about by the stimulus of the œstrogenic hormones, which increase structural growth until the endometrium is four times the non-pregnant thickness—(from $1 \cdot 5$ to $6 \cdot 2$ mm. ($\frac{1}{16}$ to $\frac{1}{4}$ inch)).

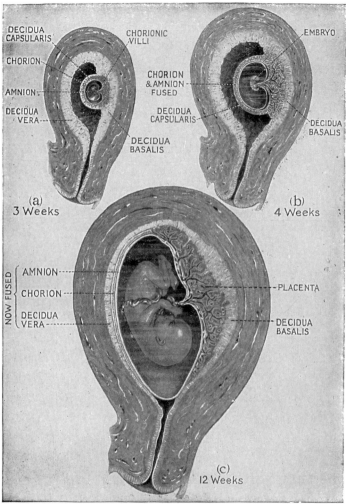

FIG. 26

THE DEVELOPING EMBRYO.

(*a*) (3 weeks).—Showing the amniotic sac, surrounded by chorion which is covered with decidua capsularis.

(*b*) (4 weeks).—Amnion is in contact with chorion: decidua capsularis is growing outwards into the uterine cavity. The placenta is seen embedded in the decidua basalis.

(*c*) (12 weeks).—The capsularis has thinned out and atrophied: the chorion is attached to the decidua vera.

(After Williams, *American Journal of Obstetrics and Gynæcology.*)

4

The hormone progesterone from the corpus luteum, under the influence of chorionic gonadotrophins, stimulates the secretory activity of the endometrial glands and increases the size of the blood vessels. The result is a soft, vascular, spongy bed in which the ovum can readily become implanted and find nutriment.

THE THREE LAYERS OF DECIDUA

(1) The compact; (2) the spongy; and (3) the basement or unaltered layer become well defined during pregnancy.

(1) The compact layer is made up of closely packed cells and the necks of glands: it is the most superficial of the three layers and is adjacent to the uterine cavity.

(2) The spongy layer is mainly formed of tortuous dilated glands and of large stroma or decidual cells. This enlargement of the stroma cells during pregnancy is known as the "*decidual reaction*" and is nature's defence against the invading propensities of the syncytiotrophoblast. The function of the decidual reaction in limiting the advance of the chorionic villi to the spongy layer can be appreciated when we consider the method by which the placenta is separated during the third stage of labour.

Throughout pregnancy the placenta remains securely embedded in the decidua, but as soon as the baby is born the placenta must be shed. If the placental attachment is limited to the loose spongy layer, it will be possible for the placenta to become separated from the decidua in much the same way as postage stamps can readily be detached at their line of perforation. Should the placenta embed too deeply, it would be morbidly adherent, and so complicate the third stage of labour.

(3) The basement layer of decidua regenerates the new endometrium during the puerperium.

THE THREE AREAS OF DECIDUA

(1) The decidua basalis is the area of decidua underneath the embedded ovum.

(2) The decidua capsularis lies over the developing ovum.

(3) The decidua vera or true decidua lines the remainder of the uterus.

As the ovum grows, the decidua capsularis distends, and at the 12th week comes into contact with the decidua vera, degenerates and disappears.

DEVELOPMENT OF THE PLACENTA

During the third week, the ovum is completely covered with chorionic villi; those next to the spongy layer of the decidua grow profusely and are known as chorion frondosum, which ultimately form the placenta. These chorionic villi penetrate the blood vessels with which they come in contact, and become bathed in a lake of maternal blood, the opened vessels being known as sinuses and the areas surrounding the villi as blood spaces.

Some of the chorionic villi are attached to the decidua—the anchoring villi—the majority float in the slowly circulating maternal blood from which they absorb nutriment. The villi on the remainder of the trophoblast degenerate, leaving the bald chorion—the chorion læve—which on its inner surface is adherent to the amnion and on its outer surface to the decidua capsularis, and after the 12th week to the decidua vera.

A chorionic villus is a branching structure arising from the chorionic membrane as a single stem, which divides and subdivides until it terminates in the fine filaments that are embedded in the decidua basalis. The outer layer of a chorionic villus is known as syncytiotrophoblast, as previously described; the inner layer of the villus—the cytotrophoblast or **Langhan's layer.** By their selective action they absorb from the maternal blood the particular substances needed for the developing embryo. The centre of the villus contains mesoderm and blood vessels, within which fetal blood circulates.

The fetus develops its own blood, just as it develops its heart, brain, eyes, etc., and it must not be thought that maternal blood circulates in the fetus. There are four

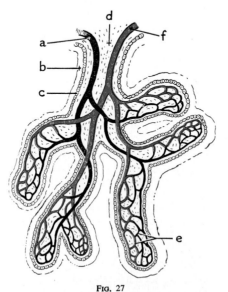

FIG. 27

DIAGRAM OF A CHORIONIC VILLUS.

(*a*) Branch of umbilical artery carrying fetal impure blood. (*b*) Syncytiotrophoblast, the outer layer of the villus. (*c*) Cytotrophoblast. (*d*) Mesoderm. (*e*) Capillaries through which the interchange between fetal and maternal blood takes place. (*f*) Branch of umbilical vein returning oxygenated blood to the fetus.

layers of tissue between fetal and maternal blood, *i.e.* syncytiotrophoblast, cytotrophoblast, mesoderm and the capillary wall. Unless some breakdown of the placenta occurs, fetal and maternal blood do not mix.

From the 12th to the 20th week the placenta weighs as much as and even more than the fetus, and this is because it must deal with the metabolic processes of nutrition, with which the fetal organs are not sufficiently developed to cope. During the later weeks of pregnancy some of the fetal organs, such as the liver, begin to function, so the cytotrophoblast and the syncytiotrophoblast gradually degenerate and disappear.

THE PLACENTA AT TERM

The placenta or afterbirth is a round, flat mass, about 22·9 cm. (9 inches) in diameter, 2·5 cm. (1 inch) thick at the centre and weighing approximately one-sixth of the weight of the baby at term.

STRUCTURE

The placenta is made up of chorionic villi and blood vessels containing fetal blood. It also consists of the decidua basalis, in which the villi embed, the chorio-decidual spaces and the maternal blood contained in them.

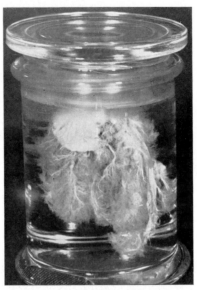

FIG. 28

COTYLEDON OF PLACENTA. Blood has been removed to demonstrate the fine chorionic villi.

The maternal surface is made up of chorionic villi, arranged in cotyledons or lobules that are separated by sulci or furrows. Maternal blood gives it a bluish-red colour, and the surface is covered by a thin layer of trophoblastic cells which were formerly thought to be decidual. Frequently the maternal surface is covered with small deposits of lime salts which feel gritty to the touch and look like finely ground egg shell. This is known as calcareous degeneration.

The fetal surface is smooth, white and shiny, and on it can be seen branches of the umbilical vein and arteries and the insertion of the umbilical cord. It is covered with two membranes, the chorion and amnion, which are continued beyond its outer edge to form the sac that contains the fetus and amniotic fluid.

PLACENTAL CIRCULATION

Blood from the fetal heart circulates through the fetus, and because of the need for oxygenation and replenishment it leaves the fetus and is carried by the arteries of the umbilical cord to the placenta. The umbilical arteries spread over the fetal surface of the placenta and subdivide until they terminate in the chorionic villi, which absorb from the mother's blood the products of digestion; *e.g.* amino-acids, glucose, minerals, vitamins, and probably fatty acids.

The process is comparable to what takes place when the villi in our intestines absorb similar substances and transfer them to the blood stream. The fetal alimentary tract does not digest food, nor do the lungs inhale oxygen, therefore the placenta carries out the functions of stomach, intestine, liver, lungs and kidneys.

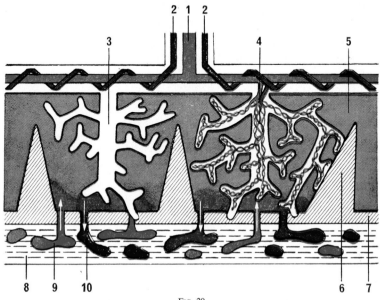

FIG. 29

DIAGRAMMATIC REPRESENTATION OF THE PLACENTA

1. Umbilical vein transporting replenished blood from placenta to fetus.
2. Umbilical artery (2) transporting impure blood from fetus to placenta.
3. Chorionic villus (blood vessels omitted to show structure); note lower tip anchored in decidua.
4. Chorionic villus containing fetal blood vessels. Interchange takes place between fetal blood in the arteries and capillaries and maternal blood in the intervillous spaces.
5. Intervillous space containing maternal blood.
6. Decidual septum between each cotyledon.　　7. Decidua.　　8. Myometrium.
9. Maternal artery providing O_2, nutrients and electrolytes. Direction of flow indicated by arrows. The pumping action of the artery sends blood towards the chorionic villi.
10. Maternal vein carrying away blood containing fetal waste products of metabolism. This is facilitated by contraction of the myometrium (Braxton Hicks contractions).

Oxygen is taken from the mother's hæmoglobin, and carbon-dioxide and other waste products are given off into the maternal blood, the interchange of substances taking place by osmosis and diffusion, as well as by the selective action of the cytotrophoblast and the syncytiotrophoblast. The replenished oxygenated blood returns to the fetus via the umbilical vein.

FUNCTIONS OF THE PLACENTA

The placenta is the means through which the fetus obtains its needs, and it not only selects and transports from the mother's blood the substances necessary for fetal life and growth; it also changes some of these so that the fetus can utilize them. The efficiency of many placental functions depends on adequate uterine blood flow. Placental functions can be classified as:

1. NUTRITIVE.	3 EXCRETORY.
2. RESPIRATORY.	4. ENDOCRINE.

5. BARRIER or INACTIVATION.

1. NUTRITIVE

The fetus requires amino-acids (proteins) for building tissue; glucose for growth and energy; calcium and phosphorus for the composition of bones and teeth; vitamins, iron and other minerals for blood formation, growth and various body processes.

Until the fetal liver is sufficiently developed to function, the placenta metabolises glucose, stores it in the form of glycogen and reconverts it into glucose as required.

The products of digestion which are present in the mother's blood pass to the fetus via the placenta, mainly by enzymatic carriers. Fatty acids are now believed to pass through the placenta; the fetus also converts glucose into fat. Minerals and vitamins are readily transported across the placenta to the fetus.

It is the mother's food which provides fetal nutriment, and only when her diet is inadequate are her tissues depleted. To meet fetal requirements and avoid maternal depletion a diet rich in the essential foodstuffs is therefore imperative during pregnancy.

2. RESPIRATORY

Actual pulmonary respiration does not take place in utero. The fetus obtains oxygen from the mother's hæmoglobin by simple diffusion and gives off carbon dioxide into the maternal blood, and although fetal respiratory movements are believed to take place there is no pulmonary exchange of gases *in utero*.

3. EXCRETORY

Excretion from the fetus is not very great as its metabolism is mainly anabolic or building up. It is the katabolic process of metabolism—the breaking down of tissue—that produces excretory products.

4. ENDOCRINE

(*a*) Human chorionic gonadotrophin (HCG) is produced in the chorionic villi. This hormone forms the basis of the immunological and other pregnancy tests. Large amounts are excreted during the 7th to 10th week but after the 12th week the peak period has passed and a low level is maintained until term.

(*b*) Progesterone is produced by the placenta from about the 12th week; the amount steadily rises throughout pregnancy and falls when the placenta is expelled.

(*c*) Œstriol is produced by the feto-placental unit from the 6th to 12th week when the amount rises steadily until term; then, after expulsion of the placenta, it falls and allows Luteotrophin (prolactin) to initiate lactation. As both placenta and fetus are concerned in the production of œstriol excreted in urine during pregnancy, the amount is an index of feto-placental function.

(*d*) Human Chorionic Somatomammotrophin (HCS). (Placental lactogen.) This hormone recently isolated affects carbohydrate metabolism and may be concerned with fetal growth.

5. BARRIER or INACTIVATION

The placenta by enzymatic function inactivates a number of undesirable substances. With the exception of certain viruses, few organisms pass through the placenta to the fetus. **The treponema pallidum** passes readily, more rarely the tubercle bacillus; the protozoa of malaria and toxoplasmosis also reach the fetal blood stream.

The virus of rubella passes through the placenta, and if the woman is infected during the eighth to twelfth week of pregnancy the infant may suffer from cardiac defects, cataract, or deaf mutism.

Antigens and antibodies are transmitted across the placenta should a leak occur. In 5 per cent of Rh negative pregnant women antigens in the red blood cells of her Rh positive fetus pass across the placenta into her blood which then produces antibodies. **Immune bodies are transmitted** from mother to fetus in maternal gamma globulin.

Every enzyme known to exist in biology has been found in the placenta.

Sedative drugs and analgesic gases do pass and act on the fetus. If morphine is given to the mother within three hours of the birth of the baby, it could depress the fetal respiratory centre and make the establishment of respiration difficult. Anæsthetics given to the mother pass into the fetal circulation. It is known that the sulphonamides and antibiotics pass; antisyphilitic drugs given to the mother have the same beneficial action on the fetus. Teratogenic drugs pass the placental barrier and cause fetal deformities.

MALFORMATIONS OF THE PLACENTA

PLACENTA SUCCENTURIATA

This is probably the most significant abnormality from the practical point of view, and consists of an accessory lobe of placental tissue, situated in the fetal sac membrane with blood vessels running to the main placenta. It is formed by hypertrophy of

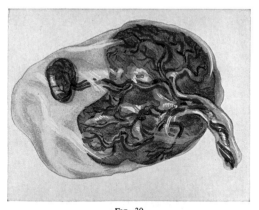

FIG. 30
PLACENTA SUCCENTURIATA.
Fetal surface—showing vessels running in the chorion from the
main placenta to the accessory lobe.

some chorionic villi in the chorion læve, which should have atrophied. Such a lobe is liable to be retained *in utero* and may give rise to profuse puerperal hæmorrhage.

If there is a hole in the membrane with blood vessels running to it, the midwife will know that a succenturiate lobe, and not a piece of membrane, has been retained.

PLACENTA BIPARTITA OR TRIPARTITA

In this placenta there are two or three complete, or almost complete, lobes. Their blood vessels unite when joining the umbilical cord, whereas the vessels of the succenturiate lobe do not directly join the cord vessels. In twin placentæ there are two cords.

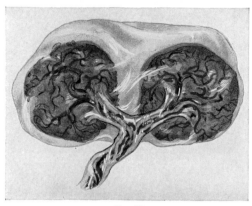

FIG. 31

PLACENTA BIPARTITA.

The umbilical vessels bifurcate at the point of insertion of the cord.

PLACENTA CIRCUMVALLATA

A double layer of amnion and chorion which has undergone infarction is seen as an opaque ring on the fetal surface. It has little significance.

DISEASES OF THE PLACENTA

Hydatidiform mole, a cystic, degenerative proliferation of the chorionic villi, is considered under complications of pregnancy.

INFARCTS

These areas of necrosed chorionic villi, red in the early stage and white later, with a solid cartilaginous consistency, are produced by increased concentration of tissue thromboplastin. They are commonly seen on the maternal surface, but may be present on the fetal aspect.

Calcareous degeneration, characterized by gritty particles that feel like sand-paper and sometimes form plaques on the maternal surface, is not infarction : it is associated with the normal degenerative processes of the placenta at term. The small white areas often present around the periphery of the placenta are fibrin nodes due to " old age " of the placenta and are not true infarcts.

Placental dysfunction.—See page 654.

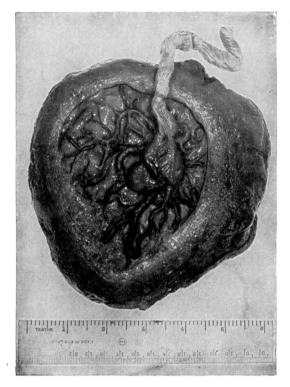

FIG. 32

PLACENTA CIRCUMVALLATA.

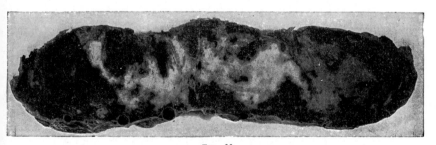

FIG. 33

PLACENTAL INFARCTIONS.

The white areas are necrosed thrombotic chorionic villi or infarcts.

SYPHILIS

On microscopic examination, changes due to endarteritis—inflammation of the wall of an artery—are seen; syphilitic placentæ are not always large, pale or greasy-looking.

Tuberculosis of the placenta is rarely seen, even in advanced cases. Tumours and cysts are extremely uncommon and have no clinical significance.

Œdema of the placenta.—The large, pale placenta with water oozing from it is associated with hydrops fetalis and is due to hæmolytic disease of the newborn, caused by incompatibility of the Rh factor.

At the Simpson Maternity Pavilion, Edinburgh, the following placentæ were seen in cases of hydrops fetalis:

Baby, 3,232 G.	(7 lb. 2 oz.)	placenta, 2,495 G.	(5 lb. 8 oz.)
Baby, 2,381 G.	(5 lb. 4 oz.)	placenta, 2,211 G.	(4 lb. 14 oz.)
Baby, 1,077 G.	(2 lb. 6 oz.)	placenta, 1,361 G.	(3 lb.)

THE FETAL SAC

The fetal sac consists of a double membrane; the outer, chorion; the inner, amnion. The fetus and liquor amnii are contained within this sac, which ruptures during labour to permit the expulsion of both.

The chorion is a thick, opaque, friable membrane, adherent to the decidua vera on its outer aspect, until the third stage of labour when it becomes detached during the expulsion of the placenta. As pieces of chorion may be retained *in utero*, it must always be carefully examined after being separated from the amnion: the chorion cannot be peeled off the fetal surface of the placenta because the placental chorionic villi are growing from it.

The amnion is a smooth, tough, translucent membrane, lining the chorion, from which it can be detached up to the insertion of the umbilical cord.

THE AMNIOTIC FLUID

The liquor amnii is the fluid in which the fetus floats and is present in the amniotic sac from the earliest weeks of pregnancy. The amount increases until at term the quantity is from 500 to 1,500 ml. It consists of 99 per cent water, is alkaline in reaction, and various mineral salts are present, including urea, which is derived from urine passed by the fetus.

A trace of protein (0·25 per cent) is usually found in liquor amnii, therefore a voided specimen of urine from a woman whose membranes have ruptured may contain a trace of protein.

APPEARANCE

It is a clear, pale, straw-coloured fluid.

A green tinge is due to the presence of meconium and should be taken as a sign of fetal distress, and the fetal heart-sounds investigated. Thick meconium during the second stage of a breech presentation may not indicate fetal distress.   breech

Golden coloured liquor is sometimes found in cases of icterus gravis neonatorum.

Epidermal cells and lanugo from the skin of the fetus are usually present. and with vernix caseosa may give it a turbid or milky appearance.

ORIGIN

The origin of the amniotic fluid is thought to be both fetal and maternal; the most likely source being the amniotic epithelium covering the fetal surface of the placenta and umbilical cord; also fetal urine from the 15th week of gestation.

Fetal malformations, monstrosities, monozygotic (uniovular) twins and diabetes are associated with an excess of fluid.

The fetus swallows liquor, and in cases where the deglutition centre in the brain is not developed, as in some cases of anencephaly, an excess of amniotic fluid is present.

FUNCTIONS

The fluid distends the amniotic sac and allows for the growth and free movement of the fetus. It acts as a shock absorber, protecting the fetus from jarring or injury.

During labour it equalizes uterine pressure and prevents marked interference with the placental circulation.

If the amount of fluid is over 1,800 ml., the condition is known as **hydramnios,** and if less than 300 ml. the term " **oligo-hydramnios** " is applied.

THE UMBILICAL CORD

The umbilical cord or funis extends from the fetal umbilicus to the fetal surface of the placenta. It is composed of an embryonic form of connective tissue, intermingled with a gelatinous substance known as Wharton's jelly, and is covered with amnion. The cord carries two arteries, which are a continuation of the hypogastric arteries, containing impure blood going to the placenta.

The umbilical arteries are empty after birth and can be felt as fibrous cords ; if one artery is shorter than the other the cord twists in a spiral fashion from left to right.

A single artery is present in some cases and is often associated with other fetal abnormalities.

The umbilical vein contains pure blood returning to the fetus after having been oxygenated, and replenished in the placenta. The vein can easily be seen, and in cases where the baby needs urgent treatment at birth, drugs may be injected into the vein and milked into the circulation.

LENGTH OF THE CORD

The average length of the cord is 55·8 cm. (22 inches), and if less than 38 cm. (15 inches) it is said to be short. Cords as short as 15·2 cm. (6 inches) have been known, but fortunately are very rare : if the cord is wound round the fetus it is relatively short. In these cases the descent of the fetus may be retarded, the placenta may be separated prematurely, causing hæmorrhage, or the cord may break. Such complications are uncommon.

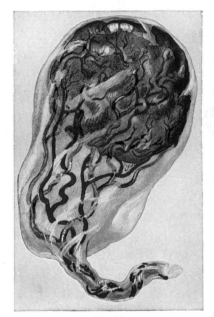

FIG. 34

Placenta velamentosa—fetal surface—showing the umbilical cord inserted in the membranes.

A long cord may become wound round the fetus, and cords of 127 to 177·8 cm.

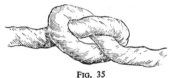

(50 to 70 inches), have been reported. It may be wound once, twice or three times round the neck, and this happens during the middle months of pregnancy, when the ratio of liquor to fetus is so great that it can move about freely.

FIG. 35

True knot in umbilical cord.

KNOTS IN THE CORD

A long cord may form loops through which the fetus can pass, thereby producing a **true knot,** which, if drawn tight when the fetus descends during labour, will lead to stillbirth due to anoxia. **False knots** are merely a heaping up of Wharton's jelly and are not significant.

INSERTION OF THE CORD

The cord is commonly inserted in the centre of the fetal surface of the placenta—a **central insertion**—one which is inserted away from the centre yet not at the edge is termed a **lateral insertion.**

Anomalies of Cord Insertion

BATTLEDORE INSERTION

In this type the cord is situated at the very edge of the placenta.

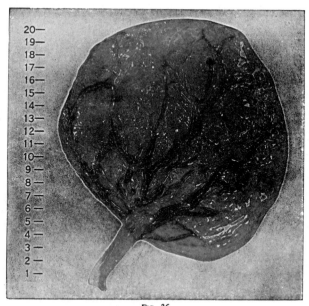

FIG. 36

BATTLEDORE PLACENTA.

Note the cord inserted at the edge of the placenta.

VELAMENTOUS INSERTION

In about 1-200 cases the cord is inserted into the membranes of the fetal sac 5·1 to 7·6 cm. (2 to 3 inches) from the edge of the placenta, rarely as much as 15·2 to 20·3 cm. (6 to 8 inches) with the umbilical blood vessels running between placenta and cord. This form of insertion is more dangerous when the placenta is situated in the lower uterine segment because the vessels may then lie over the os. (See vasa prævia below.)

VASA PRÆVIA

When the fetal blood vessels traverse the membranes and lie over the os in front of the presenting part during labour, the term vasa prævia is applied. This occurs in some cases of velamentous insertion of cord. The vessels may be compressed or may rupture with slight bleeding, but if the bleeding is severe the fetus becomes exsanguinated. In such cases it is usual to estimate the baby's hæmoglobin immediately after birth.

If there is doubt as to whether the blood passed per vaginam is fetal or maternal Singer's or Kleihauer's test is used: fetal red cells being less readily broken down in an alkali than maternal red cells.

5

QUESTIONS FOR REVISION

DEVELOPMENT OF OVUM AND PLACENTA

What term is applied to (1) The ovum: (*a*) when a ball of cells................................ (*b*) when a cavity forms in the cell mass................................. (*c*) the outer cells of the blastocyst.................................. (2) The outer layer of a chorionic villus................. .... (3) The chorionic villi which grow profusely and form the placenta ....

Which conditions might result if the following passed the placental barrier? Virus of rubella; morphine; Rh antibodies; teratogenic drugs; treponema pallidum.

Give alternative terms for the following: climacteric; rubella; placenta; liquor amnii; funis; conception; zygote.

For which main purpose does the fetus require: calcium; amino acids; iron; vitamins?

By which urine assay can feto-placental dysfunction be assessed.

Write not more than 10 lines on each of the following: conception; chromosomes; the fetal sac; amniotic fluid; the decidua.

Oral Questions

(1) What is the cause of green; golden; turbid amniotic fluid? (2) Name three harmful substances which pass through the placenta, and what the midwife could do regarding prevention. (3) Why should the amnion always be separated from the chorion when examining the placenta? (4) How would the fact that a succenturiate lobe had been retained be evident? (5) How would you recognize:—placental infarcts; a velamentous insertion of cord?

REARRANGE NUMBERS CORRECTLY:

Description	term		
(1) Cord at edge of placenta	velamentosa	(3	)
(2) Accessory lobe of placenta	bi-partita	(4	)
(3) Opaque ring on fetal surface	battledore	(5	)
(4) Two lobes of placenta	succenturiata	(2	)
(5) Thrombotic areas of placenta	circumvallata	(7	)
(6) Cord inserted in membrane	vasa prævia	(1	)
(7) Fetal blood vessels lying over os	infarcts	(6	)

C.M.B.(N. Ireland) paper.—Describe the functions of the placenta. Why are the placenta and membranes examined so carefully after delivery?

C.M.B.(N. Ireland) paper.—Describe how the placenta develops, and mention briefly abnormal forms of development.

C.M.B.(Eng.) paper.—Describe the structure of the umbilical cord. What complications involving the cord may be dangerous to the baby?

C.M.B.(Scot.) paper, 1968.—Describe the structure of the placenta. What abnormalities may occur?

C.M.B.(Eng.) paper, 1969. 50 word question.—Describe the structure of the umbilical cord.

C.M.B.(Eng.) paper, 1969. 100 word question.—Describe the succenturiate lobe of the placenta.

C.M.B.(Scot.) paper, 1970.—Describe the development, structure and functions of the placenta.

C.M.B.(Eng.) paper, 1970.—Write an essay on the functions of the placenta and the conditions which may cause impairment of these functions.

3

The Fetus

FETAL DEVELOPMENT

It is essential that the midwife should have some idea how very small the embryo is during the early weeks so that, in cases of abortion, she may know what to look for. Very seldom is the embryo of less than six weeks seen, as it is not readily detected in the blood clot, so the midwife must examine the soiled pads carefully and save everything passed, for the doctor's inspection.

THE OVUM

During the first three weeks the whole structure, including the sac is known as the ovum.

THE EMBRYO

From the 3rd to the 8th week the term "embryo" is used.

THE FETUS

From the 9th week until birth the term "fetus" is used.

THE BABY

After birth the fetus is known as a baby.

It is not always easy to estimate the age of an embryo. Length and weight, the degree of development and the period of gestation are all taken into consideration.

Three weeks.—The ovum (complete sac) is the size of a small grape and covered with fine shaggy-looking chorionic villi. No human characteristics can be recognized.

Four weeks.—The sac is 2·5 cm. (1 inch) long, about the size of a pigeon's egg. The embryo measures about 1 cm. ($\frac{3}{8}$ inch) and weighs 1 G. It is curved like a bean so that head and tail almost meet. The rudimentary eyes are visible and small buds indicate where limbs will develop. Circulation of blood in a rudimentary form exists.

Eight weeks.—The sac is the size of a hen's egg and the chorionic villi will have disappeared, leaving the chorion læve (bald chorion) except in the area where the villi are deeply embedded. The embedded villi grow profusely and are known as the chorion frondosum which ultimately form the placenta. The embryo is 3 cm. ($1\frac{1}{8}$ inch) long and weighs 4 G. amniotic fluid 5-10 ml. is present. Centres of ossification are apparent in some bones; hands and feet are recognizable. The head is large in proportion to the body.

Twelve weeks.—The sac is the size of a goose's egg and the placenta, which is now well formed, weighs more than the fetus. The length of the fetus is 8·9 cm. ($3\frac{1}{2}$ inches) and it weighs just under 57 G. (2 oz.). Fingers and toes are evident.

Sixteen weeks.—The fetus measures 15·2 cm. (6 inches) and weighs approximately 170 G. (6 oz.). The nasal septum and palate fuse, and if this fails to take place, cleft palate results. There is a good heart beat. Fetal movements occur: sex can be distinguished: meconium is present in the intestine.

Twenty weeks.—The fetus is 20·3 cm. (8 inches) long and weighs 283 G. (10 oz.). Vernix caseosa is present on the skin and there are fine downy hairs on the head and eyebrows. Finger nails can be distinguished. Fetal movement is felt by the mother (quickening) and the fetal heart can be heard on auscultation.

Twenty-four weeks.—The fetus measures 30·4 cm. (12 inches) and weighs about 690 G. (1½ lb.).

Twenty-eight weeks.—The fetus measures 35·6 cm. (14 inches) and weighs 1,134 G. (2½ lb.). Legally, the fetus is viable but only about 20 per cent of these very immature babies live.

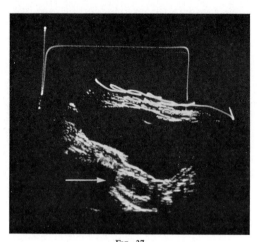

FIG. 37

ULTRASONOGRAM OF EIGHT WEEKS GESTATION SAC.

Anteverted uterus containing the sac (arrow) lying behind a very full bladder (black area above).

Queen Mother's Maternity Hospital, Glasgow

Thirty-two weeks.—The fetus measures 40·6 cm. (16 inches) and weighs 1,600 G. (3½ lb). The skin is red and wrinkled. Lanugo is less plentiful. About 60 per cent of these babies survive.

Thirty-six weeks.—The fetus is 45·7 cm. long (18 inches) and weighs 2,495 G. (5½ lb.). There is a little subcutaneous fat. The plantar creases are visible. The nails reach the finger tips and the cartilage of the ears is soft. The survival rate is good, about 94 per cent can be reared if suitable care is given.

Forty weeks.—The fetus measures 50·8 cm. (20 inches) and weighs 3,175 G. (7 lb.) but length is a better criterion of maturity than weight. The baby is well covered with subcutaneous fat and the skin is red but not wrinkled.

The figures for length and weight given above are only approximate. Wide variations can occur. The baby born at 40 weeks may weigh from 2,722 to 5,443 G. (6 to 12 lb.), male infants being slightly bigger than female, and the babies of multiparous women tend to be increasingly heavier. In a series of 40,000 deliveries at the Simpson Memorial Maternity Pavilion only six babies weighed over 5,443 G. (12 lb.) and one was 6,095 G. (13 lb. 7 oz.).

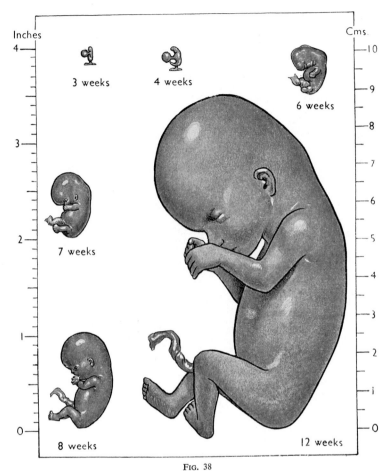

FIG. 38

Size of fetus from 3 to 12 weeks in inches and centimeters.

THE FETAL CIRCULATION

To understand the fetal circulation, the fact must be appreciated that the fetus develops its own blood and that at no time does the fetal and maternal blood mix unless some pathological process is present in the placenta. **The fetus produces its own red and white blood corpuscles.** During intra-uterine life the fetal gastro-intestinal and respiratory systems are not functioning, so from the maternal blood the fetus obtains the necessary nutriment and oxygen as explained below.

There are four temporary structures in the fetal circulation, and if the student midwife learns their functions she should obtain enough knowledge to enable her to understand how the fetal circulation differs from that of the adult, and the changes which take place at birth.

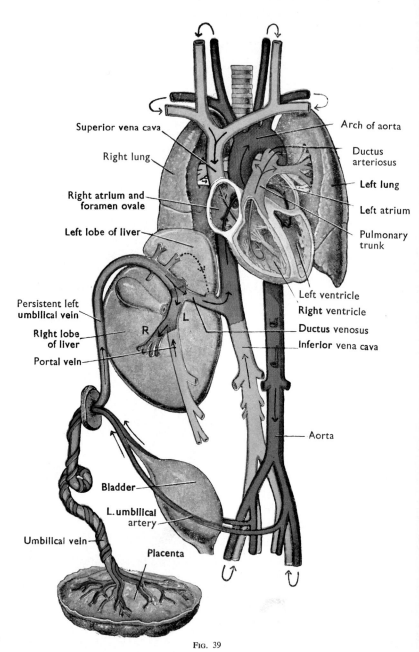

Superior vena cava

Right lung

Right atrium and
foramen ovale

Left lobe of liver

Persistent left
umbilical vein

Right lobe
of liver

Portal vein

Arch of aorta

Ductus
arteriosus

Left lung

Left atrium

Pulmonary
trunk

Left ventricle

Right ventricle

Ductus venosus

Inferior vena cava

Aorta

Bladder

L. umbilical
artery

Umbilical vein

Placenta

FIG. 39

A plan of the fetal circulation. The arrows represent the course which the blood takes in the heart
and vessels. (Gray's Anatomy.)

THE FOUR TEMPORARY STRUCTURES ARE:—

1. **The ductus venosus** (*from a vein to a vein*). This vessel from the umbilical vein to the inferior vena cava carries blood, that has been oxygenated and replenished by the placenta, to the heart for circulation throughout the fetus.

2. **The foramen ovale,** a temporary opening between the two atria in the fetal heart to allow the replenished blood to enter the left atrium and be pumped out through the aorta.

3. **The ductus arteriosus** (*from an artery to an artery*). This vessel from the pulmonary artery to the descending arch of the aorta carries the impure blood returned from the head and upper limbs thereby by-passing the pulmonary circulation.

4. **The hypogastric arteries.** These two vessels branch off from the internal iliac arteries and are known as the umbilical arteries when they enter the umbilical cord. They return impure blood to the placenta for oxygenation and replenishment.

Blood which has circulated throughout the fetus requires to be oxygenated and replenished, so it is carried by the two umbilical arteries in the umbilical cord to the placenta, where an interchange takes place between the fetal and maternal blood by a process of osmosis and diffusion, as well as by the selective action of the cytotrophoblast and the syncytiotrophoblast. Four layers separate fetal from maternal blood. These are syncytiotrophoblast, cytotrophoblast, mesoderm and the capillary wall. Carbon-dioxide and other excretory products are given off into the maternal blood; nutritional substances and oxygen are picked up. It is important to realize that the blood which circulates within the fetal, umbilical and placental vessels is fetal in origin.

The replenished blood returns to the fetus by the vein in the umbilical cord which goes directly to the liver, but, before reaching that organ, a large branch, the **ductus venosus,** is given off and empties the purified blood into the inferior vena cava which is returning the impure blood to the heart from all the vessels below the diaphragm, including the portal vein. The oxygenated blood is therefore mingled with venous blood.

Through the temporary opening, known as the foramen ovale, between the two atria of the fetal heart the oxygenated blood returning from the placenta via the inferior vena cava is shunted from the right into the left atrium and not into the right ventricle, as is the route after birth. It is thought that the force exerted by the Eustachian valve in the inferior vena cava directs the pure blood through the foramen ovale into the left atrium.

The blood then passes from the left atrium to the left ventricle where it is pumped out through the aorta. This blood has the highest oxygen content in the fetal circulation, and the major portion of it goes via branches of the arch of the aorta to the great vessels of the neck that supply the brain, and to the upper limbs. A smaller quantity passes down the descending arch of the aorta.

The impure blood from the head and upper limbs returns to the heart via the superior vena cava and passes from the right atrium to the right ventricle (as it does after birth), and leaves the right ventricle by the pulmonary artery.

The pulmonary circulation functions very slightly before birth, the major amount of blood leaving the right ventricle of the fetus is therefore diverted from the lungs via a temporary vessel—**the ductus arteriosus.** A very little blood is carried by the pulmonary artery to the lungs to nourish them and is returned by the pulmonary veins to the left atrium. The ductus arteriosus conveys the blood from the pulmonary artery to the descending arch of the aorta, where it is distributed to the abdominal and pelvic viscera and to the lower limbs, but the greater proportion of it is returned to the placenta via the **hypogastric arteries,** which are branches of the internal iliac arteries.

The two hypogastric arteries enter the umbilical cord and are then known as the umbilical arteries.

CHANGES IN THE CIRCULATION AT BIRTH

The changes which occur are not due to the tying of the umbilical cord, but rather to the establishment of respiration. **When the infant cries, the lungs expand** and their vascular field is increased: so the blood which has been passing through the ductus arteriosus to the aorta now flows through the pulmonary arteries to the lungs for oxygenation.

The ductus arteriosus ceases to function within five minutes after birth and within two months it is closed anatomically; it eventually becomes a cardiac ligament. In a very small number of cases the ductus arteriosus remains patent.

The valve-like foramen ovale closes when the increased flow of blood to the lungs reduces the pressure in the right side of the heart and increases the tension in the left side. If this does not occur, the venous blood in the right atrium will mix with arterial blood in the left atrium of the heart.

The Fetal Skull

The fetal skull is extremely important in obstetrics, not only because it contains the brain which may be subjected to great pressure while the head is being forced

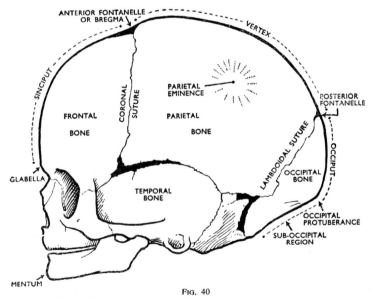

FIG. 40

Fetal skull, showing regions and landmarks of obstetrical importance.

through the birth canal, but because it is so large in comparison with the true pelvis. Obviously, some adaptation between skull and pelvis must take place during labour.

Ninety-six per cent of babies are born head first, and the head is the most difficult part to deliver, whether it comes first or last. Regions of the head may present which increase the hazards of birth for mother and child, but a sound knowledge of the landmarks and measurements of the skull will enable the midwife to recognize malpresentation or disproportion between skull and pelvis and to deliver the baby with the minimal amount of fetal and maternal trauma.

BONES

The bones that form the roof and sides of the skull are developed from membrane, whereas most of the skeleton develops from cartilage. The intra-membranous ossification of the skull bones begins as early as the second month of intra-uterine life. At term the skull bones are thin and pliable and, as ossification at their edges is not quite complete, areas of membrane persist between the bones.

SUTURES

The membranous spaces between the bones of the vault of the skull are known as sutures and during labour considerable overlapping of the skull bones takes place at these membranous spaces.

The sagittal suture lies between the two parietal bones.

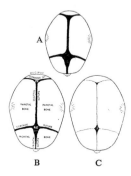

Fig. 41

FETAL SKULL SUTURES.

The three diagrams depict the sutures in premature, mature and postmature skulls. Note wide sutures and large fontanelles in the premature skull (A) and narrow sutures and small fontanelles in the postmature skull (C).

The lambdoidal suture separates the occipital and parietal bones.

The coronal suture runs between the parietal and frontal bones, crossing from one temple to the other.

The frontal suture separates the two halves of the frontal bone.

The sutures form very useful landmarks when making a vaginal examination during labour.

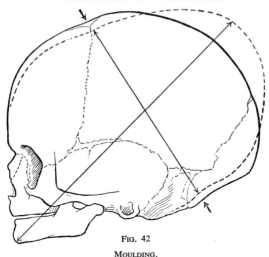

FIG. 42

MOULDING.

Arrows show direction in which the well-flexed head is being compressed. Note how it is elongated in the mento-vertical diameter.

FONTANELLES

Where two or more sutures meet, the membranous space at the junction is known
as a fontanelle. There are six fontanelles on the skull, but only two are of obstetrical
importance, the anterior and the posterior.

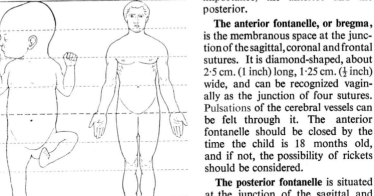

FIG. 43

Comparison of proportions of baby to adult.
Baby's head wider than its shoulders and
one-quarter of its length.

The anterior fontanelle, or bregma,
is the membranous space at the junction of the sagittal, coronal and frontal
sutures. It is diamond-shaped, about
2·5 cm. (1 inch) long, 1·25 cm. ($\frac{1}{2}$ inch)
wide, and can be recognized vagin-
ally as the junction of four sutures.
Pulsations of the cerebral vessels can
be felt through it. The anterior
fontanelle should be closed by the
time the child is 18 months old,
and if not, the possibility of rickets
should be considered.

The posterior fontanelle is situated
at the junction of the sagittal and
lambdoidal sutures; it is smaller than
the anterior fontanelle and can be
recognized vaginally as the junction
of three sutures. In shape it is
triangular and should be closed
about six weeks after birth.

We are so accustomed to the pro-
portions of a baby that we do not always realize that its head is larger than the width
of its shoulders. (The bisacromial diameter of the shoulders measures 11·4 cm. (4$\frac{1}{2}$
inches); the mento-vertical diameter of the skull measures 13·3 cm. (5$\frac{1}{4}$ inches).

MOULDING

Moulding is the term applied to the change in shape of the fetal head that takes place, due to the prolonged compression to which it is subjected, during its passage through the birth canal. This alteration in shape is possible because the bones of the vault, not being well ossified, are somewhat pliable and permit a slight degree of bending, but **the over-riding of the skull bones at the sutures** is the most important factor in moulding. The parietal bones usually over-ride the frontal and occipital bones, and the parietal bone, lying in the posterior part of the pelvic brim, is subjected to greater pressure from the promontory of the sacrum, so it goes under the anterior parietal bone.

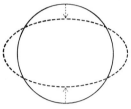

Fig. 44

Demonstration of the principle of moulding. The diameter compressed is diminished; the diameter at right angles to it is elongated

A certain amount of moulding is present on every baby's head, except in those born by elective Cæsarean section. In breech presentation compression of the head is of short duration so no moulding is evident although over-riding of the skull bones must have occurred temporarily. **During moulding the engaging diameter is compressed** and may be shortened by as much as 1·25 cm. (half an inch) and the diameter at right angles to it will be elongated. In the vertex presentation, L.O.A., the suboccipito-bregmatic diameter is reduced and the mento-vertical diameter is lengthened. It is possible to diagnose what the presentation has been by the shape of the moulded head after birth (see page 588).

In small premature babies moulding is excessive; the soft skull bones and wide sutures afford little protection to the delicate brain substance.

In postmature babies the sutures are almost closed and the head does not mould well; the hardness of the head rather than its increased size tends to make labour more difficult.

REGIONS OF THE SKULL

The skull is divided into the vault, face and base. The **vault** is the large dome-shaped compressible part made up of the two parietal, the upper parts of the frontal, occipital and temporal bones, and is the region above an imaginary line drawn from the orbital ridges to the nape of the neck. The **base** is comprised of bones firmly united to afford protection to the vital centres in the medulla.

The vertex is the area bounded in front by the anterior fontanelle, behind by the posterior fontanelle and laterally by the two parietal eminences which are seen as two prominent points on the parietal bones. Ninety-five of the 96 per cent of babies who are born head first present by the vertex.

The face, which in the newborn is very small because of the poorly developed mandible, is the area from the root of the nose to the junction of the chin and neck. The face bones are firmly united at birth and do not permit of moulding. The chin or *mentum* is an important landmark.

The brow or sinciput is composed of the frontal bones and is bounded by the orbital ridges and the coronal suture.

The occiput is the region over the occipital bone and extends from the posterior fontanelle to the foramen magnum. The suboccipital region is that part under the occipital protuberance, a prominent point on the posterior aspect of the skull.

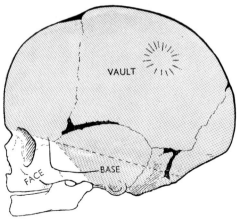

Fig. 45

Regions of the skull showing the large compressible vault,
the non-compressible face and base.

DIAMETERS

Biparietal—9·5 cm. (3¾ inches)—a transverse diameter measured between the two parietal eminences.

Bitemporal—8·3 cm. (3¼ inches)—a transverse diameter measured from the furthest points of the coronal suture (between the temples).

Suboccipito-bregmatic—9·5 cm. (3¾ inches)—is measured from below the occipital protuberance (the nape of the neck) to the centre of the anterior fontanelle or bregma.

Suboccipito-frontal—10·2 cm. (4 inches)—from below the occipital protuberance to the centre of the sinciput.

Occipito-frontal—11·4 cm. (4½ inches)—from the occipital protuberance to the glabella, a point above the bridge of the nose, see Fig. 40.

Submento-bregmatic—9·5 cm. (3¾ inches)—from where the chin joins the neck to the centre of the anterior fontanelle or bregma.

Submento-vertical—11·4 cm. (4½ inches)—from where the chin joins the neck to the highest point on the vertex.

Mento-vertical—13·3 cm. (5¼ inches)—from the tip of the chin to the highest point on the vertex (which is nearer the posterior than the anterior fontanelle).

These measurements should be learned in conjunction with the presentation with which they are associated. It is a distinct advantage for the midwife to be conversant with the most advantageous diameter in each presentation, for by promoting flexion or extension of the head she can often bring more favourable diameters over the perineum with less injury to mother and baby.

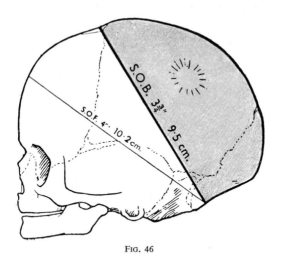

FIG. 46

Diameters concerned in a vertex presentation head well flexed.
The suboccipito-frontal diameter " sweeps the perineum."

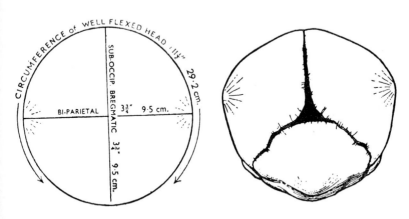

FIG. 47

Showing the diameters (and circumference) presenting in a well-flexed head.

CEPHALIC OR HEAD PRESENTATIONS

Vertex presentation.—*When the head is well flexed,* the suboccipito-bregmatic and the biparietal are the two diameters of the presenting circular area, the circumference of which is 29·2 cm. (11½ inches). This is the most favourable presentation because of its small size and circular shape. The suboccipito-frontal diameter 10·2 cm. (4 inches) will sweep the perineum.

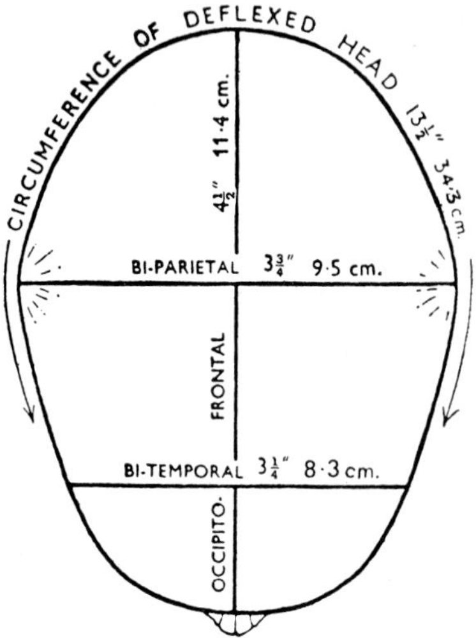

FIG. 48

Showing diameters and circumference presenting in a deflexed head.

When the head is deflexed it is erect, as in the military attitude. The engaging diameters are: occipito-frontal, 11·4 cm. (4½ inches), and transversely the biparietal, 9·5 cm. (3¾ inches) and bitemporal, 8·3 cm. (3¼ inches). The circumference measures 34·3 cm. (13½ inches), and is ovoid in shape. The occipito-frontal diameter, 11·4 cm. (4½ inches), will sweep the perineum.

Face presentation.—The face presents when the head is completely extended, and the diameter engaging is the submento-bregmatic, 9·5 cm. (3¾ inches). The submento-vertical diameter, 11·4 cm. (4½ inches), will sweep the perineum.

Brow presentation.—When partial extension occurs, the engaging diameter is the mento-vertical, 13·3 cm. (5¼ inches), with a circumference of 38·1 cm. (15 inches). Rarely can a baby be born naturally when the brow presents.

MOVEMENT OF THE FETAL HEAD

The fetal head is capable of a wide range of movement, and may be flexed until the chin is in contact with the chest, as occurs in a vertex presentation when the head is well flexed. Complete extension of the head may take place, so that the occiput is in contact with the fetal back, as occurs when the face presents. A certain amount of lateral flexion is possible and the head can also rotate on the neck two-eighths of a circle (90 degrees). These movements are of importance in the mechanism of labour.

QUESTIONS FOR REVISION

ORAL QUESTIONS

How would you recognize the anterior and posterior fontanelles P.V. ?

Which diameter distends the vulval orifice in a well flexed head ?

Which diameter sweeps the perineum during extension of the head ?

What is the benefit of a well flexed head ? When should the anterior fontanelle close ?

MATCH TERM AND DESCRIPTION BY CORRECT NUMBERS:

(1) **ovum**	fertilised cell from 3rd to 8th week	(	)
(2) **vernix:**	downy hair on newborn skin	(	)
(3) **embryo:**	fertilised cell first three weeks	(	)
(4) **sagittal suture:**	between parietal and occipital bones	(	)
(5) **lanugo:**	cheesy substance on newborn skin	(	)
(6) **suture:**	junction of membranous spaces	(	)
(7) **bregma:**	the brow	(	)
(8) **lambdoidal suture:**	between parietal bones	(	)
(9) **cephalic**	bounded by two fontanelles and bi-parietal eminences	(	)
(10) **vertex:**	the head	(	)
(11) **fontanelle:**	a membranous space	(	)
(12) **sinciput:**	the anterior fontanelle	(	)

Differentiate between the terms : ovum, embryo, fetus, baby. When is the fetus viable ?

Where are the following situated and what are their functions ? **Ductus venosus ; foramen ovale ; ductus arteriosus ; hypogastric arteries.**

C.M.B.(Eng.) paper.—Describe the fetal circulation and the changes that take place at birth.

C.M.B.(N. Ireland) paper.—Describe in detail the anatomy of the fetal skull. What benefit is this knowledge to the midwife ?

C.M.B.(Eng.) paper.—Describe the fetal skull. What changes and injuries may occur as a result of labour ?

C.M.B.(Eng.) paper.—Describe the anatomy of the vault of the fetal skull. What is moulding and why does it occur ?

C.M.B. (Scot.) paper.—Describe the fetal skull. Give a list of the important diameters and their measurements (inches or centimetres).

C.M.B.(Eng.) paper, 1968.—Describe the vault of the fetal skull. How does knowledge of this help in the conduct of labour ?

C.M.B.(Scot.) paper, 1969.—Describe the anatomy of the fetal skull.

C.M.B.(Eng.) paper, 1969.—Describe the moulding of the fetal head.

PART II: PREGNANCY

4

The Physiological Changes due to Pregnancy

A STUDY of the physiological changes that take place in the woman's body during pregnancy will explain many of the phenomena that are regarded as signs and symptoms of pregnancy, as well as affording a sound basis for the intelligent administration of prenatal care. The changes are not confined to the reproductive organs; **every tissue and organ reacts to the stimulus of pregnancy,** and the metabolic, chemical and endocrine balance of the body is altered.

THE UTERUS

Changes in the reproductive organs are, of course, predominant. The uterus must enlarge and give nourishment and protection to the growing fetus, so it increases in weight and size.

INCREASE IN WEIGHT

From 57 G. (2 oz.) to 907 G. (2 lb.). Two thirds weight increase occurs during the first 20 weeks.

INCREASE IN SIZE

From 7·6 × 5·1 × 2·5 cm. (3 × 2 × 1 inches) to 30·5 × 22·9 × 20·3 cm. (12 × 9 × 8 inches)

The uterus must also expel the fetus at a viable age, and as this process of expulsion or labour is a muscular feat the muscle coat develops in a remarkable degree: each muscle fibre increases 10 times in length and 5 times in thickness, and new fibres come into being.

THE MUSCLE COAT CONSISTS OF THREE LAYERS

The fibres of the inner layer are arranged in circular fashion, and as circular fibres guard all the orifices of the body they are plentiful in the lower pole of the uterus, allowing the lower uterine segment to stretch and the os to dilate.

The fibres of the middle layer are arranged in every conceivable direction, vertical, transverse and figure of eight. These fibres contract and retract during labour and because of their constricting action on the blood vessels during the third stage they control bleeding and are known as "*living ligatures*".

The fibres in the outer layer are arranged longitudinally and extend from the cervix, anteriorly over the fundus, down to the cervix, posteriorly. The longitudinal fibres contract and shorten during labour, causing the upper uterine segment to thicken and shorten, and at the same time they draw up and thin out the lower uterine segment.

BLOOD SUPPLY

The uterus is very richly supplied with blood during pregnancy, particularly in the area of the placental site, and it has been estimated that the uterus at term contains about 1,500 ml. of blood. **The blood vessels increase in size and number** and their tortuous arrangement allows for the rapid increase in the growth of the uterus.

The changes in the endometrium have been described under Formation of the Decidua (p. 28).

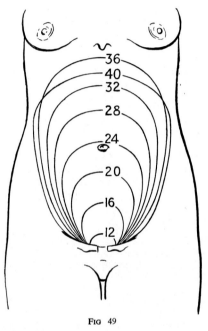

FIG 49

Fundal heights at various weeks during pregnancy in relation to the symphysis pubis.

THE LOWER UTERINE SEGMENT

This area of the uterus develops from the isthmus and at term extends upwards for 7·6 to 8·9 cm. (3 to 3½ inches) from the internal os to the upper uterine segment. The muscle fibres in the lower uterine segment are not as well developed as in the upper segment.

Because during the last weeks of pregnancy the lower uterine segment is soft and stretched the presenting part sinks further down into the uterus.

THE CERVIX

The cervix becomes softer and the cervical racemose glands secrete a tenacious mucus which forms a plug — the **operculum** — that effectively occludes the cervical canal and provides a barrier against infection.

THE GROWTH OF THE UTERUS

The uterus grows at such a regular rate that it is possible, within limits, to estimate the period of gestation by its size. There is, of course, room for error, as the uterus may contain twins, a large fetus or an excessive amount of amniotic fluid.

EIGHTH WEEK

The uterus cannot yet be palpated abdominally. On bimanual examination, it is found to be about the size of a tennis ball but more ovoid in shape, and because the ovum is embedded in the upper half of the uterus it becomes slightly more anteflexed from the 6th to the 12th week.

TWELFTH WEEK

The uterus fills the pelvic cavity and the fundus reaches just above the summit of the symphysis pubis. It is globular in shape and about the size of a small grapefruit.

6

SIXTEENTH WEEK

The uterus has risen to just less than half-way between the symphysis pubis and the umbilicus, or 7·6 cm. (3 inches) above the symphysis pubis. The shape of the uterus is more ovoid than globular and because it is in contact with the abdominal wall quickening is felt. *The uterine souffle* can be heard.

TWENTIETH WEEK

The fundus is two fingers breadth below the level of the umbilicus, or 15·2 cm. (6 inches) above the symphysis pubis. The positive signs of pregnancy—fetal heart, fetal parts and fetal movement—can be elicited without ultrasonic aid.

TWENTY-FOURTH WEEK

The fundus is at the upper margin of the umbilicus, about 19 cm. (7½ inches) and the uterus tends to lean and rotate on its axis towards the right side.

THIRTIETH WEEK

The fundus is midway between the umbilicus and xiphisternum, about 24·1 cm. (9½ inches) above the symphysis pubis.

THIRTY-SIXTH WEEK

The uterus rises to its highest level and is in contact with the xiphisternum, 30·5 cm. (12 inches) above the symphysis pubis. At the 38th week the fundus sinks down to about the level of a 34 weeks' pregnancy, and this is known as "*lightening*." (See p. 228).

FORTIETH WEEK

The uterus is ready to go into labour. The lower uterine segment is relaxed and stretched, the cervix is shortened and soft, and its canal is still closed by the operculum. The fetus lies, usually head downwards, within the amniotic sac.

THE OVARIES

The corpus luteum in the ruptured Graafian follicle degenerates after the 12th week of pregnancy and its endocrine functions are taken over by the placenta (p. 34).

THE VAGINA

There is some degree of hypertrophy of the muscle-coat of the vagina in preparation for the distension that will be necessary during labour. The greatly augmented blood supply gives rise to blue discoloration and to increased pulsation in the fornices.

All pregnant women have a white vaginal discharge which is due to the action of œstrogens and to venous engorgement.

THE BREASTS

The breasts are accessory organs of generation and changes in them occur very early, due to the stimulus of the ovarian hormones œstrogens and progesterone, so that even before a woman has missed a period she may be conscious of a prickling, tingling sensation in her breasts. Œstrogens are thought to stimulate the growth of the glandular tissue and ducts, while progesterone activates the secretory function of the breasts.

As early as the sixth week, the breasts have enlarged, they have a firm tense feeling and are sometimes tender. The growth of the breasts continues throughout pregnancy with a weight increase of about 454 G. (one pound). The nipple becomes darker in colour and more erectile.

The primary areola. At the 12th week there is darkening of the area around the nipple and its diameter, which is normally 3·8 cm. (1½ inches) extends until in some instances it may be 7·6 cm. (3 inches). It also looks moist and œdematous in comparison with the flat pink areola of the non-pregnant woman. In reddish fair-haired women the areola may remain pink, but in brunettes it becomes dark brown or even black. At this time a little clear fluid can be expressed from the breasts, but true **colostrum** does not appear until the 16th week.

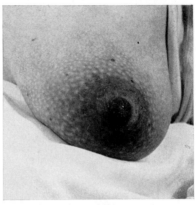

FIG. 50

Well marked pigmentation of the breast during pregnancy. The darker zone extending about 3·8 cm. (1½ inches) beyond the nipple is the primary areola. The extensive mottled area is the secondary areola.

Montgomery's tubercles.—From the 8th week onwards, 12 to 30 small nodules appear on the primary areola. They are the pouting mouths of sebaceous glands, and the sebum they secrete keeps the nipple soft and pliable.

The secondary areola is seen after the 16th week. It is a mottled zone of pigmentation, extending beyond the primary areola and sometimes covering half of the breast. This breast pigmentation may persist for 12 months after parturition.

Dilated veins can be clearly seen on the chest and breasts from the 8th week.

BREAST CHANGES IN CHRONOLOGICAL ORDER

WEEKS		WEEKS	
3 to 4	Prickling, tingling sensation.	12	Darkening of the primary areola.
6	Enlarged and tense.	12	Fluid can be expressed.
8	Surface veins are visible.	16	Colostrum can be expressed.
8	Montgomery's tubercules appear.	16	Secondary areola appears.

THE SKIN

Tiny scars, known as striæ gravidarum, appear as early as the 16th week on the lower abdomen, thighs and breasts of some pregnant women. They are thought to be due to the rapid stretching of the skin and can occur in cases of adiposity but it has been suggested that hyper-function of the anterior pituitary gland or adreno-cortical activity may play some part in their production. The deeper layer of the dermis ruptures and the epidermis is thinned out, producing little scars of a **bluish pink appearance in the present pregnancy.** From previous pregnancies, faded silvery striæ are seen intermingled with the pink ones.

The sweat and sebaceous glands are more active during pregnancy.

Pigmentation of the skin is common during pregnancy and is assumed to be due to the action of the melanin stimulating hormone of the anterior pituitary. It is more pronounced in brunettes and is often seen on the breasts and vulva. On the face it can be quite disfiguring and the bronze, blotchy areas seen on the forehead and sides of the face are known as the *chloasma* or, more commonly, the **mask of pregnancy**. In summer it is more noticeable. The linea alba, a white line between the recti muscles, becomes markedly pigmented and can be seen extending from the symphysis pubis to above the umbilicus: when pigmented it is known as the **linea nigra**. Pigmentation is sometimes seen in the striæ of multigravid women.

THE BLOOD

There is an increase of about 40–50 per cent in blood volume from the 8th week of pregnancy onwards, mainly in the plasma, but there is also a slight increase in red cells. This watery condition of the blood is known as *hydræmia*, and because of the hæmodilution, red cell counts and hæmoglobin estimations will be 10 to 15 per cent lower during pregnancy. It should be remembered that **the fetus is withdrawing iron for its immediate needs and storing iron in its liver** for future use during the lactational period. The fibrinogen content is also increased.

THE HEART AND LUNGS

During pregnancy the heart is called upon to carry an additional load, but as a rule the healthy heart can cope with this. The increased volume of blood has to be pumped with sufficient force to maintain adequate placental circulation, so the cardiac output is increased from about the 16th week of pregnancy by 20 to 40 per cent and remains elevated until delivery.

The lungs are displaced slightly upwards when the growing uterus encroaches on the thorax and restricts the free excursion of the diaphragm. Shortness of breath may be due to the deeper respirations which are necessary because of increased oxygen consumption.

THE BLOOD PRESSURE

There is no physiological rise in blood pressure during pregnancy, in spite of the increased blood volume and cardiac output: in fact it may be slightly lower than normal. This may be due to dilatation of the blood vessels which occurs under the relaxing influence of hormones. The blood pressure appears to be very labile (unstable) in some pregnant women: a slight drop in pressure, due to emotional or other causes, tends to cause fainting. Conversely, excitement or exertion may produce a transient rise.

SUPINE HYPOTENSIVE SYNDROME

A fall in blood pressure may occur in some women, when during the later weeks they lie on their backs (*as at the prenatal clinic*), due to the pressure of the uterus on the inferior vena cava delaying the return of blood to the heart: slight tachycardia occurs followed by profound bradycardia. **If a recumbent woman feels faint she should be turned on her left side immediately.**

THE BLADDER

Frequency of micturition is common from the 6th to the 12th week. This is not now considered to be due to pressure by the uterus. Investigations are proceeding. In the later weeks of pregnancy, when lightening takes place, the lax condition of all the tissues of the pelvic floor may be a contributory cause of the frequency and even of slight incontinence of urine that occurs at this time.

The ureters are liable to be compressed by the uterus when it rises out of the pelvis. After the 16th week the increased secretion of hormones, probably progesterone, produces laxity in the walls of the ureters, rendering them subject to compression and more capable of being dilated. Stasis of urine occurs in the dilated part and is believed to predispose the woman to *pyelonephritis*.

WEIGHT GAIN (based on Hytten)

A gain of about 11·340 kg. (25 lb.) is to be expected in the pregnant woman of average build and can be accounted for by the following.

FETUS .	3·175 kg.	7 lb.
PLACENTA .	0·567 ,,	1¼ ,,
AMNIOTIC FLUID	0·907 ,,	2 ,,
INCREASE IN WEIGHT OF UTERUS	0·907 ,,	2 ,,
INCREASE IN WEIGHT OF BREASTS	0·454 ,,	1
INCREASE IN BLOOD VOLUME	1·361 ,,	3 ,,
EXTRA-CELLULAR FLUID .	1·134 ,,	2½ ,,
FAT	2·722 ,,	6 ,,
Total	11·227 kg.	24¾ lb.

A pregnant woman gains on the average approximately 2·268 kg. (5 lb.) during the first 20 weeks of pregnancy. During the second 20 weeks, weight gain amounts to approximately 9.072 kg. (20 lb.). Many factors are involved, including the metabolic rate of the individual, fluid balance, and the uterine contents. (Weighing the pregnant woman is described on p. 99.)

THE SKELETON

A change in the gait of the pregnant woman is noticeable during the second half of pregnancy when the balance of the body is altered because of the enlarged uterus. The shoulders are thrown backwards and the lumbar curve is increased almost to lordosis, which, along with relaxation of the pelvic joints and ligaments during the later weeks of pregnancy, may give rise to discomfort or actual backache.

It is the bones and not the teeth that are the storehouses for calcium, so it is no longer believed that the woman's teeth decay during pregnancy because calcium is being withdrawn from them.

THE NERVOUS SYSTEM

Pregnancy is one of the three periods in a woman's life when there seems to be a lowering of the ability to cope with the emotional experiences of life. At puberty and the menopause a similar degree of instability may be manifest and in each instance the cause is probably endocrine in origin.

During pregnancy there are emotional as well as physical adjustments to be made and, even in cases where the coming baby is welcome, a mild degree of depression or irritability may be evident during the early months.

Forty years ago cravings for indigestable foods, and temper tantrums were a common occurrence, but women should be discouraged from the belief that they are a normal accompaniment of pregnancy. Longings for certain sour or tart articles of food may be due to nausea rather than to nervous instability, and the tactfal implication that cravings and tantrums are rather old fashioned is usually a sufficient deterrent.

THE GENERAL METABOLISM

During pregnancy the body is functioning at its maximal efficiency, for nature endeavours to provide an ideal environment for the nutrition and development of the fetus.

It is well known that once a woman becomes physically and emotionally adjusted to the impact of pregnancy she enjoys a feeling of well-being. Her appetite is good, she looks and feels well, but this can only be experienced if she is healthy, well nourished and not overworked.

The basal metabolic rate increases 15 to 25 per cent during the latter half of pregnancy in response to the demands of the growing fetus and maternal tissues, so the woman's fuel requirements are higher and a diet providing 2,400 calories will be necessary unless she is physically inactive.

The metabolism of carbohydrates in pregnancy is not wholly understood. Glycosuria occurs in 10 per cent of women, probably due to a lowering of the renal threshold for glucose. Normal fasting blood glucose is 80 to 100 mg. per 100 ml. of blood and the kidney does not excrete glucose in the urine of a healthy individual until the blood glucose rises to 160. During pregnancy that threshold may be lowered and the kidney excretes glucose when the blood glucose is 120.

The Endocrine Glands

The endocrine changes associated with pregnancy involve so many organs and govern so many functions that they have been discussed in various chapters throughout the book.

ŒDEMA IN PREGNANCY

PHYSIOLOGICAL ŒDEMA

About 40 per cent of pregnant women have slight ankle œdema, during the last 12 weeks of pregnancy, which disappears with rest and is rarely present in the morning. This may be due to: (a) the normal reduction of plasma proteins in pregnancy tending by osmosis to draw fluid into the tissues; (b) venous pressure in the iliofemoral veins being intensified when the erect posture is maintained for long periods because the return flow of blood from the lower limbs is slowed down by the greatly augmented venous return from the uterine veins. This may be aggravated by pressure of the enlarged uterus and by the wearing of constricting bands.

PATHOLOGICAL ŒDEMA

(a) Pre-eclampsia.—This is the cause for which the midwife must be constantly on the alert, and œdema should never be considered physiological until all pathological causes have been ruled out. Abnormal water retention may cause a marked increase in weight.

(*b*) **Cardiac disease.**—If there is circulatory inefficiency the kidneys do not function well, and when the œdema is generalized it is a sign of serious import.

(*c*) **Chronic nephritis.**—The impaired kidneys do not excrete sodium efficiently and therefore fluid is retained in the tissues.

(*d*) **Malnutrition.**—When nutrition is very poor the plasma proteins become seriously depleted. Low protein diet will therefore cause œdema.

(*e*) **Varicose veins** in the legs or vulva will give rise to œdema in those regions. When œdema is due to venous thrombosis, pain and venous engorgement are also evident. For the detection of œdema, see p. 168.

NUTRITION IN PREGNANCY

When the level of nutrition of the population is high, the number of spontaneous abortions, stillbirths and neonatal deaths is lower.

The woman's food requirements are increased during pregnancy, but more so in quality than quantity. More attention should be paid to the inclusion of the vital substances needed for growth and health, for the woman could obtain an adequate caloric intake from a most unsatisfactory diet. To avoid excessive weight gain the less active woman should not increase her food intake.

THE DIET IN PREGNANCY SHOULD PROVIDE FOR:

THE NEEDS OF THE GROWING FETUS.
THE MAINTENANCE OF MATERNAL HEALTH.
PHYSICAL STRENGTH AND VITALITY DURING LABOUR.
SUCCESSFUL LACTATION.

The expectant mother need not adhere rigidly to any special diet, but the midwife must advise and guide her in selecting proper foods, if it is evident that her diet is defective. **Advice on how to teach " nutrition " to expectant mothers** is given in the chapter on preparation for parenthood.

DAILY REQUIREMENTS	Grams				Calories
Proteins	90	×	4	=	360
Fats	90	×	9	=	810
Carbohydrates	320	×	4	=	1,280
					2,450

PROTEINS

These are absolutely essential, because they are the only substances that build tissue, and the mother has to provide for the growth of the fetus, placenta, uterus, breasts and the increased blood volume. The maintenance of a normal red cell count and hæmoglobin level is dependent on an adequate dietary intake of proteins.

A minimal daily intake of 80 G. ought to be provided during pregnancy, and 60 per cent should be first class. From the following foods, 90 G. of proteins could be obtained daily.

ONE DAY'S PROTEIN REQUIREMENTS

MILK, 900 ml. (1½ pints)	30 G.	FIRST-CLASS PROTEINS	
EGG, 1	6 ,,	,,	,,
MEAT, 113 G. (4 oz.) (raw weight) . . .	20 ,,	,,	,,
WHITE FISH, 113 G. (4 oz.) (raw weight) . .	18 ,,	,,	,,
CHEESE, 14 G. (½ oz.)	4 ,,	,,	,,
WHOLE-MEAL BREAD, 4 slices, 113 G. (4 oz.) .	12 ,,	SECOND-CLASS PROTEINS	
TOTAL	90 G.		

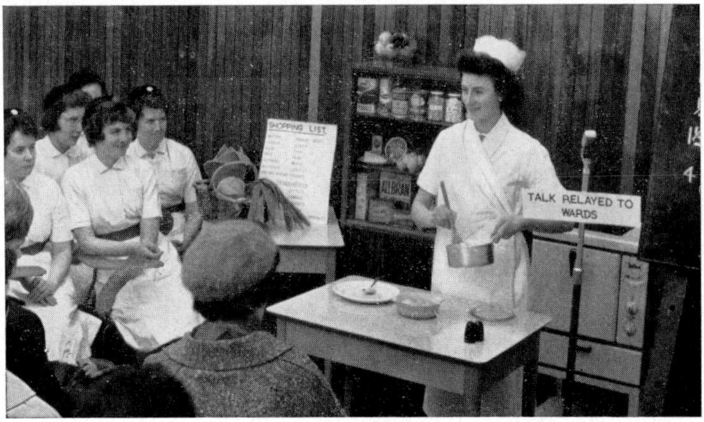

FIG. 51

Cookery demonstration and talk on suitable food for expectant mothers.   Given in Mothercraft department and relayed to wards.

(*County Maternity Hospital, Bellshill, Lanarkshire.*

CARBOHYDRATES AND FATS

Because carbohydrate is cheap and readily available the intake is usually more than adequate, and when that is so, the intake of the vital substances (proteins, minerals, vitamins) may be dangerously low.   Abnormal weight gain may be due to ingesting an excessive amount of sugar in foods such as cakes, biscuits, jam, ice-cream, sweets and chocolate.

Fat should consist mainly of the animal type, which contains vitamins A and D. A daily quota of 90 G. of fat would be a reasonable amount.   An excessive fat intake will produce weight gain as when foods such as pastry, fat meat or bacon, and cream are eaten, and where frying is the main method of cooking meat and fish.

Some authorities advocate controlling the weight by dietary measures and limiting the total weight gain to 10·8 kg. (24 lb.).   A diet with adequate proteins and containing the essential minerals and vitamins found in fresh fruits and vegetables will help to produce a healthy mother and baby.   Sugar and starchy foods should be curtailed, fat foods limited.

WEIGHT-CONTROL DIET

(*Approx.* 1,760 *calories*, 95 *G. proteins*)

Breakfast. Orange ; porridge or flakes and milk with no added sugar ; egg ;
one slice 28 G. whole-meal bread ; 7 G. butter ; coffee or tea .   .   .   milk
                                                                        240 *ml.*

Mid-morning. Milk, flavoured if desired .   .   .   .   milk
                                                                        240 *ml.*

Lunch. 210 ml. milk-soup ; 113 G. lean meat or liver or fowl or kidney or
sweetbreads ; one average-size potato ; cooked green or root vegetable or
salad ; 7 G. butter ; raw or stewed fruit .   .   .   .   .   .   milk
                                                                        210 *ml.*

Tea. One slice whole-meal bread ; 7 G. butter ; tomato, lettuce, cress or
grated raw carrot ; slice plain cake (no icing or cream filling) .   .   .   milk
                                                                        30 *ml.*

Supper. 113 G. fish or tripe cooked with milk, or egg or 14 G. cheese ; one
slice bread ; 7 G. butter ; apple or other raw fruit .   .   .   .   milk
                                                                        240 *ml.*

Bed Time. Milky drink .   .   .   .   milk
                                                                        240 *ml.*

At each main meal, meat, fish, egg or cheese and fresh fruit or vegetable should be taken.
Dried and canned fruits contain sugar. By skimming 1,200 ml. (2 pints) milk 300 calories
can be removed. *Unfortunately meat and fruit are expensive articles of diet.*

MINERALS

Iron, an essential component of hæmoglobin, ranks very high in importance for
the pregnant woman: the fetus requires iron, not only for its immediate needs but
for the lactational period, so iron is stored in its liver during the last 10 weeks of
intra-uterine life. The woman's diet should contain 15 mg. iron per day.

Foods rich in iron are: Liver, kidney, beef, blood sausage, eggs, prunes, raisins,
green vegetables, black treacle. Six slices of whole-meal bread provide half the day's
iron requirements.

Folic acid is a coenzyme necessary in the formation of blood cells in the bone
marrow. Foods rich in folic acid are dark green vegetables, liver and kidney.

Calcium is needed in the formation of fetal bones and teeth. The teeth are forming as early as the 6th week of pregnancy, but the calcium need is greatest in the
last 12 weeks when rapid ossification of the fetal skeleton is taking place. The pregnant woman needs 1·5 G. of calcium daily.

Six hundred ml. of milk contains 0·68 *G. of calcium.* Cheese is also a good source.
The calcium in milk is very readily absorbed and utilized, whereas the calcium in
tablet form is not.

VITAMINS

During pregnancy a vitamin deficiency may be due to imperfect absorption, or
persistent nausea and vomiting, as well as an insufficient intake. Vitamins are present
in nearly all fresh animal and vegetable foods.

Vitamin A (Retinol equiv.). The chief sources are butter, milk, liver, egg-yolk and
particularly fish-liver oils. A pregnant woman needs 750 μg. daily (2,250 i.u.).

Vitamin B₁.—During pregnancy the demand for vitamin B_1 is increased fivefold, to about 700 to 800 units, or 2 to 2·5 mg. daily. The chief sources are whole-meal bread, meat, liver and yeast.

Vitamin C—ascorbic acid—is required during pregnancy for the growing fetus. It is also concerned in blood formation and the absorption of iron. The daily intake of ascorbic acid during pregnancy should be 100 mg.

Vitamin D is the anti-rachitic vitamin produced by the body when exposed to sunlight. Certain animal products are good sources, *e.g.* milk, butter, eggs, cheese, herring and salmon.

Vitamin K is essential in the formation of prothrombin, which is necessary for the coagulation of blood. The pregnant woman's diet should contain foods which are good sources, such as cabbage, cauliflower, lettuce, carrots.

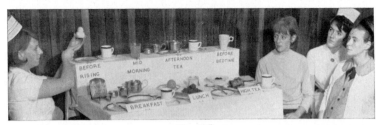

FIG. 52

Mothercraft Sister giving lesson on diet in pregnancy: demonstrating suitable meals for one day.
(*County Maternity Hospital, Bellshill, Lanarkshire.*)

THE DAILY MENU SHOULD INCLUDE

Milk, 900 ml. (1½ pints).	Porridge or other whole-grain cereal.
Egg, 1.	Orange, grape-fruit, or tomato.
Meat, average helping.	Two vegetables, one green (raw).
Fish.	Potatoes.
Wholemeal bread.	Butter, or margarine (fortified).

If these foods are taken, the woman can make up the remainder of her diet with whichever foods she prefers so long as they are wholesome and digestible . **Liver is a valuable food** and should be taken once a week if available. All the necessary factors can be obtained within a comparatively small range of well selected foods; proteins, minerals and vitamins frequently being present in one food.

Fluid.—Two glasses of water, in addition to milk, tea, coffee, etc., will provide the necessary amount.

Whether the baby's birth weight can be lessened by decreasing the mother's intake of food during pregnancy has not yet been satisfactorily proved. It is more likely to result in the birth of an infant of such poor vitality as to be incapable of withstanding the hazards of birth or of surviving the risks of the neonatal period.

QUESTIONS FOR REVISION

THE PHYSIOLOGICAL CHANGES IN PREGNANCY

FUNDAL HEIGHT—fill in correct week

Level	week
(1) Midway between symphysis and umbilicus 12	( )
(2) At summit of symphysis pubis 16	( )
(3) When lightening occurs 36	( )
(4) At the umbilicus 30	( )
(5) In contact with xiphisternum...............................38	( )
(6) Midway between umbilicus and xiphisternum............24	( )

(7) When do the following appear in the breast ?

Montgomery's tubercles...............Colostrum ....
Darkening of primary areola............Surface veins............
Give examples of pigmentation. What are striæ gravidarum ?

ORAL QUESTIONS

Which conditions may influence fundal height levels ? What is the average weight gain for a pregnant woman ? State the average weekly weight gains. How would you deal with syncope from supine hypotensive syndrome ? Why look for œdema in the pregnant woman ?

Practical Application

1. Which physiological changes are used as probable signs of pregnancy ?
2. How soon should a pregnant woman wear a supporting brassière ?
3. What can a midwife surmise from seeing silver striæ ?
4. Why does the hæmoglobin fall in pregnancy ?
5. Give causes of œdema.

C.M.B.(N. Ireland) paper.—What are the changes that appear in the breasts during pregnancy ? What advice would you give a pregnant woman about the care of her breasts ?

C.M.B.(N. Ireland) paper.—At the 36th week of pregnancy a woman has swollen feet and legs. To what may this be due and how are these conditions treated ?

C.M.B.(Scot.) paper.—Describe the anatomy of the uterus in a pregnant woman approaching term.

C.M.B.(Eng.) paper.—What are the aims of antenatal care ? At what intervals should a healthy pregnant woman be examined ?

C.M.B.(Eng.) paper, 1969.—Describe the anatomy of the female breast. What changes occur in the breasts during pregnancy ?

C.M.B.(Eng.) paper, 1969. 50 word question on Glycosuria in pregnancy.

C.M.B.(Eng.) paper, 1970.—Describe the anatomy of the uterus. What changes does it undergo during pregnancy ?

C.M.B.(Scot.) paper, 1970.—Describe the physiological changes associated with pregnancy up to the onset of labour.

NUTRITION IN PREGNANCY

What is the reason why the following are necessary: Proteins—iron—calcium—vitamins ?

	Protein	Iron	Calcium	Vit. A	Vit. C
Red meat Milk Liver Butter Fish Cheese Orange					

Use + signs to indicate the nutrients contained in the above foods.

Outline a diet for one day containing at least 80 G. protein. Which foods are rich in iron ? Which foods cause excessive weight gain ? Mention foods you would recommend in language the woman could understand: for breakfast, lunch, supper.

C.M.B.(Scot.) paper.—What advice regarding diet would you give to a primigravida ? What modifications are required in a mild case of hyperemesis gravidarum and mild preeclampsia ?

C.M.B.(N. Ireland) paper.—What advice would you give a patient about her diet during pregnancy, with special reference to weight gain ?

C.M.B.(Eng.) paper, 1969.—Describe the diet you would recommend a pregnant woman to take, and give reasons for your advice.

C.M.B.(Eng.) paper, 1969.—What advice should be given to an expectant mother concerning hygiene and diet during pregnancy ?

C.M.B.(N. Ireland) paper, 1969.—Discuss the importance of diet in pregnancy. Give the essential elements of a suitable diet for an expectant mother.

5

The Signs and Diagnosis of Pregnancy

When a healthy married woman who has been menstruating regularly misses a period she suspects pregnancy and in 98 per cent of cases she is correct.

The use of immunological pregnancy tests and ultrasonic devices has eliminated the need to rely on the more inaccurate presumptive and probable signs of pregnancy.

PRESUMPTIVE SIGNS AND SYMPTOMS

AMENORRHŒA.	MORNING SICKNESS.	SKIN CHANGES.
BREAST CHANGES.	BLADDER IRRITABILITY.	QUICKENING.

AMENORRHŒA

Almost invariably amenorrhœa accompanies pregnancy, and the sudden cessation of menstruation is most significant. Very slight bleeding may take place during the implantation of the ovum, which might be mistaken for menstruation: hence the need to inquire whether the last menstrual period was normal in length and amount. Change of environment; emotional disturbances; serious illness may also cause suppression of menstruation. When the contraceptive pill is discontinued a short period of amenorrhoea may ensue. At the menopause, because of increase in body weight and delayed periods, women often erroneously think they are pregnant.

BREAST CHANGES

These have been described on page 58, and are only significant in the primigravid woman. Slight tingling may be experienced by non-pregnant women, and fluid can be expressed from the breasts when ovarian cysts or fibroids are present: pigmentation may persist after parturition.

MORNING SICKNESS

About 50 per cent of pregnant women are sick in the morning during the 4th to the 14th week, but other conditions may give rise to vomiting. Although morning sickness is not considered to be a definite symptom, in conjunction with amenorrhœa it is very suggestive of pregnancy.

BLADDER IRRITABILITY

This usually consists of frequency of micturition without pain or burning, occurring before the 12th week. The cause is not understood.

SKIN CHANGES

Pigmentation of the skin, manifest as the chloasma, linea nigra, darkening of the primary areola and the formation of the secondary areola of the breasts, is a useful but not indisputable sign of pregnancy. The presence of striæ on the abdomen thighs and breasts is an equally indefinite sign.

QUICKENING

This term is applied to the movements of the fetus in utero when first recognized by the mother, and is usually felt between the 16th and 20th week. The fetus is, of course, alive from the moment of conception, but in the early months the fetal limbs are not well developed and their movements are sluggish. Not until the uterus has risen out of the pelvis and is in contact with the abdominal wall will any feeling of movement be perceptible by the woman.

There is no sense of touch in the uterus, and the kicking must be transmitted to the abdominal wall before the woman is conscious of it. Non-pregnant women sometimes imagine they feel fetal movement, so the symptom is not dependable.

PROBABLE SIGNS

HEGAR'S SIGN.	SOFTENING OF CERVIX.
CHANGES IN UTERUS.	BRAXTON HICKS' CONTRACTIONS.
JACQUEMIER'S SIGN.	UTERINE SOUFFLE.
OSIANDER'S SIGN.	ABDOMINAL ENLARGEMENT.

INTERNAL BALLOTTEMENT.

The majority of these signs are elicited by the doctor, mainly by vaginal examination: the midwife must ensure that the patient's bladder has first been emptied.

Hegar's sign—6*th to* 12*th week*—is one of the early signs, seldom now employed unless facilities for pregnancy tests are not available. Two fingers are inserted into the anterior fornix of the vagina, and the other hand is placed behind the uterus abdominally. The fingers of both hands almost meet, because of the softness of the isthmus which is marked at this period. Rough handling of the uterus should be avoided.

Changes in the uterus—8*th week onwards*—In size the uterus enlarges: the consistency is soft: the shape globular rather than pear.

Jacquemier's sign—8*th week onwards*—is the violet blue discoloration of the vaginal mucous membrane, and is due to pelvic congestion. It may also be present, in cases of retroversion and pelvic cellulitis.

Osiander's sign—8*th week onwards*—is the increased pulsation felt in the lateral vaginal fornices, due to the marked vascularity. It may also be present in pathological conditions that cause pelvic congestion.

Softening of the cervix—10*th week onwards*—The consistency of the cervix is comparable with that of the lips, while the cervix of the non-pregnant uterus feels like the tip of the nose.

Braxton Hicks' contractions—16*th week onwards*—are the painless uterine contractions felt on abdominal palpation, occurring about every 15 minutes and increasing in intensity after the 35th week. These contractions facilitate the circulation of blood in the placental site and also play some part in the development of the lower uterine segment.

The uterine souffle—16*th week onwards*—is a soft blowing sound, heard on auscultation and synchronous with the mother's pulse. The uterine souffle is best heard in the lower lateral borders of the uterus where the blood vessels are largest. The uterine souffle can be heard two or three weeks previous to the fetal heart, but is is also heard when fibroid tumours are present and during the puerperium.

Abdominal enlargement—16*th week onwards*—No other condition makes the uterus enlarge so rapidly and so progressively. Abdominal enlargement may, however, be due to fat, gaseous distension of the bowel, a full bladder, tumours or ascites.

Internal ballottement—16*th to* 28*th week*—is most useful in cases of obesity during mid-term and is performed with the patient in the semi-recumbent position. Two fingers are inserted into the vagina, and the uterus is given a sharp tap just above the cervix, which causes the fetus to float upwards in the liquor amnii. The left hand, which is placed on the fundus uteri, detects the gentle impact of the fetus. The fetus sinks back again and is felt by the fingers in the vagina; this **rebound is known as ballottement.**

None of these signs is positive, as there are fallacies, mostly gynæcological in origin, that prevent them from being conclusive. The probable signs are more reliable than the presumptive signs.

IMMUNOLOGICAL PREGNANCY TESTS (*Hobson*)

The most reliable tests are those which depend upon the presence of chorionic gona-dotrophin in the urine. This hormone is excreted soon after the fertilised egg has implanted and continues to be found in the urine in varying amounts throughout pregnancy and also in the puerperium. Biological methods like the Aschheim Zondek and Hogben tests have now been superseded by immunological tests for pregnancy.

Immunological tests for pregnancy are of two types, hæmagglutination inhibition tests such as Pregnosticon (Organon Ltd.) and Prepuerin (Burroughs Wellcome & Co.) and latex particle tests like Gravindex (Ortho Pharmaceutical Ltd), Planotest (Organon Ltd.) and Prepurex (Burroughs Wellcome & Co.). These tests are available as kits containing all the reagents needed to do a test. In the Pregnosticon and Prepuerin tests the reagents and the urine to be tested are mixed together in a tube or ampoule.

A positive reaction, inhibition of hæmagglutination, appears as a brown ring or button at the bottom of the ampoule or tube.

A negative reaction, hæmagglutination, shows up as a uniformly yellow-brown precipitate at the bottom of the tube.

In the latex particle inhibition tests the reagent and urine are mixed together on a glass slide. A positive result is one in which there is no agglutination of particles and a negative result is one in which agglutination occurs within 2 minutes of the reagents being mixed together.

The hæmagglutination tests Pregnosticon and Prepuerin are very accurate and can be expected to give the correct answer in about 99 per cent of cases. The slide tests being less sensitive are less accurate and will give the right answer in 96 to 98 per cent of cases. Results are more reliable if the tests are done on urines collected 10 to 14 days after the missed but expected period.

A positive pregnancy test is not synonymous with the presence of a viable fetus. Immunological tests like biological tests measure chorionic gonadotrophin and will be positive when urines from women who are pregnant, who have a hydatidiform mole, invasive mole or choriocarcinoma are tested.

For these tests an early morning mid stream specimen of urine 15 ml. is required: the vulva should be swabbed with water (without antiseptic). The specimen must be labelled accurately, kept cool and sent to the laboratory as soon as possible.

POSITIVE SIGNS

FETAL HEART. FETAL PARTS. FETAL MOVEMENT. ULTRASONIC AND RADIO-LOGICAL EVIDENCE.

HEARING THE FETAL HEART

This is a most convincing sign of pregnancy and can with acute hearing be detected as early as the 20th week. When the abdominal wall is thick, the amount of liquor amnii excessive, or the examining room noisy, the heart sounds may be inaudible; but inability to hear the fetal heart does not necessarily exclude pregnancy or denote fetal death although it may arouse suspicion.

FETAL PARTS

These can be felt about the 22nd week, but fibroids may be mistaken for fetal parts. After the 28th week it becomes increasingly easy to map out and distinguish head, back and limbs.

FETAL MOVEMENT

Movements felt by the examiner about the 22nd week, should not be confused with quickening which is felt by the mother and is only a presumptive sign of pregnancy. Often, when listening to the fetal heart, the thud of fetal kicking is felt. In cases after the 28th week where no fetal heart is heard, the fact that the fetus is alive can be elicited by percussing the uterus and so stimulating fetal movement.

ULTRASONIC EVIDENCE

As early as 6 weeks amenorrhoea the gestation sac can be seen on the oscilloscope screen or recorded by a polaroid camera as an ultrasonogram (see Fig. 466).

The Doptone and the Sonicaid. Ultrasonic detectors pick up the fetal blood flow or pulse (not the FH sounds) at 14 weeks and have done so at 10 weeks.

RADIOLOGY

Demonstration of the fetal skeleton by X-rays can be made at the 16th week of pregnancy, but as other diagnostic methods are available X-rays are not used at this early stage because of the radiation hazards.

SIGNS OF A PREVIOUS PREGNANCY

It is desirable for practical reasons that the midwife should be aware whether the pregnant woman has previously given birth to a child. The second stage may be very rapid in a multiparous woman and if the midwife is under the impression that the woman is a primigravida she may not be " scrubbed up " for delivery in time. Women do not always admit, for reasons best known to themselves, that they have already had a baby, and the midwife must accept the woman's statement without question and keep her opinion to herself. In fair-headed women whose skin is elastic, evidence of a previous pregnancy is scarcely obvious, especially if the child to which they had given birth was small.

The following signs are suggestive of previous childbirth :

THE BREASTS

The breasts are more flabby and the nipples prominent in women who have breast-fed their infants, and pigmentation of the areola may still persist in brunettes.

THE ABDOMEN

The abdominal muscles are more lax and the skin loose, so that there may be anterior obliquity of the uterus and bulging of the colon at the sides of the abdomen. The woman may on that account volunteer the information that she is much bigger than in her previous pregnancy.

The uterine wall is less rigid and the contour of the uterus is broad and round rather than ovoid. The fetus is more easily palpated.

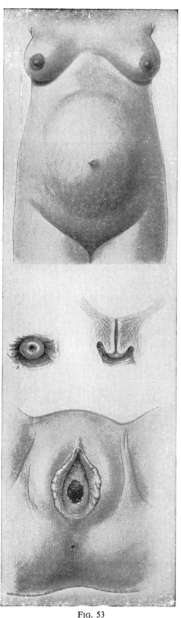

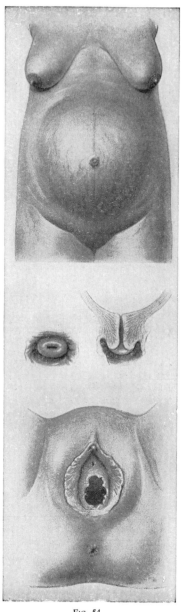

Fig. 53

PRIMIGRAVIDA

Breasts firm; uterus ovoid; abdominal muscles firm; os, round opening; os admits finger-tip; vulva not patulous; hymen partly evident; perineum firm, no scars.

Fig. 54

MULTIGRAVIDA

Breasts flabby; uterus round; abdominal muscles flabby; os, transverse slit; os admits one finger; vulva patulous; carunculæ myrtiformes present; perineum may be lax; scars may be present.

7

Old striæ gravidarum are silvery-white in appearance, but when due to the present pregnancy they are pink. Some pigmentation of the linea alba and striæ may be present from a previous pregnancy.

THE VULVA

The **vulva gapes** and is more patulous: the labia minora tend to project below the labia majora and are darker in colour and leathery in texture. The vaginal orifice is larger and a cystocele may be evident.

Carunculæ myrtiformes (*tags of hymen*) **are present.** A lax or deficient perineum and the *scars* from previous laceration or episiotomy may be seen.

The vagina is more roomy and the cervical os *is a slit* which admits one or more fingers, whereas in the primigravida it is a small pinhead opening at the beginning of pregnancy but may admit one finger-tip during the last month.

PSEUDOCYESIS

Phantom or false pregnancy are terms applied to the condition in which a woman shows several of the signs and symptoms of pregnancy, such as breast changes and enlarged abdomen, firmly believes she is pregnant and yet no pregnancy exists. Such patients are usually infertile married women who have an overwhelming desire to give birth to a baby. Obstetric examination reveals the **absence of any positive signs.**

THE DURATION OF PREGNANCY

The actual duration of pregnancy is believed to be about 265 days from the date of conception, but there is no accurate method of calculating this. Ovulation usually occurs 14 days previous to the first day of the menstrual period but it may be delayed. The ovum is only capable of fertilization for 48 hours, but conception has been known to take place at other times during the menstrual cycle.

The question sometimes arises as to the length of the period of gestation which can be considered legitimate when a child is born more than 280 days after the death or absence of the putative father. In Gt. Britain and the United States there is no legal limit to the length of pregnancy; each case is considered on its merits. In the English courts, during the year 1921, a gestational period of 331 days was allowed, in 1948 one of 340 days was not allowed. The Scottish courts have allowed a period of 305 days.

CALCULATION OF THE DATE OF CONFINEMENT

For practical purposes the date of the last menstrual period has proved by experience to be a reliable guide. By adding seven days to the first day of the last menstrual period and counting back three months or forwards nine months, **a total of 280 days,** the expected date of delivery is arrived at. (*Printed obstetric calculators are available.*) But the baby may be born one week before or after that date and yet be at term.

It has been estimated that only 5 per cent of women go into labour on the calculated day, 20 per cent after the end of the 41st week and 10 per cent after the 42nd week. Expectant mothers should be aware of this, as they tend to get perturbed when the expected date of confinement is passed.

In cases where the menstrual periods are irregular or when the woman forgets the date of her last period, 22 *weeks are added to the date of quickening.* **The height of the fundus** can also be used as a means of assessing the period of gestation, but the fallaciousness of this method must be kept in mind (p. 108).

The Relationship of the Fetus to the Uterus and Pelvis

Certain terms are used to describe the relationship of the fetus to the uterus and pelvis, and the student midwife ought to be familiar with them before learning how to palpate the abdomen. This relationship determines which part of the fetus will enter the pelvic brim first, and governs the mechanism by which the fetus will pass through the birth canal.

The terms are:

1. **LIE.**	3. **PRESENTATION.**	5. **POSITION.**
2. **ATTITUDE.**	4. **DENOMINATOR.**	6. **PRESENTING PART.**

1. LIE

Lie is the relation of the long axis of the fetus to the long axis of the uterus (not to the abdomen or spine). It should be longitudinal, and is so in 99·5 *per cent* of cases, but it may be transverse. The fetus and uterus are both longer than they are broad, and when the fetus *in utero* lies with its length parallel to the length of the uterus the lie is longitudinal, and the head or the breech will occupy the lower pole of the uterus.

The longitudinal lie is usual because the uterine cavity is ovoid in shape, but any condition, such as lax uterine walls or an excessive amount of amniotic fluid, making the uterine cavity round instead of ovoid, would reduce the likelihood of the fetus adopting the longitudinal lie.

When the lie is transverse, the shoulder occupies the lower pole of the uterus and the long axis of the fetus lies across the long axis of the uterus.

2. ATTITUDE

Attitude is the relation of the fetal limbs and head to its trunk, and should be one of *flexion*. It concerns the fetus only. The back is bent, the head is flexed with the chin on the chest, the arms are flexed on, or alongside the chest, the thighs are flexed

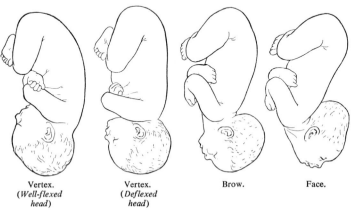

Vertex.	Vertex.	Brow.	Face.
(*Well-flexed head*)	(*Deflexed head*)		

FIG. 55

VARIETIES OF CEPHALIC OR HEAD PRESENTATION.

on the abdomen and the legs on the thighs. The fetus, therefore, forms a snug compact, ovoid mass, which accommodates itself admirably to the uterine cavity and can be expelled en masse during labour.

Any deviation from this normal attitude of flexion will give rise to difficulty during labour ; *e.g.* if the head is not well flexed a larger circumference will have to engage in the pelvic brim ; if extended, the face presents.

3. PRESENTATION

Presentation refers to the part of the fetus which lies at the pelvic brim or in the lower pole of the uterus. There are five presentations : the vertex, breech, shoulder, face and brow, in that order of frequency :

1. THE VERTEX presents in approx. 96 per cent of cases
2. THE BREECH   ,,   ,,   3·3   ,,   ,,
3. THE SHOULDER ,,   ..   0·4   ,,   ,,   1 per 250
4. THE FACE   ,,   ,,   0·2   ,,   ,,   1 per 500
5. THE BROW   ,,   ,,   0·1   ,,   ,,   1 per 1000

Vertex, face and brow are all head or cephalic presentations. When the head is flexed the vertex presents : when it is extended the face presents, and when neither

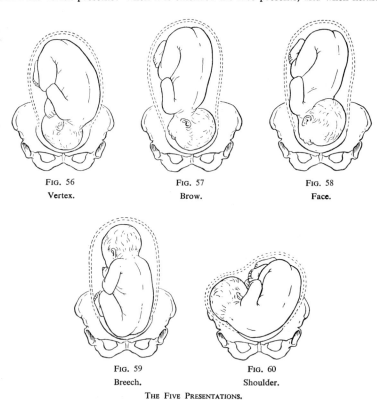

Fig. 56   Fig. 57   Fig. 58
Vertex.   Brow.   Face.

Fig. 59   Fig. 60
Breech.   Shoulder.

THE FIVE PRESENTATIONS.

well flexed nor properly extended it is midway between vertex and face, so the brow presents (see Fig. 57). The reason for the greater number of head presentations is explained mainly by the **law of accommodation.** The uterine cavity is ovoid in shape during the later months of pregnancy and its walls, being contractile, tend to cause the fetus to accommodate its ovoid shape to that of the uterus. The bulky breech of the fetus finds greater space in the fundus which is the widest diameter of the uterus, and the head lies in the narrower lower pole.

The tonicity of the fetus also plays a part in maintaining the vertex presentation: a dead fetus has no tone so the normal presentation and attitude are not maintained.

Anything which interferes with the natural accommodation of the fetus in the uterine cavity will cause a malpresentation, *e.g.* when the fetal head is unduly large, as in hydrocephaly it may occupy the roomy fundus, causing the breech to present.

4. THE DENOMINATOR

The denominator is the part of the presentation that indicates or determines the position.

(*a*) **The denominator** in vertex presentation is the **occiput.**

(*b*)	,,	,,	breech	,,	,,	**sacrum.**
(*c*)	,,	,,	face	,,	,,	**mentum.**
(*d*)	,,	,,	shoulder	,,	,,	**acromion process.**

5. POSITION

Position is the relation of the denominator to six areas of the pelvic brim. The areas of the brim are:

RIGHT POSTERIOR.	LEFT POSTERIOR.
RIGHT LATERAL.	LEFT LATERAL.
RIGHT ANTERIOR.	LEFT ANTERIOR.

In the vertex presentation the occiput is the denominator. If the occiput points to the left anterior the position is left occipito-anterior.

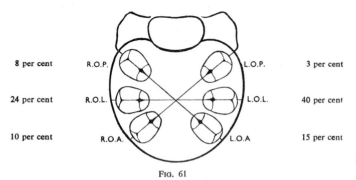

8 per cent	R.O.P.	L.O.P.	3 per cent
24 per cent	R.O.L.	L.O.L.	40 per cent
10 per cent	R.O.A.	L.O.A	15 per cent

Fig. 61

Diagrammatic representation of the six vertex positions and their relative frequency.

POSITIONS IN VERTEX PRESENTATION

LEFT OCCIPITO-ANTERIOR (L.O.A.)

The occiput points to the left ilio-pectineal eminence on the left anterior area of the pelvic brim; the sagittal suture is in the right oblique diameter of the brim.

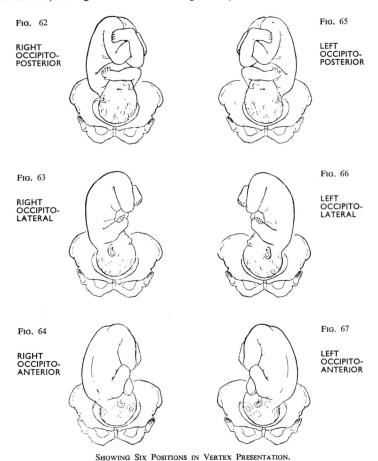

FIG. 62

RIGHT
OCCIPITO-
POSTERIOR

FIG. 65

LEFT
OCCIPITO-
POSTERIOR

FIG. 63

RIGHT
OCCIPITO-
LATERAL

FIG. 66

LEFT
OCCIPITO-
LATERAL

FIG. 64

RIGHT
OCCIPITO-
ANTERIOR

FIG. 67

LEFT
OCCIPITO-
ANTERIOR

SHOWING SIX POSITIONS IN VERTEX PRESENTATION.

	Right Ant.	Right Lat.	Right Post.	Left Ant.	Left Lat.	Left Post.
VERTEX	R.O.A.	R.O.L.	R.O.P.	L.O.A.	L.O.L.	L.O.P.
BREECH	R.S.A.	R.S.L.	R.S.P.	L.S.A.	L.S.L.	L.S.P.

LEFT OCCIPITO-LATERAL (L.O.L.)

The occiput points to the left side of the pelvic brim midway between the left ilio-pectineal eminence and the left sacro-iliac joint; the sagittal suture is in the transverse diameter of the brim.

LEFT OCCIPITO-POSTERIOR (L.O.P.)

The occiput points to the left sacro-iliac joint, the left posterior area of the pelvic brim; **the** sagittal suture is in the left oblique diameter of the brim.

RIGHT OCCIPITO-ANTERIOR (R.O.A.)

The occiput points to the right ilio-pectineal eminence on the right anterior area of the pelvic brim; **the** sagittal suture is in the left oblique diameter of the brim.

RIGHT OCCIPITO-LATERAL (R.O.L.)

The occiput points to the right side of the pelvic brim midway between the right ilio-pectineal eminence and the right sacro-iliac joint.   The sagittal suture is in the transverse diameter of the brim.

RIGHT OCCIPITO-POSTERIOR (R.O.P.)

The occiput points to the right sacro-iliac joint in the right posterior area of the pelvic brim; the sagittal suture is in the right oblique diameter of the brim.

Anterior positions are more favourable than posterior positions, because when the fetal back is in front it conforms to the concavity of the mother's abdominal wall and can therefore flex better.   When the back is flexed, **the head tends also to flex** and a smaller diameter engages.   There is also more room in the anterior part of the pelvic brim for the broad biparietal diameter of the head.

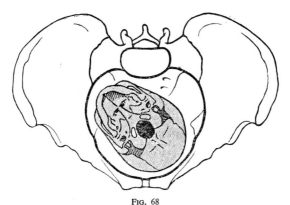

FIG. 68

Vertex—left occipito-anterior, showing the advantage of an anterior position.   The biparietal diameter is in the roomy anterior part of the pelvic brim.

6. PRESENTING PART

The presenting part is the part that lies over the os during labour and on which the caput forms.   The term is often used erroneously, when the word " presentation " is meant.   The situation of the presenting part differs in each position:

In an L.O.A. it is the posterior area of the right parietal bone.

In an R.O.A. it is the posterior area of the left parietal bone.

In an R.O.P. it is the anterior area of the left parietal bone.
In an L.O.P. it is the anterior area of the right parietal bone.

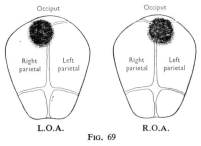

L.O.A.   R.O.A.

FIG. 69

Showing position of caput succedaneum in vertex
presentation.

The practical significance of the presenting part is that, should the baby's head be born before there has been time to diagnose the position of the fetus by abdominal examination, and the caput is situated on the right parietal bone posteriorly, this will indicate that the position is left occipito-anterior. Such knowledge facilitates management of the delivery of the shoulders.

QUESTIONS FOR REVISION

DIAGNOSIS OF PREGNANCY

State whether the following signs are positive, probable, or presumptive:

1. Morning sickness............................
2. Amenorrhœa ....
3. Uterine enlargement........................
4. Fetal heart heard ....
5. Quickening...................................
6. Fetal movement felt ....
7. Immunological test ....
8. Uterine souffle heard ....
9. Braxton Hicks' contractions............
10. Fetal parts on palpation ....

At which weeks do the following signs and symptoms occur:

1. Quickening...................................
2. Colostrum ....
3. Fetal heart ....
4. Uterine souffle ....
5. Enlargement of breasts.....................
6. Abdominal enlargement..................
7. Primary areola.............................
8. Bladder irritability ....
9. Fetal parts felt ....
10. Tingling of breasts ....

At 2, 6, 10, 16, 20, 22 weeks amenorrhœa state which of the following give positive signs of pregnancy: fetal parts; radiography; ultrasonogram; chorionic gonadotrophin test; Sonicaid; hearing fetal heart.

How would you recognize that a woman was a multigravida from :

(*a*) Abdominal examination ?   (*b*) Vulval and vaginal examinations ?

C.M.B.(Eng.) paper.—What is the normal duration of pregnancy and how do you estimate the expected date of delivery ? What observations during pregnancy may assist you in estimating the date and how may errors arise ?

C.M.B.(Eng.) paper.—A woman comes to you thinking that she may be pregnant. On examination a swelling reaching 2·5 cm. (1 inch) above the umbilicus is found. How would you decide whether she is or is not pregnant ?

C.M.B.(Scot.) paper.—Describe the signs and symptoms of pregnancy during the first three months.

C.M.B.(Eng.) paper.—What signs of pregnancy may be detected at the 24th week of pregnancy in a primigravida ?

C.M.B.(Scot.) paper.—Describe the signs and symptoms of pregnancy under the following headings : (*a*) Presumptive ; (*b*) Certain.

C.M.B.(N. Ireland) paper.—Describe the early diagnosis of pregnancy.

RELATIONSHIP OF THE FETUS TO THE UTERUS AND PELVIS

What is the presentation when the lie is transverse ? Name two presentations produced by faulty attitude of the head. What are the advantages of the vertex presentation ? Why are the anterior vertex positions more favourable than posterior positions ?

Rearrange numbers

Description			Term
(1) Part that lies over os.	(	)	Presentation.
(2) Relation of fetus to the long axis of the uterus.	(	)	Attitude.
(3) Relation of limbs and head to the trunk.	(	)	Lie.
(4) Part that lies at the pelvic brim.	(	)	Presenting part.
(5) Part of presentation that determines position.	(	)	Position.
(6) Relation of fetus to certain areas of mother's pelvis.	(	)	Denominator.

ORAL QUESTIONS

What is quickening ? How can you estimate the expected date of delivery by knowledge of quickening ? When does (*a*) the primigravid (*b*) the multigravid woman recognize it ? On what symptoms does a married woman suspect pregnancy ? What do you mean by a quantitative gonadotrophin test and when is it used? How many days are there in pregnancy ? In transverse lie what is the presentation ? Why is this a serious state of affairs ?

Differentiate between: cephalic and vertex presentation; quickening and lightening; presentation and presenting part; face and brow presentation; primigravida and multigravida.

6

Prenatal Care

Prenatal care is one of the more recent developments in the history of obstetrics, and it may be difficult for the modern midwife to realize that until about 1915 few pregnant women came under the care of doctor or midwife until they actually went into labour. The results were often disastrous to both mother and baby; the maternal and fetal death rates were high, and many women who survived childbirth suffered from some disability or discomfort which incapacitated them or made life miserable.

As a stimulus to further endeavour, it is fitting that we should recall the work of the pioneers in this field. Dr J. W. Ballantyne, who has been called " the father of antenatal care," was lecturer in antenatal pathology at the University of Edinburgh. He wrote a paper deploring how little progress had been made in antenatal pathology and urged that a " pre-maternity " hospital was necessary. The anonymous gift of £1,000 to endow a bed in the Royal Maternity and Simpson Memorial Hospital enabled him, in the year 1901, to set apart the *first bed ever to be used* for the study of the pregnant woman.

During the same year, in Boston, U.S.A., visits were paid to some patients in their homes, and the first antenatal clinic was opened there in 1911, others in Sydney during 1912 and in Edinburgh during 1915.

The passing of the Notification of Births (Extension) Act, 1915, and the Maternity and Child Welfare Act, 1918, gave additional impetus to the movement by placing the responsibility for making provision for the health and care of expectant mothers and young children on Local Authorities. Antenatal and child welfare clinics were set up in the towns throughout Great Britain; but in rural areas antenatal supervision was given by local doctors and midwives. Health visitors also visited pregnant women in their own homes.

ADMINISTRATION OF THE MIDWIFERY SERVICE IN GREAT BRITAIN

The National Health Service Act which came into force in July 1948 placed responsibility for the administration of the midwifery service in the hands of three bodies.

1. **The Regional Hospital Boards** provide maternity hospitals, the services of obstetric-specialists; blood transfusion, radiological, family planning, laboratory services, and **in Scotland, ambulances.** Prenatal clinics are run in connection with maternity hospitals, and to these clinics general practitioners and midwives may refer their patients for specialist opinion.

2. **Local Health Authorities** also are responsible for administering maternity and child welfare services; they therefore provide the domiciliary midwifery service in their areas. Each domiciliary midwife visits her patients during pregnancy in their own homes, and also examines them at the prenatal clinics which the Local Health Authorities may provide. Pregnant women are seen by a doctor every 4 weeks until he 28th week, every two weeks until the 36th week and every week until term, and by an obstetrician when necessary. **Ambulances are provided in England by the** Local Health Authorities.

3. **Local Executive Councils** administer the general practitioner services. They provide panels of doctors who desire to undertake domiciliary midwifery. **In England there are also panels of general-practitioner-obstetricians** who have had special midwifery experience. Prenatal care can be given by the doctor in the patient's home, at his surgery, or at the clinics which may be provided by the Local Health Authority.

Under the General Practitioner Co-operation Scheme normal patients who attend the hospital prenatal clinic may be referred to their family doctor for routine care after the first visit until the 34th week.

THE AIMS OF PRENATAL CARE

The modern conception of prenatal care is CONSTRUCTIVE AND COMPREHENSIVE IN CHARACTER and has a positive approach to the subject. To realize this, all the aspects of prenatal care will have to be developed; **social, psychological** and **educational,** as well as **medical** and **obstetrical.** The inauguration of a scheme on these lines will embrace all the aims of prenatal care, which have been summarized as follows:

1. **To promote and maintain good physical and mental health during pregnancy.** Health education including good nutrition is of primary importance.

2. **To ensure a mature, live, healthy infant.** This also includes the prevention of congenital abnormalities due to virus infection, drugs and other causes.

3. **To prepare the woman for labour,** lactation and the subsequent care of her child from the physical, psychological, social and educational points of view.

4. **To detect early and treat appropriately conditions, medical and obstetrical,** that would endanger the life or impair the health of mother or baby.

The mother must get the best possible care, and this can be most easily accomplished when there is continuity of supervision by those who are to be responsible for the confinement.

THE SOCIAL ASPECT OF PRENATAL CARE

If prenatal care is the root of the tree of preventive medicine, the social aspect is the soil in which it grows. The pregnant woman cannot be dissociated from the conditions under which she lives, and it has been proved by various investigators that social factors profoundly influence the processes of childbearing and rearing.

The expectant mother's health and skeletal structure may be adversely affected by poor nutrition during her infancy, childhood and adolescence. The perinatal mortality rate is high in social groups that are financially unable or intellectually incapable of providing a good standard of living, and particularly when the mother's health is poor. Premature labour is more common in these circumstances, therefore the prevention of prematurity has social as well as obstetrical implications.

SOCIAL TRENDS

The improved standard of living, family planning and **married women in industry,** have altered the way of life for British mothers; husbands are now expected to participate in domestic duties including care of the children.

The increased number of hospital confinements also reflects a social trend, and early discharge presents a problem that will require the co-operation of hospital as well as domiciliary midwives. The inauguration of a follow-up service to care for and supervise mothers and babies discharged prematurely from hospitals is urgently needed. More home helps are required on an hourly basis, and at reasonable cost.

The family unit is the basis of the social structure of the nation, and setting up such a unit under modern conditions almost invariably requires, by sheer economic necessity, that the wife must also go out to work. Social and financial adjustments have to be made, on the advent of a baby in the home, with which young parents in lower income groups are sometimes unable to cope. They may be immature and unable to meet the responsibilities of parenthood. Disorganization of domestic routine, loss of sleep and additional financial commitments may give rise to friction and impose a severe strain on the marital situation.

THE ROLE OF THE MIDWIFE

Midwives should be qualified to advise parents on how to meet their responsibilities for the welfare and happiness of the family group, *e.g.* budgeting economically for baby equipment, planning baby's day, reorganizing housework, avoiding and coping with jealousy in the toddler, making the best of the situation by cultivating pleasures that can be enjoyed within the home.

The midwife is concerned with the health-education of expectant mothers, but this should begin prior to marriage; in fact, by trying to ensure conditions that contribute to the welfare and vitality of the fetus *in utero* she is helping to lay the foundations of good health in the next generation of parents.

The domiciliary midwife is an important member of the Public Health team and vitally concerned in the promotion of the health of the nation. She should be permitted to organize and direct the instruction given to individual, and groups of, expectant mothers as well as closely supervising and teaching baby-care during the first 10 days of life.

HOME CONDITIONS

The domiciliary midwife has an obligation to visit her patients during pregnancy to see whether the house is suitable for confinement and, if not, she must notify the Local Supervising Authority : she must also advise the woman regarding preparations for home confinement.

It is equally essential that the hospital midwife should have some knowledge of the home conditions of patients who are in the lower income groups so that she may better understand the difficulties with which they have to contend.

Living in overcrowded, inconvenient houses, in dirty, drab surroundings, saps the physical and mental vitality, and it takes will-power, energy, pride and some intelligence to manage a home and family successfully and to rise above such conditions.

Admittedly, the solution of many social problems is outside the sphere of the midwife but she should be aware of them and ready to advise when the opportunity presents. She should know where and to whom she should refer patients with social problems. The midwife should know that unsatisfactory housing conditions which have not been rectified by the landlord should be reported to the Local Authority, and that where overcrowding exists this authority will endeavour to provide adequate accommodation if another child is expected.

BENEFITS PROVIDED BY THE STATE

The midwifery service is part of the National Health Service, and every woman in Great Britain is entitled to the services of a doctor and midwife during pregnancy, labour, and the puerperium. The confinement may take place at home or in hospital, and in both instances it is free.

Provisions made by the State for mother and child may be summarized as follows:

1. CLINICS

Prenatal; postnatal; child health; special clinics, *e.g.* dental, chest, cardiac, diabetic, hæmatological, urological, leucorrhœa, venereal disease, family planning, infertility.

2. FOR HOSPITAL CONFINEMENT

Obstetricians; physicians; pædiatricians; anæsthetists; radiologists; bacteriologists; midwives. Ambulances are provided when necessary.

3. FOR HOME CONFINEMENT

Doctor; consultation by obstetrician; midwife; mobile obstetric and pædiatric resuscitation units: home help (charge made). Maternity packs with sterile supplies (issued free).

4. WELFARE FOODS

Free milk and vitamin tablets are available to expectant and nursing mothers and their children under school age in families in receipt of supplementary benefits (see leaflet W 11). Free milk is also available for an expectant mother **regardless of income** if she has two children under school age. The claim form is obtainable from her doctor, midwife or health visitor. Expectant mothers can purchase 2 packets of A, D and C Vitamin tablets every 13 weeks at welfare food distribution centres.

5. FINANCIAL

Maternity Grant, £25.00, is paid to all mothers giving birth to a live or stillborn child after 28 weeks' gestation. It is claimed on their own or their husband's insurance, but not both; application for the grant being made between 9 weeks before the baby is expected and 3 months after he is born.

In cases of multiple births an extra £25.00 grant may be paid for each additional baby who is alive 12 hours after birth.

Maternity Allowance.—This is £5.00 per week for 18 weeks, beginning 11 weeks before the expected week of confinement, and is claimed by the employed woman who has paid the required number of contributions. **She must cease paid work during this period.**

Pregnant women should obtain leaflet N.I. 17A and the claim form from the local Department of Health and Social Security office not later than 14 weeks before the expected date of confinement.

Family Allowance of 90p weekly is paid for a second child and £1.00 weekly for each subsequent child during the period until the child reaches the 15th birthday.

Supplementary Allowances are granted in necessitous cases, on application to the local Department of Health and Social Security office.

6. OTHERS

The Local Health Authority provides: clinic medical officers; midwives; health visitors; social workers; residential and day nurseries; holiday homes for mothers and babies; ambulances (England); immunization facilities. The Social Worker of the Local Authority can make arrangements for care of orphan infants, and for adoption, and undertakes the supervision of foster-mothers, child minders and of boarded-out children.

EMPLOYMENT OF PREGNANT WOMEN

The opinion of the midwife may be asked as to whether a pregnant married woman should continue to work beyond mid-term. The need for extra money is sometimes urgent, but it is an unwise measure in the long run for only the strongest type of woman can keep house successfully and carry on a full-time job as well. Pregnancy superimposed on such a situation is more than the average woman can cope with.

An industrial nurse may have to approach the factory personnel officer on behalf of a pregnant woman, regarding the suitability of a job which involves heavy work. Occupations necessitating exposure to certain chemical or radio-active substances may be safe for the non-pregnant woman, but hazardous during pregnancy. A doctor should be consulted.

Although the Factory Act does not forbid a woman to work during the latter weeks of pregnancy, she should be dissuaded from doing so. The maternity allowance paid to employed persons after the 28th week is intended to enable them to cease work then.

THE UNMARRIED MOTHER AND HER CHILD

The term " unsupported mother " is sometimes used to include pregnant women who are single, divorced, separated or widows.

Some 8·4 per cent of births in Great Britain are illegitimate, and this amounts to about 70,000 annually with a marked increase in young teenage unwed mothers. The unmarried mother has a problem which is acute and complicated; she is emotionally distressed and in dire need of guidance and help; but there are so many aspects of her problem that expert handling is essential for their solution.

The midwife should put the girl in touch with the social worker employed by the Local Authority or maternity hospital. The worker will, if the support of the girl's family is not forthcoming (*and this occurs now less frequently*), make the necessary contacts with the most suitable organization to help the unwed mother, and will follow up the case until the social problem has been solved.

Voluntary organizations such as the National Council for the Unmarried Mother and her Child, and religious bodies often employ specialized social workers and may provide homes for the unmarried mother and her child.

Legal aid may be required if it is necessary to raise an action of *affiliation* (proof of paternity) or of *alimony* (maintenance allowance). But, even when the father admits paternity and is willing to make payment towards the upkeep of the child, the arrangement should be made through the court.

ADOPTION

Adoption must always be arranged through a registered adoption society, or the Local Authority, to whom the midwife should refer her patient. The social worker of this authority will help to make arrangements or recommend getting in touch with a registered adoption society. The midwife would be well advised to refrain from using her influence either for or against adoption and to leave the solution of the problem in the hands of those who have greater knowledge and experience of all its aspects.

No action will be taken until the child is born. The infant must be at least six weeks old before the mother can give her consent to adoption, although the infant may be placed with prospective adopters before this age. Sometimes the mother remains with her baby in a mother and baby home until she decides about adoption. In other instances, if the mother is unable to look after her infant but has not made up her mind about adoption, the infant may be taken into care by the Local Authority.

The adopters must notify the Local Authority when they intend to apply for an adoption order. They must also have had the child in their care for three consecutive months before they apply to the court for an Adoption Order, which makes the transaction legal and binding. The parent or parents of the child give their written consent and relinquish all further claim on the child.

Classes in preparation for parenthood for adoptive parents are held at some maternity hospitals.

INVESTIGATIONS

The character, health and financial status of the adopters are investigated; the home must also be satisfactory.

The mentality, physical health, including Wassermann test, and parental background of the baby are also investigated. The baby must (*under the Adoption Act*) be examined for congenital dislocation of hip and phenylalanine in the blood (see Guthrie Test p. 799) which gives evidence of a defect that causes mental subnormality.

FOSTER MOTHERS

Any person who undertakes to look after a child under 15 years of age, for payment, must notify the Local Authority seven days before doing so. The social worker will first inspect the home, and in the majority of cases will continue to visit, in order to ensure that the child is being properly cared for.

MARITAL DIFFICULTIES

A pregnant married woman may have an urgent social problem and the midwife should refer her to a social worker or to the Local Authority, who will get in touch with such agencies as the National Council of Social Service or the Family Welfare Association. When financial help is required, they will recommend the appropriate association or advise application for a supplementary allowance.

If the marriage is in danger of breaking up, the Marriage Guidance Council may be consulted. Legal advice will be arranged for in such instances as neglect, cruelty or desertion.

THE PSYCHOLOGICAL ASPECT

It is now accepted that, for the successful practice of obstetrics, understanding of the psychological aspect of childbearing is as essential as knowledge of the physical aspect. Undoubtedly we must concern ourselves with the woman's health and obstetric well-being, but we must be equally concerned about her emotional welfare. Attitudes are just as important as knowledge and skills. The tendency to become so engrossed in obstetrics *per se* should be resisted, in case the woman as an individual is relegated to second place.

The advent of a first pregnancy produces a certain degree of emotional turmoil in the mind of any thinking woman. Emotions, such as mother-love and pride in creation, induce a feeling of tranquillity and gladness, for the woman is about to enter on one of life's most enriching experiences. But these emotions may be counter-balanced by others of a disturbing nature such as fear and resentment.

Not all women are well balanced or emotionally mature, and their reactions to pregnancy will depend on such factors as temperament, intelligence and education, health, age and the marital situation. Whether the child is wanted or not dominates almost everything else.

All babies are not planned or wanted at the time of conception but the majority of married women adjust to the situation and when born the baby is welcomed.

THE ATTITUDE OF THE HUSBAND

Being sustained by the care and consideration of a kindly husband is essential for the happiness and emotional stability of the pregnant woman.

It seems reasonable to expect the husband to have some understanding of the emotional demands pregnancy makes on his wife, and it should be his responsibility to ensure that life does not become intolerably drab with the burden of repeated childbearing and rearing. By taking an active interest in her physical well-being, particularly in regard to nutrition, rest and recreation, he is also meeting her psychological needs, because he is demonstrating his protective rôle and showing his concern for her welfare.

The discomforts of pregnancy may make her petulant at times, but the husband should **exercise** forbearance on such occasions. **She needs his steadying influence and** will respond to understanding and kindliness rather than logical argument.

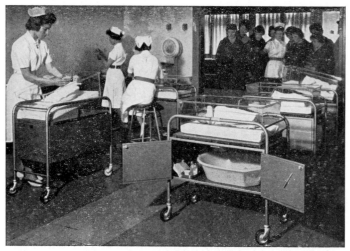

FIG. 70

"PREPARATION FOR PARENTHOOD" CLASS HAVING A GLIMPSE OF THE NURSERIES.

Trolley cots with cupboards for individual equipment. (*Hoskins & Sons Ltd., Upper Trinity Street, Birmingham.*)

(*Photographed at County Maternity Hospital, Bellshill, Lanarkshire.*)

THE INFLUENCE OF THE MIDWIFE

The midwife must try to appreciate the heightened sensitivity of the expectant mother, and endeavour to inculcate in her patients an attitude of mind that brings the higher emotions into play, for when a woman can anticipate the birth of her baby with courage and serenity, fear is subordinated. She should keep in front of her patients the idea that childbearing is a natural event and try to foster a cheerful outlook.

Motherhood and happy family life should be depicted as the most desirable and satisfying life for a woman.

The midwife must also be aware of the conflicts and fears that can be so disturbing to the expectant mother's peace of mind; her willingness to listen and give sympathetic advice will often help the woman to face and overcome her difficulties. **Tact and**

resourcefulness are needed, so that her approach and advice may be acceptable to all types of women.

Invariably the successful midwife is one with certain qualities of character that are apparent in her kindly manner and friendly interest in human beings; she expresses her interest in the woman as an individual as well as a patient.

FEAR OF LABOUR AND HOW TO ELIMINATE IT

Even when a woman is delighted at the prospect of motherhood and eagerly awaiting the birth of her baby, her peace of mind may be upset by vague fears, some real, some imaginary, but none the less real to her. These can be counterbalanced by confidence in the hospital, doctor and midwife as well as by education.

She dreads the unknown experience, so the process of labour should be explained in simple language, telling her what to expect and in what way she can help herself. Fear of death no doubt crosses the mind of every pregnant woman at some time, but it is not a dominant fear. It could be likened to the fleeting fear that may precede a journey by sea or air.

The expectant mother should be reminded that thousands of women give birth to babies, simply and easily, every day, and her thoughts directed away from labour and focused on the *baby's birthday*—a happier thought. A few mothers worry about some hereditary taint in case it be transmitted to their babies. Many such fears are groundless.

Fear of pain looms large on the horizon of the pregnant woman. She can be taught how to relax, shown the apparatus for the relief of pain, and told that everything possible will be done for her comfort, as long as it does not harm the baby or unduly retard labour (see " Relief of pain," p. 251). With such assurance, the woman's fear is diminished and she gains confidence in herself and her midwife. *It should not be forgotten that what the midwife feels as a uterine contraction the woman feels as pain.*

KNOWLEDGE

Practically every method of preparation for childbirth includes giving knowledge of labour. When the woman is aware of what is going to happen she gains confidence in her ability to cope with the situation.

This must not be interpreted as meaning that the expectant mother will be less afraid if given a detailed description of the anatomy of the pelvic organs and the physiological processes of labour. The pregnant woman is more concerned regarding what she will experience and how she will react than with anatomical details.

Knowledge of labour must be presented in an elementary fashion and judiciously applied in a practical rather than theoretical way to elaborate some point concerning the management of labour or to explain the processes of labour as they affect the woman's feelings and reactions.

The knowledge she needs most of all is the assurance that she will be physically safe and psychologically secure under the care of a competent team who are interested in her welfare, willing to alleviate discomfort, mental or physical, and eager to relieve pain.

If by her understanding of the psychological aspect of pregnancy the midwife can bring a woman into labour in a serene, courageous frame of mind, she is making a valuable contribution to obstetrics.

THE EDUCATIONAL ASPECT

No matter how excellent the medical and obstetrical care is, it cannot be completely effective without the active co-operation of the mother. It is she, personally, who will

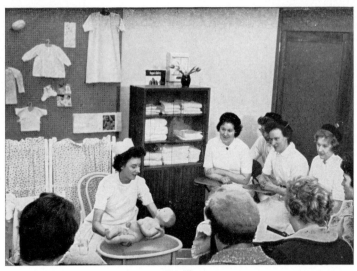

Fig. 71

Bathing demonstration to expectant mothers and student midwives in Mothercraft Department.
(*County Maternity Hospital, Bellshill, Lanarkshire.*)

observe the rules of health to keep herself fit during pregnancy and in preparation for labour.

Every prenatal clinic should be a school for expectant mothers; every midwife a teacher. The mother-to-be is eager to do what is best for her baby and this attitude should be fostered; she is in a most receptive frame of mind and midwives should be prepared to talk to mothers individually or in groups.

Suitable talks are set out in the Preparation for Parenthood Section.

HEALTH EDUCATION

The midwife has an excellent opportunity for the promotion of good health : the need for inaugurating a programme of health education, over and above what may be included in parenthood teaching, is urgent.   The maintenance of physical fitness during pregnancy has a profound influence on the health and vigour of the baby before, during and after birth.

Anæmia is still more common among childbearing women than it ought to be and an active campaign for its prevention is long overdue.   Foods rich in iron are given on page 65.

Mothers need guidance regarding immunization of their babies, advice in the prevention of home accidents, as well as in rearing a healthy baby.

MENTAL HEALTH

Promoting mental health is just as important as promoting physical health. Not all pregnant women have the emotional stability that is fostered by being reared in a secure happy home and strengthened further by a happy marriage.

Midwives should endeavour to prevent or alleviate some of the factors that give rise to mental strain and emotional tension (see Pregnancy (p. 88), Labour (p. 249)). Fewer tranquillizing drugs are now being prescribed for pregnant women because of the detrimental effect of some on the fetus so midwives should make an effort to meet the psychological needs of the pregnant women in their care.

The recorded incidence of psychosis in obstetric patients is considerable.

GOOD HUMAN RELATIONSHIPS

Interest should be shown in the woman as a person; not only in her blood pressure, pelvis and fetus, important though they be. She should be made aware that what she feels and thinks regarding pregnancy, labour and the baby matters. Getting to know the woman as an individual is time consuming but it is an integral part of good prenatal care.

Most women approach labour with some degree of apprehension and this aspect deserves more attention. Midwives should be qualified and allowed time to give the necessary emotional support, viz. :

DURING PREGNANCY

Giving sympathetic understanding, listening, offering advice, answering questions.

DURING LABOUR

Providing patient, kindly care and companionship: instilling confidence; reducing mental trauma and physical suffering.

DURING PUERPERIUM

Proffering guidance and encouragement rather than direction regarding care of the baby. Discussing personal questions such as family planning.

PREVENTION OF CONGENITAL MALFORMATIONS

Health education includes giving advice to promote the health of the fetus *in utero*.

The lethal time for the fetus is during the first eight weeks, but most women do not come under the care of doctor or midwife during this period. It should be made widely known that early booking is essential.

Midwives should at this time advise mothers-to-be regarding the avoidance of infection, drugs, or other substances known to cause congenital malformation.

THE MEDICAL ASPECT

The need for medical, as apart from obstetrical, supervision should be clearly appreciated. Far too many childbearing women are below par physically; they are anæmic, tired, flabby, prematurely old; they lack the physical and emotional stamina needed during labour.

Every effort should be made to maintain the woman's health at a high level, for the good health of the mother has an important bearing on the prevention of obstetrical complications and on ensuring the future well-being of the child. It could be argued that it is too late to start a scheme for physical fitness during pregnancy, but if we presume that the fetus *in utero* is a potential parent, then we are truly laying the foundations of good health for the next generation.

The midwife should encourage the woman to be seen early in pregnancy by the doctor, so that he can assess her general health and give advice before any existing disease has been aggravated by pregnancy. The routine blood and chest examinations provide a means of recognizing early such conditions as cardiac disease, anæmia, diabetes, syphilis and tuberculosis, the prompt treatment of which may avert disaster.

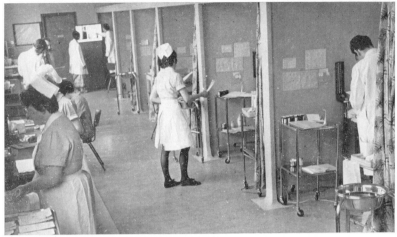

Fig. 72

The prenatal clinic, Simpson Memorial Maternity Pavilion, Edinburgh.

THE OBSTETRICAL ASPECT

The purely obstetrical aspect of prenatal care cannot be separated from the other aspects, they dovetail into each other and all have obstetrical significance. In the narrow sense, it is concerned with the supervision and management of pregnancy, the making of provision for labour, the puerperium and the newborn child, as well as the prevention, diagnosis and treatment of complications.

This involves investigation, examination, supervision, advice and treatment: these are described in subsequent chapters.

TAKING THE HISTORY

It should be kept in mind that the purpose of taking a history is not merely for the recording of facts and statistics; it is a means of assessing the health of the woman and bringing to light any defect which would adversely affect childbearing.

THE SOCIAL HISTORY

The midwife must satisfy herself that the patient is financially capable of procuring the necessary nourishment and rest during pregnancy, and of making adequate preparation for her confinement and the care of the young baby.

THE FAMILY HISTORY

This should be inquired into, as some families have a predisposition to certain diseases such as psychiatric disorders, cardiac disease, diabetes and essential hypertension. The tendency to produce twins also runs in families. If parent, brother or sister is dead, the cause should be ascertained without giving rise to distress in doing so.

THE MEDICAL HISTORY

It is necessary to have some knowledge of the woman's previous health, as former illnesses may have damaged certain structures or organs, and this might give rise to complications during pregnancy or labour. Anterior poliomyelitis, or tuberculosis of the spine and hip may cause deformities; rheumatic infection or chorea may leave cardiac impairment. Diseases, such as chronic nephritis, tend to be aggravated by childbearing: diabetes and cardiac disease may seriously complicate pregnancy and labour: syphilis and diabetes both endanger the life of the child. Previous accidents or pelvic operations may affect parturition.

Inquiries should be made regarding blood transfusions given at any time, including childhood, because of the possibility of Rh iso-immunization occurring in an Rh negative woman.

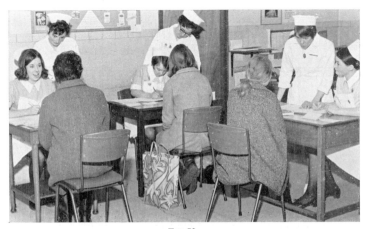

FIG. 73
Student midwives taking histories under supervision.
(Simpson Memorial Prenatal Clinic, Edinburgh.

THE OBSTETRICAL HISTORY

Is the woman pregnant for the first time?

A record of what happened in previous pregnancies, labours and puerperia will often give a clue as to what may be anticipated in the present instance. Certain conditions may recur, and it may be possible to give advice or institute treatment to avert them.

1. PREVIOUS PREGNANCIES

The majority will have been normal, but an account of any complications should be obtained. Particulars of abortions should be included, with a statement of the month at which they occurred and the cause, if known. Any previous history of excessive sickness, pyelonephritis or pre-eclampsia will necessitate close supervision during this pregnancy.

2. PREVIOUS LABOURS

Was labour premature or postmature; if induced, why?

Most labours are straightforward. The length of labour is important, and, if over 24 hours, the woman should be asked if the contractions (pains) were short or if they went off for long periods, as would occur in hypotonic uterine action.

The baby's weight, and the fact that forceps had been necessary, would give an idea as to whether delay was due to cephalo-pelvic disproportion. A woman, who has previously given birth spontaneously to a baby weighing 3,402 or 3,629 G. (7½ or 8 lb.) is likely to have a normal pelvis.

If a Cæsarean section has previously been performed (the scar would be evidence), all subsequent labours ought to be conducted in hospital, on account of the risk of rupture of the uterine scar.

A previous third degree perineal tear would suggest the need for an episiotomy to avoid its recurrence.

A history of postpartum hæmorrhage or adherent placenta would necessitate hospitalization in case such an accident be repeated.

3. PREVIOUS PUERPERIA

Progress during the puerperium can best be assessed by asking the woman whether she felt well during this period. Complications, such as mastitis, venous thrombosis, or puerperal sepsis, usually come to light with shrewd questioning.

4. PREVIOUS BABIES

A record of normal-sized babies, born alive and well, is usual, but when the weight of a previous baby is stated to have been over 4,082 G. (9 lb.) it is usual to examine the urine for glucose to rule out diabetes, some do a glucose tolerance test. The unreliability of spring-balance scales used in domiciliary practice should also be kept in mind.

A history of stillbirth would demand careful questioning if no record was available, and the **cause of neonatal deaths should be investigated.** If there is no living child, or in cases of repeated premature births, or of severe jaundice, the doctor should be informed; he will recommend delivery in hospital where prompt skilled treatment and the facilities available may save the baby's life.

Should infant deaths appear to be due to lack of good mothercraft, additional instruction ought to be given by the midwife, who will get in touch with the health visitor before ceasing to visit the woman, or on her discharge from hospital.

THE PRESENT PREGNANCY

The first question when taking the history is usually in regard to (a) the **date of the last menstrual period** to establish the period of gestation, (b) whether it was normal in length and amount and if the woman had been menstruating regularly. If there is any doubt regarding the last menstrual period, the woman should be told to note and record the date of quickening (see p. 69). The length of time married is important in cases of infertility.

Enquiry should be made as to whether she has felt well since becoming pregnant, and if not the cause should be sought and appropriate action taken. Exposure to rubella during or immediately prior to pregnancy is very significant (see p. 200).

Drugs taken. Some authorities enquire regarding drugs taken during pregnancy and six weeks prior to conception because of their possible teratogenic effects. Antidepressive drugs such as Nardil may potentiate the action of pethidine.

The obstetrician and anæsthetist ought to know if the woman has had corticosteroid therapy within 2 years.

THE GRANDE MULTIPARA

This term is applied to the woman who has given birth to six or more children, in order to stress the hazards of such a situation. With each succeeding birth after the third the maternal mortality and stillbirth rates rise steeply and even more so when the woman is over 30 years of age. Severe anæmia is common because of repeated childbearing and poor nutrition; many of these women are over-worked and worn out. Because of their age the cardio-vascular system is often impaired. Hypertension and obesity accentuate the risks of high parity.

Midwives ought to pay special attention to these women, advising them regarding the need for rest and suitable food and referring them to the Local Authority who will arrange for a home help or other means of lightening the domestic burden. They should be delivered in hospital for the incidence of malpresentation, rupture of uterus and postpartum hæmorrhage is very much greater in the grande multipara.

THE OLDER PRIMIGRAVIDA

Age is important, particularly if this is her first baby and she is over 30. To such a patient the term " older primigravida " is applied and women of that age often worry regarding their ability to go through the processes of child-bearing safely so much assurance accompanied by careful supervision throughout pregnancy and labour is essential. It may be, if she has been married for a number of years, that she is relatively infertile so special precautions are taken to prevent abortion and to secure a live child. For example, postmaturity is not permitted to develop and Cæsarean section is performed four times more frequently than in the younger woman. Pre-eclampsia and prolonged labour increase the dangers to the fetus.

The maternal mortality rate is only slightly increased but the morbidity rate is rather high because of pre-eclampsia, essential hypertension, venous thrombosis and uterine fibroids: uterine dysfunction and rigidity of the soft tissues of the birth canal accentuate the need for delivery by forceps.

The perinatal mortality rate is doubled in women over 35 and the possibility of Down's syndrome is always present. Midwives should, when the opportunity arises, advise women not to defer their first pregnancy too long beyond the optimal child-bearing age of 18 to 25 years.

DIET HISTORY

If there is no dietitian, the midwife should inquire into the type of meals the woman is having, in order to make sure she is getting the necessary substances for the baby's and her own well-being (*body building foods, minerals, vitamins*), and that she is procuring the food supplements available (see Nutrition, p. 85). Dietary advice is given when weight gain is excessive, but in cases of gross obesity specialist advice is essential, also in certain medical complications of pregnancy (*see under appropriate headings*).

METHOD OF TAKING THE HISTORY

Great patience and infinite tact are needed when taking the history of a new patient, especially a primigravida, to whom the experience may seem to be something of an ordeal. The midwife should be kindly in her approach, and by her reassuring manner convey the impression that having a baby is a happy event and a natural process.

The woman's name, address, age and **occupation** are recorded. Patients are often forgetful in regard to dates and past illnesses; they may even neglect to mention a surgical operation until their attention is drawn to the presence of a scar.

Questions should be asked in such a way as to avoid creating the impression that you suspect the woman is suffering from some particular ailment. To ask an expectant mother outright if there is tuberculosis or psychiatric disorders in her family might well alarm her; it would be better to inquire whether her father and mother were in good health and if there had been any serious illnesses in the family.

Unless the prenatal record provides a list of questions to be asked, the midwife should have some system of questioning that will elicit the required information, *e.g.*:

1. **Illnesses.**—Which did you have as a child? Since you grew up?
2. **Accidents.**—Have you had any?
3. **Operations.**—Have you had any?
4. **Blood transfusion.**—Have you ever had one?

Simple, non-technical language should be used, as terms very familiar to the midwife may be unknown and even frightening to the woman, and wrong answers may be given because of lack of understanding. By listening to an experienced midwife taking histories the student midwife learns the terminology which suits the mentality of different patients.

QUESTIONS FOR REVISION

PRENATAL CARE

THE SOCIAL ASPECT

Define what is meant by: (*a*) a voluntary organization; (*b*) supplementary allowances; (*c*) a home help; (*d*) a foster mother; (*e*) adoption order; (*f*) alimony; (*g*) an unsupported mother; (*h*) suitable employment in pregnancy.

C.M.B.(Eng.) paper, 1969. 50 word question.—What are the essential differences between placing a baby with foster parents and placing a baby for adoption ?

C.M.B.(Eng.) paper, 1969. 50 word question.—What is: (*a*) a maternity allowance ? (*b*) a maternity grant ?

C.M.B.(Eng.) paper, 1969.—What services are available to an unmarried mother and her child ?

C.M.B.(Eng.) paper, 1969. 50 word question.—What statutory benefits are available to a pregnant woman ?

C.M.B.(Eng.) paper, 1970.—What help and information would you give to the mother who wishes to have her baby adopted ?

C.M.B.(Eng.) paper, 1970. 50 word question.—Maternity Benefits.

C.M.B.(Eng.) paper, 1970. 50 word question.—What services are provided by the local authority child welfare clinics ?

C.M.B.(Scot.) paper, 1970.—What services are available for the unsupported woman and her child before and after delivery ?

ORAL QUESTIONS

How could you give emotional support to a pregnant woman ? What advice would you give if asked about adoption ? How could you try to prevent congenital abnormalities ? How much does National dried milk cost ? State the amount of the maternity grant; maternity allowance.

Write not more than 10 lines on each of the following: Taking the obstetrical history. The older primigravida. Health education. Good human relationships at the clinic. The influence of the midwife.

TAKING THE HISTORY

In taking the obstetrical history, why are the following facts significant ? (*a*) Length of labour ; (*b*) weights of babies ; (*c*) stillbirths or neonatal deaths ; (*d*) instrumental delivery ; (*e*) previous Cæsarean section.

C.M.B.(Eng.) paper.—What questions would you ask a woman early in her second pregnancy who states that her first child was stillborn ? How may this information be of value in preventing a further stillbirth ?

C.M.B.(Scot.) paper.—What questions concerning her previous pregnancies and labours would you ask a multipara ? How might the information obtained help in the management of the present pregnancy and labour ?

C.M.B.(N. Ireland) paper.—In booking a multigravida one gives attention to the history of her previous confinements : of what value may this be ?

C.M.B.(Eng.) paper, 1969.—What information do you seek when taking the history of a multiparous patient and what are your reasons ?

C.M.B.(N. Ireland) paper, 1970.—Define " grande multiparae ". What factors make this group especially important in midwifery.

C.M.B.(Scot.) paper, 1970.—What particular complications do you associate with pregnancy and labour in the grande multipara ?

AIMS OF PRENATAL CARE

C.M.B.(Eng.) paper.—How can antenatal care benefit the unborn child ?

C.M.B.(Eng.) paper.—What are the main features of antenatal care in the last three months of pregnancy ?

C.M.B.(Scot.) paper.—Discuss the ways in which good antenatal care can prevent complications of labour.

C.M.B.(Scot.) paper.—Describe three clinical examples to illustrate the value of antenatal care.

C.M.B.(N. Ireland) paper.—Discuss the aims of antenatal care. Indicate briefly the complications likely to be detected during the middle trimester (middle three months) of pregnancy.

C.M.B.(Eng.) paper.—What are the aims of antenatal care? At what intervals should a healthy pregnant woman be examined?

PSYCHOLOGICAL ASPECT

C.M.B.(Eng.) paper.—What anxieties and fears may beset pregnant women ? How would you seek to allay them ?

7

Examination of the Pregnant Woman

The examination of the pregnant woman can be carried out entirely by the doctor, or it may be shared by the midwife. There are, however, certain procedures which midwives are not qualified to undertake, and it is only right that every woman should reap the benefit of any investigation or examination that makes childbirth safer for mother and child.

A friendly atmosphere should prevail in the prenatal clinic, and scientific investigation, essential though it is, should not obtrusively dominate the situation. **The woman needs helpful advice** and friendly counsel as well as professional supervision, for her concern is mainly about the minor disorders which make her life miserable and her lack of knowledge regarding labour and the care of babies. The midwife can do much to remedy this.

Zeal should not outstrip discretion, for a woman can be upset to the verge of tears when interviewed and examined by too many people; she is so confused that she cannot remember the advice she has been given. The appointment system has reduced waiting time; further organization will, by postponing some of the investigations to the second or third visit, eliminate much unnecessary emotional and physical stress.

THE FIRST VISIT

The woman usually goes to her doctor or the clinic when she has missed one or two menstrual periods, and as she walks into the examining room observation begins, for **small stature, deformity or a limp** are more readily detected when the woman is on

Fig. 74

PLAYROOM AT PRENATAL CLINIC MANNED BY THE WOMEN'S ROYAL VOLUNTARY SERVICE.

(Aberdeen Maternity Hospital.)

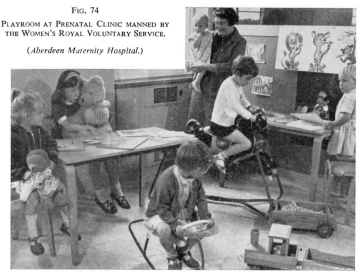

98

her feet. An impression of health and vitality can be gained by her bearing; the tired malnourished woman looks apathetic, her shoulders droop and she lacks energy.

HEIGHT

The woman of good physique is unlikely to have a contracted pelvis, and as a general but not infallible rule few women over 1·60 m. (5 feet 3 inches) in height are found to have abnormal pelves. Short stature is more significant when due to disease or malnutrition than when occurring in the petite type of woman with small bones who is more likely to give birth to a small baby.

WEIGHT

The woman should be weighed early in pregnancy (at her first visit) in order to determine her normal weight; the procedure being repeated on each subsequent occasion. She should be undressed and given a washable dressing-gown to wear, because the difference in the weight of clothing may be considerable during the three seasons over which pregnancy extends. Recording the weight in graph form draws attention to any marked increase or decrease.

A gain of 11·3 kg. (25 lb.) can be accounted for physiologically during pregnancy (p. 61). Women who are apparently healthy have gained as little as 4·5 kg. (10 lb.) and as much as 15·8 kg. (35 lb.). (*A weight control diet is given on p. 65.*)

URINE ANALYSIS

This is carried out at every visit, and includes *inspection, reaction, specific gravity,* and testing for protein and glucose. Great importance is attached to finding protein in the urine, as it is one of the signs of pre-eclampsia, a condition which must be treated promptly to avert more serious developments. Proteinuria may also be caused by such conditions as pyelonephritis and chronic nephritis.

Glycosuria is fairly common during pregnancy, and if more than a trace of glucose is present on two occasions a blood glucose test is done after breakfast and if necessary a glucose tolerance test is carried out ; but in the absence of clinical signs of diabetes the blood glucose is usually found to be normal.

OBTAINING A MIDSTREAM SPECIMEN (*at Clinic*)

Seven per cent of pregnant women have asymptomatic bacteriuria. If urinary infection is suspected a " clean catch " specimen of urine is obtained. The woman standing over the " toilet " passes some urine then obtains a specimen directly into a 60 ml. universal container with screw top, or a plastic carton; a 300 ml. metal measuring jug is convenient for the woman to hold but the urine must then be poured into the laboratory container. Some recommend swabbing without an antiseptic, others, separation of the labia.

Unless the urine reaches the laboratory within one hour it must be kept in a cool place at 4·4° C. (40° F.) or the bacterial count will be inaccurate.

EXAMINATION BY THE DOCTOR

During the first trimester of pregnancy it is mainly the medical aspect that requires supervision. Obstetrical complications, such as pre-eclampsia, malpresentation and disproportion, occur later. The cardiovascular and respiratory systems are examined as early in pregnancy as possible: when conditions such as diabetes, tuberculosis or cardiac disease are diagnosed the woman is referred to the appropriate clinic or specialist.

BLOOD TESTS

The following blood tests are carried out :

WASSERMANN (OR OTHER SEROLOGICAL TESTS)

These should be made on all pregnant women.   At the Simpson Maternity Pavilion 1-2,000 are found to be positive.

BLOOD GROUPS ABO

Because of the risk of hæmorrhage in obstetrics it is a wise precaution to know the woman's blood group, so that compatible blood can be given without delay should transfusion be necessary.

RHESUS FACTOR

The blood of every pregnant woman should be examined for the Rh factor because of the possibility of isoimmunization.

HÆMOGLOBIN

Childbearing women often suffer from anæmia, and if the hæmoglobin is below 12·6 G. (85 per cent) iron and vitamins B_1 and C are prescribed.   If below 8·9 G. (60 per cent) further blood investigation is carried out.

Sickle cell haemoglobin tests are made in certain immigrant women (see p. 199).

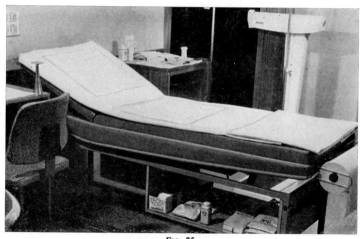

FIG. 75
EXAMINATION COUCH AT PRENATAL CLINIC.
(*Aberdeen Maternity Hospital.*)

Vaginal Examination

At the first visit some doctors make a vaginal examination, not only to confirm the diagnosis and duration of pregnancy but to exclude any pelvic abnormality. Conditions such as retroversion, fibroids, ovarian or vaginal cysts, double uterus and septate vagina will be detected.   Other authorities consider that the procedure is not warranted because the findings are so often negative.

Cervical cytology is done in many prenatal clinics at this visit.

The midwife provides draping and privacy to avoid unnecessary embarrassment to the woman.

EXAMINATION BY THE MIDWIFE

The woman lies comfortably on a firm bed or couch, and before beginning the examination, the midwife should ask her a few simple questions such as, how she is feeling, whether she sleeps well, if she goes out every day, in order to show interest in her as an individual. An inquiry as to whether she is eating well, will lead to the giving of advice about a suitable diet with adequate body building foods, fruit, vegetables and milk.

Much helpful advice can also be offered about the minor disorders, such as constipation, heartburn and morning sickness, if necessary.

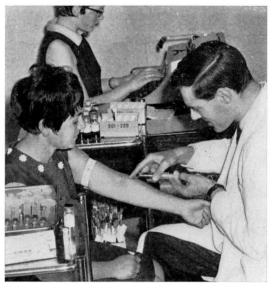

FIG. 76

Venepuncture is employed to procure blood for all tests. The finger prick is painful and subject to the error of dilution of the blood specimen by tissue fluid when squeezing is employed to obtain a free flow of blood.

Secretary types in triplicate lists for the departments of Hæmatology, Bacteriology and Blood Transfusion Service.

(*Prenatal Clinic, Simpson Memorial Maternity Pavilion, Edinburgh.*)

THE BLOOD PRESSURE

The blood pressure should be estimated at the first visit to find out the usual level and then at each subsequent visit because a rise in blood pressure, manifest during the second half of pregnancy, is one of the earliest signs of pre-eclampsia. The blood pressure tends to be lower than normal during pregnancy (p. 60).

A blood pressure of 130/80 is viewed with suspicion, and 140/90 is considered to be pathological. But a steadily rising blood pressure may be significant, even although it has not reached 130/80.

In some pregnant women the blood pressure is very unstable, and excitement or exertion may cause a temporary increase which subsides with rest. The woman should be recumbent when the test is made, and if her pulse is rapid and her blood pressure raised it may be due to nervousness, but some consider this to be a significant warning rise. The test should be repeated 20 minutes later.

PHYSICAL EXAMINATION OF THE WOMAN

The examination should be carried out systematically, so that no point is omitted, always beginning at the head.

THE HEAD

Facial appearance gives a general impression of physical and mental well-being. The woman may look healthy, well-nourished and happy, or she may be malnourished, ill, or apprehensive. Pallor of gums, lips and conjunctiva may denote the presence of anæmia, but a red conjunctiva does not preclude anæmia.

Œdema of the face is a grave sign (*not usually seen at the prenatal clinic*) most commonly found in serious cases of pre-eclampsia. Other signs of ill-health, such as swollen glands of the neck, cyanosis, breathlessness or persistent cough, would be apparent; and if the midwife detects any abnormality at the first or any subsequent examination she must obtain medical advice.

The mouth is inspected for dental caries, and arrangements made for the woman to see the dentist when necessary.

THE BREASTS

They are examined for signs of pregnancy (p. 58), and if any condition exists that would create difficulty in lactation appropriate advice should be given.

THE VULVA

The presence of a vaginal discharge that is profuse, purulent, irritating, green and frothy or blood-stained should be reported.

Œdema or varicose veins, vulval warts, or lesions suggesting syphilis—such as chancre or condylomata lata—would necessitate getting medical advice.

THE LOWER LIMBS

They are examined for deformities; bending of the tibia would be suggestive of rickets. The size and width of the foot may give a clue to pelvic capacity, size three or less in shoes being abnormally small.

The tissue over the tibia near the ankle should be tested for œdema (*pre-tibial œdema*) at every visit, but, if present during the first half of pregnancy, is not due to pre-eclampsia.

Varicose veins, unless very slight, should be reported to the doctor so that suitable advice may be given (see p. 132).

PELVIC CAPACITY

The majority of pelves are adequate for the safe passage of an average-sized baby, but the midwife must be constantly on the alert for any deviation from normal, so that arrangements can be made for labour and delivery to be conducted in hospital.

No matter how normal the woman's physique and stature may be, pelvic capacity should be estimated, for a small pelvis may be present in a woman of average proportions.

PELVIS AND FETAL HEAD

The pelvis must also be considered in relation to the size of the fetus *in utero.* It has been aptly said that " **the fetal head is the best pelvimeter,**" for, unless the pelvis is large enough to accommodate the head of the fetus, the fact that the pelvis is of average size and shape is of no value. But not until the 36th week of pregnancy has the fetal head grown sufficiently large to judge whether it will enter the pelvic brim or whether disproportion exists. Some pelves are so small or deformed that a 3,175 G. (7 lb.) baby could not be born naturally and Cæsarean section would be necessary.

A minor degree of pelvic contraction may be difficult to diagnose.

The midwife will, of course, realize that it is not possible by pelvimetry to determine that the fetal head will pass safely through the pelvis. The strength of the uterine contractions, the " give " of the pelvic joints and the degree of over-riding of the skull bones, all influence the outcome of labour.

THE ASSESSMENT OF PELVIC CAPACITY

1. **RADIOGRAPHY.**
2. **INTERNAL PELVIMETRY,** by digital examination *per vaginam.*

RADIOGRAPHY

This is the most precise and accurate method, but X-rays are not employed for pelvimetry unless there are clinical indications of contracted pelvis because of the radiation hazards involved.

The critical measurements are the antero-posterior diameter of the inlet and the bi-spinous transverse diameter of the outlet.

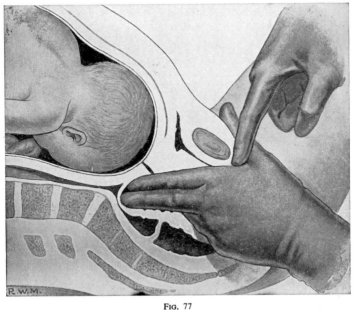

Fig. 77

Taking measurement of the diagonal conjugate.

INTERNAL PELVIMETRY

Internal pelvimetry is probably the most widely used method, and an experienced obstetrician can usually give a very good estimate of pelvic capacity by vaginal examination. The size of the obstetrical conjugate can be assessed by measuring the diagonal conjugate.

DIAGONAL CONJUGATE

The diagonal or internal conjugate is measured from the lower border of the symphysis pubis to the centre of the promontory of the sacrum and is usually 12·1 to 13·3 cm. (4¾ to 5¼ inches). To allow for the depth of the pubic bone 1·3 to 1·9 cm. (½ to ¾ inch) is subtracted; the result is the measurement of the obstetrical conjugate. This measurement may be taken in every primigravida and in multi-gravid women who have had a difficult labour with normal-sized babies.

It is usually done between the 32nd and 36th week of pregnancy as the vagina and pelvic floor are softer then, causing less discomfort to the woman and making it easier for the examiner.

Method

The woman lies in the dorsal position with knees drawn up, the bladder having previously been emptied. The vulva is swabbed with antiseptic, *e.g.* Hibitane 1-2,000 and the thighs draped. The two fingers of the gloved left hand are lubricated with obstetric cream and inserted into the vagina. An effort is made to reach the sacral promontory, and if bone is encountered the fingers should be directed farther upwards. No bone is felt above the promontory because the fifth lumbar vertebra recedes.

The point where the left hand is in contact with the lower border of the symphysis pubis is marked by the right forefinger (Fig. 77) and after withdrawal the distance

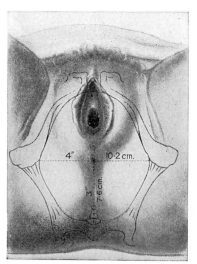

between that point and the tip of the middle finger is measured with ruler or calipers. On subtracting 1·9 cm. (¾ inch) the measurement of the obstetrical conjugate is obtained.

ASSESSMENT OF THE PELVIC OUTLET

The ischial spines are palpated to see if they are unduly prominent, which would indicate diminution of the bi-spinous transverse diameter of the outlet. Two fingers are placed in the sacro-sciatic notch to determine if it is adequate. The curve of the sacrum is noted, and before removing the fingers the pubic arch is examined to see whether it is acute. Two fingers can usually be accommodated in the apex of the pubic arch.

The intertuberischial or transverse diameter of the lower outlet, the distance between the ischial tuberosities, is 10·2 cm. (4 inches) on the bony pelvis, but the fat and tissue of the buttocks lessen the diameter by at least 1·3 cm. (half an inch).

FIG. 78

Intertuberischial diameter of the pelvic outlet.

It is practically impossible to measure this diameter with any degree of accuracy but a general impression of size can be obtained by inserting the closed fist between the ischial tuberosities. Fists vary in size, but after the midwife has estimated the size of the outlet in a large series of patients it is possible for her to judge whether the intertuberischial diameter is average, small or large; and, if small, medical advice is necessary.

Method

The patient lies on her left side with her knees well drawn up. The midwife places the knuckle of her middle finger on the posterior border of the anus, and the middle joints of the gloved fist are inserted between the ischial tuberosities and directed slightly backwards.

ABDOMINAL EXAMINATION

The midwife should be thoroughly proficient in abdominal examination, not only for the purpose of diagnosis during pregnancy but also for the conduct of labour. Considerable practice is needed in order to acquire manual dexterity and to develop the essential sense of touch.

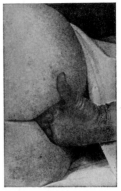

FIG. 79

Assessing the intertuberischial diameter by inserting the fist between the ischial tuberosities.

EXAMINATION DURING THE FIRST HALF OF PREGNANCY

Abdominal examination is usually carried out to corroborate the diagnosis of pregnancy and the period of gestation. It is not always easy to palpate the uterus before the 16th week, and the presence of obesity or a rigid abdominal wall exaggerates the difficulty. If doubt exists, the woman should be referred to the doctor who will perform a bi-manual examination, when, by feeling the size, shape and consistency of the uterus, it may be possible to substantiate the diagnosis.

It is usual to ascertain whether the size of the uterus corresponds with the period of amenorrhœa.

At about the 18th week the fundus will be mid-way between the symphysis pubis and the umbilicus. At this time the woman will detect fetal movement (*quickening*); the multiparous woman, having had previous experience, will recognize this, one or two weeks earlier than the primigravida.

Although the umbilicus is usually taken as a landmark to assess fundal height its situation in the abdomen may vary as much as 3·8 cm. (1½ inches) in different women depending on their height and build.

Fetal parts can be felt about the 20th week.

The fetal heart will sometimes be heard if the stethoscope is placed in the midline, half-way between the umbilicus and symphysis pubis. But, unless the room is absolutely quiet and the examiner has very acute hearing, the fetal heart is not likely to be heard until the 24th week. An ultrasonic pulse detector, the Sonicaid or the Doptone, will pick up the fetal blood flow at 14 weeks; sometimes as early as the 10th week.

METHOD OF ABDOMINAL EXAMINATION

The woman should be comfortable so that she can relax physically and mentally.
Her arms ought to lie limply by her sides and her back should sink into the couch so
that she can relax her abdominal muscles. An interested inquiry about her family
or her own welfare and a few words of advice on how to relax are usually sufficient
to put her at ease.

Her bladder should be empty.

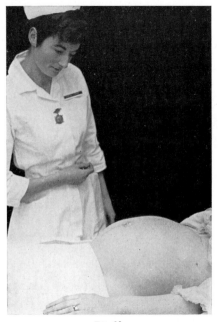

FIG. 80

Abdominal inspection.

The blanket should be folded down once to knee level, and the sheet folded in a
similar manner to just above the level of the symphysis pubis, as it is impossible to
examine the abdomen properly with a mound of bedclothes in the way. *Patients
should never be exposed unnecessarily.*

It is a good habit to stand on the patient's right side, for the same reason that all
nursing procedures are done on the right: most people are right-handed and become
expert when one method is used. From the left side, the procedure is often done in
a perfunctory manner.

Three senses are used, visual, tactile, auditory, and the examination should be
carried out systematically by (1) **inspection,** (2) **palpation** and (3) **auscultation,** in that
order.

ABDOMINAL INSPECTION (after 30th week)

1. SIZE OF THE UTERUS

(a) PERIOD OF GESTATION

Although it is possible to make a rough estimate of the period of gestation by inspection it is by no means reliable without palpation for a distended colon or a thick abdominal wall gives the impression of undue size.

(a) TWINS OR HYDRAMNIOS

These increase the length and breadth of the uterus whereas a large baby increases the length.

2. SHAPE OF THE UTERUS

(a) LIE OF THE FETUS

When the lie of the fetus is longitudinal as occurs in 99·5 per cent of cases, the shape of the uterus is ovoid longitudinally (longer than it is broad). When the lie of the fetus is transverse the uterine shape is ovoid transversely (low and broad).

(b) MULTIPARITY

The uterus lacks the snug ovoid shape of the primigravid uterus.

(c) POSITION

Occasionally it is possible to diagnose the anterior or lateral position of the fetus by seeing the prominent back on one or other side of the abdomen. In posterior positions of the vertex a saucer-like depression is seen at or below the umbilicus.

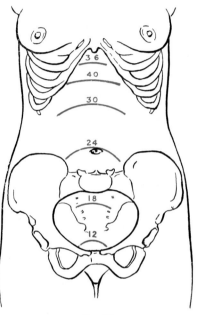

FIG. 81

Growth of the uterus, showing the fundal heights at the 12th, 18th, 24th, 30th, 36th and 40th weeks.

3. FETAL MOVEMENT

This is evidence that the fetus is alive; it also aids in the diagnosis of position, as the back will be on the opposite side to that on which movement is seen.

4. CONTOUR OF ABDOMINAL WALL

(a) A pendulous abdomen is more commonly seen in the multigravid woman and can be more readily detected when she is standing. It is due to laxity of the abdominal muscles which allows the uterus to sag forwards, sometimes known as anterior uterine obliquity.

In primigravid women pendulous abdomen is of serious import and necessitates medical investigation as it may be due to pelvic contraction or spinal deformity.

(*b*) **The umbilicus becomes less dimpled** as pregnancy advances and during the later weeks may protrude above skin level.

(*c*) **Full bladder.**—This is more evident during the later weeks of pregnancy.

5. SKIN CHANGES

(*a*) **Striæ gravidarum** are frequently seen: silvery streaks suggest a previous pregnancy; pink streaks occur in the present pregnancy.

(*b*) **Linea nigra** is the dark line of pigmentation seen running longitudinally in the centre of the abdomen above and below the umbilicus. It is of interest as a presumptive sign of pregnancy.

(*c*) **Operation scars.**

ABDOMINAL PALPATION (after 30th week)

HOW TO PALPATE THE UTERUS

The hands should be clean and warm: cold hands do not have the necessary acute sense of touch; they tend to induce contraction of the abdominal muscles and the patient resents the discomfort of them.

Arms and hands should be relaxed and the pads—not the tips—of the fingers used with delicate precision, the hands being moved smoothly over the abdomen without lifting them. Erratic dipping of the fingers, sudden pressure and rough manipulation are irritating to the abdominal wall and the uterus, causing contractions that make the detection of fetal parts impossible.

UPPER OR LOWER POLE ?

The traditional method of palpation is to start at the fundus, and should be used by the novice, until sufficient experience has been obtained to become proficient in diagnosis, but the practice of beginning with pelvic palpation is popular.

The advantage of palpating the lower pole first is that the important part of abdominal palpation—finding out what lies at the pelvic brim—can be determined before contractions have been stimulated by handling the upper pole of the uterus.

The disadvantage is that having made what is believed to be the correct assessment by pelvic palpation, the midwife neglects to palpate the fundus and so misses the opportunity of correcting any erroneous diagnosis.

1. ESTIMATING THE PERIOD OF GESTATION

The following system of assessing the period of gestation is open to fallacy, because the size, number of fetuses and amount of liquor amnii vary, but it is a convenient, useful method so long as its limitations are appreciated.

(*a*) ASSESSING FUNDAL HEIGHT

As many fingers (*not the tips*) of the left hand, as can be accommodated, are laid flat between the upper border of the fundus and the xiphisternum; the distance between fundus and xiphisternum is estimated in fingers breadth. At 36 weeks no fingers can be inserted. When lightening takes place three or four fingers can be inserted.

(b) SIZE OF THE UTERUS

This can be assessed by measuring the girth of the abdomen with a tape measure at the level of the umbilicus; the circumference in a woman of average size being about 71·1 cm. (32 inches) at the 34th week; 96·5 cm. (38 inches) at the 40th week. Measuring the circumferences is of no diagnostic value prior to the 34th week.

When the girth increases slowly after the 34th week the small baby syndrome is suspected (see p. 546).

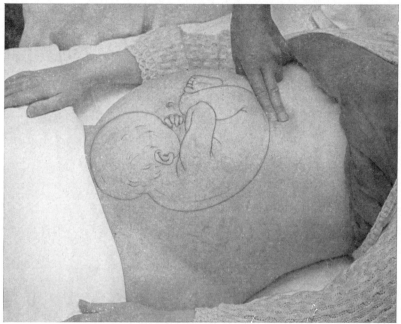

FIG. 82

Assessing the fundal height in fingers-breadth below the xiphisternum.

UTERUS UNDULY LARGE

Twins or hydramnios may be suspected: in some cases it might be due to a large baby or, more rarely, fibroid tumours.

The uterus of the woman of short stature appears to be more prominent than the uterus of the tall woman.

UTERUS SMALLER THAN AVERAGE

That the woman is mistaken in the date of her last menstrual period is the most likely explanation when the uterus is smaller than the estimated period of gestation warrants.

8A

Fetal death may have occurred: this can be verified on auscultation.

In cases of pre-eclampsia the fetus may be small due to placental dysfunction.

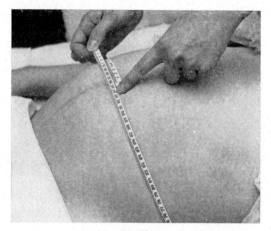

Fig. 83

Measuring abdominal girth at umbilical level.

2. FUNDAL PALPATION

This manœuvre will help to determine whether the presentation is cephalic or podalic, and the lie longitudinal or transverse. In 95 per cent of cases the breech will be in the fundus and this denotes a cephalic presentation, commonly the vertex. When the head is in the fundus the presentation is podalic (breech).

When breech or head is in the fundus the lie is longitudinal. If neither can be palpated in the fundus further investigation is required in case the lie is transverse.

Method

The midwife stands on the patient's right with her thighs against the couch and her body, turned at the waist, facing the woman's head. Both hands are laid on the sides of the fundus, fingers held close together and curving round the upper border.

Gentle yet deliberate pressure is applied using the palmar surfaces of the fingers as well as the tips to determine the soft consistency and indefinite outline that denotes the breech. Sometimes the buttocks feel rather firm but they are neither as hard, smooth nor well defined as the head.

With a gliding movement the position of the hands is changed in an endeavour to grasp the fetal mass, which may be in the centre or deflected to one or other side, and assess its size and mobility.

The breech cannot be moved independently of the body as can the head.

The head is much more distinctive in outline being hard and round; it can be ballotted between the finger-tips of the two hands, or between the thumb and finger of one hand, because of the free movement at the neck. If the diagnosis is in doubt the

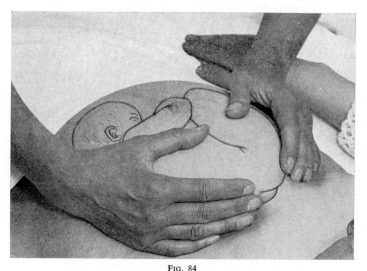

Fig. 84

FUNDAL PALPATION.

Palms of hands on either side of the fundus, fingers held
close together palpate the upper pole of the uterus.

finger-tips should be pressed deeply into the abdominal wall over what is thought
to be the head and by giving a sharp tap the bony hardness of head will be readily
detected.

3. LATERAL PALPATION

This manœuvre is useful to locate the fetal back as an aid to diagnosis of position.
Obesity, and an excess of amniotic fluid increase the difficulties in palpation.

Method

While facing the woman's head (or feet) the hands are placed on both sides of the
uterus at about umbilical level. Pressure is applied with the palms of alternate hands
to differentiate the degree of resistance between the two sides of the uterus.

**One hand is used to steady the uterus and press the fetus over towards the examining
hand** which determines the presence of the broad resistant back or the small parts
that slip about under the examining fingers. If the back cannot be palpated readily
and small parts are evident over a wide area occipito-posterior position may be
suspected.

By using a rotary movement of the fingers the back may be mapped out as a continuous smooth resistant mass from the breech down to the neck, where the resistance
disappears.

" **Walking the finger tips** " of both hands over the abdomen from one side to the
other is an excellent method of locating the back (see Fig. 86). The fingers should be
dipped into the abdominal wall deliberately and fairly deeply and the firm back can

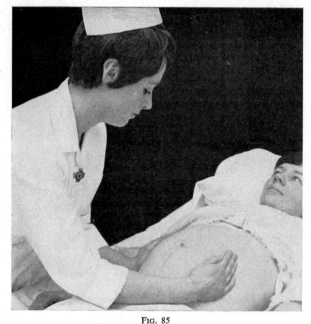

FIG. 85

LATERAL PALPATION.

Hands placed at umbilical level on either side of the uterus. Pressure is applied alternately with each hand.

be distinguished from the fluctuating liquor amnii and the receding knobbly small parts.

The back in an L.O.A. will be felt 2·5 cm. (1 inch) left of the midline.

    ,,   ,,   **L.O.L.**   ,,   **7·6 cm. (3 inches)**   ,,   ,,

    ,,   ,,   **L.O.P.**   ,,   **10·2 cm. (4+inches)**   ,,   ,,

To make the back more prominent fundal pressure can be applied with the left hand, and the right hand used to " walk " over the abdomen.

THE ANTERIOR SHOULDER

The anterior shoulder can be located by palpating from the neck upwards and inwards. When the head is high the shoulder will be about 12·7 cm. (5 inches) above the symphysis pubis; about 5·1 cm. (2 inches) when the head is engaged, and just above **the symphysis when the head is engaged deeply in the pelvis.**

4. PELVIC PALPATION

This is the most important manœuvre in abdominal palpation because of its value in the diagnosis of presentation of the fetus, position, engagement of the fetal head **and disproportion between** head and pelvis.

Method

To relax the abdominal muscles the woman's knees should be slightly raised: she can assist still further by opening her mouth and breathing steadily and quietly. The midwife stands with her thighs against the couch, her body, turned at the waist, facing towards the woman's feet.

The sides of the uterus just below umbilical level are grasped snugly between the palms of the hands; the fingers, held close together, pointing downwards and inwards. If the hands are placed correctly the first joints of the little fingers will be on a level with the anterior superior iliac spines, and the outstretched thumbs will meet at about the level of the umbilicus (see Fig. 87).

DIAGNOSIS OF CEPHALIC OR HEAD PRESENTATION

The fingers are directed inwards and, if the head is presenting, a hard mass with a distinctive round smooth outline will be detected. To determine if the vertex is presenting the two cephalic prominences, the occipital and sincipital, are located. The higher one will, if on the opposite side from the fetal back, be the sincipital and this denotes a vertex presentation, head flexed.

In face presentation the higher cephalic prominence will be on the same side as the fetal back.

DIAGNOSIS OF POSITION

With the hands grasping the lower pole of the uterus, the finger tips palpate both sides of the head and are arrested on the higher cephalic prominence which may be at a level of 5·1 to 7·6 cm. (2 or 3 inches) above the prominence on the other side.

The higher cephalic prominence is the sincipital and, in vertex presentation, it is always on the side of the woman's abdomen opposite to that on which the fetal back is located. The lower and less definite cephalic prominence is the occipital and the position of the fetus in relation to the pelvic brim is determined according to which of the six areas of the brim the occiput points.

The position will be one of the following:

Right occipito posterior	Left occipito posterior
„ lateral	„ lateral
„ anterior	„ anterior

PAWLIK'S MANŒUVRE

This method of palpating the lower pole of the uterus is most effective when the head is not engaged. By this manœuvre it is easy to locate the round, hard head and to judge its size, flexion and mobility.

Method

The midwife, standing on the patient's right, faces the woman's head and, using the right hand, grasps the lower pole of the uterus with the thumb on the woman's right side and the fingers on the left side of the uterus (Fig. 89). Fingers and thumb must be sufficiently far apart to accommodate the fetal head. The woman is asked to take a deep breath and let it escape slowly through her open mouth. In carrying out this manœuvre great gentleness should be exercised.

An excellent diagnostic procedure is falling into disrepute because it is being done roughly and therefore causing pain. No matter where the head is situated or how it is grasped undue pressure applied to it will be painful for the expectant mother.

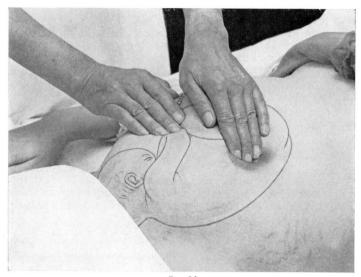

FIG. 86

"Walking " the finger tips across the abdomen to locate the position of the back.

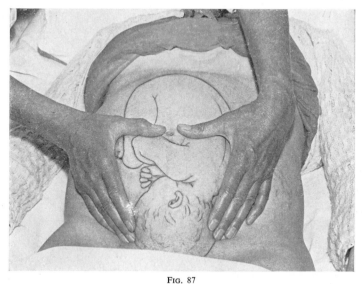

FIG. 87

PELVIC PALPATION.

If the hands are in the correct position the outstretched thumbs will meet at about umbilical level. **The fingers are directed inwards and downwards.**

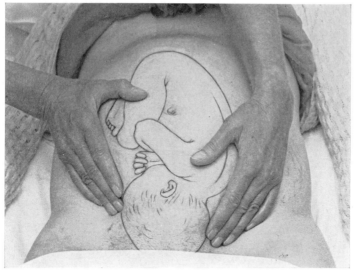

FIG. 88

Method of pelvic palpation to determine position in a vertex presentation. The higher cephalic prominence (the sincipital) will be on the opposite side to the back; on the right in an L.O.A.

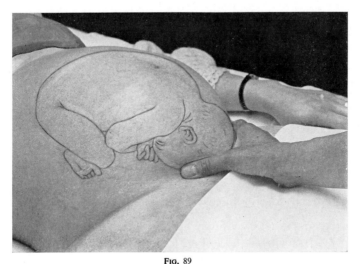

FIG. 89

PAWLIK'S MANŒUVRE.

The lower pole of the uterus is grasped with the right hand, the midwife facing the woman's head.

THE COMBINED GRIP

This manœuvre can be used when there is doubt regarding whether head or breech is presenting. It is an excellent method of comparing the contour and consistency of what is in the upper and lower poles of the uterus.

Method

While facing across the woman's body the right hand grasps the lower pole of the uterus as in Pawlik's manœuvre and the left hand grasps the fundus in a similar manner.

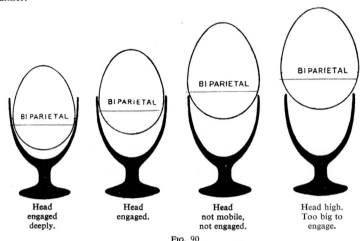

Head engaged deeply.	Head engaged.	Head not mobile, not engaged.	Head high. Too big to engage.

FIG. 90

Diagrammatic representation of engagement of the fetal head by the use of egg-cups and eggs.

ENGAGEMENT OF THE HEAD

An engaged head is one in which the largest presenting diameter (the bi-parietal in the well-flexed head) has passed through the pelvic brim.

Deciding whether the head is engaged or not requires, as well as manual dexterity, judgment in assessing the clinical findings for no one manœuvre or observation is conclusive.

FINDINGS WHEN HEAD IS ENGAGED

1. The greater bulk of the head is not palpable above the brim.

2. The head is not mobile.

3. The higher cephalic prominence will be felt less than 5·1 cm. (2 inches) above the brim.

4. The anterior shoulder would be little more than 5·1 cm. (2 inches) above the symphysis pubis.

Method

When grasping the head as in pelvic palpation it cannot be moved from side to side nor can the fingers displace it upwards. The amount of head accommodated within the two hands is less than with a non-engaged head. While the woman is breathing out, the fingers are directed further down because more of the head is in the pelvis.

To reach the lower cephalic prominence the finger tips, descending steeply, are dipped well down, in a somewhat backward direction, depending on how deeply the head has descended into the pelvic cavity. The higher cephalic prominence will be less pronounced than in the non-engaged head.

The head should be engaged in a primigravid woman at the 38th week of pregnancy and, if not, the cause must be investigated so medical aid should be sought. Engagement does occasionally occur in multigravid women who have firm abdominal muscles but more commonly not until after the onset of labour.

HEAD ENGAGED DEEPLY IN THE PELVIS

On rare occasions the head is not palpable abdominally because it is engaged so deeply in the pelvis that the vertex has reached the level of the ischial spines.

The finger tips are dipped well down into the pelvis while the woman " breathes out " and by giving a sharp tap the hard head may be detected. The anterior shoulder in these circumstances will lie immediately above the symphysis pubis and may be thought to be a breech presentation. When doubt exists a vaginal or rectal examination will reveal the deeply engaged head.

Terminology that should be abolished

In the past the word " fixed " has been used to designate an engaged head. It is true that the engaged head is fixed but conversely the fixed head is not necessarily engaged. This has given rise to misunderstanding and confusion. If the student midwife considers a fixed head to be engaged cases of minor degree disproportion will be missed.

The word " fixing " or " engaging " is used by some to describe cases in which the head is neither mobile nor considered to be engaged; but the head is either engaged or it is not engaged and no intermediate stage should be countenanced diagnostically. The midwife must seek medical advice if the head is not engaged when it ought to be.

FINDINGS WHEN HEAD IS NOT ENGAGED

1. The head may be high and freely movable.

2. The higher cephalic prominence—the sincipital—may be 7·6 cm. (three or more inches) above the brim.

3. The greater bulk of the head is above the brim.

There is no difficulty in diagnosing a non-engaged head that is high because it will be mobile. But the non-engaged head is not always high and movable: it may partly settle into the pelvic brim and be immobile although the parietal eminences have not passed through the brim.

The hydrocephalic head could mould during labour and partially enter the brim: it would not be mobile, but it could not engage. A duck's egg could partly enter an ordinary egg-cup; it would not be movable yet its largest presenting diameter could not pass through the rim of the egg-cup.

Method

The mobile head is most easily detected by using Pawlik's manœuvre (Fig. 89).

When the head is not mobile and the question of engagement is in doubt the midwife should make an attempt to find out whether the head will engage temporarily or not.

9

While grasping the head with the two hands, as in pelvic palpation, steady yet gentle pressure is applied in a downward, backward direction, keeping in mind the inclination of the plane of the pelvic inlet. If a feeling of " yield " or " give " is experienced the outlook is good. The left hand grip (p. 121) can also be used.

If doubt still exists the woman must be seen by a doctor.

CAUSES OF NON-ENGAGEMENT OF THE HEAD

1. **Failure of the lower uterine segment and lower birth canal to soften** and so allow the head to sink into the pelvis.

2. **Larger diameters of the deflexed head** which present in posterior positions of the vertex.

3. **Faulty assessment of period of gestation:** dates probably wrong.

4. **Cephalo-pelvic disproportion** due to contracted pelvis, large head, or a combination of both: brow presentation; hydrocephalus.

5. **Twins and hydramnios.**

6. **Full bladder.**—This cause ought not to exist: the woman should be required to empty her bladder prior to abdominal examination.

7. **Placenta prævia.**

8. **Tumours and ovarian cysts** are uncommon but significant causes.

AUSCULTATION

The fetal heart-sounds are heard over the area at which the fetal left scapula and ribs come in contact with the uterine wall. They should be listened for at every visit after the 20th week of pregnancy.

Fetal heart-sounds have been likened to the ticking of a watch under a pillow but the suggestion of the dull thud of a small motor is also helpful. Other sounds may be heard, such as fetal movement, intestinal rumbling, uterine and, rarely, funic souffle.

A rate of 120 to 140 is usual and the novice should count the mother's pulse rate for comparison. (*Confusion in rates is more likely in cases where the mother's heart-beat is rapid.*)

The Sonicaid or the Doptone, ultrasonic fetal pulse detectors, will pick up fetal blood flow (not the FH sounds) as early as the 10th week.

DIAGNOSTIC VALUE OF HEARING THE FETAL HEART

1. **A positive sign of pregnancy** not manifest until after the 20th week (see p. 71).

2. **Proof that the fetus is alive** (see p. 120).

3. **Corroboration in the diagnosis of presentation and position.**

Method

Pinard's stethoscope is commonly used and the hand should not touch it while listening, or extraneous sounds are produced. Closing the eyes is an aid to concentration. The ear must be in close, firm contact with the stethoscope and care taken that it is held at right angles to the point over which it is directed, otherwise the abdominal wall moves causing the stethoscope to slip sideways.

The area on the mother's abdomen on which the fetal heart is heard most clearly is known as the point of " maximal intensity " and the fetal stethoscope should

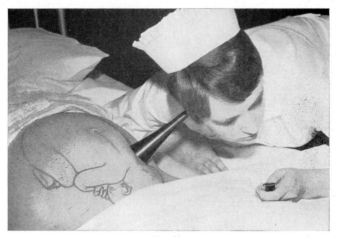

FIG. 91

Auscultation of the fetal heart. Vertex left occipito-anterior.

be moved about until that point is located. The point of maximal intensity varies according to fetal presentation and position, and is high or low depending on whether the fetal head is engaged or not. An experienced midwife having palpated the abdomen can usually place the stethoscope on the correct spot.

LOCATING THE FETAL HEART-SOUNDS

From the 20th to 28th week of pregnancy the fetal heart is heard most clearly in the midline well below the umbilicus.

From about the 30th week onwards

VERTEX L.O.A. POSITION

The heart-beat will be best heard at a point midway between the umbilicus and the left anterior superior iliac spine.

VERTEX L.O.L. POSITION

The heart-beat will be heard about 5·1 cm. (2 inches) further to the left than in the L.O.A.

VERTEX R.O.A. POSITION

The point of maximal intensity is on the right but nearer the midline than in an L.O.A. (*By placing the doll in the pelvis this can be demonstrated.*)

VERTEX R.O.P. POSITION

The heart-sounds will be heard in the mother's right flank and as the muscles there are thick the sounds may be muffled. Should the fetus be in the military attitude with the chest thrown forwards the fetal heart will be heard in the midline (through the fetal chest wall) and just below umbilical level, because the head will be high.

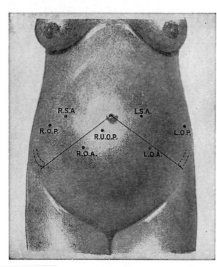

COMPLETE BREECH

The heart-sounds will be heard at or above the level of the umbilicus.

BREECH WITH EXTENDED LEGS

If the breech is engaged the heart-sounds will be lower than in the complete breech, and a mistaken diagnosis of vertex presentation is sometimes made.

FIG. 92

Showing the points of maximal intensity of the fetal heart-sounds in vertex and breech presentation.

The Uterine Souffle

This is a soft blowing sound which is synchronous with the maternal pulse, heard mainly on the lower lateral borders of the uterus where the large uterine vessels are (see p. 70).

The Funic Souffle

This high-pitched sound synchronous with the fetal heart-beat is believed to be caused by interference with the circulation in the umbilical cord. Occasionally it may be heard during the latter weeks of pregnancy or during labour, but in these instances the fetal heart is usually satisfactory. It will only be heard if the cord is in such a situation that the stethoscope can be placed directly over it.

IS THE FETUS ALIVE ?

The absence of fetal heart-sounds, or the woman not feeling fetal movement when previously having done so, is suspicious but not diagnostic of intra-uterine death. The mother need not be told, as it may be possible to hear the fetal heart one week later and if not medical aid should be sought. Cases are known in which the woman states that she feels fetal movement and the baby is subsequently born in a macerated condition. The movement experienced by the woman was probably due to the shifting of the dead fetus *en masse* that occurred when she altered her posture. *For causes and signs of intra-uterine death see Chapter* 34.

VAGINAL EXAMINATION

This is usually carried out at the 34th to 36th week in primigravidæ to determine pelvic size and shape (see diagonal conjugate, p. 104). Septate vagina, double uterus or other abnormality in the lower birth canal will also be detected if present.

CEPHALO-PELVIC DISPROPORTION

Disproportion means that the head is too big for the particular pelvis through which it must pass: there is a misfit. It is a relative term, and disproportion can be pelvic or cephalic in origin, due to a small pelvis, a large fetus or a combination of both. It cannot be diagnosed until the 36th week, because before then the fetal head is too small for comparison with the pelvis.

There are three degrees of disproportion:

MINOR DEGREE
The anterior parietal bone is level with the anterior border of the symphysis pubis

MODERATE DEGREE
The head slightly overlaps the anterior edge of the symphysis pubis.

MAJOR DEGREE
There is a pronounced bulge of head over the anterior edge of the symphysis pubis.

It is considered to be a fairly good working rule that if there is no disproportion at the 36th week the head will engage during labour, but this is not infallible so the patient should be seen every week to make sure.

The circumference of the head increases by about 2 mm. per week from the 36th to the 40th week, but this additional growth is compensated for during labour by head flexion, over-riding of the skull bones, good uterine contractions, as well as by the " give " of the pelvic joints.

It is not the duty of the midwife to determine the degree of disproportion but to obtain medical assistance when any condition exists which suggests disproportion between head and pelvis.

METHODS OF DETERMINING DISPROPORTION

1. BY PELVIC PALPATION.
2. LEFT HAND GRIP.
3. BY SITTING THE PATIENT UP.
4. CHASSAR MOIR'S METHOD.
5. MUNRO KERR'S METHOD.

1. BY PELVIC PALPATION
The head is grasped, as described for pelvic palpation (Fig. 87), and pressure exerted on it, in a downward and backward direction, remembering that the plane of the brim makes an angle of about 30 degrees with the bed. If a sense of " give " is experienced and there is no overlap, cephalo-pelvic disproportion is not present.

2. LEFT HAND GRIP
While facing the woman's feet, the left hand grasps the fetal head, the thumb being on the patient's right side, and when the head is pushed in a downward-backward direction " give " can be recognized. The first two fingers of the right hand assess any overlap at the symphysis pubis.

3. BY SITTING THE PATIENT UP
The midwife grasps the fetal head using her right hand as in Pawlik's manœuvre, with the ulnar border of that hand resting on the symphysis pubis. The woman is asked to sit up without assistance and to lean forwards for a short time. Her diaphragm and

abdominal muscles tend to press the fetus downwards, and sitting forwards enlarges the antero-posterior diameter of the pelvic brim.

The right hand, grasping the fetal head and resting on the symphysis pubis, acts as a brace directing the head into the pelvic inlet. As the woman lies down again, pressure may be applied to the fundus in a further endeavour to cause the head to engage temporarily. The right hand remains in position throughout the procedure and when no cephalo-pelvic disproportion exists no overlap is palpable.

If the head remains above the brim, the patient is referred to the doctor who will estimate the degree of disproportion.

4. CHASSAR MOIR'S METHOD

The midwife straightens her left arm until it is rigid and, using the ulnar border of her hand, presses the head in a downward and backward direction in the axis of the pelvic inlet. The first two fingers of the right hand are used to estimate the degree of overlap at the symphysis pubis.

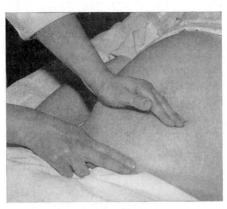

FIG. 93
CHASSAR MOIR'S METHOD OF DETERMINING THE DEGREE
OF OVERLAP.

5. MUNRO KERR'S METHOD

Munro Kerr's modification of Müller's method is employed by the doctor to determine the degree of disproportion when there is doubt as to whether vaginal delivery is possible. The patient is placed in the lithotomy position. Two fingers of the gloved hand are inserted into the vagina, with all antiseptic precautions. The other hand grasps the head abdominally and applies downward pressure to it, and the amount of descent is detected by the fingers in the vagina. The thumb of the hand in the vagina assesses the degree of overlap at the summit of the symphysis pubis.

FUTURE VISITS

To provide good prenatal care the woman should be seen frequently during the period of the possible onset of pre-eclampsia, the 20th to 30th week.

EVERY FOUR WEEKS until the 20th week⎫
EVERY TWO WEEKS until the 30th week ⎬ and more frequently if necessary.
EVERY WEEK until she is delivered ⎭

Under the General Practitioner Cooperation Scheme normal patients who attend the hospital prenatal clinic may be referred to their family doctor for routine care until the 34th week.

FOLLOW UP OF DEFAULTERS
At the Simpson Memorial Maternity Pavilion, Edinburgh

A letter is sent to each defaulter within 24 hours asking her to attend the clinic the following week or give reason for not being able to do so. If the letter is ignored a home visit is paid.

If the woman is a diabetic or has a cardiac or any other condition requiring close supervision and she fails to attend the clinic her family doctor is requested by telephone to visit her.

THE MIDWIFE'S RESPONSIBILITY

The domiciliary midwife should take responsibility for the examination of women, at the times stated above, for whose home confinement she is booked unless specifically told otherwise by the doctor in charge of the case. The welfare of the woman and her unborn child depends on close cooperation between family doctor, clinic and midwife.

Domiciliary midwives in Scotland are required to examine their patients fortnightly until the 32nd week and weekly thereafter, or more frequently if circumstances of the case so demand. The blood pressure should be taken and the urine examined at every visit and the findings recorded. (C.M.B.(Scot.) rule.)

Midwives must tell pregnant women of the importance of these frequent prenatal examinations, and persuade them to attend regularly.

QUESTIONS FOR REVISION

EXAMINATION OF THE PREGNANT WOMAN

As a midwife how would you conduct a physical examination ? What would you suspect from: (1) small stature, limp or deformity; (2) œdema of hands or face; (3) breathlessness on slight exertion.

ORAL QUESTIONS

How would you put a woman at ease in a busy clinic ?

Why is the woman weighed at each visit ?

Name the various blood tests ? Why are they carried out ?

What do you consider to be an abnormal rise in blood pressure ?

What reasons would you give a woman to encourage her to attend the prenatal clinic early and regularly ?

For what type of vaginal discharge would you seek medical aid ?

Which investigations are made at every visit ?

If pregnancy was in doubt what test would be made ?

Why should the bladder be empty prior to abdominal examination ?

What is the purpose of cervical cytology ?

What is the value of routine weighing and urine testing during the prenatal period ?

What can be learned from examination of: (1) the head; (2) the breasts; (3) the vulva; (4) the lower limbs.

Demonstrate how you would palpate the abdomen: (a) fundal; (b) lateral; (c) pelvic; (d) Pawlik's manœuvre; (e) for disproportion.

How would you diagnose: (a) vertex, L.O.A., R.O.P.; (b) an engaged head; (c) location of FH in R.O.A., L.O.P.; (d) well flexed head.

Differentiate between the diagnosis of: (a) twins and hydramnios; (b) vertex and breech presentation; (c) three degrees of disproportion.

WRITE NOT MORE THAN 10 LINES ON

(a) Asymptomatic bacteriuria; (b) internal pelvimetry; (c) glycosuria; (d) proteinuria; (e) auscultation; (f) causes of a high head in a primigravida at term.

STATE WHEN

(1) The head engages in a primigravid woman.

(2) A clean catch specimen of urine should reach the laboratory.

(3) Fetal heart is first heard with Pinard's stethoscope.

(4) Fundus reaches the (a) umbilicus; (b) xiphisternum.

(5) Disproportion can first be diagnosed.

(6) Internal pelvimetry is carried out.

(7) The patient is seen from 30-36 weeks.

(8) The patient is seen from 36-40 weeks.

What arrangements could a midwife make to teach " preparation for labour " ?

How would you encourage a pregnant woman to discuss her fears and to ask questions.

C.M.B.(Eng.) paper.—Enumerate the causes of non-engagement of the head in a primigravida 38 weeks pregnant. Discuss the possible investigations of this condition.

C.M.B.(Scot.) paper.—Enumerate the causes of undue enlargement of the uterus in pregnancy. Discuss the possible dangers associated with the conditions mentioned.

C.M.B.(N. Ireland) paper.—A patient is found to have a girth of 40 inches at the 34th week of pregnancy. Discuss the possible causes.

C.M.B.(Scot.) paper.—What is meant by " engagement " of the fetal head ? In what circumstances may this be delayed ? What possible dangers to mother and child may such delay indicate ?

C.M.B.(Eng.) paper.—Describe your antenatal examination of a primigravida at 36 weeks. To what points would you pay particular attention at this stage in pregnancy ?

C.M.B.(Scot.) paper.—Give the causes of non-engagement of the fetal head at term. How may these causes influence labour ?

C.M.B.(Eng.) paper.—Describe the examination of the abdomen of a pregnant woman at term. What may be the significance of the findings ?

C.M.B.(Eng.) paper.—At what intervals should a pregnant woman be examined? What special observations should be made in the last month of pregnancy and what advice may be needed ?

C.M.B.(Eng.) paper.—Give a list of the common disorders that may be revealed during antenatal care. What advice would you give to prevent any three of these becoming major disorders ?

C.M.B.(N. Ireland) paper.—Protein is found in the urine at the 32nd week of pregnancy. What may be the cause of this and what investigations should be made ?

C.M.B.(N. Ireland) paper.—What particular points would be noted on an antenatal visit at the thirty-sixth week of pregnancy ?

C.M.B.(Eng.) paper.—What complications of child bearing may a patient avoid by attending an antenatal clinic at regular intervals ?

C.M.B.(Eng.) paper.—At the 36th week a primigravida is found to have a vertex presentation which is not engaged. Discuss the possible causes and the investigations which should be made.

C.M.B.(Eng.) paper.—What abnormal constituents of the urine may be found in pregnancy ? What may be their significance ?

C.M.B.(Eng.) paper.—At what intervals should a pregnant woman be examined ? To what particular points would you pay attention during the last month of pregnancy ?

C.M.B.(Scot.) paper.—Give an account of the causes of weight gain in pregnancy.

C.M.B.(Scot.) paper.—Discuss the value of the examination of urine during pregnancy and labour.

C.M.B.(Scot.) paper.—Discuss the value of hæmoglobin estimation in pregnancy and labour.

C.M.B.(N. Ireland) paper.—What information may be obtained from examination of the patient's blood during pregnancy ? Describe the management of one abnormality which may be detected.

C.M.B.(Eng.) paper.—50 word question.—Engagement of the fetal head.

C.M.B.(Eng.) paper.—What blood tests should be carried out during pregnancy and what is their purpose ?

C.M.B.(Eng.) paper. 50 word question.—Maternal hæmoglobin levels in pregnancy.

8

Advice to the Pregnant Woman

A woman pregnant for the first time has much to learn, and is usually eager and willing to do what is best for her baby. Advice may be given to individual women or to groups, and should be presented in a simple attractive manner, the matter being sound as well as practical.

Expectant mothers should be encouraged to ask questions and to discuss obstetric or parentcraft subjects regarding which they are in doubt or worried.

HYGIENE OF THE PREGNANT WOMAN

FRESH AIR: SUNSHINE.	**CLOTHING.**	**BATHING.**
EXERCISE: RECREATION.	**BOWELS.**	**SMOKING.**
REST: SLEEP.	**TEETH.**	**MARITAL RELATIONS.**
RELAXATION.	**BREASTS.**	**DIET** (*see Nutrition, p.* 63).

FRESH AIR AND SUNSHINE

The pregnant woman should be **advised to spend two hours a day in the fresh air,** if possible away from busy streets and preferably walking or sitting in the garden or

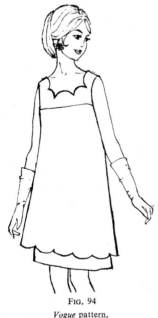

park. If reminded that baby needs a daily airing before birth as well as after, she will be more likely to go out when she might not otherwise do so.

EXERCISE AND RECREATION

Exercise **out-of-doors is, of course, ideal,** and pregnant women need to be encouraged to continue with such out-door recreation as they have been accustomed to, so long as it does not cause jolting, as would occur with riding or tennis.

Games should not be strenuous, nor should they be carried to the stage of exhaustion. A good brisk walk is excellent. It provides a change of scene, stimulates the circulation, and gives a feeling of well-being besides whetting the appetite, aiding elimination and inducing sleep. During the later months the woman's activities will be curtailed to some extent by her ungainliness, so that she is unlikely to indulge in any harmful pursuit. Housework, such as making beds, sweeping and polishing brings many, but not all, muscles into play, so exercises have been devised to keep the muscles to be used during labour in good trim and the pelvic joints flexible. At some clinics, classes are held where keep fit exercises are practised and the women shown how to maintain good posture.

Fig. 94
Vogue pattern.

126

The pregnant woman should not lift heavy weights, as this may predispose to abortion in susceptible cases. Constant standing may aggravate any predisposition to varicose veins. The woman should not climb to reach high shelves, because of the likelihood of over-balancing and her tendency to faint.

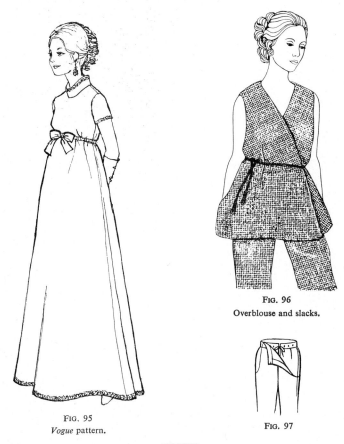

FIG. 95
Vogue pattern.

FIG. 96
Overblouse and slacks.

FIG. 97

TRAVEL

The advice of the midwife may be sought as to whether a long rail or car journey should be undertaken. The woman should be warned that during the first three months the jarring and the excitement may induce abortion; the possibility of premature labour should be mentioned.

The majority of international airlines do not permit pregnant women to fly after the 32nd week. After the 28th week a statement of fitness to fly must be obtained from the woman's doctor.

REST AND SLEEP

During the second half of pregnancy the expectant mother is carrying a constant load, which increases to 10·8 kg. (24 lb.) or more, and towards the end of the day she becomes fatigued and her legs may ache. She should be advised to have short rests with her feet up throughout the day, and to lie down and relax or sleep for one or two hours during the afternoon. This is not always easy where there is a family to be looked after, but, if overworked, she will only become exhausted and irritable.

At least nine hours sleep should be obtained every night, and some women need more than that. The minor disorders and the petty frustrations of life are felt more acutely at this time, and nervous exhaustion should be avoided at all costs. Sleep is the great restorer. The gentle tiredness induced by outdoor recreation, a warm bath and a glass of hot milk are natural sedatives.

The weight of the uterus may create discomfort and sleeplessness, but a small pillow tucked under the abdomen when lying on the side usually gives relief.

Near term, sleep may be disturbed by false pains, and, if persistent, it may be necessary to see the doctor so that a sedative can be prescribed.

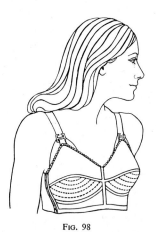

FIG. 98

Maternity Bra. Broad shoulder straps, lower half of cups reinforced. Deep lower border.

RELAXATION

The ability to relax at will is of inestimable value, both during pregnancy and labour: if a woman can relax completely she will obtain more benefit from her rest periods. By conserving nervous energy she will be able to keep calm in times of stress, and sleep will be more easily induced; all of which will be invaluable during labour.

SUITABLE CLOTHES

These are a necessity, not a luxury, and their psychological value should not be underestimated. When dressed in comfortable, becoming, maternity garments, the woman has a feeling of assurance that combats her inclination to be self-conscious about her figure. She can be just as feminine and elegant as at any other time and there is no reason why she should not enjoy a normal social life throughout the whole of pregnancy, as long as it does not interfere with rest and sleep.

It is essential that the expectant mother goes out every day for fresh air and change of environment, so she ought to have clothes to wear in which she feels inconspicuous and happy.

An uplifting brassière, reinforced on its under-surface and with broad shoulder straps, should be worn as early as the 12th week because of the enlargement of the breasts, which may increase the bust measurement by as much as 7·6 to 10·2 cm. (3 to 4 inches). The brassière ought not to be tight enough to depress the nipples.

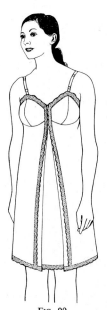

FIG. 99

A maternity belt need not be worn until after the 20th week and, although many primigravidæ have good abdominal muscles and do not require support, they appreciate the comfort of a maternity roll-on during the last twelve weeks. Tight corsets are harmful and must not be worn.

Multigravid women frequently have lax abdominal muscles which allow the uterus to lean forwards. The shoulders have then to be held back to counteract the anterior obliquity, so the lumbar curve of the spine is increased, giving rise to backache and fatigue which could be eliminated by wearing an adjustable supporting belt or corset. Women should be advised not to wear constricting bands on the legs; they impede the venous circulation and increase any susceptibility to varicose veins and œdema.

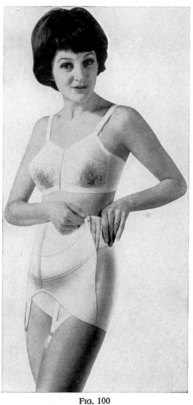

FIG. 100
Camp maternity belt No. 3030.

Sensible shoes should be worn, with a 4·4 cm. (1¾-inch) heel having a broad base. Narrow high heels cause fatigue in maintaining good posture, and increase the likelihood of stumbling or overbalancing which is common in pregnancy. If the foot muscles are in poor tone, the additional weight during pregnancy may strain the muscles supporting the arches and cause pain.

THE BOWELS

The bowels should move every day without having to resort to laxatives. Simple wholesome remedies, such as a glass of warm water on rising in the morning and the regular habit of defæcation after breakfast will often help matters. Adequate fluid should be taken between meals, and drinking two glasses of water daily, either plain or flavoured with orange juice, may promote bowel action. Strong tea is better avoided because of the constipating effect of tannin. Plenty of roughage ought to be included in the diet, and wholemeal bread, fruit, vegetables, prunes, raisins and figs are excellent for the purpose.

CARE OF THE TEETH

It was previously believed that the withdrawal of calcium from the mother's teeth occurred because of the fetal demands for calcium, but it is from the mother's bones and not her teeth that calcium is withdrawn during pregnancy. For tooth extraction a local anæsthetic is administered to avoid cyanosis. (**Dental treatment in Gt. Britain is free during pregnancy.**)

Care of the breasts is discussed under lactation (p. 508).

BATHING

The skin is an excretory organ which should be kept active during pregnancy. A daily tub-bath or shower is ideal, but hot baths are exhausting and may cause fainting. Unless the patient is very vigorous and accustomed to sea-bathing, it is better that she should not indulge in it round the shores of Great Britain where the water is very cold.

SMOKING

The welfare of the unborn child may be an effective inducement in persuading women to break the habit or curtail the daily number of cigarettes. Unfortunately many heavy smokers prefer cigarettes to food and as a result are thin and malnourished. It has been found that nicotine passes through the placenta and diminishes the weight of the fetus by about 227 G. (8 ounces). As few as 5 per day will affect fetal growth.

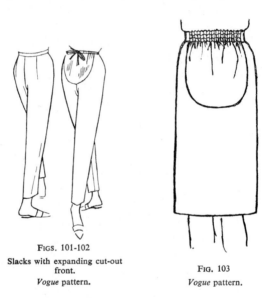

FIGS. 101-102
Slacks with expanding cut-out front.
Vogue pattern.

FIG. 103
Vogue pattern.

MARITAL RELATIONS

In women who have a history of abortion, coitus should be prohibited during the early months of pregnancy.

WARNING WITHOUT FRIGHTENING

It is necessary to tell pregnant women to report any unusual symptoms promptly because, if treated in the early stages, a major complication may be averted. This should be done in a matter-of-fact, almost casual, manner without giving the impression that their occurrence is anticipated. The woman should be told to go to her doctor or midwife if she thinks things are not quite right, or to send for her doctor if she feels ill or has any **vaginal bleeding, swelling of her face or hands, or severe headache.** It would not be wise to mention too many possible danger signals.

THE MINOR DISORDERS OF PREGNANCY

MORNING SICKNESS.	**BACKACHE.**	**ITCHING OF THE SKIN.**
HEARTBURN.	**VARICOSE VEINS.**	**FAINTING.**
CONSTIPATION.	**HÆMORRHOIDS.**	

Although the minor disorders do not endanger life, they must not be ignored or treated lightly, for by interfering with nutrition, sleep and outdoor recreation they may undermine the woman's health. They can make life very miserable and often distress the woman far more than the more serious disorders of pregnancy. The midwife should ensure that women do not accept the minor disorders as an inevitable accompaniment of pregnancy and she should endeavour to cure or alleviate them.

MORNING SICKNESS

About 50 per cent of pregnant women vomit between the 4th and the 14th week of pregnancy. It usually occurs immediately after getting up in the morning, and at this time retching and the vomiting of mucus, sometimes bile-stained, takes place. The sickness is usually accompanied by nausea which may persist throughout the day and impairs the appetite. If the vomiting of food continues, the mother's nutrition suffers. The condition should never be ignored, for if " nipped in the bud " the serious complication of hyperemesis gravidarum would seldom occur.

The vomiting may be endocrine in origin. It is more common in women who have a " sensitive " nervous system, but there appears to be some disturbance in the metabolism of glucose with increased production of ketone bodies. The ensuing ketosis causes vomiting and this is likely to occur when the intake of glucose is low, as occurs during the night. Some authorities believe that the sudden assumption of the upright position plays a part.

Treatment

To maintain the glycogen supply, a light sweet meal should be eaten before retiring: a glass of milk and biscuits would be suitable. Extra sugar should be taken, and it may be expedient to prescribe some specific product, *e.g.* barley sugar, or treacle. Foods with a high fat content, like butter, cream, pastries and those that are fried ought to be restricted.

The woman should have a cup of tea and toast with marmalade-jelly or a biscuit before getting up in the morning, and although a thermos flask could be utilized it seems to be more efficacious if freshly made tea is brought to her, preferably by the husband. After lying still for half an hour, the woman should dress slowly and breakfast can usually then be taken and retained. Nausea may be extremely troublesome, and the avoidance of hunger by having some easily digested food every two hours may help. The odour of cooking can induce nausea and in persistent cases it might be advisable to make arrangements for the woman to get away from this for a few days.

It is important that the woman should eat food, and a savoury may tempt the appetite when sweet foods are refused. Vomiting may deplete the blood chlorides and reduce the intake of vitamin B_1, so Marmite, which is usually acceptable will help to replace both. An adequate fluid intake is essential and in mild cases treated at home the woman should be told to report if her urine is dark in colour. Constipation results because of dehydration and the lack of food.

WARNING REGARDING DRUGS

Pregnant women should be warned regarding taking drugs for morning sickness unless prescribed by the doctor. The embryo is at risk during the first 12 weeks.

HEARTBURN

This is probably the most usual and the most intractable minor disorder of pregnancy, particularly during the last 12 weeks, because the enlarged uterus displaces the stomach upwards. At night, when the recumbent position is adopted, it is likely to be troublesome. The burning sensation is due to irritation caused by the reflux of gastric juice into the œsophagus. The cardiac sphincter of the stomach is relaxed and this may be due to the action of progesterone. The idea that heartburn is due to an excess of acid in the stomach is not valid, for gastric analyses have shown that in the majority of cases hypochlorhydria rather than hyperchlorhydria exists.

Treatment

Greasy, highly seasoned, or indigestible foods should be eliminated from the diet.

Raising the head of the bed 22·9 cm. (9 inches) and an extra pillow may help. No infallible cure exists, although many simple remedies seem to give relief. Sips of milk or hot water, peppermint, liquorice and the proprietary alkaline lozenges are reputed to be efficacious.

A teaspoonful (5 ml.) of Aludrox or milk of magnesia may be beneficial, also Nulacin; and 4 ml. of magnesium trisilicate is sometimes prescribed in stubborn cases. The practice of ingesting repeated doses of sodium bicarbonate is neither rational nor advisable: it inhibits digestion, causes flatulence, hinders the absorption of vitamin B, and in some women may produce œdema.

CONSTIPATION

There is a tendency to constipation during pregnancy which may be due to the relaxing effect of progesterone, on the muscle coat of the intestine, diminishing peristalsis. The pressure of the enlarged uterus may also play some part. Drugs will have to be resorted to if diet is not sufficient to treat the condition; Senokot. Dulcolax or any mild vegetable laxative being suitable.

BACKACHE

Slight backache may be due to faulty posture and is more common in tired multigravid patients whose muscle tone is poor. Lax abdominal muscles produce anterior obliquity of the uterus and this causes the woman to hold her shoulders too far back in order to support the uterus and to keep her balance. The increased lumbar curve amounts to lordosis and gives rise to strain of the muscles of the back, resulting in fatigue and backache.

A firm supporting maternity corset and a reasonable amount of rest are needed. Good posture, sensible shoes and a comfortable bed that does not sag will do much to prevent backache.

Sacro-iliac strain may be troublesome during the last months when the uterus is heavy and the joints are relaxed, and it may be necessary to provide firm support in the sacro-iliac region. Backache is, of course, one of the early signs of labour.

If backache is severe and persistent medical advice must be sought.

VARICOSE VEINS

The tendency to varicose veins is increased during pregnancy, and about 10 per cent of pregnant women are found to have varicosities of the legs in greater or lesser degree. The relaxing effect of progesterone on plain muscle may account for the lack of tone in the walls of the veins, causing them to dilate; the venous return from the lower limbs is impeded in the common iliac veins by the increased flow of blood from the uterus.

The woman complains of a dull aching pain in her limbs, and the superficial veins are often seen to be in a state of engorgement. The limbs may be œdematous in severe cases.

Medical advice must be obtained when varicose veins are troublesome or serious.

Injury may lead to hæmorrhage or to ulceration of the skin, but the most vital risk is that varicose veins predispose to vein thrombosis.

Varicose veins tend to subside after parturition, but frequently recur, and are aggravated by each succeeding pregnancy.

Treatment

No tight bands that would impede the circulation of the lower limbs should be worn. The woman is advised to avoid long periods of standing and when reading or knitting to sit with her feet raised as high as possible; the ankle joints should be moved freely while sitting.

If the aching causes her to be disinclined for walking out of doors, she should be advised to lie down for an hour, with her feet higher than her head, to relieve the congestion and the pain before going out. The wearing of an elastic stocking or crepe bandage supports the column of blood, relieves the aching and gives considerable comfort.

The bandage should be applied from well below the varicose veins and always removed during the night. Before putting on the bandage or stocking, the legs should be elevated at right angles to the body for a few moments previous to getting out of bed in the morning. In serious cases absolute rest in bed, the foot of which is raised, may be necessary.

VARICOSE VEINS OF THE VULVA

They can be very painful and if so the doctor may inject them but, as a rule, wearing a firmly applied perineal pad for support, and resting with the hips raised, give relief. In serious cases they might rupture during delivery of the baby.

HÆMORRHOIDS

External hæmorrhoids are varicose veins on the anal margin. The avoidance of constipation and the application of some soothing, hæmorrhoidal ointment are sufficient in mild cases; suppositories, e.g. Anusol, are frequently prescribed. Cold compresses may be tried and in some instances a warm sitz bath, to which magnesium sulphate crystals have been added, will reduce the engorgement. The hæmorrhoids should then be lubricated and an attempt made to replace them gently.

ITCHING OF THE SKIN

The stretching of the skin of the abdomen and breasts may give rise to intense itching, but occasionally the itching is generalized over the whole body (scabies, of course, should be kept in mind and can usually be diagnosed). The cause is not understood and may be endocrine, toxic, or due to some nervous element. Simple remedies, such as the application of lanoline or cold cream, can be tried. Soothing substances, such as calamine lotion or concentrated sodium bicarbonate solution, can be dabbed on, but sodium bicarbonate is drying when used repeatedly. The clothing worn next to the skin should be non-irritating; water should be taken freely and the bowels kept open.

PRURITUS VULVÆ

Itching of the vulva may be very distressing. If due to irritation from vaginal discharge or lack of cleanliness, the remedy is soap and water. It may be due to glycosuria and, if so, further investigation is necessary to rule out diabetes. *Vaginal thrush* gives rise to intense itching of vagina and vulva, accompanied by a white flaky discharge (see p. 204). The application of Nystatin ointment is helpful.

FAINTING

This is a frequent source of anxiety to the patient and her relatives, but if cardiac impairment is absent she can be assured that the condition is not serious. Fainting in pregnancy is thought to be due to the instability of the vaso-motor centre in the medulla which controls arterial tone, and if a rapid fall in blood pressure takes place the woman faints. It may also be due to pressure of the uterus on the inferior vena cava (see supine hypotensive syndrome, p. 60).

Sudden changes in posture, as from the recumbent to the upright, or standing for long periods, particularly in hot weather, may cause fainting. Fatigue or excitement may instigate an attack, as well as stuffy rooms or crowded halls. Tight corsets should not be worn and meals that overload the stomach or cause flatulence should be avoided.

WHEN THE WOMAN'S COMPLAINTS SUGGEST MORE THAN A MINOR DISORDER SHE MUST BE REFERRED TO THE DOCTOR.

QUESTIONS FOR REVISION

ORAL QUESTIONS

If a pregnant woman sought your advice on the following matters what reasons would you give to convince her:

1. (a) Entering a strenuous sports contest; (b) travelling by air.
2. The amount of rest and sleep needed during pregnancy.
3. The benefit of attending relaxation classes.
4. How to treat (a) morning sickness; (b) heartburn.
5. (a) Excessive aching in her legs; (b) backache.
6. Is fainting a sign of heart disease ?
7. How to apply a crepe bandage for varicose veins.

Why should a pregnant woman (a) have a daily walk out of doors ? (b) curtail the daily number of cigarettes ? (c) be told to report any vaginal bleeding ?

Write not more than 10 lines on the value of:
(a) Weighing the pregnant woman. (b) Taking blood tests in pregnancy.
(c) Obtaining a clean catch specimen of urine.
(d) Taking the blood pressure. (e) Examining the lower limbs.

C.M.B.(Eng.) paper.—Mention some of the commoner minor disabilities of pregnancy and the advice you would give for their relief. What would make you decide to advise medical aid ?

C.M.B.(Scot.) paper.—What advice would you give a primigravid woman in regard to (a) diet; (b) clothing; (c) exercise; (d) care of the breasts ?

C.M.B.(N. Ireland) paper.—Discuss the treatment of vomiting in early pregnancy. What clinical findings show that the patient is seriously affected by the vomiting ?

C.M.B.(Scot.) paper.—What advice and guidance would you give to a young primigravida at her first attendance at an antenatal clinic ?

C.M.B.(Eng.) paper.—What advice would you give if your patient complained during pregnancy of (a) morning sickness ? (b) constipation ? (c) heartburn ?

C.M.B.(Scot.) paper.—What advice would you give a patient about her mode of life during pregnancy ? State briefly how antenatal care may help to avoid difficulties in labour.

C.M.B.(Eng.) paper.—What instructions should be given to the patient during the antenatal period which would help her during her pregnancy and labour ?

C.M.B.(Eng.) paper. 50 word question.—What are the risks to mother and child of smoking during pregnancy ?

9

Conditions associated with Bleeding in Early Pregnancy

All vaginal bleeding during the prenatal period should be reported to the doctor, for prompt treatment will often save the pregnancy and prevent serious loss of blood. The midwife should instruct her patients to report any bleeding, however slight, but such advice should be given in a matter-of-fact way, without creating the impression that bleeding is anticipated.

CAUSES

1. IMPLANTATION BLEEDING	4. ECTOPIC GESTATION
2. CERVICAL LESIONS	5. HYDATIDIFORM MOLE
3. ABORTION	

1. IMPLANTATION BLEEDING

Slight vaginal bleeding may occur when the trophoblast erodes the endometrium during the process of embedding. This may simulate the menstrual period that would be anticipated at about this time and if the implantation bleeding is erroneously thought to be a menstrual period calculation of the expected date of delivery will be incorrect.

2. CERVICAL LESIONS

(a) EROSION

This may produce a slight blood-stained mucoid discharge; treatment is seldom required during pregnancy.

(b) MUCOUS POLYPUS

This is a tiny growth, rather like a small cherry with a short stalk. It can be very readily snipped or twisted off.

(c) CARCINOMA OF THE CERVIX

This is a rare but very serious condition, which is dealt with in Appendix I.

3. ABORTION

The commonest cause of bleeding in early pregnancy is abortion, which can be defined as " *the interruption of pregnancy before the 28th week of gestation,*" after which period the fetus is viable (*capable of living a separate existence*).

FREQUENCY

It is believed that about 15 per cent of pregnancies terminate in abortion, and this occurs more frequently in multigravid women; the majority take place during the second month and relatively few after the third month.

Abortions can be divided into two main groups: **spontaneous** and **induced**. Further sub-divisions are tabulated below:

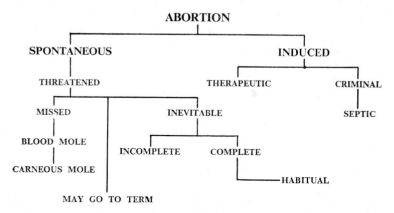

CAUSES

Abortion may be due to a combination of factors, particularly conditions that interfere with the embedding, development or nutrition of the embryo ; chromosomal anomalies have been found in 30 per cent of first trimester spontaneous abortions. In 60 per cent of cases no cause is found.

FETAL CAUSES

Maldevelopment or disease of the fertilized ovum, and in 30 to 40 per cent of early abortions the embryo is found to be malformed.

The normal development of the embryo may be affected by anoxia resulting from separation of and damage to the placenta.

MATERNAL CAUSES

1. *General Conditions*

(*a*) **Infections.**—Acute febrile conditions such as influenza may cause death of the fetus.

(*b*) **Disease such as chronic nephritis.**

(*c*) **Effect of Drugs.**—Drugs such as phosphorus cause necrosis of the decidua; lead affects the placenta; quinine and ergot are ecbolic in action. The large doses necessary to induce abortion are poisonous.

(*d*) **Extreme Emotion,** such as fright or grief, in susceptible women.

(*e*) **Endocrine Dysfunction.** No convincing proof. (Progesterone deficiency is the secondary effect of feto-placental damage, not the cause.)

2. *Local Conditions*

(*a*) **Implontation of the ovum in the lower uterine segment.**

10A

(*b*) **Trauma.**—Criminal interference; accidents; violent exercise; stimulation of the uterus such as might be due to some necessary abdominal operation.

(*c*) **Incompetent cervix** (see p. 143).   (*d*) **Uterine malformations;** fibroid tumours.

SIGNS AND SYMPTOMS

1. **Vaginal bleeding** is the earliest sign and is due to partial detachment of the embedded ovum.

2. **Pain,** which is usually felt low in the abdomen, intermittent in character and often accompanied by backache, is due to uterine contractions.   They are miniature labour pains.

3. **Dilatation of the os** is present when the abortion is inevitable.

THREATENED ABORTION

Threatened abortion is one in which the disturbance is so slight that it is possible for the pregnancy to continue to term. **Bleeding is not severe.** Backache may be present, the **Os is closed** and the **Membranes intact.** Very occasionally, intermittent pain is felt low in the abdomen.

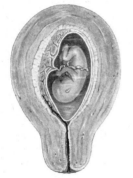

Fig. 104

THREATENED ABORTION.

Slight placental separation: slight bleeding: membranes intact: os closed.

Possibilities in the Outcome of a Threatened Abortion

1. **The pregnancy goes to term** if the signs and symptoms subside.

2. **The abortion becomes inevitable** when free bleeding continues, and painful uterine contractions are present.

3. **Missed abortion** occurs when the fetus **dies** and is retained *in utero* (p. 143).

TREATMENT OF THREATENED ABORTION

(*a*) **The patient is put to bed,** reassured, and kept quiet.

(*b*) **Medical assistance** is obtained. (C.M.B rule.)

(*c*) **All vaginal discharge, pads, stained clothing and linen are kept** for the doctor's inspection. (The relatives should be instructed to save everything passed vaginally during the midwife's absence.)

(*d*) **Vulval swabbing is carried out twice daily** while the brownish discharge persists.

(*e*) **Sedatives are usually ordered.**

Panasorb, tabs 2, for slight pain.

Pethidine, 100 mg. or D.F. 118 dihydrocodeine tartrate, 30-60 mg., if pain is troublesome or promazine (Sparine) 25 mg.   Amylobarbitone sodium (Sod. Amytal) 200 mg. may be ordered for night sedation.

(*f*) **Vaginal and cervical smears** may be taken to determine prognosis and treatment, but some think that hormonal deficiency reflects failure of the pregnancy rather than causing this.

(*g*) **A pregnancy test** may be ordered, and, if negative, it is probable that the fetus is dead. The Sonicaid (ultrasound) will detect fetal vascular pulsation at 10 to 12 weeks gestation.

(*h*) **Purgatives and enemata** should not be given in case the uterus be reflexly stimulated to contract. If constipation exists, the doctor may order small doses of a mild aperient: suppositories may be employed. It has been suggested that 48 hours should elapse before any attempt is made to stimulate the bowel actively.

(*i*) **The pulse and temperature** are taken and recorded twice daily in non-febrile cases; otherwise every four hours.

(*j*) **Physical and mental rest is considered advisable** and to ensure this the patient is kept in bed until 48 hours after bright red bleeding has ceased. (*Some do not believe that rest in bed will prevent abortion.*)

(*k*) **A speculum examination is made** to exclude cervical lesions. The opportunity is taken to detect early cancer by taking a Papanicolaou smear (see Appendix I).

(*l*) **Diet.**—A diet rich in proteins, with supplementary iron and vitamin C, is given.

(*m*) **Advice on discharge.**—The patient is advised to take extra rest, to restrict her activities within reasonable limits and to avoid heavy lifting, strenuous exercise, fatigue and excitement. Coitus is contra-indicated for 2 or 3 weeks. She should go to bed immediately, if bleeding starts again, and call her doctor.

INEVITABLE ABORTION

In this case it is not possible for the pregnancy to continue.

Free bleeding usually means that a considerable part of the placenta has become detached.

Intermittent uterine contractions, accompanied by pain, constitute a reliable sign.

If the membranes rupture and the **ovum protrudes** through the dilating os, abortion must take place.

Treatment

The midwife should treat an inevitable abortion as " threatened," until the arrival of the doctor, unless the bleeding is severe when she should give ergometrine 0·5 mg. or Syntometrine 1 ml. intramuscularly. Everything passed vaginally is kept for the doctor's inspection. Pethidine 100 mg. is given for pain.

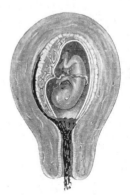

Fig. 105

INEVITABLE ABORTION.

Placental separation: moderate bleeding: membranes ruptured: os dilated.

In hospital an oxytocin drip is usually given, especially after the 16th week. If not successful, the uterus is evacuated digitally, aided by the use of swab-holding forceps, under general anæsthesia. Some consider it advisable to explore the uterus in all cases, unless the abortion appears to be complete, to ensure that no placental tissue has been retained. *Preparation for evacuation of the uterus* is described on page 142. Ergometrine, 0·5 mg., is usually administered when the evacuation is completed.

COMPLETE ABORTION

Before the 8th week an abortion is more likely to be complete because the feta sac is expelled intact. When an abortion is complete, **bleeding is reduced to a mere staining, pain ceases, the cervix closes** and involution of the uterus takes place.

After the 20th week milk may come into the breasts; if so, a firm uplift binder should be applied.

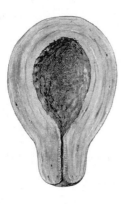

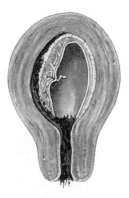

FIG. 106

COMPLETE ABORTION.

Fetus and placenta expelled: bleeding scanty: os closed.

FIG. 107

INCOMPLETE ABORTION.

Fetus expelled: placenta partially separated: free bleeding: os dilated.

INCOMPLETE ABORTION

The fetus has been expelled, but the whole or part of the placenta and membranes has been retained *in utero*. The patient is usually more than 12 weeks' pregnant because then the placenta is firmly embedded and the slender cord breaks.

Lochia continue and bleeding may be profuse.

Pain may or may not be present.

The os partly closes, but not completely; the cervix is patulous.

Involution does not take place.

Treatment of Hæmorrhage by Midwife on District

The midwife must immediately send for the doctor (C.M.B. rule).

ADMINISTRATION OF ERGOMETRINE

If medical aid is not readily available the midwife should give Syntometrine, 1 ml., or ergometrine, 0·5 mg., intramuscularly: this can be repeated in 10 minutes or even in 5 minutes if hæmorrhage is profuse, but the second dose is seldom necessary.

If bleeding is profuse the midwife should send for the " flying squad " who will deal with the emergency.

Resuscitative measures are always employed prior to removing the patient by ambulance. A blood transfusion, to which 5 to 10 units oxytocin are added, will probably be given.

Subjecting a shocked or exsanguinated woman to an ambulance journey may be the cause of her death. The midwife will, of course, accompany her patient to hospital and report on treatment and drugs administered.

WHEN NO MEDICAL AID IS AVAILABLE

In desperate cases when bleeding endangers life and the home is in a remote area the midwife will have to cope with the situation alone.

A second dose of Syntometrine or ergometrine is given as mentioned on page 140.

Retained products must be removed as bleeding will continue otherwise, so hands and vulva must be cleansed quickly: antiseptic obstetric cream is applied to the gloved right hand.

With her left hand on the abdomen the midwife will antevert and press the uterus downwards. With the right index finger the retained products are removed.

PACKING MAY BE NECESSARY IN REMOTE AREAS

Packing could be condemned as an out-of-date measure and if the uterus has been evacuated properly it should not be necessary but it may be the only means of controlling severe hæmorrhage in the absence of medical aid in remote areas.

A pack made of 91·4 cm. (36 inch) folded gauze. Six perineal pads smeared with obstetric cream could be used. The number inserted must be recorded to ensure their entire removal.

The bladder should always be emptied before inserting a vaginal pack.

With the patient in Sims' left lateral position and the fingers of the left hand used as a perineal retractor the fornices are packed firmly and the vagina tightly filled until the pack protrudes at the vulva. A perineal pad applied firmly will increase the pressure. The pack should be removed within six hours.

To treat shock the foot of the bed is raised and 300 ml. of tap water given rectally.

TREATMENT IN HOSPITAL

If the patient is not suffering from the effect of blood loss Syntometrine, 1 ml., or ergometrine, 0·5 mg., is given intramuscularly; the blood is typed and hæmoglobin estimated; a high vaginal swab is taken. The uterus is evacuated vaginally. The woman may be discharged 24 hours later if there are no reasons for further treatment.

WOMAN COLLAPSED FROM LOSS OF BLOOD

She is received into a warm bed, the foot of which is then elevated. Ergometrine 0·5 mg. is given intravenously. While waiting for cross-matched blood, dextrose 5 per cent with Ringers lactate solution is given to combat circulatory failure; Syntocinon 10 units may be added to the dextrose drip or to the blood transfusion.

The pulse is taken and recorded every 5 minutes, the blood pressure every 15 or 30 minutes. The central venous pressure is monitored.

When the patient's condition is satisfactory the uterus is evacuated under general anæsthesia. Pentothal may be adequate. To ensure against further hæmorrhage, a gauze pack may be inserted into the uterus; the remainder fills the vagina, thus

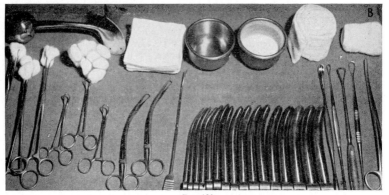

Fig. 108

INSTRUMENTS FOR EVACUATION OF UTERUS.
(*Simpson Memorial Maternity Pavilion, Edinburgh.*)

Prepacked

INSTRUMENTS	LINEN: DRESSINGS
3 Swab holding forceps.	Gowns, caps, masks.
3 Towel clips.	2 Leggings.
1 Auvards speculum.	2 Towels.
2 Volsellum forceps.	10 Gauze swabs (2 bundles of 5).
1 Uterine sound.	20 Wool swabs.
1 Set cervical dilators.	1 Vaginal pack, 1·3 m. (1½ yard)
1 Spoon curette.	long ×91 cm.
3 Loop curettes.	2 Gallipots.

MISCELLANEOUS EQUIPMENT

Prepacked disposable gloves.	Drugs:
Prepacked latex catheter	Ergometrine and Syntometrine.
Kidney basin for urine	Pitocin or Syntocinon.
Extra packs of swabs.	Methedrine, Nikethamide.
Extra vaginal pack.	Hydrocortisone.
Tray with syringes and needles.	Hibitane Cream.

Central venous pressure manometer, fluid to combat circulatory failure e.g. 5 per cent Dextrose and Ringers lactate: Cross-matched blood.

stimulating good uterine contractions. Syntometrine, 1 ml., or ergometrine, 0·5 mg., is given intramuscularly. Pulse and blood pressure are recorded every half hour until satisfactory—temperature 4 hourly. The pack is removed in 6 hours. Anæmia if present is dealt with.

The woman is discharged, if her condition warrants this, on the 4th or 5th day after evacuation.

HABITUAL OR RECURRENT ABORTION

When a woman has had three consecutive spontaneous abortions, the term " habitual abortion " is used. The cause is obscure in many cases.

A very thorough investigation is carried out between pregnancies, to exclude diseases such as diabetes, nephritis, hypothyroidism. A pelvic examination is made to diagnose uterine abnormalities, displacements or fibroids. Cervical erosion, laceration, incompetence or infection are dealt with, if present.

MANAGEMENT

Husband and wife are both advised to take a well balanced diet, especially proteins, minerals and vitamins (see p. 63), and another pregnancy may be started as soon as the woman is in good health. She reports to the clinic when she thinks she is pregnant, and is given the same advice as on discharge following threatened abortion (p. 139). The fact is stressed that coitus should not take place during early pregnancy.

Adequate rest is essential; a minority recommend admission to hospital during the first half of pregnancy. Women with home responsibilities should not undertake outside employment or heavy work in the home.

Psychological support is needed by certain personality types and when no cause of abortion is apparent, repeated encouragement regarding a successful outcome and reassurance (weekly visits to doctor or clinic) may be effective. Any emotional stress should be enquired into and suitable advice given. A mild sedative may be necessary.

CERVICAL INCOMPETENCE

Abortions occurring at about mid-term may be due to incompetence of the cervix allowing the membranes to rupture. A purse-string suture of heavy non-absorbable material is inserted after the 12th week, e.g., braided Mersilk. Mersilene (5 mm.) is non-irritating but expensive.

Cervical assessment is made by some authorities prior to suture and, if a No. 8 dilator passes easily into the cervix it is incompetent.

WARNING REGARDING REMOVAL OF SUTURE

Midwives should be aware that the cervical suture must be removed at the 38th week, or sooner if the woman goes into premature labour, otherwise severe damage will be inflicted on the dilating cervix.

In certain cases of bad obstetric history the suture is inserted prior to pregnancy, left in situ and Cæsarean section performed.

MISSED ABORTION

This term is used when the fetus dies and is retained in utero.

Signs of threatened abortion arise and then subside; the uterus does not increase in size.

The breasts become soft and the other signs of pregnancy disappear.

The woman has a brownish vaginal discharge, but no pain.

The ultrasonic Doppler cardioscope has been used to confirm the absence of fetal blood flow.

The uterus may retain the fetus for long periods, in one case for as long as 14 months. Certain authorities do not believe in interfering because of the risk of sepsis, but few women are willing to suffer the discomfort of a constant vaginal discharge, and they also object to having a dead fetus in utero.

Blood coagulation disorders may develop in cases of missed abortion which persist for over six to eight weeks, therefore plasma fibrinogen level estimations are made weekly.

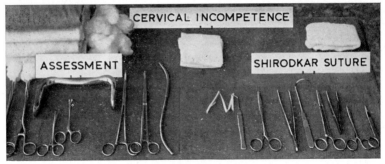

FIG. 109

Prepacked requirements for cervical assessment and modified Shirodkar's Suture.
(*County Maternity Hospital, Bellshill, Lanarkshire.*)

FOR ASSESSMENT

Instruments

2 Sponge forceps.
2 Towel clips.
1 Sims' speculum.
2 Ring forceps.
1 Cervical dilator No. 8.

Linen and dressings

1 Doctor's gown and cap.
1 Lithotomy sheet or leggings.
1 Waterproof paper sheet.
20 Wool swabs; 5 gauze swabs; 1 perineal pad.

FOR SUTURE

Instruments

1 Blunt aneurysm needle.
1 Spencer Wells forceps, 17·8 cm. (7 inches).
1 Spencer Wells forceps, 12·7 cm. (5 inches).
1 Non-toothed dissecting forceps, 17·8 cm. (7 inches).
1 Non-toothed dissecting forceps, 12·7 cm. (5 inches).
1 Sharp aneurysm needle.
1 Needle holder. 1 Stitch scissors.
Braided mersilk. Mersilene is non-absorbable and non-irritating, but is expensive.

BLOOD MOLE

Rarely, a blood mole forms. This is a brownish red mass, about as big as a medium-sized orange, that arises in cases of missed abortion when the decidua capsularis remains intact and permits the ovum to be surrounded with layers of blood. The mole forms before the 12th week and if it is retained *in utero* for a period of months, the fluid is extracted from the blood and the fleshy firm hard mass is known as a carneous mole. When cut, it resembles a miniature placenta at first glance, but what appear to be cotyledons are raised blebs of amnion with blood underneath. A tiny embryo, less than 1·25 cm. (half an inch) long, may be seen hanging by a short cord.

Treatment

HIGH DOSAGE OXYTOCIN DRIP

Give 10 units Syntocinon in 540 ml. dextrose 5 per cent at 1·2 ml (20 drops) per minute. Increase by 0·3 ml. (5 drops) every 30 minutes until 2·4 ml. (40 drops) are being given.

If no response: start a new bottle with double the amount of Syntocinon = 20 units at 1·2 ml. (20 drops) per minute and increase by 5 drops every 30 minutes to 2·4 ml. (40 drops).

If no response: double the number of units to 40, start with 1·2 ml. (20 drops) and increase to 2·4 ml. (40 drops) per minute.

If no response: the doctor may review the situation before giving 80 and 160 units. Some give as much as 200 units.

Vigilant observation is essential. A careful collection of urine is made and if the output is low the infusion should be stopped.

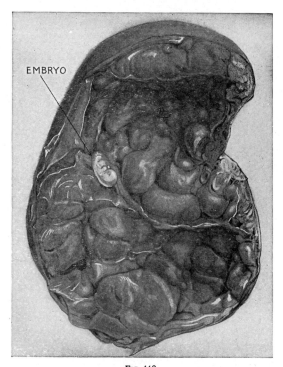

EMBRYO

FIG. 110

CARNEOUS MOLE.

The mole cut open shows the embryo and the blebs formed by blood collected between the amnion and chorion. The outer surface is smooth. Measurement (unopened) 7·6 × 8·9 cm. (3 inches × 3¼ inches).

(*Specimen in student midwives' classroom, Simpson Memorial Maternity Pavilion, Edinburgh.*)

INDUCED ABORTION

Induced abortions are divided into two classes, therapeutic and criminal.

THERAPEUTIC ABORTION

Therapeutic abortion consists in the evacuation of the uterus, carried out by a qualified medical practitioner as treatment in the interest of the mother's life or of her total well-being. The abortion may be legally carried out in Great Britain only in a National Health Service Hospital or a Nursing Home recognized for this purpose.

11

Husband and wife must both give written consent, and the duty of obtaining such signatures as well as permission to operate is usually delegated to the ward sister to avoid unnecessary delay. In certain religious beliefs therapeutic abortion is not sanctioned, but the priest should be informed when the question arises.

Before the 12th week it is usual to evacuate the uterus vaginally following dilatation of the cervix under a general anæsthetic.

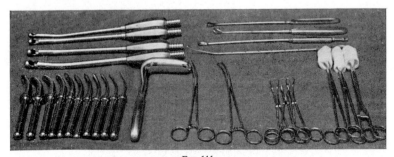

FIG. 111

Instruments for vacuum aspiration of embryo and placenta.

Termination of pregnancy by aspiration technique may be carried out using an electric vacuum pump up to 12 weeks (8 weeks being the optimal time). At 12 weeks a large cannula No. 14 Hegar size is necessary: the conception material being broken up and sucked out.

Abdominal hysterotomy may be performed when the fetus is large (16 to 28 weeks), and for the dangerously ill patient the shortness of the abdominal operation is in her favour.

THE ABORTION ACT, 1967

The provisions of the Act are briefly as follows:—If two registered medical practitioners are of the opinion that a pregnancy should be terminated under the following conditions they shall not be guilty of an offence under the law relating to abortion: That the continuance of the pregnancy would involve a risk to the life of the pregnant woman or of injury to her physical or mental health, or any existing children of her family; or a substantial risk that the child when born would suffer from such physical or mental abnormalities as to be seriously handicapped.

The woman's actual or reasonably foreseeable environment may be taken into account when determining the risk of injury to health should the pregnancy be allowed to continue.

The termination must be reported to the Chief Medical Officer, Ministry of Health and Social Security (Eng.) and Home and Health Department (Scot.).

Difficulty may be encountered in stimulating the uterus to expel its contents after the 12th week of pregnancy. On this account some older measures have again been resorted to: *i.e.*

(1) **Utus paste** 20 ml. is introduced slowly into the uterus. Because of the danger of embolism the patient should be conscious in order that any shoulder pain may be felt. If there is no response in 36 to 48 hours a high dosage oxytocin drip is given (see p. 144).

(2) **Hypertonic saline,** 20 per cent, has been injected transabdominally into the amniotoc sac usually between the 16th to 20th week. The woman must be conscious therefore 20 mg. papaveretum and a local anæsthetic are administered. The procedure is contraindicated in cardiac or renal disease. Potential dangers are sepsis

and vascular collapse. A number of maternal deaths have been recorded from Japan and elsewhere.

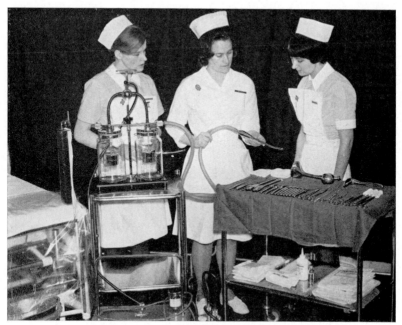

FIG. 112

Non-sterile set up for clinical instruction. Electric vacuum pump for evacuation of uterus in therapeutic abortion. (*Simpson Memorial Maternity Pavilion, Edinburgh*)

CRIMINAL ABORTION

A criminal abortion is one performed when the conditions set out in the Abortion Act, 1967, as described on page 146, are not fulfilled. As the name implies, the procedure is *illegal* and is punishable by imprisonment. Drugs are sometimes employed, but abortionists usually resort to vaginal interference. Many are unqualified persons having little knowledge of asepsis, and the fact that the procedure is carried out surreptitiously increases the risk of sepsis. Abortion has now become an important cause of maternal mortality and illness and there are good grounds for believing that it is criminal abortions which are largely responsible for this.

The midwife must, therefore, under no circumstances give advice or information which could result in an illegal abortion; neither should she assist any person to perform an illegal abortion.

DANGERS

Injuries such as perforation of the pouch of Douglas and laceration of the uterus have been known to be inflicted.

Sudden death due to the introduction into the uterus of soap solutions and pastes and from air embolism. **Sepsis and acute** renal failure **may cause death.**

Acute renal failure has resulted from forcible douching with soap solution as an abortifacient; this causes blood hæmolysis and destruction of the tubular epithelium of the kidney. (For Treatment see p. 203.)

SEPTIC ABORTION

This serious condition is usually associated with incomplete abortion, and particularly if it has been induced criminally. The condition is similar to *puerperal sepsis* following childbirth and is a *notifiable disease* in Scotland. Infertility and ill health may ensue; the mortality rate is high. In some of these cases the doctor is not called until sepsis is well developed, therefore antibiotics are not given early enough to combat the infection and prevent complications.

SIGNS AND SYMPTOMS

Uterus.—Tender on palpation.	**Pulse.**—Rapid.
Lochia.—Offensive and profuse.	**Temperature.**—Raised.

Abdominal pain may or may not be present.

Management

Isolation. When a patient who is in the process of aborting develops an elevated temperature or rapid pulse, or is admitted to hospital with these signs, barrier nursing should be instituted immediately, or, better still, she should be removed to a single room until the diagnosis is confirmed, when she will be transferred to an isolation hospital.

Clinical, bacteriological and hæmatological investigations, including the degree of leucocytosis, are made as in puerperal sepsis. A blood culture is made in serious cases. *Cl. Welchii* or *E. Coli* may be the causal organism.

Ampicillin, 500 mg., may be given, followed by 250 mg. 6 hourly. A blood transfusion is given if necessary. (*After* 24 *hours when the bacteriological report is received the appropriate antibiotic is administered.*)

Vaginal interference is usually avoided, unless severe bleeding occurs, until the infection is controlled.

Electrolyte control is necessary, daily.

The medical and nursing treatment is similar to what is necessary for puerperal sepsis.

Acute renal failure. After the first 12 hours the main concern is the kidney. A careful watch must be kept on renal function: an accurate fluid balance chart being kept. (See acute renal failure, p. 203.)

BACTERAEMIC (ENDOTOXIC) SHOCK

In obstetrics endotoxic shock is most frequently associated with septic criminal abortion. When a patient suffering from severe septicæmia exhibits a low cardiac-output-state this is usually due to the endotoxins released into the circulation from Gram negative organisms, commonly *E. Coli*.

SIGNS AND SYMPTOMS

The degree of hypotension is always greater than any blood loss warrants: the blood pressure may be unrecordable.

Tachycardia, cyanosis, cold moist skin.

The temperature may or may not be high.

Oliguria is a serious sign.

Mental confusion and coma are terminal manifestations.

Treatment

1. **Blood and urine are cultured:** cervical and throat swabs are taken.

2. **Blood gases and electrolytes** are monitored.

3. **Full doses of a wide spectrum antibiotic** are prescribed.

4. **Intravenous infusion of blood and glucose** 5 per cent is administered to maintain cardiac output.

5. **Electrolytes are given** to correct the metabolic acidosis.

6. **Corticosteroids** may be given for a few days to combat circulatory failure.

7. **The central venous pressure** is noted.

8. **The amount of urine secreted** is monitored.

9. **The administration of oxygen** is controversial.

4. ECTOPIC GESTATION

The word " ectopic " means " out of place." Therefore, if the fertilized ovum or zygote embeds outside the uterus, the condition is known as an ectopic or extrauterine pregnancy. Most commonly it is tubal, but it may occasionally be abdominal and very rarely ovarian.

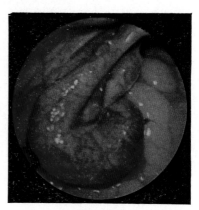

Fig. 113

INTACT TUBAL PREGNANCY.

Diagnosed by abdominal laparoscopy.

(*Courtesy of Mr. Patrick C. Steptoe, F.R.C.O.G. Oldham.*)

If the passage of the zygote is delayed by the effects of previous salpingitis, or by spasm, or the kinking of a long tube, it will embed in the Fallopian tube. When the chorionic villi penetrate blood vessels the hæmorrhage that occurs greatly distends the tube.

Three possible terminations of a Tubal Pregnancy

(1) TUBAL ABORTION

The lining of the tube ruptures, the ovum and blood escape into the lumen of the tube and are then expelled through the fimbriated end into the peritoneal cavity.

(2) TUBAL MOLE

It is similar to a uterine blood mole (p. 144) and develops when the ovum dies and becomes surrounded by layers of blood clot.

(3) TUBAL RUPTURE

Rupture may occur into the peritoneal cavity, or more rarely between the folds of the broad ligament, and usually takes place between the sixth and tenth week.

When the zygote embeds in the ampulla, any of the three terminations just mentioned may take place, but when embedding takes place in the narrow isthmus, rupture of the tube usually occurs about the sixth week.

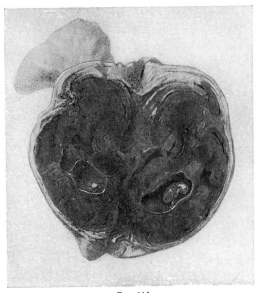

FIG. 114

TUBAL MOLE.

Tubal pregnancy, in which the embryo has died and is surrounded
with blood clot. The distended Fallopian tube is opened length-
wise. Ovary attached.

(*Specimen in student midwives' classroom, Simpson Memorial
Maternity Pavilion, Edinburgh.*)

SIGNS OF TUBAL PREGNANCY

The early signs of tubal pregnancy are very similar to those of threatened abortion,
but in abortion, bleeding precedes pain and is more profuse than in ectopic gestation.

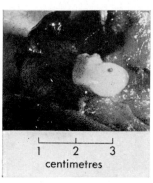

FIG. 115

TUBAL PREGNANCY.

Recurrent spasmodic pain, low on one side of the
abdomen, which is increased during defæcation
and often accompanied by nausea and faintness.

A history of having missed one or two periods
is elicited in 60 per cent of cases; and the early
signs of pregnancy such as breast changes
and morning sickness may be present.

Slight dark brown vaginal discharge (which
comes from the decidua).

It is the midwife's duty to get medical assistance
for any abnormality in pregnancy, and if these
early warning signs are overlooked the prognosis
will be more grave.

SIGNS OF TUBAL RUPTURE

1. **The general condition of the patient is always
worse than the slight vaginal bleeding warrants.**

2. **Severe abdominal pain.**
3. **Signs of internal hæmorrhage:**
>   (*a*) Fainting or collapse.   (*c*) Low blood pressure.
>   (*b*) Cold clammy skin.   (*d*) Pallor.
>   (*e*) Rapid thready pulse.

Treatment

Should such a catastrophe occur, the midwife will send for medical aid, treat the patient for shock by the application of blankets and by raising the foot of the bed. If the need for blood transfusion is obvious the " flying squad " should be called. The patient will be transferred to hospital for immediate salpingectomy, blood transfusion being given before, during and following operation as is necessary.

In only 60 per cent of cases will tubal rupture give rise to the acute signs described above; when rupture is gradual signs of internal hæmorrhage and shock may not be obvious.

ABDOMINAL PREGNANCY

Abdominal pregnancy is very rare, and occurs when the intact fetal sac is expelled from the tube into the abdominal cavity and the chorionic villi become attached to omentum, intestine, or perimetrium and re-embed. If the fetus subsequently dies, it may become surrounded with lime salts and form a **lithopædion** or stone fetus. Should the fetus live, the abdominal pregnancy may go to term, when an abdominal section will be necessary. A few cases have been recorded in which the baby was born alive.

In view of the grave risk of hæmorrhage as there are no " living ligatures " to control bleeding from the placental site, it is usual to leave the placenta *in situ*, where it will be absorbed by the lymphatics and peritoneum.

OVARIAN PREGNANCY

The spermatozoon fertilizes the ovum before it has been expelled from the ruptured Graafian follicle—bleeding into the substance of the ovary occurs. The signs and symptoms are similar to those of tubal pregnancy, but the Fallopian tube is found to be intact at laparotomy.

5. HYDATIDIFORM OR VESICULAR MOLE

A hydatidiform mole is a mass of vesicles resulting from cystic proliferation of chorionic villi. Some are simple, a few are malignant. The centre of each villus degenerates and the distended villi form vesicles varying in size from a pin-head to a small grape. This process begins about the sixth week of pregnancy, and the embryo is absorbed. The exuberant growth of the chorionic villi gives rise to the production of excessive quantities of **chorionic gonadotrophin,** and large amounts are excreted in the urine.

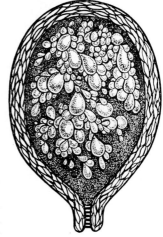

Fig. 116

Uterus with hydatidiform mole *in situ.*

SIGNS AND SYMPTOMS

Vaginal bleeding, beginning about the 12th week, is the earliest sign, and the discharge may be bright red and profuse, or brown due to the presence of old blood. The vesicles, which have been likened to " white currants in red currant juice," are rarely found until actual expulsion of the mole is taking place.

Undue enlargement of the uterus occurs in the majority of cases and a woman with 12 weeks' amenorrhœa may have a uterus the size of a 24 weeks' pregnancy. But if the mole becomes detached from the uterine wall the uterus may be normal in size or even less than normal.

Fetal movement will not have been felt.

Fetal parts will not be detected on palpation.   The fetal heart-beat is not heard.

The uterus has an elastic consistency; pain and tenderness, if present, are due to its excessive distension by the mole or blood clot.

Pre-eclampsia occurs in about 30 per cent of cases.

Vomiting is often present.

DIAGNOSIS

A quantitative chorionic gonadotrophin test is a valuable aid to diagnosis, and when the Pregnosticon test is positive in dilutions of 1 in 500, this is diagnostic.

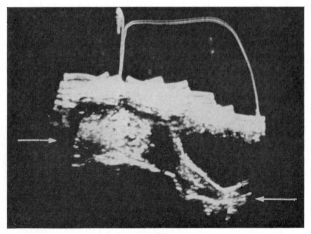

FIG. 117

HYDATIDIFORM MOLE. ULTRASONOGRAM.

White speckled area indicates the mole (left arrow). (Lower arrow indicates the cervix.)
(*By courtesy of Professor Ian Donald, Queen Mother's Maternity Hospital, Glasgow*)

The Diasonograph (diagnostic ultrasound) is used with greater certainty than any other method (see Fig. 117). The Doppler effect cardioscope has also been used to rule out the presence of a live fetus.

Treatment

1. **The patient is admitted to hospital and kept in bed.**
2. **Routine blood examination and urine analysis** are carried out.
3. **The vulva is shaved** and swabbing carried out twice daily.
4. **Pads are carefully inspected.**

A high dosage intravenous oxytocin drip preceded by a suppository or enema, is given and if not successful the bladder is emptied and the cervix dilated by the use of graduated metal dilators (see p. 144).

Because of the risk of perforation of the uterus, ovum forceps and curette are not used. Sponge-holding forceps may sometimes be employed to remove the mole which has been loosened with the gloved finger. Vacuum aspiration is sometimes used.

If intravenous ergometrine does not control severe hæmorrhage a gauze pack may be inserted into the uterus and removed within six hours. Cross-matched blood should be at hand.

Hysterotomy is sometimes performed to ensure more complete removal of the mole, particularly when large; blood loss is less and the risk of perforation reduced.

Hysterectomy is frequently performed in the woman over 40 to lessen the risk of chorion epithelioma at this age.

After operation the midwife must keep a close watch on the patient's pulse and also for vaginal bleeding.

DANGERS

1. **Hæmorrhage** which, before, during and after evacuation, may be sudden and profuse.

2. **Sepsis,** which is combated by strict aseptic technique and prevention of blood loss.

3. **Erosion of the uterine wall.**—The chorionic villi may erode through the uterus, and the uterine wall may be so dangerously thin that it is readily perforated during evacuation of the mole.

4. **Chorion epithelioma.**—Because of the risk of this malignant growth, which ensues in about 6 per cent of cases, repeated quantitative immunological tests are carried out. (Chorionic gonadotrophin excretion in the urine will be high when chorion epithelioma is present.) The test should be negative four weeks after the mole is completely evacuated; and, if so, it is repeated every month during the first six months and every three months during the next 18 months. The woman is told to report at once any vaginal bleeding other than a menstrual period.

Diagnostic curettage (*endometrial biopsy*) is done if an immunological test is positive or should irregular bleeding occur. If chorion epithelioma is diagnosed, hysterectomy may be performed.

CYTOTOXIC CHEMOTHERAPY

Cytotoxic chemotherapy has been used with 80 per cent success in cases of chorion epithelioma treated early. Methotrexate 25 mg. in one litre isotonic saline and 2000 i.u. heparin daily in divided doses is administered by an intra-arterial infusion pump for 3 to 6 days and repeated at intervals until 6 to 8 weeks after normal gonadotrophin excretion levels are obtained. Folinic acid 6 mg. is also given. Those who do not respond may be given Actinomycin-D. (Hysterectomy is not usually performed under this treatment.)

QUESTIONS FOR REVISION

VAGINAL BLEEDING

Mention the various causes of bleeding early in pregnancy:
FROM THE CERVIX (3); MOLES (3); VARIOUS TYPES OF ABORTION (6); OTHER CAUSES (3).

Define ectopic gestation and describe the signs of tubal pregnancy before and after rupture of the tube.

C.M.B.(Scot.) paper.—A patient who is two months pregnant complains of vaginal bleeding. Outline the possible causes.

C.M.B.(Scot.) paper.—A patient complains of vaginal bleeding at the 12th week of pregnancy. Discuss the possible causes and describe the treatment of any one obstetric cause.

ABORTION

Give reasons why the following procedures are necessary in cases of threatened abortion: (a) No ENEMA is given for 48 hours; (b) PREGNANCY test is done; (c) ALL VAGINAL DISCHARGE is saved for inspection.

Give three general and three local causes of abortion. What are the signs and dangers of hydatidiform mole?

What drugs and equipment would you anticipate might be used in cases of: (1) missed abortion; (2) ruptured ectopic; (3) insertion of Shirodkar's suture; (4) vesicular mole; (5) evacuation of uterus for incomplete abortion.

Differentiate between: inevitable and incomplete abortion; blood mole and carneous mole; uterine, ectopic and abdominal pregnancy.

Give alternative names for: vesicular mole; abortion; fleshy mole; tubal pregnancy.

What special investigations are made in: (a) missed abortion; (b) septic abortion; (c) hydatidiform mole; (d) habitual abortion.

Write not more than 10 lines on: cervical incompetence; therapeutic abortion; bacteræmic shock; chorionic epithelioma.

What questions would you ask a woman who has slight vaginal bleeding in early pregnancy? What first aid treatment would you give for serious bleeding from an inevitable abortion?

What are the midwife's responsibilities: (a) when a Shirodkar's suture has been inserted? (b) in dealing with severe hæmorrhage from an incomplete abortion in a remote area?

C.M.B.(N. Ireland) paper.—Define the terms (a) therapeutic abortion; (b) criminal abortion; (c) missed abortion. Pending the arrival of the doctor, how would you treat a patient (a) who was threatening to abort; (b) who was bleeding freely from an incomplete abortion?

C.M.B.(Scot.) paper.—Enumerate the main varieties of abortion, and describe the clinical features and nursing treatment of any one of those.

C.M.B.(Scot.) paper.—Describe the clinical features of a case of inevitable abortion at the third month of pregnancy. In the presence of severe bleeding while the patient is still at home, what emergency treatment would you carry out pending the arrival of medical assistance?

C.M.B.(N. Ireland) paper.—Discuss the diagnosis and management of a case of threatened abortion.

C.M.B.(N. Ireland) paper, 1970.—Write short notes on: (a) threatened abortion; (b) inevitable abortion; (c) missed abortion.

10

Hydramnios—Uterine Displacement—Fibroids

In hydramnios the amount of liquor in the amniotic sac exceeds the normal quantity of 500 to 1,500 ml. but is not as a rule clinically apparent until the amount is over 3,000 ml. During a period of 10 years in the Simpson Memorial Maternity Pavilion five patients had over 12 litres of fluid, the maximum being 15·6 litres. Hydramnios occurs in about 1 in 200 pregnancies.

The cause is unknown, but hydramnios is associated with monozygotic (uniovular) twins and with pathological conditions, both fetal and maternal.

FETAL CONDITIONS ASSOCIATED WITH HYDRAMNIOS

Monstrosities and malformations such as anencephaly and spina bifida are common, and it is possible that in these conditions transudation of cerebro-spinal fluid, through the exposed meninges, occurs into the amniotic sac. The fact that hydramnios occurs when the œsophagus is imperforate, give credence to the idea that the inability of the fetus to swallow liquor amnii may be a causative factor. Fetal diseases, such as hydrops fetalis, are also associated with hydramnios.

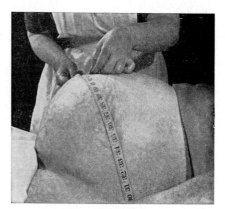

FIG. 118

Measuring abdominal girth in a case of hydramnios.

MATERNAL CONDITION

About 25 per cent of pregnant diabetic women have marked hydramnios; a number having it in lesser degree.

CLINICAL TYPES

1. **Acute hydramnios is very rare.** It usually occurs just prior to mid-term, comes on suddenly, and in three or four days' time the uterus is so excessively distended that the fundus reaches the xiphisternum. **monozygotic twins or some fetal abnormality** are usually present but the uterus may be so tense that it is impossible to detect fetal parts. Abdominal pain may be severe, vomiting troublesome and if pressure symptoms are causing distress the membranes are punctured. The most common outcome is spontaneous abortion.

2. **Chronic hydramnios** is the common type, which comes on slowly, usually about the 30th week. When the amount of fluid is excessive, the term " **polyhydramnios** " is applied, and in such a case it is usual to find some gross fetal malformation.

155

SIGNS AND SYMPTOMS

1. *On Inspection*

(a) **The uterus is large,** and at term the girth is over 1 m. (39·3 inches) (the author having seen a case in which the girth was 1·37 m. (54 inches)).

(b) **The shape of the uterus is globular** rather than ovoid.

(c) **The abdominal wall is thin and tense,** the skin shiny with prominent veins and marked striæ gravidarum.

2. *On Palpation*

(a) **Palpation of the fetus is difficult,** because it recedes from the examining fingers, but can be balloted between the two hands. To facilitate palpation the woman may be turned on her side or placed in the knee-elbow position, and by deep percussion of the dependent part of the abdomen, fetal parts can be detected.

(b) **A fluid thrill** can be elicited by laying the palm of the left hand in close contact with one side of the uterus, and on giving a sharp flick or tap on the other side of the uterus with the fingers of the right hand the wave of fluid transmitted is felt by the left hand.

3. *On Auscultation*

The fetal heart-beat is muffled and may be inaudible because of the density of fluid.

4. ON X-RAY

It is usual to X-ray the abdomen after the 30th week in order to detect the presence of twins or fetal monstrosities. If there are twins the mother will want to know, so that she can prepare for two babies; if a monstrosity is present the doctor will almost certainly induce premature labour. The excess of fluid makes the film milky or blurred in appearance; the large uterine outline can be seen.

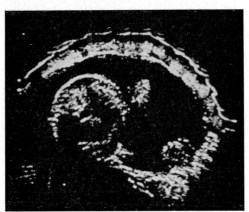

Fig. 119

HYDRAMNIOS. 30 WEEKS. ULTRASONOGRAM.

Showing anterior placenta, two floating limbs, large round area to the left is fetal buttocks.
(*Aberdeen Maternity Hospital*)

Ultrasonics reveal hydramnios as clear areas containing blob-like echo complexes (floating fetal limbs).

THE EFFECT OF HYDRAMNIOS ON PREGNANCY

Pressure symptoms may be intense and distressing.

1. **Œdema of the vulva** and lower limbs is present in severe cases.

2. **Dyspnœa and palpitation** may be disturbing, especially at night, interfering with rest and sleep. Extra pillows will give some relief, but a sedative may be necessary.

3. **Vague abdominal discomfort** and pain in the region of the lower ribs may be complained of.

4. **Indigestion,** heartburn and constipation are more troublesome.

5. **The weight of the uterus** and general ungainliness may incapacitate the woman if distension is severe, and extra rest in bed should be advised.

The urine should be examined for glucose because of the possibility of diabetes.

Very rarely, abdominal amniocentesis is carried out to relieve extreme discomfort, but unfortunately the fluid accumulates again very rapidly and in some cases the procedure tends to induce labour. A 50 ml. syringe, two-way stop-cock and spinal needle are required; as much as 3,000 ml. may be withdrawn, but 600 to 1,200 ml. is more usual. **The bladder must first be emptied.**

EFFECT ON LABOUR

The following conditions may arise:

1. **Prolapse of cord.**—If the membranes are allowed to rupture spontaneously the cord is usually swept down with the rush of fluid. A vaginal examination should be made immediately.

2. **Malpresentations** are common, because the fetus can move freely *in utero*.

3. **Labour is likely to be premature,** which increases the danger to the fetus.

4. **Hypotonic uterine action** may occur because of the over-distended uterus. (*Some authorities do not believe this to be so.*)

5. **Postpartum hæmorrhage** may take place because of the over-stretched and ineffectual uterine muscle. (*Some doubt this.*)

Treatment

Treatment is directed towards avoiding or dealing with the complications. In view of the risks involved and the high perinatal mortality rate, the woman should be delivered in hospital, and it is advisable to admit her for complete rest during the last two weeks of pregnancy, or earlier if possible.

PUNCTURE OF MEMBRANES AND OXYTOCIN DRIP

The membranes are punctured prior to or when labour starts (*any malpresentation having first been rectified*) for the following reasons:

1. **In order to reduce the size of the uterus** so that contractions will be more effective.

2. **To allow the presenting part to sink into the lower pole of the uterus,** in order to stimulate the cervical nerve endings.

Method

The woman empties her bladder. A sedative is usually given.

After cleansing the vulva amniotomy forceps are used to puncture the fore-waters. *The hind waters are not punctured as frequently as formerly.* Some insert a metal

12

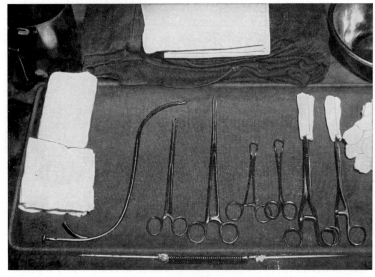

Fig. 120

PUNCTURE OF MEMBRANES.

(*Simpson Memorial Maternity Pavilion, Edinburgh.*)

LINEN: DRESSINGS	INSTRUMENTS: METAL WARE
1 Lithotomy sheet.	2 Swab holding forceps : 2 Mayo towel clips.
2 Dressing towels.	1 Goodwin's, or Stiles'
20 Wool swabs.	amniotomy forceps, or Drew
5 Gauze swabs.	Smythe's catheter.
1 Perineal pad.	1 Swabbing lotion bowl : 1 Litre measuring jug.

1 Goodwin's, or Stiles' amniotomy forceps, or Drew Smythe's catheter. } To puncture membranes.

Pack, with gown and hand towel; gloves.

NON-STERILE SHELF

Obstetric antiseptic cream; fetal stethoscope.

catheter to drain the amniotic fluid into a measuring jug; others introduce a gauze pack into the vagina or insert the hand to surround the cervix and stem the rush of fluid, *for the following reasons.*

Prolapse of cord is less likely to occur.

Fetal and maternal distress are avoided; the fetal heart being carefully noted.

Premature separation of the placenta (antepartum hæmorrhage) **does not occur so readily** when the size of the uterus is slowly reduced.

An oxytocin drip is given simultaneously; starting cautiously with 0·5 units in 540 ml. dextrose 5 per cent at 1·2 ml. (20 drops) per minute and increasing 0·3 ml. (5 drops) every half hour to 2·4 ml. If no response a new bottle with 2 units is begun and increased as formerly. When labour is established no increase in rate or dosage is made (see p. 610).

The baby should be held upside down at birth to drain the fluid from the respiratory passages; a No. 8 œsophageal catheter is passed into the stomach and fluid is aspirated with a syringe to avoid its regurgitation and inhalation. The passage of the œsophageal catheter is a necessary means of diagnosing the œsophageal atresia which may be present

OLIGOHYDRAMNIOS

In this rare condition there is a gross deficiency in the amount of liquor amnii, the total being probably less than 60 ml. It is associated with congenital absence of

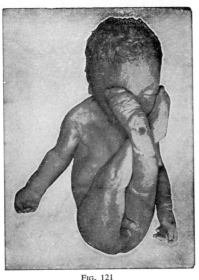

FIG. 121

Fetus in case of oligohydramnios. Compression of fetus with deformities of legs and toes.

the kidneys. Certain deformities, such as talipes, may develop because of pressure on the fetus: amputation of limbs due to adhesions between the amnion and the tiny embryo are sometimes attributed to this cause. The baby's skin is dry and leathery in appearance.

DISPLACEMENTS OF THE PREGNANT UTERUS

RETROVERSION

Causes.—Retroversion may be congenital or it may be a sequela of previous child-bearing, during which the uterine ligaments and the pelvic floor have been over-stretched.

No attempt is made to rectify a backwardly displaced uterus during pregnancy unless it is giving rise to discomfort or pain.

There are two possibilities in the outcome of retroversion in pregnancy:

1. **Spontaneous rectification** is the more likely. At the 12th week the uterus, now globular in shape, rises above the pelvic brim, and becomes anteverted.

2. Incarceration of the retroverted gravid uterus is a rare condition in which the backwardly displaced pregnant uterus becomes imprisoned in the pelvic cavity and does not rise above the pelvic brim after the 12th week.

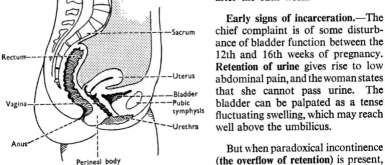

FIG. 122

The non-pregnant uterus in the normal position of anteflexion and anteversion.

Early signs of incarceration.—The chief complaint is of some disturbance of bladder function between the 12th and 16th weeks of pregnancy. **Retention of urine** gives rise to low abdominal pain, and the woman states that she cannot pass urine. The bladder can be palpated as a tense fluctuating swelling, which may reach well above the umbilicus.

But when paradoxical incontinence **(the overflow of retention)** is present, the inexperienced midwife may not associate it with an over-distended bladder.

Treatment

The midwife should send for medical assistance. While awaiting his arrival, she ought to pass a fine plastic disposable catheter to withdraw the urine slowly: if the rectum is loaded an enema should be given. The doctor will manually correct the displacement and insert a Hodge pessary, which is worn for four or six weeks. Except in very mild cases, the woman is admitted to hospital for a few days; a self-retaining catheter is inserted for 48 hours (with closed drainage system or air-sealed polythene bag to reduce the risk of infection).

The results of incarceration, i.e. sacculation of the anterior wall of the uterus, exfoliative cystitis, rupture of bladder are extremely rare and would only occur in areas where doctors and qualified midwives were not available to recognize and deal with incarceration.

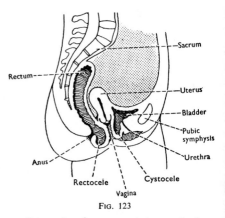

FIG. 123

Retroversion of non-pregnant uterus, cystocele and rectocele.

Note: Uterus lies in the same axis as the vagina and can readily prolapse. Compare with uterus in Fig. 122.

ANTEVERSION AND ANTEFLEXION

In multiparous women, the abdominal wall may be so lax, because of repeated childbearing, that it fails to provide the necessary support for the pregnant uterus. When the fundus leans forwards and the abdomen is unduly prominent this is known as **anterior obliquity** of the uterus.

EFFECT ON PREGNANCY

Sometimes the rectus muscles are widely separated and the uterus leans so far forwards that it hangs downwards, giving rise to a *pendulous abdomen.* To relieve pain and discomfort in walking, and to support the weight of the uterus, a well-fitting maternity corset should be worn.

EFFECT ON LABOUR

Such obliquity may give rise to malpresentation during labour. The force of the uterine action will also be misdirected and labour will be prolonged. To avoid this a firm binder should be worn during labour and the woman advised to lie on her back until the head has entered the pelvis.

Anteversion of the uterus in a primigravida is a serious matter, usually indicating pelvic contraction or spinal deformity which so limits the accommodation for the pregnant uterus that it is forced outwards. In such a case the woman should be seen by an obstetrician.

PROLAPSE OF THE PREGNANT UTERUS

This type of displacement is very rare because the woman with a prolapsed uterus does not usually become pregnant.

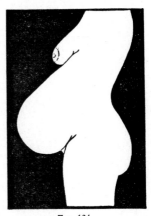

Fig. 124

Pendulous abdomen.

A ring pessary is inserted, and worn until the uterus rises out of the pelvic cavity. In cases where the cervix protrudes outside the vulva, the woman should be confined to bed and any cervical abrasions treated. Strict aseptic precautions must be observed because of the risk of sepsis.

THE EFFECT OF FIBROID TUMOURS ON CHILDBEARING

Fibroids are most commonly found in older primigravidæ. The situation of these tumours has an important bearing on the outcome, depending on whether they are in the upper or lower uterine segment and into which of the three coats of the uterus they permeate. From 5 to 50 small fibroids may be scattered throughout the uterine wall, and **infertility** may exist when they encroach on the endometrium. The large fibroid can be palpated as a firm mass during pregnancy and after the expulsion of the baby.

EFFECT ON PREGNANCY

1. **Abortion may take place.**

2. **Red degeneration of the fibroid may occur** and give rise to pain and uterine tenderness: palliative measures are often successfully employed—rest in bed and sedatives.

3. **Pressure symptoms.**—Very rarely in pregnancy is a fibroid so large as to cause real distress, and if so, myomectomy is sometimes performed; unfortunately the operation tends to induce abortion.

EFFECT ON LABOUR

1. **Malpresentation.**—A fibroid in the lower pole of the uterus may cause malpresentation.

2. Weak uterine contractions.—The presence of a number of small fibroids in the muscle coat of the uterus may interfere with its action. The fibroids may inhibit good retraction of the uterine muscle in the third stage and predispose to postpartum hæmorrhage.

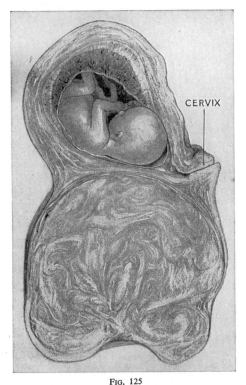

FIG. 125

FIBROID TUMOUR IN PREGNANT UTERUS.

The fibroid being in the lower segment of the uterus and measuring 11·4 to 12·7 cm., (4½ to 5 inches) would have filled the pelvic cavity and obstructed labour.

(*Specimen in student midwives' classroom, Simpson Memorial Maternity Pavilion, Edinburgh.*)

3. Obstruction.—Very rarely does a fibroid tumour obstruct labour. When situated in the corpus, it rises out of the true pelvis with the growing uterus, but if situated in the lower pole, obstruction may occur.

EFFECT ON THE PUERPERIUM

During involution the fibroids become reduced in size, but if they have been bruised during labour they may cause subinvolution and profuse red lochia.

OVARIAN CYSTS

The presence of a fluctuating swelling alongside the uterus would necessitate seeking medical aid. Pressure symptoms will exist if the cyst is large, and torsion may occur during pregnancy or the puerperium, giving rise to acute pain and vomiting. Very rarely a *pedunculated ovarian cyst* will occupy the pelvic cavity, preventing engagement of the head, and if not diagnosed will obstruct labour.

BICORNUATE UTERUS

The bicornuate or double uterus is a rare malformation due to a developmental error, and in some cases there is complete duplication of uterus, cervix and vagina.

POSSIBLE OUTCOME

When pregnancy occurs in one horn, the other also enlarges and forms a decidua. Abortion is common. If the septum extends only part way down the centre of the uterus, a transverse lie may be present, the fetus lying with its head in one horn, breech in the other. Attempts at external version do not succeed in such cases.

DIAGNOSIS

The condition is usually diagnosed on vaginal examination during pregnancy, but the author recalls one case being diagnosed during labour, in which the os was

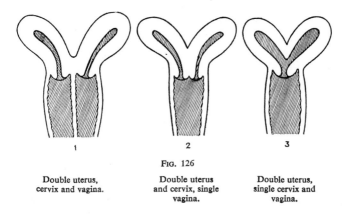

FIG. 126

| Double uterus, cervix and vagina. | Double uterus and cervix, single vagina. | Double uterus, single cervix and vagina. |

said to be "fully dilated" by one midwife and cervix "not taken up" by the other; each having inserted her fingers into different halves of a septate vagina. The labour was completed spontaneously.

The course of labour may not be affected, but if the non-pregnant horn fills the pelvic cavity it will obstruct labour. In order to avert such an outcome Cæsarean section would be performed.

QUESTIONS FOR REVISION

COMPLETION TEST

Give the term for:

1. **insufficiency of amniotic fluid**...
2. **an excessive amount** of amniotic fluid..
3. **withdrawing fluid** through the abdominal wall...
4. **an œsophageal catheter is passed** in the baby to diagnose..............................
5. **retroverted uterus imprisoned** in the pelvic cavity ....
6. **double uterus**..

HYDRAMNIOS

Why is it advisable ?
1. To examine the urine for glucose in cases of hydramnios ?
2. To make a vaginal examination when the membranes rupture ?
3. To drain off the liquor slowly ?
4. To puncture the membranes at the onset of labour ?

How could the midwife help to alleviate the discomforts of hydramnios ? Why should delivery take place in hospital ?

How would you differentiate between hydramnios and multiple pregnancy ?

C.M.B.(Scot.) paper.—How is hydramnios recognized ? What abnormal conditions are associated with it ? Outline the treatment.

C.M.B.(Eng.) paper.—How can hydramnios be recognized in the antenatal period? What is the significance of this condition ?

C.M.B.(Eng.) paper.—What would make you suspect that a patient had hydramnios ? With what conditions may hydramnios be associated ? How may hydramnios be treated ?

C.M.B.(Scot.) paper.—What are the clinical features and complications of hydramnios ? Discuss its management.

C.M.B.(Scot.) paper.—Discuss the differential diagnosis of undue enlargement of the abdomen in the latter part of pregnancy.

C.M.B.(N. Ireland) paper.—Describe the clinical features of hydramnios. What effect can this condition have (*a*) on pregnancy ? (*b*) on labour.

RETROVERSION

Give the causes of retroversion of the uterus, and state which symptoms would indicate the necessity for medical assistance.

C.M.B.(Scot.) paper.—What complications may arise when pregnancy occurs in a retroverted uterus ?

C.M.B.(Eng.) paper.—What conditions may cause retention of urine during pregnancy and the puerperium ? What dangers may result from it ?

11

Disorders due to Pregnancy

HYPEREMESIS GRAVIDARUM

Hyperemesis differs from morning sickness in that the vomiting persists throughout the day and the woman's health becomes impaired. The combination of vomiting, nausea and anorexia can produce an undesirable state of malnutrition, which results in a profound metabolic disturbance that may be fatal. **Women are very apt to neglect morning sickness** and many cases of hyperemesis might have been " nipped in the bud " had the woman sought advice sooner.

The midwife refers cases of hyperemesis to the doctor.

There is no satisfactory explanation as to why normal pregnant women should vomit or why it only occurs in 50 per cent of cases; nor is it understood why in some women the vomiting becomes pernicious. There is little doubt but that the emotions play an important part in the production and aggravation of sickness in pregnancy. In women who have a " sensitive " nervous system, morning sickness is more likely to develop into hyperemesis. It is known that the emotions stimulate the sympathetic nervous system which in turn probably influences the endocrine system.

All the pathological changes which take place in the liver, kidneys, heart and brain can be explained as being due to deprivation of certain constituents of food, as well as the **ketosis, dehydration, avitaminosis and electrolyte imbalance** that are present.

Potassium deficiency causes muscle weakness particularly of the cardiac muscle. Vomiting produces potassium deficiency and this induces further vomiting.

SIGNS AND SYMPTOMS

These vary according to the length of time vomiting has persisted, and the severity of the condition. In a moderately severe case the woman usually gives a history of persistent nausea and vomiting for a week or more, and in some cases, intermittently for three or four weeks.

The patient is apathetic, weak and miserable. The eyes are dull and sunken.

The skin is dingy and inelastic. **The tongue is brown,** thickly coated or red and raw.

The teeth are covered with sordes, the lips cracked and sore.

The breath is offensive and smells of acetone.

The urine:—dark in colour, high specific gravity, contains ketones, low chlorides.

Constipation is present, due to starvation and dehydration.

ADMISSION TO HOSPITAL

All but the mildest cases should be admitted to hospital, and this appears to have a beneficial effect. probably because of the psychological factor which seems to predominate. The home surroundings are associated with nausea and retching, and relatives may have been too sympathetic or too indifferent.

On admission the patient is seen by the doctor, who takes her history and carries out a physical examination. Serum electrolytes are estimated. Other causes of vomiting are excluded.

The room should be airy, bright and single if possible, for in a large ward the meals and toilet of other patients may induce vomiting in a woman already nauseated.

Treatment

The vital substances of which the woman has been seriously depleted—fluid, glucose, sodium chloride and vitamins B and C must be replaced. No food is given by mouth for at least 24 hours, in order to rest the stomach, and as these patients are usually constipated an enema is given. Dulcolax suppositories are preferred by some.

Fluid is urgently needed, and in all but the mildest cases the intravenous route is chosen.

Dextrose is essential to counteract the ketosis, protect the liver and overcome the prostration.

Salt is required to replenish the blood chlorides. **Potassium is added** to the I.V. drip if the serum potassium is low.

When marked dehydration or ketosis is present, it is usual to give 2,500 to 3,000 ml. of 5 per cent dextrose and isotonic saline intravenously daily for two or three days (2 bottles 5 or 10 per cent dextrose and one of isotonic saline).

A fluid balance record is kept and vomitus should not be charted under output, but recorded in a separate column.

DRUGS

The vitamin B complex is required in the metabolism of carbohydrate and for the health of nerve tissue. Parentrovite can be given intramuscularly once daily when food is not retained.

Calcium gluconate, 20 ml. of a 10 per cent solution, may be given (*intravenously or intramuscularly*) daily to protect the liver.

Promazine (Sparine), 50 mg., administered 8 hourly has proved effective. **Meclozine** (Ancolan), **buclizine hydrochlor** (Vibazine) and **promethazine** (Avomine) are sometimes used.

Certain antihistamine and anti-emetic drugs are not now given because of the possible harmful effects on the developing embryo during the first twelve weeks of pregnancy.

The patient is usually worn out with retching and from lack of sleep, but the opium derivatives tend to induce vomiting, so should not be used.

NURSING CARE

The psychological aspect.—The impression that recovery is assured should be created and the patient told that she is past the worst and not likely to vomit much more. The idea of vomiting should be banished from her mind, and the best way to do so is to remove the vomit bowl. *Subtle suggestion* is needed, and the personality of the midwife in charge is of paramount importance, for a judicious blending of kindness, firmness and optimism is needed.

Temperature—pulse.—These should be taken and recorded twice daily, and in serious cases four-hourly, as the slightest increase may be significant.

The blood pressure is taken twice daily, but it is low blood pressure that is being watched for—a sign of myocardial weakness—and on that account student midwives should be warned, when getting convalescent patients up for the first time, to be on the lookout for any signs of faintness.

Urine analysis.—The urine is examined on admission and twice daily for specific gravity, ketones, chlorides, and once daily for protein and bile. In serious cases these tests are done more frequently.

Weight.—The patient is weighed on admission, and if able to be out of bed, every second day.

DIET

If nausea and retching persist, 48 hours may elapse before food is retained, and an effort should then be made to get the patient to take some solid food. The secret of success lies in pushing up the diet quickly, for the stomach is more likely to retain solid food than fluids.

Meals should be served every two and a half hours or so, because an empty stomach contracts more violently than one which contains food. As most women enjoy a cup of tea, it is the first meal given, along with crisp toast or a water biscuit and marmalade jelly. Marmite or Bovril drinks may be acceptable. Tinned orange juice is preferable, being high in potassium; glucose may be added to it, but too many cold sweet drinks are irritating to the stomach. If the patient has a preference for something savoury rather than sweet, her wishes should be gratified.

First few days.

Horlick's, Ovaltine, milk puddings, fruit jellies, steamed white fish.

The tray should be immaculate and as attractive as possible. Fresh fruit and salads are valuable for their colourful appearance, as well as their vitamin content.

Rich and greasy foods must be avoided for some time.

After three or more days—the sooner the better—the following articles of food can be served:—Cold chicken or small lean grilled lamb chop; baked or mashed potato; sieved vegetable; baked apple. Thin sandwiches of tomato, lettuce or cress, and a very little butter mixed with equal parts of Marmite.

SERIOUS SIGNS

It is the duty of the midwife to watch for and notify the doctor of serious signs, for they may indicate that the pregnancy should be terminated before irreparable damage has been done.

1. **When the pulse is over 100,** this is a warning sign, and when over 120, weak or irregular, it denotes serious myocardial weakness.

2. **Temperature over 37·2° C. (99° F.).**

3. **Jaundice or the presence of bile in the urine.**   4. **Persistent proteinuria.**

5. **Cerebral signs are a late manifestation,** and the following should be reported immediately:—dimness of, or double vision, nystagmus, squint, low muttering delirium and loss of memory. *Korsakoff's syndrome* (see Glossary). Drowsiness may supervene and the patient sinks into coma.

Hyperemesis gravidarum is amenable to early treatment, and **the midwife should be aware of its tragic possibilities.** Her sphere lies in prevention, and this involves the careful supervision of every woman during the early months of pregnancy. Fortunately, therapeutic abortion is seldom necessary and a fatal outcome rare because patients are now sent to hospital in the early stages when the prognosis is good.

On discharge the patient is advised regarding her diet, to avoid constipation and to report any further vomiting, as a recurrence of the condition is looked on as unfavourable.

PRE-ECLAMPSIA: ECLAMPSIA
ESSENTIAL HYPERTENSION

PRE-ECLAMPSIA

This disease is peculiar to pregnancy, usually becoming manifest after the 30th week, and rarely prior to the 24th week. It occurs more commonly in primigravidæ, and the incidence is increased in cases of multiple pregnancy, essential hypertension, diabetes and hydatidiform mole. Reduced uterine blood flow is a feature of pre-eclampsia.

Pre-eclampsia is associated with placental dysfunction (see p. 654) and if so intra-uterine growth retardation is likely to occur.

THE CAUSE IS STILL UNKNOWN

Increased resistance in the arterioles, due to vasospasm, is characteristic: this produces hypertension and also affects the brain, liver and kidneys. Sodium retention occurs in some cases.

Theories as to its causation are so manifold as to be outside the scope of this book. Intensive research has been conducted, all over the world, for many years: endocrine, metabolic, biochemical, physiological and obstetrical investigations having been made.

SIGNS

MODERATE	SEVERE
BLOOD PRESSURE, 140/90.	BLOOD PRESSURE, 160/110.
ŒDEMA OF ANKLES.	ŒDEMA OF HANDS AND FACE.
PROTEINURIA UNDER 0·5 G./litre	PROTEINURIA OVER 1 G./litre.

The figures given above as moderate and severe are only generalizations and not strict criteria of the severity of the condition. Individual variations occur, *e.g.* eclampsia or fetal death can occur with proteinuria 0·5 G./litre, slight œdema or moderate hypertension.

HYPERTENSION

Raised blood pressure is one of the cardinal signs of pre-eclampsia, therefore to detect an incipient rise the woman's blood pressure should be taken early in pregnancy in order that her usual pressure is known. At 20 weeks 138/80 is considered the dividing line between normal and abnormal blood pressure: 140/90 during the last 4 weeks of pregnancy. The height of the diastolic pressure is of greater prognostic significance than the systolic, *i.e.* a blood pressure of 140/100 is more serious than one of 150/90. When over 160/100 the fetus is in danger.

An increase of 10 mm. Hg. is an indication for close supervision: the doctor should be notified and the woman given the appropriate advice regarding rest and diet (avoiding excessive salt intake).

ŒDEMA

Occult œdema may be suspected when there is a marked increase in weight, but this may, of course, be due to causes other than tissue-fluid retention.

All pregnant women should be weighed every two weeks from the 16th to the 30th weeks of pregnancy, and if, during this critical period, 1,361 G. or more (3 lb.) are gained in any two weeks, the increase is excessive. This should be an indication for close supervision; the woman being weighed and examined weekly; her diet ought to be one with moderate salt, low carbohydrates, high proteins: additional rest should be taken.

ŒDEMA OF THE ANKLES

If œdema of the ankles is of slight degree it may be confused with the ankle œdema seen in about 40 per cent of pregnant women which tends to disappear with rest over night. Œdema extending up the leg, can be taken as a more definite sign.

The following are more serious than ankle oedema:—

The hands and fingers feel stiff, especially in the morning, because of the swelling; the wedding ring is tight. On palpating the pads of the fingers the midwife will note their firm, tense consistency. In severe cases the backs of the hands are massively swollen; the wedding ring is almost submerged.

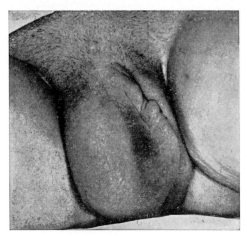

Fig. 127
Œdema of the vulva.

Puffy eyelids and bagginess under the eyes may be present in the morning only; in serious cases the features are coarse and bloated, the eyes almost closed.

Over the sacral region œdema can frequently be detected when the œdematous pre-eclamptic woman is confined to bed.

When gross œdema is present the skin has a pearly appearance: Pinard's stethoscope leaves a deep indented ring on the abdominal wall.

Labial swelling is not common but can be excessive. In one case seen by the author each labium was the size of a large clenched fist. (*No delay occurred during the perineal phase of delivery.*)

PROTEINURIA

Proteinuria is a late and usually a serious sign of pre-eclampsia.

All pregnant women with proteinuria, however slight in a mid-stream specimen of urine should be admitted to hospital for investigation, close supervision, complete rest and dietary measures.

The amount of protein is frequently taken as an index of the severity of the condition, and when eclampsia supervenes the urine may contain as much as 12 G. of protein per litre. But eclampsia may occur with only 0·5 G./litre of protein in the urine.

PROPHYLAXIS

Prenatal visits are being made more frequently and greater vigilance directed toward detecting early manifestations of the disease.

It is highly desirable that every primigravid woman should be seen

EVERY FOUR WEEKS UNTIL THE 20TH WEEK ⎫ *More often if*
EVERY TWO WEEKS UNTIL THE 30TH WEEK ⎬ *necessary*
EVERY WEEK UNTIL DELIVERED ⎭

Particular attention is being paid to cases of multiple pregnancy, diabetes and essential hypertension as such patients are more liable to suffer from pre-eclampsia.

A scheme whereby women are made aware of the necessity for keeping their regular clinic appointments, and an efficient system for getting in touch promptly with defaulters should be in operation (see p. 123).

Promising results have been obtained by restricting carbohydrates in the diet of pregnant women and increasing proteins and iron. This requires much individual instruction and persuasion of expectant mothers.

THE MIDWIVES' RESPONSIBILITY

Modern prenatal care requires that urine analysis for protein is carried out, blood pressure estimated, and the woman weighed and examined for œdema at each prenatal visit. Domiciliary midwives must co-operate in encouraging women to attend for the frequent examinations now considered essential. Merely visiting a pregnant woman in her home to enquire about her health, without carrying out the measures mentioned above, does not constitute competent prenatal care.

The necessary examinations must be made, and in remote areas the midwife can transport bathroom scales in her car. Albustix reagent strips for the detection of proteinuria are available. Uristix strips detect protein and glucose simultaneously.

The fact that a doctor is booked for the case does not relieve the midwife of her share of responsibility.

C.M.B.(Scot.) Rule 1965. When engaged to attend a domiciliary confinement a midwife must: (*e*) Examine the patient fortnightly until the 32nd week, and weekly thereafter or more frequently if the circumstances of the case so demand. The blood pressure should be taken and the urine examined at every visit and the findings recorded.

DANGERS OF PRE-ECLAMPSIA

MATERNAL	FETAL
1. Eclampsia.	3. Intra-uterine death.
2. Abruptio Placentæ in 8 per cent of cases.	4. Neonatal death (often associated with low birth weight and light for dates babies.

The fetus may die during pregnancy because of placental dysfunction: during labour an insufficient placental oxygen reserve may cause fatal anoxia.

Management of Pre-Eclampsia

All patients with pre-eclampsia, however slight, should be admitted to hospital for the close supervision that is so essential.

1. REST IN BED

Rest in bed is one of the most important measures in the management of pre-eclampsia. The blood pressure falls, œdema is diminished and the uterine blood flow is improved. When the woman lies on her side the output of urine and sodium is increased.

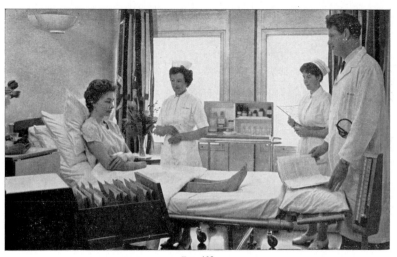

Fig. 128

Note drop-end trolley bed.   Chart cabinet, sphygmomanometer and medicine cabinet are portable.

(*County Maternity Hospital, Bellshill, Lanarkshire.*)

To facilitate rest, sedatives are usually prescribed and only mild cases should be in wards having more than two beds.   Ambulation for toilet facilities may be permitted after one week if there is no proteinuria and the diastolic pressure is not higher than 100.   Visitors should be limited when the blood pressure is high and proteinuria present.   Freedom from worry is essential.

2. ADMINISTRATION OF DRUGS
(a) SEDATIVES

MILD CASES—

In order to procure mental serenity it is customary for the doctor to order a sedative such as **chlordiazepoxide** (Librium) **5 mg.**, three times daily.   To ensure sound sleep at night **amylobarbitone sodium** (Sodium Amytal), **200 mg.**, is prescribed.

SEVERE CASES—

Amylobarbitone sodium (Sodium Amytal), **200 mg.** 6 or 8 hourly for 36 to 48 hours

Some prescribe the Lytic cocktail (see p. 176), 20 drops per minute for 15 minutes every 6 or 8 hours.

(b) ANTI-HYPERTENSIVE DRUGS

Anti-hypertensive drugs are used by some in severe cases of pre-eclampsia prior to viability of the fetus and when eclampsia is imminent, also during induction of and throughout labour. They do not prevent intra-uterine death nor do they have any effect in reducing proteinuria.

Methyldopa (Aldomet), 250 mg. orally t.i.d., is being administered with success in selected cases when the blood pressure is unduly high. The dose may be increased: drowsiness should be reported to the doctor.

Protoveratrine (Puroverine).—This alkaloid of veratrum, used only on rare occasions, may be given intramuscularly or intravenously. Orally the dose is 0·25 to 1 mg. When given in 300 ml. dextrose 5 per cent I.V. by mechanical syringe pump steadier control of blood pressure is obtained than by the I.M. route.

N.B.—**All derivatives of veratrum may cause a marked fall in blood pressure** with fainting and slow pulse rate. The patient must be observed closely and the blood pressure recorded hourly, at least, during parenteral administration until the desired response is attained. Nausea and vomiting may occur.

(c) DIURETICS

Oral diuretics are now used less frequently. They do not improve the pre-eclampsia nor the prognosis for the fetus. Chlorothiazide (Saluric) or frusemide (Lasix) may be prescribed for a period of days in cases of persistent or massive œdema.

3. DIET

In mild and moderate cases the woman is given the ordinary diet for a pregnant woman containing 90 G. of protein daily: milk is an excellent source and 1,200 ml. contain 40 G. of first class proteins. Minerals are essential, particularly iron, so fresh fruit and green vegetables are served: it is advisable to give iron and vitamins A, B, C, in tablet form to augment the diet.

A low carbohydrate diet reduces the calories and helps to control excessive weight gain.

Foods high in salt are excluded and no salt added at table.

Foods high in salt are:—tinned fish and meat, smoked fish, ham, tongue, bacon, sausage-meat, meat-pastes, cheese, Bovril, ketchup.

THE FLUID INTAKE

Pre-eclamptic patients are usually allowed fluid *ad lib.*; some limit the fluid intake to 1,200 ml. when œdema is marked. **When inducing labour** by I.V. drip the amount of fluid should be carefully controlled by syringe pump.

THE BOWELS

The bowels should move every day but strong purgatives should not be used Senokot, Dulcolax are suitable laxatives.

4. OBSERVATION

(a) URINE

A mid-stream specimen of urine is obtained on admission and daily, examined for protein and if present an Esbach's or other more accurate quantitative test is set up.

Urinary œstriol assays are made in some centres on two consecutive days every 1 or 2 weeks after the 30th week to assess the degree of feto-placental dysfunction, and so to determine whether labour should be induced. In serious cases urinary œstriol would be estimated twice (or oftener) weekly. If the excretion is below 5 mg. per 24 hours at 30 weeks and 10 mg. at 38 weeks the danger level for the fetus is reached.

(b) BLOOD PRESSURE

This is recorded twice daily in mild cases and four-hourly when the condition is severe. The doctor should be informed if the diastolic pressure rises to 110: sedation and hourly blood pressure recording may then be prescribed.

(c) ŒDEMA

The amount of œdema is assessed and recorded each day with a series of plus signs (see p. 185). The sacral region should be examined in recumbent patients.

(d) WEIGHT

Every second day the woman is weighed on special armchair bedside scales.

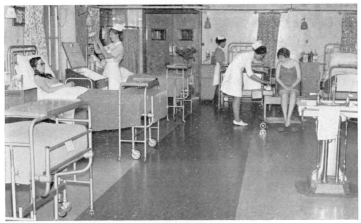

Fig. 129
PRENATAL WARD, ARMCHAIR BEDSIDE SCALES.
(*Simpson Maternity Pavilion, Edinburgh*)

(e) FLUID BALANCE

The fluid intake and output is measured and recorded daily.

(f) Temperature, pulse and respirations are recorded b.i.d.

(g) ABDOMINAL PAIN

The midwife should be fully aware of the causes of abdominal pain in the woman suffering from pre-eclampsia. These are :—

1. **Epigastric pain.** See serious signs, page 174 (9).

13

2. **Abruptio placentæ.** This serious condition is sometimes associated with pre-eclampsia: the pain is constant and excruciating, the uterus tender and board-like.

3. **Labour may have commenced.** The onset is gradual, pain intermittent, and other signs of labour will be present.

5. SERIOUS SIGNS AND SYMPTOMS

The midwife must be constantly on the alert for the development of serious signs which are danger signals of the onset of eclampsia. The doctor must be notified at once as immediate heavy sedation is imperative.

1. **Sharp rise in blood pressure.** 2. **Definite increase in proteinuria.**

3. **Marked increase in œdema.** 4. **Severe headache, usually frontal.**

5. **Visual disturbances:**—(*a*) Dimness or blurring of vision; (*b*) Flashes of light, coloured spangles; (*c*) Specks floating in front of the eyes.

6. **Vomiting is a significant sign.** 7. **Drowsiness.**

8. **Urinary output diminished** to less than 600 ml. in 24 hours.

9. **Epigastric pain.**—**This is a particularly ominous sign,** probably due to distension of the liver within its capsule. The patient may describe the pain as acute indigestion, and this symptom is the one most frequently misinterpreted.

6. NURSING CARE OF SERIOUS CASES

When serious signs or symptoms of pre-eclampsia develop the patient should be nursed as an eclamptic:—

(*a*) **The woman should be in a quiet, single room, with sufficient light to observe her colour.**

(*b*) **The lateral or semi prone position is recommended.**

(*c*) **The requirements to deal with an eclamptic fit should be at hand,** including oxygen and a polythene or other face mask. **Dentures are removed.**

(*d*) **A midwife should be on constant " special " duty.**

(*e*) **Heavy sedation must be achieved. Lytic cocktail** may be administered (see p. 176) and if the blood pressure rises again it may be given intermittently at 40 drops per minute for 30 minutes 6 or 8 hourly until the blood pressure is satisfactory.

(*f*) **Each specimen of urine is examined for protein.**

(*g*) **The blood pressure is recorded every one, two or four hours** depending on the severity of the case and if rising.

(*h*) **The diet consists of milk and fresh orange juice.** (*i*) **Fluid balance chart is kept.**

(*j*) **Magnesium trisilicate** 4 ml., orally, every 4 hours, will reduce the acidity of the gastric juice which may inadvertently be inhaled.

7. OBSTETRIC MANAGEMENT

(A) INDUCTION OF LABOUR

1. **When serious signs are manifest such a state of affairs is not allowed to pesist beyond 6 to 12 hours,** and should no improvement be apparent in that time the pregnancy is terminated.

2. **In severe cases, even with no signs of imminent eclampsia,** pregnancy would be terminated if no improvement is manifest after 36 to 48 hours treatment in hospital.

3. **When hypertension and proteinuria persist** labour is induced at the 37th week.

4. **Because of placental dysfunction the patient is not permitted to go beyond term.**

5. **Anti-hypertensive drugs may be prescribed** if the blood pressure is high.

6. **Puncture of membranes will be carried out,** and an intravenous oxytocin drip employed. The amount of fluid given should be carefully regulated when œdema is present. The Palmer syringe pump (see p. 610) is useful for slow injection.

7. **Cæsarean section may be preferred** in the older primigravida, and for the patient whose uterus does not respond to surgical induction and oxytocin drip.

(B) CARE OF THE PRE-ECLAMPTIC WOMAN IN LABOUR

1. **A midwife or student midwife should remain in constant attendance** because of the danger of an eclamptic fit occurring.

2. **Every specimen of urine is examined for protein.**

3. **The blood pressure is taken and recorded hourly.**

4. **A fetal heart record is kept in graph form.**

5. **The woman is well sedated** to minimize the likelihood of a convulsive seizure Early in labour she is given amylobarbitone sodium (Sodium Amytal) 200 mg., or cyclobarbitone, 200 mg.

6. **Chlormethiazole (Heminevrin)** is hypnotic, sedative and anticonvulsant; it has been used successfully in Aberdeen Maternity Hospital in 100 moderate or severe cases of pre-eclampsia in labour; an intravenous infusion of 0·8 per cent solution being given. The drug is not anti-hypertensive so protoveratrine may be necessary. As it is not analgesic, pethidine 100 mg. and Entonox are prescribed for labour pain. The perinatal mortality rate is low. Superficial phlebitis occurred at the infusion site when administration exceeded 8 hours. There were no convulsions.

7. **Epidural anæsthesia** is used in some centres, the hypotensive effect being advantageous.

8. **An episiotomy may be made and low forceps applied** under nitrous oxide gas (66 per cent), and oxygen to avoid the effort of " pushing " which may raise the blood pressure and also initiate an eclamptic fit. A muscle relaxant, *i.e.*, suxamethonium, is administered by continuous injection or drip. Endotracheal intubation is essential.

9. **Some authorities consider that ergometrine should not be administered in the** absence of bleeding (less than 300 ml.) because of its vasopressor action. Five units of Syntocinon is sometimes preferred.

(C) AFTER LABOUR

The first and only convulsion may occur soon after the completion of labour.

All patients with pre-eclampsia are given a sedative after delivery, i.e. morphine 15 mg.: in severe cases the woman may be given amylobarbitone sodium, 500 mg., I.M.I. before being transferred to the puerperal ward where she is nursed in a single, quiet room with a midwife in constant attendance for the first 12 hours.

Papaveretum (Omnopon) 20 mg. may be given four-hourly or t.i.d. (depending on the height of the blood pressure) with amylobarbitone sodium, 250 mg., I.M.I. at night.

The blood pressure is recorded at the completion of labour and, if giving rise to concern, every half-hour; then every four hours for 24 hours, then daily.

Eclampsia

Eclampsia, an acute condition characterized by convulsions and coma, is a more advanced stage of serious pre-eclampsia.

20 per cent of cases occur antepartum. ⎫

45 per cent occur intrapartum.   ⎬ *approx.*

35 per cent occur postpartum, usually during the first 12 hours. ⎭

SIGNS AND SYMPTOMS

The prodromal signs of eclampsia are those described as " serious signs " of pre-eclampsia (p. 173); the more immediate precursors of eclampsia being: **vomiting, intense headache, epigastric pain.**

These prodromal signs may be absent in the fulminating type of eclampsia which comes on suddenly but is very rare.

THE STAGES OF AN ECLAMPTIC FIT

PREMONITORY STAGE (lasts from 10 to 20 seconds)

The patient is restless and her eyes roll sideways or upwards, the head may be drawn to one side and **twitching of the facial muscles occurs.**

TONIC STAGE (lasts from 10 to 20 seconds)

The whole body is rigid, in a state of muscular spasm, and may be arched in the opisthotonos position. The teeth are tightly clenched, eyes staring, and because the diaphragm is in spasm, **respiration is checked and cyanosis ensues.**

CLONIC STAGE (lasts from 60 to 90 seconds)

Violent contraction of the muscles produces convulsive movements, which may be so severe as to throw the patient out of bed. The rapid movement of the jaw churns up the profusely secreted saliva and causes foaming at the mouth, which may be blood-stained if the tongue is bitten. **The face is congested and horribly distorted.** The woman is unconscious, her breathing stertorous and the pulse full and bounding. Gradually the convulsion subsides.

STAGE OF COMA

Stertorous breathing continues and coma may persist for minutes or hours; further convulsions sometimes occur without the patient regaining consciousness.

MEDICAL TREATMENT

The main principle of treatment is to prevent the occurrence of fits, and if this can be achieved, recovery is more likely.

SEDATION

When the patient is first seen it may be necessary to administer narcotics *intravenously* in order to bring the convulsions quickly under control.

Morphine, 15 mg., may be given intravenously on district if a more suitable narcotic is not available but should not be repeated because of producing respiratory depression with subsequent cyanosis, diminished secretion of urine and vomiting.

" Lytic cocktail." A combination of 50 mg. chlorpromazine (Largactil); 50 mg. promethazine (Phenergan) and 50 mg. pethidine in 250 ml. 5 per cent dextrose is

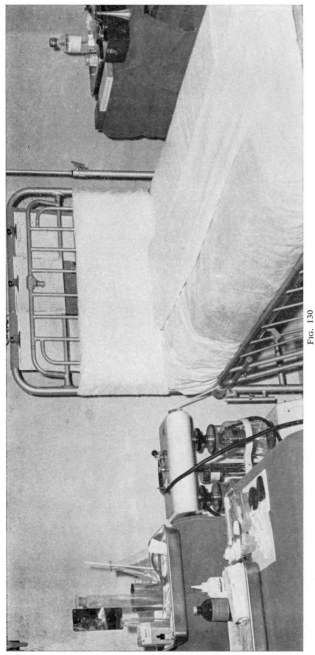

Fig. 130

Room Set Up for the Admission of an Eclamptic Patient.

Oxygen on tap; electric suction apparatus with disposable catheters; oral hygiene tray; rubber teeth wedge; airways; vaginal examination pack; Hibitane 1-2000; obstetric antiseptic cream; gloves; emergency delivery pack; sphygmomanometer; binaural stethoscope; fetal stethoscope; disposable fluid administration set; drip stand; drugs, syringes and needles. Head of bed padded with two bolsters and draw sheet.

(Simpson Memorial Maternity Pavilion, Edinburgh.)

given intravenously: the first half is run in quickly, the second half at 13 ml. (200 drops) per minute. **A second solution containing 100 mg. chlorpromazine; 50 mg. pethidine** in 250 ml. of 5 per cent dextrose is given intravenously at 2·6 ml. (40 drops) per minute. **Two hours later** 50 mg. chlorpromazine and 50 mg. pethidine may be given intramuscularly every 4 to 6 hours for 48 hours. The fetal condition must be closely supervised.

The prescribing of drugs is the doctor's responsibility, but the midwife must report to him when the narcotics administered do not produce the necessary degree of narcosis. Restlessness ought not to be allowed to develop, and as soon as the effect of the drug is wearing off (usually in about three hours) the dose is repeated or some other sedative given.

BROMETHOL

Avertin

Avertin is used when the onset of convulsions seems imminent and in cases of established eclampsia prior to, during, or after labour. It is given rectally.

DOSAGE AND EFFECT OF AVERTIN

The dose of Avertin is 0·1 ml. per kg. body-weight and the amount necessary is calculated on the assessed weight of the woman. The usual dose of Avertin fluid for an average-sized pregnant woman 63·5 kg. (140 lb.) is approximately 6 ml.

Avertin takes effect in about 10 to 15 minutes and the patient usually sleeps quietly for three or four hours.

The second dose is given when the woman becomes restless and moves when spoken to, but not within three hours of the first dose; it may not be necessary to give a third dose for a period of six or eight hours and a total of four doses is usually adequate. As a rule the acute phase has passed within 48 hours, so the administration of Avertin is rarely prolonged beyond that period.

Avertin does not produce excitement during the induction, and other sedative drugs can be used in conjunction with it. The blood pressure falls, and this is of great value in eclampsia. It does not diminish kidney secretion, nor produce respiratory depression and cyanosis or vomiting. **Further convulsions seldom occur.**

Requirements:

1 **Bottle Avertin.**
1 **Jug tap water, 500 ml.**
1 **Graduated glass measure, 150 ml.**
1 **Graduated glass measure, 10 ml.**
Rectal catheter and funnel.

1 **Empty flask 1,000 ml. to mix and shake solution.** 1 **Solution thermometer.**
1 **Bottle Congo red 1 in 1,000.**
1 **Minim dropper for Congo red.**
1 **Test tube for Congo red test.**

Avertin is diluted 1 in 40 with water at not less than 32·2° C. (90° F.) and not more than 40° C. (104° F.) then vigorously shaken. Five millilitres of the diluted solution should be tested by adding a few drops of Congo red 1 in 1,000 before the remainder of the solution is administered. If the result is orange red the solution is suitable, but if bluish it has been overheated or it contains products of decomposition and should not be used.

Avertin must be given before it cools as it does not remain in solution below 32·2° C. (90° F.).

Methylamphetamine (Methedrine), 10 to 20 mg., should be available to counteract any rapid fall in blood pressure.

To avoid moving the woman unnecessarily the injection may be given, and success-fully retained, when she is lying on her right side, if the foot of the bed is raised. A pad is held over the anus for five minutes after the rectal catheter is withdrawn. It is not essential to give an enema prior to the administration of Avertin.

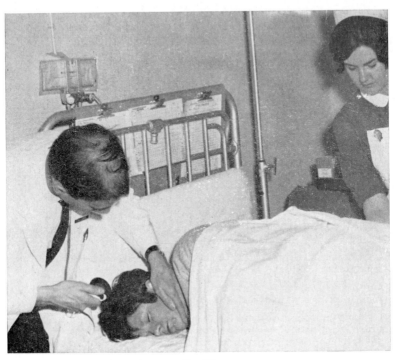

Fig. 131

Note rubber wedge in doctor's hand to insert between the teeth should a convulsion occur.
Cotton wool in patient's ears to exclude noise.
(*Simpson Memorial Maternity Pavilion, Edinburgh.*)

DRUGS AND SUBSTANCES THAT MAY BE ORDERED

The total fluid given in 24 hours should not exceed 2,000 ml. and in oliguric patients and in the presence of pulmonary œdema it should be restricted to 500 ml. per day.

Magnesium sulphate is rarely used now (intravenously or intramuscularly).

Anti-hypertensive drugs are used less frequently.

Protoveratrine (Puroverine) may be given by intramuscular injection or intravenous drip infusion: close supervision is essential. **When giving veratrone derivatives the blood pressure must be recorded hourly** and the doctor notified if it falls below 140 systolic or should vomiting or bradycardia occur.

Antibiotics are administered, when necessary, to combat respiratory infection.

Cardiac and respiratory stimulants may be required, and should be at hand, *e.g.*

Methylamphetamine (Methedrine), 10 to 30 mg.   Digoxin, 0·5 mg.

Nikethamide, 2 to 4 ml.

EQUIPMENT REQUIRED

Sphygmomanometer and binaural stethoscope.   Pinard's fetal-heart stethoscope.

Oxygen and polythene face mask.   Suction apparatus.

Blocks for foot of bed.   Kidney basin and gauze wipes for vomitus.

Tracheostomy set.   Mechanical syringe pump

Anæsthetic tray with spatula, airways, swab-holders and gauze swabs.

Intravenous pack—sterile syringes and needles for giving large and small injections. Flasks of dextrose; distilled water.

A feeding cup, water and fruit juice are needed for the conscious patient.

It is advisable to deliver the woman in the quiet room in which she is being nursed, so a trolley with emergency delivery supplies and a cot should be at hand, as well as equipment for resuscitation of the baby.

TRANSFER OF THE PATIENT TO HOSPITAL

The " flying squad " is summoned and it is a distinct advantage when the obstetrician and midwife have had special experience in dealing with eclamptic patients.

A sedative should be administered 30 minutes before moving the patient; she must be deeply under the effect of bromethol (Avertin) or morphine.

Adequate preparations for the journey should be made, because lack of sedation, warmth or equipment may prejudice the woman's chance of recovery.

To ensure warmth, the stretcher is brought into the house; blankets and pillows heated. The doors of the ambulance ought to be closed and the heater turned on during this time. The ambulance driver is instructed to drive carefully over rough roads.

Dentures and hair pins are removed.

Equipment for the journey.—The midwife should take with her a basin and towels in case the woman should vomit, a padded spoon, and her delivery bag.

The midwife must accompany her patient to hospital, and no one can absolve her from that professional and moral duty. The author is aware of three cases in which unconscious eclamptic patients arrived in hospital by ambulance with only a relative in charge, and in one instance dentures had not been removed.

ADMISSION OF AN ECLAMPTIC PATIENT

1. **No treatment should be carried out until the newly admitted patient is under the influence of sedatives or narcotics ordered by the doctor.**

2. **The blood pressure,** temperature, pulse and respirations are taken and recorded.

3. **The vulva is shaved or clipped and swabbed.**

4. **A self-retaining catheter is inserted** (with closed drainage system or air-sealed polythene bag to reduce the risk of infection). **A specimen of urine is obtained and examined for protein, bile, casts and red cells. Esbach's proteinometer is set up.**

5. The mouth is cleansed.

6. No enema or suppository should be given until the acute convulsive stage is under control, which is usually within 48 hours.

7. The full admission bed-bath is postponed for 24 hours or longer.

OBSTETRICAL MANAGEMENT

Many patients go into labour spontaneously after the onset of eclampsia, and delivery is usually accomplished quickly and easily. Low forceps are sometimes applied to shorten the second stage or to eliminate the need for pushing which may instigate another convulsion.

Induction by Syntocinon drip may be necessary; accurately controlled by syringe pump.

Cæsarean section may be considered advisable.

The anæsthetic commonly used in hospital is nitrous oxide and oxygen given by an obstetric anæsthetist; sodium thiopentone 0·25 G. (Pentothal) may be used to induce anæsthesia.

AFTER DELIVERY

The woman is deeply sedated for 24 hours. A sedative such as amylobarbitone sodium (Sodium Amytal) 500 or papaveretum 20 mg. may be given on the completion of labour. Some give the drug that was administered during labour, *e.g.* bromethol (Avertin), " Lytic cocktail ". A nurse should be in constant attendance until the acute stage is past and all serious signs have abated; the woman should also be conscious, and 48 hours ought to have elapsed with no convulsions.

Mental confusion and impairment of vision may exist for a few days.

Breast feeding is contra-indicated.

The period of convalescence should be extended until the blood pressure and proteinuria are much reduced, although both may persist for some weeks.

NURSING CARE

Good nursing is an important factor in saving the patient's life, and in few instances are experience, efficiency and devotion to duty more necessary than in nursing the woman with eclampsia.

Quietness is essential.—A single room should be set up for the nursing of an eclamptic patient and must be well removed from the telephone bell and other noises. The locker top and all trays are covered with towels. The midwife must work and speak quietly. **Cotton wool plugs in the patient's ears will help to exclude noise until adequate sedation is achieved.**

Sufficient light for observation of changes in the patient's condition should be provided. If the room is too dark, lights must be flashed on in order to carry out treatment, and this is likely to provoke fits. The unconscious or sedated woman is not disturbed by ordinary light nearly so much as by noise.

PROTECTION FROM INJURY

The top of the bed should be padded, and two bolsters, held securely in position with a draw-sheet pinned at the back, are most efficient. If the midwife is alone, it would be advisable for her to push the bed alongside the wall and to place pillows down that side. Any attempt to limit the convulsive movements should be by guiding rather than forcibly restraining them.

The woman must never be left alone for one instant, in case she might take a fit; she may also roll out of bed while in her confused state of mind.

To prevent biting of the tongue, a rubber wedge is useful, and should be placed between the back teeth during the premonitory phase of the fit and before the jaws are clenched. Rubber has sufficient elasticity to prevent jarring. Two wooden spatulæ, bound with a gauze bandage, make a useful substitute; in an emergency the handle of a spoon wrapped in a towel can be used. An unpadded metal spatula

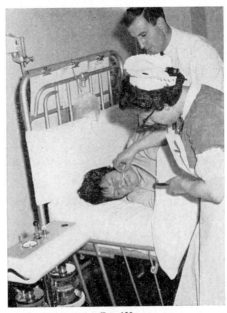

FIG. 132

USE OF ELECTRIC SUCTION TO KEEP AIRWAY CLEAR.
Simpson Memorial Maternity Pavilion, Edinburgh.)

or spoon is too hard, and care must be taken to avoid breaking the patient's teeth by not forcing them apart while clenched. A pencil, cork, or substance that can be bitten off should not be used, in case part of it is inhaled into the trachea.

It is not advisable to pull the tongue forwards with forceps, as it will then be bitten; neither should a mouth gag be used, in case the jaw might be dislocated, and because saliva cannot be swallowed when the mouth is wide open.

Dentures should have been removed; pins in the hair ought to have been taken out.

KEEPING THE AIRWAY CLEAR

During and after a convulsion the woman may inhale saliva, so she should be propped over on to her right side, to allow the saliva to drain out of her mouth. If on her back, her tongue may block the larynx and produce asphyxia; cyanosis must also be avoided for the sake of the fetus.

Suction apparatus is excellent and a Guedel airway facilitates the removal of mucus : if not available a swab on a swab-holder is used to mop out the fluid that collects between cheek and teeth.

SUMMARY OF CARE DURING A FIT

Place a rubber wedge or substitute between the patient's teeth.

Send for medical aid without leaving the patient.

Turn the woman on her right side; pillow behind shoulders.

Keep a clear airway; use suction apparatus or mop out saliva.

Do not forcibly restrain the convulsive movements.

Oxygen should be given.

PULMONARY ŒDEMA

Pulmonary œdema is not caused by the inhalation of saliva but is due to failure of the heart and of the pulmonary circulation as well as to a generalized state of œdema.

In serious cases of pulmonary œdema the woman is propped up. If necessary a tracheostomy is performed, an endotracheal tube passed and fluid withdrawn by very brief periods of suction (short sharp sucks). Oxygen may be given by positive pressure.

Frusemide (Lasix). 20 mg. I.V. is efficacious in acute pulmonary œdema.

NURSING CARE AFTER A FIT

Oxygen is given for five minutes after each fit, or longer if cyanosis persists, to meet the needs of the fetus and to relieve the right side of the heart.

1. POSITION OF THE PATIENT

The woman is drowsy, dazed, or comatose, so she is placed in the right semi-prone position, obliquely across the bed, with her head at the edge of the mattress. In this position saliva can drain out, for with deep stertorous breathing there is grave danger of the inhalation of mucus and saliva. The jaw is held forwards if necessary.

The patient is turned at intervals of at least 2 hours to avoid hypostatic congestion of the lungs.

2. WORK SHOULD BE PLANNED

Any necessary treatment ought to be carried out immediately after a fit, while the patient is unconscious, or postponed until half an hour after a sedative has been administered. Incessant handling is not good nursing, and all non-essential treatment should be eliminated.

She should not (unless specifically told to do so) take the blood pressure oftener than every hour, the fetal heart rate oftener than every one or two hours. Work should be carried out expeditiously yet gently, two midwives (*sometimes three*) being required for major nursing procedures.

3. ORAL HYGIENE

The mouth and nostrils should be cleansed after each fit, or every three hours, because a septic mouth increases the risk of aspiration pneumonia.

4. THE BLADDER

A self-retaining catheter (with water seal or air-sealed polythene bag) may be inserted for the following reasons:

(*a*) **It causes less disturbance to the patient** than repeatedly passing catheters, changing wet beds, or trying to get a semi-conscious woman to pass urine.

(*b*) **The kidney output can be accurately measured.**

(*c*) **A specimen of urine can be obtained for analysis as required.**

An Esbach's or a biochemical quantitative test for protein is carried out daily.

5. THE BOWELS

Neither enema, suppository nor laxative is given until the acute convulsive stage is under control, which is usually within 48 hours.

6. BED-BATHING

Although a daily sponge bath is desirable for many reasons, it is wise to postpone the first bath until at least 24 hours after admission. During this time, face, hands, groins and buttocks can be washed. Every precaution is taken to avoid chilling the patient.

7. NO FLUID BY MOUTH

Not even one teaspoonful to moisten the tongue should be given to an unconscious patient; the swallowing reflex may be absent, and the fluid will run into the trachea. **Any necessary fluid is given intravenously.**

8. OBSERVATION

The midwife must note the following:

    (*a*) CONVULSIONS.

    (*b*) SIGNS OF LABOUR.

    (*c*) THE GENERAL CONDITION of the woman, including serious signs.

(*a*) **The premonitory signs** of an eclamptic fit are described on page 176. **The number, length, severity and time of occurrence must be recorded.**

(*b*) SIGNS OF LABOUR

    (1) **Restlessness** or moaning when accompanied by uterine contractions can be taken as a sign of labour.

    (2) **Show,** and rupture of the membranes.

    (3) **On vaginal or rectal examination, the os will be dilated.** (*It is usual for labour to start soon after convulsions occur, unless the woman is very heavily sedated.*)

(*c*) THE GENERAL CONDITION OF THE WOMAN

The midwife must note and record the following points, but there is no agreement among obstetricians as to how frequently such observations should be made.

    (1) **The pulse** should be taken every 15 minutes, as this can be done without disturbing the patient.

    (2) **The temperature** is usually taken every four hours and may rise to 38·8° C. 102° F.) after a succession of fits or if respiratory infection is present.

    (3) **The respirations** are charted every 15 minutes.

Slow Respirations (below 12) may be due to cerebral hæmorrhage.

Rapid Respirations may indicate a pulmonary infection, especially if associated with a rising temperature and pulse.

Moist Respirations may be a sign of pulmonary œdema.

(4) **Blood pressure.**—Every one or two hours would seem a reasonable time, but when a drug is given which causes the blood pressure to fall, or when it is very high, estimations may be made more frequently. The arm band can be left loosely in position. A fall in blood pressure may denote an improvement in the woman's condition, and this often follows death of the fetus. If accompanied by cyanosis and cold extremities, it indicates cardiac failure.

(5) **The fetal heart rate** may be taken every one, two or three hours, but the woman should not be disturbed unnecessarily to do so, as very little can be done if fetal distress occurs.

(6) **The colour of the woman** may be dusky, due to cyanosis, and is an indication for the administration of oxygen. An icteric tinge may be due to liver damage.

(7) **Urine.**—The colour of the urine may be dark brown because of its high concentration and the presence of blood.

(8) **Fluid balance.**—An exact record of kidney output must be kept, as well as the intake by mouth or intravenously, and when gross œdema is lessening, the output may be double or treble the amount of the intake for a few days. Bladder distension should be looked for at this period of diuresis. An output of 800 ml. in 24 hours is considered to be a favourable sign.

Anuria is a serious sign, and may indicate the onset of acute renal failure. For treatment, see page 203.

(9) **Œdema** is recorded by a series of + signs, *e.g.*:

Date		7th	8th	9th	10th
O	Face	++	+	trace	trace
E	Hands	+++	++	+	trace
D of	Feet	++++	+++	+++	++
E	Legs	+++	++	++	+
M	Sacrum	+++	+++	+++	++
A					

SERIOUS SIGNS OF ECLAMPSIA

1. **Over 20,** or **rapid fits.** (Patients have recovered who have had 40 fits.)
2. **Pulmonary œdema.**   3. **Jaundice.**
4. **Pulse over 120**—thready.   5. **Anuria.**
6. **Temperature over 39·4° C. (103° F.).**

SUMMARY OF COMPLICATIONS OF ECLAMPSIA

1. **Cerebral:** hæmorrhage, thrombosis, mental confusion.
2. **Hepatic:** liver damage.
3. **Injuries:** to tongue, fractures.
4. **Cardiac:** myocardial failure.
5. **Renal:** acute failure.
6. **Visual:** temporary blindness.
7. **Respiratory:** asphyxia, pulmonary œdema, broncho-pneumonia.
8. **Fetal:** anoxia; stillbirth.

THE CAUSE OF DEATH

Death is most commonly due to **cerebral hæmorrhage, myocardial failure, pulmonary œdema** or **acute renal failure.** The woman may die of aspiration broncho-pneumonia or from asphyxia during a convulsion, but in both these instances the midwife can do much to prevent their occurrence.

The maternal mortality rate depends on the severity of the condition and whether treatment is started promptly. With expert care the death rate will be as low as 2 per cent, but when prenatal supervision is perfunctory and the treatment of eclampsia unsatisfactory the mortality will range between 12 and 15 per cent.

The perinatal mortality varies between 10 and 30 per cent.

IT SHOULD BE THE AIM OF EVERY MIDWIFE TO PREVENT THE OCCURRENCE OF ECLAMPSIA.

ESSENTIAL HYPERTENSION

Essential hypertension may be defined as an elevation of blood pressure over 140/90 present on two or more occasions prior to the 20th week of pregnancy, which is not due to any apparent pathological condition. It seems to be an inherited characteristic in about 80 per cent of cases.

The hypertensive woman is liable to develop pre-eclampsia. Fetus and placenta may both be small.

MANAGEMENT

MILD CASES

When the blood pressure is not over 150/90 the woman may be treated at home. She is advised regarding the great need for additional rest, *i.e.* two hours during the day and 10 hours at night. To ensure sound sleep a sedative is usually prescribed: salt restriction and the necessity for weight control is explained.

The woman ought to be seen and weighed every week, a careful check on blood pressure being maintained. The development of signs of pre-eclampsia or a sudden rise in blood pressure would indicate the need for admission to hospital.

All patients with essential hypertension are admitted to hospital not later than the 38th week of pregnancy.

SEVERE CASES

The woman may have to spend long periods in hospital to ensure complete bed rest, weight control and salt restriction.

Urinary œstriol assays are made weekly in some centres on two consecutive days after the 30th week, to detect feto-placental dysfunction.

Sedatives are prescribed to promote emotional tranquillity during the day and sound sleep at night.

Anti-hypertensive drugs may benefit the patient but they do not reduce the peri-natal loss. *Methyldopa* (Aldomet), dose 250 mg. orally t.i.d., is useful when the blood pressure is unduly high.

INDUCTION OF LABOUR

The likelihood of intra-uterine death is kept in mind when the blood pressure remains persistently high. For the multigravid woman with a bad obstetric history, labour is usually induced at the 36th week. Puncture of membranes and oxytocin intravenous drip are usually employed.

Early in labour. Amylobarbitone sodium (Sodium Amytal), 200 mg., or cyclobarbitone, 200 mg., may be prescribed.

Care during labour is similar to that given in pre-eclampsia: ergometrine is not usually prescribed; any amylobarbitone sodium (Sodium Amytal), 200 mg. or morphine 15 mg., is administered on the completion of labour.

The older primigravida may be delivered by Cæsarean section at 36 to 37 weeks to ensure a live infant.

QUESTIONS FOR REVISION

HYPEREMESIS GRAVIDARUM

Define hyperemesis gravidarum. What could a midwife do to prevent it ?

State why the following substances are prescribed in hyperemesis: (1) fluid; (2) glucose; (3) isotonic saline; (*d*) promazine hydrochloride; (*e*) calcium gluconate; (*f*) vitamin B; why should vomitus not be recorded under " output ".

Outline a suitable diet for the first day when feeding is recommenced. What records should be kept ? **Give five serious signs.**

C.M.B.(N. Ireland) paper.—A patient is admitted to hospital with vomiting in early pregnancy. Describe the nursing care and treatment which will be carried out.

C.M.B.(N. Ireland) paper.—Define hyperemesis gravidarum. Indicate the signs and symptoms which would cause concern. Outline the treatment.

C.M.B.(Scot.) paper.—Give the management of a case of Hyperemesis.

PRE-ECLAMPSIA—ECLAMPSIA

Give six sites where œdema may be detected. **Give six** prodromal signs of eclampsia.

Name three conditions in pregnancy often associated with pre-eclampsia

What effect does placental dysfunction have on the fetus ?

How do you set up an Esbach's test for proteinuria ?

What precautions would you take prior to transferring a patient suffering from eclampsia to hospital ?

How would you suspect that an unconscious woman was in labour ?

What nursing care may be necessary in cases of pulmonary œdema ?

Pre-eclampsia may occur prior to the .... week; more commonly from the .... to the .... week.

Urinary œstriol assays are made after the .... week on .... consecutive days every .... or .... weeks.

Pre-eclampsia affects about .... per cent of pregnant women. Uterine .... is reduced placental .... and I.U.G.R. are common.

State why the following are prescribed: rest in bed,...............................; sedation ....; low carbohydrate diet ....; œstriol assay ....

What should be reported to the doctor when the following drugs are being administered ? Methyldopa; morphine; bromethol (Avertin); Protoveratrine.

STATE " WHY "

1. You would suspect that an unconscious woman was in labour.

2. An eclamptic patient should not be nursed in a dark room.

3. **Postmaturity is dangerous** in cases of pre-eclampsia.

4. (*a*) **Oxygen is given following a convulsion**; (*b*) the right semi-prone position is preferred after a fit; (*c*) the patient's ears are plugged; (*d*) **a mouth gag should not be used**; (*e*) **rubber is an ideal substance for a wedge to place between the teeth.**

Write not more than 10 lines on:

1. Care of an eclamptic patient (*a*) during the journey by ambulance; (*b*) during and immediately after labour; (*c*) during and immediately after a convulsion.

C.M.B.(N. Ireland) paper.—A patient, 36 weeks pregnant, is admitted following an eclamptic fit. Describe your preparations for the admission of this patient and her subsequent nursing care.

C.M.B.(Scot.) paper.—Describe an eclamptic fit. How would you manage a case of eclampsia pending the arrival of a doctor?

C.M.B.(Eng.) paper, 1969.—What are the signs of pre-eclampsia ? What are the dangers of this condition and how may they be avoided ?

C.M.B.(Scot.) paper, 1969.—What is pre-eclampsia ? Describe the management of a patient with this condition.

C.M.B.(Scot.) paper.—Describe an eclamptic fit and outline briefly the management of a patient with eclampsia.

C.M.B.(Eng.) paper, 1970.—What are the dangers of raised blood-pressure to the mother and the fetus during pregnancy ?

12

Diseases associated with Pregnancy

Systemic diseases may become aggravated during pregnancy and so endanger the Woman's life that the pregnancy must be terminated; others cause abortion or stillbirth. They are responsible for a considerable number of maternal deaths.

CARDIAC DISEASE

The main causes of heart disease in childbearing women are rheumatic infection, and congenital lesions. During pregnancy the increased blood volume and body weight put a severe strain on an impaired heart, so that a certain amount of deterioration may be anticipated in the majority of cases.

THERE ARE FOUR FUNCTIONAL GRADES :

GRADE 1

These women make no complaint; the heart lesion is found on physical examination.

GRADE 2

These patients are breathless on moderate exertion. Palpitation and dyspnœa are troublesome and fatigue easily induced; anginal pain may occur. They are unable to do heavy household tasks.

GRADE 3

These patients are distressed on slight exertion such as walking. Climbing stairs or ordinary housework is beyond their capacity. Anginal pain may occur. They are comfortable at rest.

GRADE 4

These patients are in varying degrees of congestive heart failure, they are distressed and breathless, with anginal pain even when at rest in bed. The slightest physical activity increases their discomfort.

MANAGEMENT OF PREGNANCY

These patients are referred to the Cardiologist; radiological and electrocardiographic evidence give accurate information re the cardiac lesion

The main causes of deterioration in cardiac patients are anæmia, respiratory infections, insomnia, overweight and overwork. Such conditions must therefore be avoided. For the common cold Grades 1 and 2 should go to bed; Grade 3 should be admitted to hospital. Dental extractions should be avoided.

Weight control is essential in all cases.

Sleep and rest are of fundamental importance for ambulant patients, *i.e.* 10 hours at night and two hours during the afternoon being necessary. No heavy work should be attempted and exercise that induces breathlessness or exhaustion must be avoided.

Anæmia is treated by the administration of a ferrous preparation which is well tolerated, *e.g.* Fersamal, and if the hæmoglobin level is below 10·3 G. (70 per cent) the woman should be admitted to hospital.

Induction of premature labour is not advocated as no additional cardiac stress occurs during the last four weeks of pregnancy.

Mitral valvulotomy has been successfully performed in certain patients, the pregnancy having subsequently continued to term. Recent advances in surgical and anæsthetic techniques have considerably lessened the danger of operating after the 12th week.

GRADES 1 AND 2

Women who are in Grades 1 or 2 are seen every one or two weeks at the cardiac clinic by the obstetrician and cardiologist, admitted for one week's rest prior to term and delivered in hospital.

GRADE 3

Those who are in Grade 3 should have their ordinary activities curtailed. Complete bed rest is essential from the 23rd to the 32nd week when the strain on the heart is greatest. They remain in hospital for delivery.

GRADE 4

For Grade 4 patients complete rest in bed is imperative. They will spend most of their pregnancy in hospital, and will be delivered there.

SIGNS AND SYMPTOMS OF ACUTE HEART FAILURE:

1. INTENSE BREATHLESSNESS.
2. CYANOSIS.
3. RAPID OR IRREGULAR PULSE.

4. COLD SWEATING EXTREMITIES.
5. COUGH WITH BLOOD-STAINED SPUTUM.
6. PULMONARY ŒDEMA.

Treatment of Acute Heart Failure

Maintenance doses of digoxin or digitoxin are administered. When œdema is present **frusemide** (Lasix), 80 mg., may be given daily or on alternate days. For attacks of breathlessness frusemide and oxygen are prescribed. Aminophylline, 250 mg., given slowly intravenously is useful to relieve bronchospasm.

For pulmonary œdema the patient is propped up: morphine, 15 mg., and oxygen are usually necessary. The mechanical aspirator is useful to remove frothy mucus and maintain a clear airway.

Obstetrical operative treatment is never carried out during acute heart failure; Cæsarean section is rarely advocated unless indications other than cardiac disease are manifest; sterilization, if indicated, is usually performed during the puerperium.

NURSING CARE

This is similar to what is given to non-pregnant patients in congestive heart failure and includes suitable diet, warmth and the avoidance of any exertion.

A **single room is an advantage,** and two midwives should assist with all major nursing procedures; a back-rest and arm-pillows are usually necessary but the woman should be allowed to adopt the position in which she is most comfortable.

Sedatives are imperative, such as papaveretum (Omnopon), 20 mg., or amylo-barbitone sodium (sodium amytal), 200 mg., to ensure sound sleep at night. To produce mental calm and physical comfort during the day dichloralphenazone 1·3 G. (Welldorm) is useful.

Fluid may occasionally be restricted to 1,200 ml. daily, and a fluid balance chart kept; a salt-poor diet is served when œdema is present.

The apex beat is recorded hourly or as directed by the physician.

To prevent venous thrombosis anæmia is treated; the physiotherapist gives gentle massage and encourages leg movement in long-term cases.

Simple remedies are often efficacious in treating the minor ailments which add so much to the woman's discomfort, *i.e.*, nausea, heartburn and flatulence.

MANAGEMENT OF LABOUR

Labour tends to be shorter in cardiac patients, particularly the second stage: prolonged or difficult labour should not be permitted.

THE FIRST STAGE

Dichloralphenazone (Welldorm) 2 G. is given early in labour to allay anxiety. Pethidine, 100 mg., is usually prescribed, but morphine or papaveretum (Omnopon) may be necessary to provide adequate sedation. Continuous epidural anaesthesia has been used with success.

Serious signs should be reported; such as severe breathlessness or increased cyanosis, a pulse over 110 and respirations over 24. (*The pulse and respirations should be recorded every* 15 *minutes in graph form.*)

THE SECOND STAGE

The patient should adopt the position she prefers, but should be sitting up if she is distressed, and given oxygen continuously. Pushing will embarrass the heart, so it should not be permitted; an episiotomy is made under local anæsthesia to shorten the perineal phase. The doctor will apply low forceps for distress or delay, preferably under pudendal nerve block or perineal infiltration. The lithotomy position increases the load on the heart, so ought to be avoided. Nitrous oxide and oxygen should be administered by an obstetric anæsthetist.

THE THIRD STAGE

To avoid the collapse which sometimes follows expulsion of the baby, the hand is laid firmly on the abdomen, above the umbilicus, to increase abdominal pressure. Drugs such as nikethamide, digoxin and methylamphetamine hydrochlor (Methedrine) should be at hand. Collapse may also occur when the retracted uterus returns blood to the general circulation and temporarily overloads the heart. Ergometrine is usually only administered when needed to control hæmorrhage. (Some believe that the administration of 0·25 mg. ergometrine I.M. is less hazardous than severe blood loss.)

Sedatives are essential after labour and morphine, 15 mg., is usually given. In order to procure rest and quietness the woman should be nursed in a single room; further sedation and vigilant, skilful, nursing care is necessary.

THE PUERPERIUM

To avoid bacterial endocarditis, puerperal sepsis and respiratory infection must be prevented. The temperature should be taken four-hourly during the first few days in order to detect sepsis early.

Movement of the legs is encouraged as soon as possible and graduated exercises are given by the physiotherapist.

Mild cases are ambulant in 5 or 6 days and when heart failure is present, one week after it has cleared up. A period of convalescence should be arranged and help provided with domestic duties when they are resumed.

Contraceptive advice is given to allow the lapse of two years (or longer) between pregnancies. Sterilization may be recommended.

DIABETES

Diabetes is found in about 1 in 200 pregnant women at the Simpson Maternity Pavilion, Edinburgh, most being referred from the diabetic clinic. It may appear for the first time during pregnancy; in fact, pregnancy is one of the factors that may precipitate the onset of diabetes in women genetically predisposed to the disease.

Since the introduction of insulin, the diabetic woman can go through pregnancy and labour in comparative safety, provided she is under the combined care of an obstetrician and a diabetic specialist.

Unfortunately the perinatal rate still remains high, but when strict supervision during pregnancy, delivery at 36 to 38 weeks by induction or Cæsarean section, the services of a pædiatrician and **skilful nursing care are employed,** the perinatal mortality rate should not exceed 8 per cent.

DIAGNOSIS

1. **Obstetric History.**—When a woman has given birth to babies weighing over 4,536 G. (10 lb.) or has had two or more late intra-uterine deaths, investigation of the blood glucose curve is necessary.

This potential diabetic state may indicate that the woman will eventually develop clinical diabetes.

2. **Glycosuria** occurs in approximately 10 per cent of pregnant women (see p. 62), and when more than a trace of glucose is present on two occasions a breakfast containing 100 G. carbohydrates is given and a blood sample withdrawn 2 hours later. Should this contain more than 120 mg. of glucose per 100 ml. a full glucose tolerance test is done. **The glucose tolerance test shows the typical diabetic curve.**

3. **Polyuria** and thirst are diagnostic symptoms. (The woman should be asked if she requires to drink during the night or has a dry mouth in the morning.)

4. **Pruritus vulvæ** is suggestive, but not diagnostic.

THE EFFECT OF DIABETES ON CHILDBEARING

1. *Hydramnios* of slight degree is evident in a large number of cases, and of marked degree in about 25 per cent: when severe the fetal prognosis is poor. Close supervision in hospital is essential.

2. **The incidence of pre-eclampsia** is 3 times higher and may be a factor in causing intra-uterine death. If pre-eclampsia is severe pregnancy is usually terminated.

3. *Large babies* over 3,629 G. (8 lb.) occur in approximately 40 per cent of cases due to the passage of maternal insulin-antagonists through the placenta; this stimulates fetal over-production of insulin which causes increased growth and adiposity of the fetus.

4. **Small babies** under 2,722 G. (6 lb.) are also common due to placental dysfunction.

5. *Intra-uterine death* of the fetus occurs in a number of cases after the 36th week.

6. **The incidence of fetal abnormalities** is said by some to be 5 times higher.

7. *Vaginal moniliasis* may be present.

8. **Ketosis** and diabetic coma may occur, because the woman's glucose tolerance and insulin requirements may change rapidly during pregnancy. But if she has been properly taught how to adjust her own insulin doses according to the results of her home urine tests such complications are rare.

MANAGEMENT

PREGNANCY

The woman is admitted to hospital for reassessment of diabetic control about the 12th week; in many patients the insulin requirements are increased. She should be seen weekly, after the 16th week, by an obstetrician and a diabetic specialist conjointly, and because of the serious consequences of some of the minor disorders of pregnancy it may be necessary for her to come into hospital for such conditions as colds or morning sickness.

A good protein diet is essential.

The woman is again hospitalized not later than the 32nd week or earlier, if required *e.g.* for pre-eclampsia, hypertension or hydramnios, as day-to-day observation is so important from this time onwards. Weekly œstriol assays are made.

An abrupt fall of insulin requirements from the 30th-37th week is an ominous sign; i.e. of impending fetal death.

In pregnancy the renal threshold for glucose may fall, in which case the insulin dosage should be adjusted to keep the urine tests showing ½ to ¾ per cent glycosuria. More reliance is placed on blood glucose than on urine glucose.

CÆSAREAN SECTION

This operation is performed at the 36th to 38th week in the older primigravida, in the multigravid woman with a bad obstetric history, or if the fetus is unduly large. (72 *per cent of diabetic women had Cæsarean section at the Simpson Maternity in* 1969.)

On the day prior to Cæsarean section long-acting insulin is changed to soluble for more precise control. No food, glucose or insulin is given on the morning of operation. An intravenous drip with dextrose and soluble insulin is given; the blood glucose being kept at 120-180 mg. per 100 ml. Ketosis must be avoided. A pædiatrician is present to take charge of the baby.

The mother's blood glucose concentration is determined and during the period between completion of the operation and next morning 120 to 150 G. carbohydrates is given as fluid and light meals. If unable to take food by mouth a 5 per cent dextrose intravenous drip is administered.

Somatomammotrophin (H.C.S.) (placental lactogen), which antagonises insulin from the 8th week of pregnancy, falls 6 hours after delivery so very small doses of insulin, based on blood glucose measurements, are required.

LABOUR

Induction of labour is usual at the 36th to 38th week in the young primigravida and in the multigravid woman whose past and present obstetric history is satisfactory.

Procedure—No breakfast is given. At 8.00 hours the membranes are punctured and an oxytocin drip started. A second drip (in the other arm) administers the prescribed amount of dextrose and insulin depending on the blood glucose level. (Hypoglycaemia must be avoided.)

Sedatives and analgesics that depress the fetal respiratory centre should be avoided.

Delay in labour, i.e. over 12 hours is more serious in the diabetic woman. Should the woman not be approaching delivery at 17.00 hours the situation is reassessed and Cæsarean section considered.

Diabetic women are usually advised to have not more than 3 children.

Care of the Baby (see p. 549).

PULMONARY TUBERCULOSIS

The number of pregnant women found to have pulmonary tuberculosis requiring observation or treatment is now below 0·1 per cent. Routine radiography of pregnant women has now been abandoned in many centres, but if chest radiography is indicated during pregnancy, a large film is to be preferred because of its smaller radiation exposure.

DURING PREGNANCY

These patients should be under the care of an obstetrician and a chest physician who will supervise the chest condition and give such advice as is indicated. A combination of streptomycin, para-aminosalicylic acid (PAS) and isoniazid is still the recommended standard anti-tuberculosis treatment. Two new drugs—ethambutol and rifampicin—appear to be highly effective, and, if further study confirms this, one or other may replace PAS in standard treatment. For secondary anæmia, present only in acute cases, the woman is given the appropriate treatment. A home help will be arranged for and food supplements provided if necessary.

The modern tendency is to allow pregnancy to continue. It has been proved that pregnancy, labour and the puerperium very rarely have any adverse effect on pulmonary tuberculosis, and modern methods rapidly bring under control any deterioration which may occur.

Therapeutic abortion is exceedingly rarely advocated even in advanced cases; severe dyspnœa due to gross destruction of lung tissue, squalid home conditions and exceptional circumstances in which the woman is grossly overworked looking after her family may sometimes be taken into consideration. If evacuation of the uterus is imperative it must be carried out before the 12th week.

The woman in hospital, if the disease is infectious, should be isolated during pregnancy, labour and the puerperium in a bright airy room.

DURING LABOUR

An endeavour should be made to provide maximal rest with the minimum of effort.

Exhaustion must be avoided.—Pethidine may be given, but inhalational analgesia must not be administered by midwives without permission from the chest physician in charge. Special anæsthetic care is required if bronchitis or bronchiectasis is present. Epidural anæsthesia may be employed if a difficult forceps delivery is anticipated.

To eliminate the need for strenuous pushing, an episiotomy is performed under local anæsthesia, and, if necessary, forceps are applied under pudendal nerve block, or perineal infiltration.

Blood loss during the third stage should be minimal.

B.C.G. VACCINATION

If the mother is infectious she should not handle the infant, and he should be segregated until B.C.G. (Bacille Calmette-Guérin) vaccination has been successful or until the mother is non-infectious.

A baby is rarely infected with tuberculosis before birth, so he will be Mantoux negative. After vaccination a small superficial nodule appears on the arm (*which need not be bandaged*) in two or three weeks' time. The presence of a papule is sufficient evidence of successful vaccination, there being no need to carry out a confirmatory tuberculin test at six weeks.

The infant may be discharged after B.C.G. vaccination when the Mantoux test is converted from negative to positive, usually in six or eight weeks, but if the Mantoux test is not positive within three months the vaccination is repeated.

In situations where separation of mother and baby is impossible, the infant may be given isoniazid, 25 mg. in syrup twice daily and immunized with isoniazid-resistant B.C.G. vaccine.

THE SOCIAL ASPECT

Tuberculosis is a social and economic problem. Although the woman may give birth to two or three children without deterioration in her condition, the hard work involved in child-rearing may prove to be even more detrimental than childbearing. Extra help in the home is necessary for 3 months. It may be desirable that contraceptive advice is given, or sterilization may be performed after the birth of 2 or 3 children depending on the extent of the disease.

The possibility of infection of the baby when the father at home suffers from active pulmonary tuberculosis is a problem that requires attention.

ANÆMIA

Anæmia is common in childbearing women, and particularly in multiparæ of the lower income group. Many are anæmic before they become pregnant, so it is essential that the condition is diagnosed at the beginning of pregnancy and treated effectively.

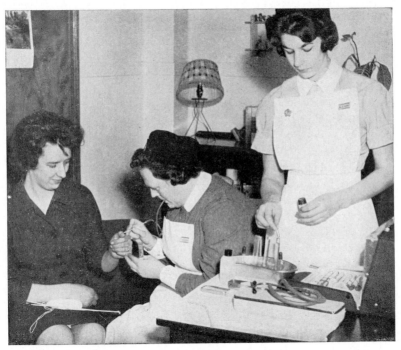

FIG. 133

DISTRICT SISTER TAKING BLOOD: STUDENT MIDWIFE EXAMINING URINE IN PATIENT'S HOME.

With a hæmoglobin pipette 0·02 ml. of blood is withdrawn and mixed with 4 ml. of 0·04 per cent ammonia or cyanmethœmoglobin solution in a stoppered glass tube. Subsequently read by photoelectric colorimeter.

(*Simpson Memorial Maternity Pavilion, Edinburgh.*)

HÆMOGLOBIN ESTIMATION IS MADE

1. When the woman first comes to book and at each subsequent visit if necessary.

2. At the 32nd week and at the 36th week as a check that the hæmoglobin is at a safe level for labour.

A minimal hæmoglobin of 10·3 G. (70 per cent) is the usual standard for anæmia.

A 10 per cent reduction in hæmoglobin occurs during pregnancy because of the physiological increase in blood plasma; the pregnant woman also loses 500 mg. of iron to the fetus and placenta.

Most authorities consider that all pregnant women should receive iron, *e.g.* ferrous sulphate, 180 mg. (gr. 3) t.i.d., throughout pregnancy, others give iron when the hæmoglobin level is below 12·6 G. (85 per cent) and repeat the hæmoglobin test at each subsequent visit until a satisfactory level is reached.

MINOR DEGREES OF FOLIC ACID DEFICIENCY

Minor degrees of folic acid deficiency occur in 26 per cent of pregnant women particularly the multigravida over 30 years of age and in cases of multiple pregnancy.

Folic acid is necessary for the normal development of red blood cells in bone marrow; liver, kidney and green vegetables in the diet are good sources.

At many prenatal clinics folic acid, 0·5 mg., is prescribed daily, in addition to iron throughout pregnancy as a prophylactic measure.

Fefol contains ferrous sulphate, 150 mg., and folic acid, 0·5 mg., one capsule daily.

EFFECTS OF ANÆMIA

(1) **It undermines the woman's general health,** saps her vitality and deprives her of the energy needed for her household duties and outdoor recreation.

(2) **Other complications of pregnancy are rendered more severe.**

(3) **Oxygen transport at placental level is impaired.**

(4) **Signs of exsanguination ensue after normal blood loss.**

(5) **Collapse occurs more readily** following moderate hæmorrhage.

(6) **Shock, whatever the cause, is more severe.**

(7) **Venous thrombosis is predisposed to.**

(8) **The morbidity rate is increased.**

(9) **It is a contributory cause of maternal deaths.**

MICROCYTIC OR IRON DEFICIENCY ANÆMIA

CAUSES

1. **Menstrual loss** between pregnancies, especially if profuse.

2. **Dietary deficiency,** *e.g.* low protein and iron intake.

3. **Imperfect absorption of iron,** often associated with hypochlorhydria, which is aggravated by the ingestion of alkalis, *e.g.* for heartburn.

4. **Withdrawal of iron by the fetus** for its immediate and future needs.

5. **Loss of blood during third stage of labour.**

6. HOOK WORM INFECTION

This cause of anæmia is found in malnourished immigrants from tropical countries. The hook worm enters the tissues through the sole of the foot (when shoes are not worn) and the larvæ find their way to the intestine. When ova are found in the patient's stool Alcopar is prescribed: one sachet, 5 G. in water by mouth, repeated on three successive days if necessary. Food is withheld for 2 hours after giving Alcopar. Oral iron is continued for 3 months after the hæmoglobin has reached normal levels.

SIGNS AND SYMPTOMS OF ANÆMIA

1. **Pallor of mucous membranes.**   4. **Palpitation** and rapid pulse in some cases
2. **Lassitude** (always tired).   5. **Poor appetite,** gastro-intestinal upsets.
3. **Breathlessness.**

Treatment

Mild cases of anæmia respond well to the oral administration of medicinal iron but digestive disturbances and constipation may occur. *All iron tablets should be taken after meals with a little water.* A diet rich in first class proteins, vitamins C and B$_2$, iron and other minerals should also be partaken. The need for fresh air and sunshine ought to be stressed.

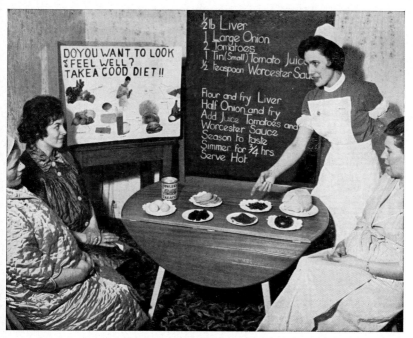

FIG. 134

Staff nurse giving talk-demonstration in prenatal ward sitting-room to patients being treated for anæmia. Foods exhibited :—Liver: red meat: brown bread: eggs: prunes: raisins: treacle: green vegetable. (*Royal Maternity Hospital, Rottenrow, Glasgow.*)

Ferrous sulphate tablets, 180 mg. t.i.d., are effective and cheap: some give one daily dose of folic acid, 300 μg. throughout pregnancy.

Ferrous iron 40 mg., folic acid 200 μg. one tablet t.i.d.

Ferrous gluconate (Cerevon), ferrous succinate (Ferromyn) and ferrous fumarate (Fersamal) are readily absorbed, and well tolerated. **Rarical** contains iron, calcium and aneurin. Pregfol contains ferrous sulphate 200 mg. and folic acid 0·5 mg.: one daily = prophylaxis.

Pregamal, which contains ferrous fumarate, 200 mg., and folic acid, 100 μg. (one tab. t.i.d.), is given as a prophylactic measure for folate deficiency in some centres throughout pregnancy.

When the hæmoglobin is below 9·6 G. (65 per cent) more detailed expert blood investigation is required and the woman admitted to hospital.

Intravenous Imferon

In cases where the hæmoglobin is below 10·3 G. (70 per cent) and response to oral iron is poor or time limited a total dose of iron dextran is given by intravenous infusion. Any other form of iron therapy is withheld for two days prior to the administration of imferon.

The woman is admitted to hospital for one day, six to eight hours being required for the infusion and one hour for supervision afterwards.

Imferon is administered in sterile i otonic saline and if the dose exceeds 25 ml. it is divided equally between two vacolitres of 540 ml. saline. The first 100 ml. are administered slowly (20 drops per minute) as a test dose and if no reaction occurs increased to 45 drops. Isotonic saline, 200 ml., is given following the Imferon infusion.

A transfusion of whole blood or packed cells is always given when the hæmoglobin is dangerously low, especially when the time of labour is approaching, *i.e.* at about the 36th week of pregnancy. Slow administration and careful supervision is necessary.

THE MIDWIVES' RESPONSIBILITY

Midwives have an important part to play in the prevention of iron deficiency anæmia.

1. **By taking blood in the homes to test the hæmoglobin,** anæmia can be detected (see Fig. 133).

2. **Explaining to pregnant women some of the reasons why they become anæmic:** how they can try to prevent this by taking a wholesome diet with adequate amounts of body-building foods and those rich in iron such as liver, meat and brown bread, as well as vitamin C in citrus fruits and green vegetables: urging them to take regularly the tablets prescribed by the doctor.

3. **Doing their utmost to avoid excessive blood loss** during the third stage of labour.

4. Encouraging puerperal women to continue taking iron pills for one month.

MEGALOBLASTIC ANÆMIA OF PREGNANCY

This severe form of anæmia, due to insufficiency of folic acid, results from the demands of the fetus or some factor interfering with the absorption or metabolism of folic acid. It tends to occur when the hæmoglobin is below 7 G. (50 per cent), therefore the administration of iron prophylactically should significantly reduce the incidence of megaloblastic anæmia.

Patients with anæmia that fails to respond to iron therapy in four weeks and cases in which the hæmoglobin is less than 10 G. (70 per cent) should have blood investigation made to determine if megaloblastic anæmia is present.

Pallor is marked, the woman complains of extreme weakness, vomiting, dyspnœa and sometimes diarrhœa and persistent swelling of the ankles.

Treatment

A striking improvement is evident following the administration of folic acid 5 mg. three times daily with iron throughout pregnancy and continued six weeks postpartum. Rest in bed, and a light diet, high in proteins, iron, and other minerals, are essential.

A blood transfusion will be necessary if anæmia is severe or if in untreated cases delivery is imminent: extreme care is exercised with this procedure.

SICKLE CELL ANÆMIA

This condition is now being diagnosed in immigrant pregnant negroes but is rare in other races. An abnormal hæmoglobin S which changes the shape of the red blood cells is inherited in the genes from one or both parents.

Alarming hæmolytic crises, which may be fatal, may occur in the last trimester of pregnancy: the treatment being blood transfusion. Multiple painful capillary thromboses sometimes occur, hæmaturia may be manifest. Anæmia in such cases should be treated by an expert: there is no response to iron or folic acid. Infections must be treated promptly. Flying above 4,000 ft in non-pressurised aircraft is contra-indicated.

NEURITIS

Neuritis may occur, both during pregnancy and the puerperium; the woman complaining of pain, numbness and loss of power, usually in one limb. It may be due to deficiency of the vitamin B complex, but is occasionally of cerebral origin. The response to proprietary preparations of vitamin B is usually very good.

CARPAL TUNNEL SYNDROME

This condition is fairly common during pregnancy (68 *cases occurred at The Simpson Maternity in* 1969). Tingling, numbness and pain are felt in the thumb and fingers during the night, due to compression of the medial nerve in the carpal tunnel at the wrist. The fluid retention of pregnancy is believed to give rise to pressure on the nerve

Rest and night-splinting may help: diuretics and low salt diet have been tried The condition disappears spontaneously after delivery.

ACUTE INFECTIONS

By their toxic effect and possibly the high temperature acute infectious diseases may cause abortion, premature labour and stillbirth.

PNEUMONIA

Pneumonia and severe influenza of the respiratory type are grave complications during the later months of pregnancy. The disease is treated as in the non-pregnant woman; oxygen is essential to counteract cyanosis. Fifty per cent will go into premature labour, but the induction of labour is contra-indicated. Forceps, if required, are applied under pudendal nerve block or perineal infiltration.

SMALLPOX

Vaccination is not recommended during pregnancy unless contact with smallpox has occurred: babies of vaccinated mothers have been born with generalized vaccinia.

ANTERIOR POLIOMYELITIS

Because of the suspected increased severity of poliomyelitis associated with pregnancy, polio immunization of expectant mothers is advocated but not before the 16th week of pregnancy when the embryo is at risk. The Sabin-type vaccine is commonly used. The dangers of poliomyelitis are similar to those in the non-pregnant woman and 75 per cent of deaths occur in the over-15 age group. Spontaneous delivery of the baby is possible even when the abdominal and pelvic floor muscles are paralysed.

RUBELLA

This disease is a menace when contracted by the pregnant woman because of its harmful effect on the fetus *in utero*. If infection occurs during the first 12 weeks, and particularly during the first eight weeks, the placenta is not sufficiently developed to provide an adequate barrier, and the fetal organs (eyes, ears, heart and brain) are in an early embryonic state with little resistance to infection. The child may be born with one or all of the following congenital defects: cataract (30 per cent), deafness (50 per cent), heart disease (50 per cent), mental subnormality (1 per cent).

Prophylaxis

Women should be made aware of the danger so that they know to avoid contact with the disease during pregnancy, and to report exposure to infection without delay.

The injection of convalescent serum or gamma-globulin to non-immune women within five days of contact with infection has been found to confer a degree of passive immunity in some cases. Therapeutic abortion is considered justifiable by certain authorities if the woman develops Rubella during the first 12 weeks of pregnancy.

Cendevax rubella vaccine is now available and is given to schoolgirls prior to puberty. Pregnancy, or the likelihood of becoming pregnant within two months, is an absolute contraindication to being inoculated with this new rubella vaccine (consisting of live attenuated rubella virus).

URINARY TRACT INFECTION

Pyelonephritis occurs in about 2 per cent of pregnant women, especially primigravidæ, from approximately the 16th to the 26th week of pregnancy.

PREDISPOSING FACTORS

During pregnancy the ureters lack tone because of the relaxing effect of the hormone progesterone on unstriped muscle. The flaccid ureters are therefore more readily dilated, kinked or compressed, and this causes stasis of urine with subsequent risk of the multiplication of organisms; the right ureter being more commonly affected because the pregnant uterus leans and rotates on its axis towards the right side.

Compression by the pregnant uterus on the ureter where it enters the pelvic brim is most marked from the 16th to the 24th week.

SOURCE OF INFECTION

The predominant infecting organism in about 80 per cent of cases is the *Escherichia coli,* but the staphylococcus, streptococcus or *ps. aeruginosa* may also be the causal organism. There is some doubt as to how the *Esch. coli* gains access to the kidney. It may be because the right kidney lies in such close proximity to the colon and there is a lymphatic connection between the two.

Recent work suggests ascending infection, so catheterization should never be used for diagnostic purposes: mid-stream (*or clean catch*) specimens of urine are obtained.

The reflux of urine that occurs from the bladder to the ureters during pregnancy favours ascending infection.

Asymptomatic Bacteriuria

Seven per cent of pregnant women have asymptomatic bacteriuria (a count of 100,000 or more organisms in one ml. of urine on two occasions) and about 20 per cent of these women will develop pyelonephritis during pregnancy if the existing bacteriuria is not treated.

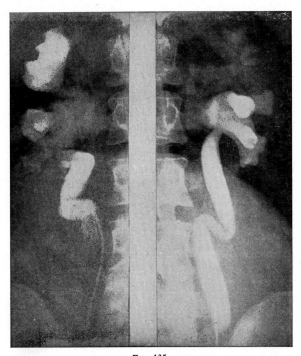

FIG. 135

Case of pyelonephritis of pregnancy showing dilatation and marked kinking of ureters.

SIGNS AND SYMPTOMS OF PYELONEPHRITIS

These will vary, depending on whether the condition is mild or acute. In mild cases the most pronounced features may be loss of appetite, nausea and vomiting which are sometimes mistaken for hyperemesis gravidarum.

The onset in acute cases is usually sudden, and abdominal pain, commonly on the right side, is severe. Abdominal tenderness and rigidity are sometimes present and in conjunction with the other signs and symptoms the condition is somewhat similar to appendicitis. In other cases the patient complains of dull backache and pain radiating **down to the groin.** The temperature ranges from 38·3 to 38·8° C. (101° to 102° F.) and the pulse from 110 to 130. **The patient complains of feeling shivery** and sometimes actual rigors occur.

The urine looks turbid, and is commonly acid. It contains protein and has a high specific gravity.

DIAGNOSIS

Medical advice must of course be obtained, and the doctor will make the diagnosis. Eliciting tenderness in the loin of a patient with pyrexia, whose urine contains over 100,000 organisms per ml., suggests that active urinary infection is present; finding pus cells is diagnostic but the absence of pus cells does not rule out pyelonephritis.

Treatment

The patient is put into a warmed bed, and as she will usually perspire freely, chilling must be avoided, so bathroom privileges are not allowed until the temperature has been normal for some days.

Before treatment is begun and 48 hours after a course of antibiotics is completed a mid-stream specimen of urine is obtained, sent for culture and bacteriological investigation.

Specimens should reach the laboratory within one hour of passing urine or be kept at a temperature of 4·4° *C.* (40° *F.*), otherwise the organisms multiply and give an excessively high bacterial count. The laboratory may give a tentative report in 6 hours, causal organism in 15 hours and antibiotic sensitivity in 24 hours.

A fluid balance chart is kept.

Temperature and pulse are taken and recorded every four hours.

These patients are usually constipated so an enema or suppository is given on admission. Only mild laxatives should be employed.

DRUG THERAPY

The appropriate antibiotic will be prescribed as indicated by the bacteriological sensitivity tests, *e.g.* ampicillin (Penbritin), 500 mg., six to eight hourly for 10 to 14 days.

A course of sulphonamides, 30 G., may be given unless the organisms are known to be sulphonamide resistant. Many strains of *E. coli* are sensitive to sulphonamides but prolonged administration may have a harmful action on the fetus. The more effective ones are sulphadimidine, sulphatriad and sulphamethizole, 2 G. followed by 1 G. every 4 or 6 hours for 10 to 14 days. Some continue treatment on a reduced dosage basis throughout pregnancy. The fluid intake should be 2,000 ml. daily.

Nalidixic acid (Negram) has been used with some success against gram-negative organisms, especially *E. Coli* and *B. proteus vulgaris:* relapse may occur.

Kanamycin (Kannasyn). A short course is occasionally given in staphylococcal infections resistant to other antibiotics.

Cycloserine may be prescribed under expert urological supervision in persistent cases of *E. coli* infection (after the 12th week). Renal function must first be assessed and plasma Cycloserine concentration measured throughout treatment. Cycloserine is not given to patients with epilepsy.

THE RELIEF OF PAIN

Heat is usually effective in relieving pain, and as it is advisable to have the patient lying on the non-affected side to encourage good drainage: an electric pad, hot water bottle or Kaolin plaster can be conveniently maintained in position; flexing the knees may also give relief. If the pain is acute the prone position can be adopted and it may be necessary to give an analgesic such as dihydrocodeine (D.F. 118), 30 to 60 mg. or Buscopan, 20 mg., Codis tablets (2) or pentazocine (Fortral) tablets 25-50 mg.

The nutritional needs of the pregnant woman must not be forgotten, and her general health should be built up as soon as possible. A diet adequate in first-class proteins, calcium, iron and vitamins, supplemented by multiple vitamin tablets and ferrous sulphate, is essential and should be given as soon as her appetite returns.

Urological investigation. If the infection recurs or bacteriuria persists, radiological examination, cystoscopy and renal function tests are necessary. This should be postponed until twelve weeks after delivery.

RENAL DISEASE

When patients with established renal disease become pregnant, features such as proteinuria, hypertension, œdema, or an elevated blood urea level are present prior to the 20th week. Primary renal disorders complicate about 1 in every 1000 pregnancies, and pre-eclampsia may be superimposed on the pre-existing disease.

If kidney dysfunction is slight, the pregnancy is allowed to continue. When renal function is impaired, or where sudden deterioration takes place, termination should be considered. Intra-uterine death may occur so, because of this, delivery at 36 weeks may be resorted to by Caesarean section for primigravidæ and induction of labour for multigravidæ.

ACUTE RENAL FAILURE

This serious condition, when it occurs in obstetric practice, more commonly follows septic abortion, abruptio placentæ and postpartum hæmorrhage with severe shock. Oliguria is the outstanding sign (less than 500 ml. urine daily) and this must be reported to the doctor without delay.

It is mandatory that an accurate fluid balance record is kept in patients who have been subjected to the above predisposing causes: blood urea estimations and potassium determination usually being carried out for 3 days.

MANAGEMENT

The patient is treated if possible in a renal intensive care unit with single rooms to limit the possibility of extraneous infection.

Fluids must be carefully regulated, a fluid balance record is kept and 400 ml. per 24 hours plus the volume lost in urine and vomitus during the previous 24 hours is given. A protein free fluid with a high carbohydrate content, i.e. 20 per cent lactose, should be given to provide calories. If this is not tolerated intravenous fluid 20 per cent fructose is administered. Parentrovite is given daily. Overhydration is avoided during the oliguric stage and dehydration during the diuretic stage. (Recovery has taken place in patients who have had oliguria for 4 weeks.)

Control of the electrolytes is necessary because potassium and sodium are not being excreted by the kidneys; daily estimations of serum, potassium and sodium as well as urea and bicarbonate are made. Hycal glucose syrup (flavoured) is useful being high calorie, low fluid, low electrolyte.

Calcium resonium is specific in removing potassium from the body and may be given, 30 G. rectally, when the potassium level is found to be rising.

If the blood urea or serum potassium rise rapidly—as is the case in most infected patients with acute renal failure—conservative measures will not be sufficient to maintain life until kidney function returns. In these circumstances dialysis is used.

Dialysis therapy will allow a patient to survive even if renal function takes several weeks to return. If the oliguric phase lasts for more than four or five days the use of dialysis with a 50 G. protein diet may be safer than the rigorous starvation involved in prolonged conservative therapy.

NON-VENEREAL VAGINAL INFECTIONS

TRICHOMONIASIS

The trichomonas vaginalis, a protozoon, thrives when the vaginal secretion is less acid. Trichomonas vaginitis is found in 45 per cent of pregnant women who have sufficient vaginal discharge to necessitate medical investigation.

SIGNS AND SYMPTOMS

The woman complains of a profuse green or yellow discharge, with burning and irritation of the vulva. The vagina looks red, and a profuse purulent discharge, some-times frothy or blood-stained with a stale offensive odour, is seen exuding from it.

Treatment

Metronidazole (Flagyl) oral tablets, 200 mg., t.i.d., for seven days are sometimes used. Metronidazole should not be given while the embryo is at risk, *i.e.* the first 12 weeks of pregnancy: *some do not prescribe Flagyl during pregnancy*. The husband may also be treated.

The vagina is mopped dry with wool swabs, which in severe cases are moistened with sodium bicarbonate solution to remove the discharge. The doctor may paint the vagina and vulva with an aqueous solution of gentian violet, 1 per cent, to allay irritation, but the staining of linen is a disadvantage. (Because of the grave danger of air embolism when insufflating the vagina with powder during pregnancy, such a procedure is not used.) **Penotrane pessaries have been found to be very effective** in relieving irritation and counteracting the offensive odour of the discharge. They are inserted into the upper part of the vagina at night, and the woman should lie with her buttocks elevated on two pillows for at least half an hour after their insertion.

Conotrane cream, containing penotrane and silicone is suitable for local application to excoriated areas.

MONILIASIS
Vaginal Thrush

This yeast infection is caused by the Candida (monilia) albicans, a fungus found in the vagina of 28 per cent of all pregnant women, and if the vaginal flora is slightly more acid than normal, thrush may develop.

SIGNS AND SYMPTOMS

The woman complains of intense itching of the vulva and vagina and a white or yellow vaginal discharge, which may not be profuse. On the insertion of a speculum, the vagina is seen to be coated with a grey, whitish or yellow curd-like substance which is adherent to the epithelium and on removal leaves an abraded area.

DIAGNOSIS

Yeast spores and branching filaments are seen on slides prepared from the plaques of white substance on the vaginal walls.

Treatment

The vagina is swabbed, as described for trichomoniasis: 1 per cent gentian violet is useful for the immediate treatment of vaginitis but repeated application is not advocated.

Nystatin pessaries, two inserted at night for one or two weeks and one for a further week are very effective. Pruvagol pessaries, two or three times weekly, may be used.

Nystatin ointment is useful for local application to the vulval skin.

VULVAL WARTS

Vulval warts are **not necessarily due to syphilis or gonorrhœa,** although they are sometimes seen in such cases. They are caused by a virus and they may spread extensively in the vulval region during pregnancy, particularly if the woman has a trichomonal discharge. It is important to find out whether the husband has penile warts as the disease can be spread sexually. A few lesions, ranging from the size of a pinhead to that of a walnut, may be present, and in rare cases they grow profusely to form a large, foul-smelling, fungating mass, which covers the entire vulva and may extend to the thighs and pubes.

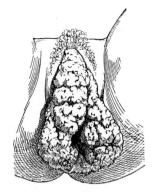

FIG. 136

VULVAL WARTS are due to a viral infection.

Treatment

The first requisite is the diagnosis and treatment of any accompanying discharge. **Cleansing with soap and water is essential.** Small warts are treated by touching them with collodion salicylate or podophyllin resin, 25 per cent in liquid paraffin, and in order to prevent the resin from coming in contact with the surrounding skin, zinc ointment is smeared on. The application is repeated four or five days later. Extensive warts are removed by the electro-cautery under local anæsthesia.

SYPHILIS

Syphilis tends to be latent during pregnancy, but unless the infection is acquired during or after conception, rarely are signs of syphilis manifest in pregnant women; the diagnosis being made by taking routine serological tests for syphilis during pregnancy. These tests should include the Wassermann Reaction, the Venereal Disease Reference Laboratory test (VDRL) and the Reiter's Protein Complement Fixation test. Cases with doubtful serological tests may require further investigation which should include a Fluorescent Treponemal Antibody test or a Treponema pallidum immobilization test.

Student midwives should be warned that *false positive Wassermann reactions* do occur in pregnancy and that the term " syphilis " or " V.D. clinic " should not be used when talking to patients. The doctor only should inform the woman of the result of such tests or discuss their implications.

14

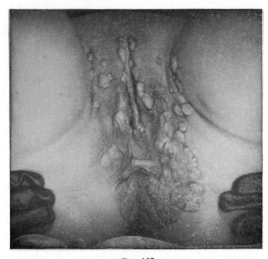

Fig. 137

Condylomata lata on vulva and around anus.

THE EFFECTS OF UNTREATED SYPHILIS ON CHILDBEARING

1. **Abortion may occur after the 20th week.** 2. **Labour may be premature.**
3. **The fetus may be stillborn (macerated).**   4. **The child may be born with syphilis.**

The untreated syphilitic baby who shows clinical manifestations of the disease soon after birth usually dies, but the less severe cases may recover.

Treatment

Prophylaxis is the best form of treatment, and the routine examination of the blood of all pregnant women by serological tests is one of the finest examples of preventive medicine.

Penicillin therapy is used almost exclusively ; ideally treatment should begin before the 20th week but results are good even when the treatment is started as late as the 28th week. The woman may be admitted to hospital, though out-patient treatment is adequate in the latent stage of the infection. Triplopen 1·25 mega units daily for 14 days is adequate. If the patient is sensitive to penicillin, Cephaloridine is a possible alternative. When treated as an in-patient, crystalline penicillin 1 mega unit 8 hourly for 10 days will produce levels adequate to cure. Vaginal moniliasis is not uncommon as a side effect of such treatment.

The baby is almost certainly non-syphilitic at birth but may have positive blood tests caused by passive transfer of reacting substance from the mother's blood. The tests usually become weak positive or negative within three months.

When infective lesions are present the midwife takes the necessary precautions to protect herself by wearing gown and gloves, and the other patients by segregation of dishes and equipment. Care in the disposal of dressings is necessary until the lesions are non-infectious, which is within 48 hours after intensive penicillin therapy is begun.

After the birth of the baby the woman continues to attend the clinic, where blood tests are made every three months for two years: the spinal fluid is also examined. Further treatment is given if required.

CONGENITAL SYPHILIS

No baby has been born at the Simpson Maternity Pavilion with congenital syphilis during the past 18 years

An infant with strongly positive serological tests (WR; VDRL; RPCFT) may appear to be normal in every way. Midwives seldom see a newborn baby with signs of syphilis, as these do not usually develop until after the first month of life, neither is the placenta always large and unhealthy-looking, unless the infant is stillborn and macerated. Jaundice may occur.

Skin lesions, if present at birth, give rise to suspicion, especially when there are blebs on the palms and soles (syphilitic pemphigus). Various skin rashes may develop during the first month, and the napkin area is particularly vulnerable.

The baby is not born with a saddle nose; such a deformity becomes apparent near the end of the first year, due to necrosis of the nasal bones, and is preceded by a profuse purulent blood-stained nasal discharge which seldom exists prior to the second month.

If the larynx is affected the cry has a peculiar, cracked or hoarse quality. Fissures in the centre of the lips, the angles of the mouth and around the anus leave permanent scars known as **rhagades.**

DIAGNOSIS

Cord-blood may contain maternal antibodies which make the interpretation of the infants' serology difficult. Not until the infant is six weeks old can a positive or negative result be accepted as such; a heel stab is made and sufficient blood obtained for the test.

Treatment

Isolation of the infant is wise until penicillin has been given for 48 hours.

If the mother was untreated or inadequately treated, the infant is given procaine penicillin, 150,000 units, by intramuscular injection daily for 10 days. If blood tests are not negative within one month a second course is given.

GONORRHŒA

The diagnosis and treatment of gonorrhœa during pregnancy is important because of the risk of the baby's eyes being infected by the gonococcus during birth.

SIGNS AND SYMPTOMS

In the majority of cases the symptoms are slight. Most pregnant women have leucorrhœa, but when the vaginal discharge is greenish, profuse, offensive, or irritating, the midwife should inform the doctor, who will investigate the cause.

Gonorrhœa may co-exist with other vaginal infections, such as trichomoniasis and moniliasis, or in conjunction with syphilis. Acute gonorrhœa is infrequently found, and in such a case the vaginal discharge is greenish or yellow and profuse, giving rise to œdema of the labia. The woman complains of frequency and burning pain on micturition.

14 A

EXAMINATION OF PATIENT

1. The woman is told not to pass urine for two hours prior to examination and the vulva must not be swabbed.

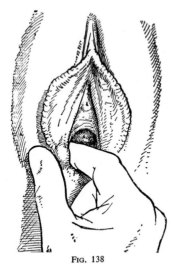

FIG. 138

Showing chronic infection of Bartholin's gland. This is not always due to the gonococcus.

2. The patient is placed in the lithotomy position.

A platinum loop is used to collect discharge from the urethra, cervix and from Bartholin's ducts; if infected, smears and cultures are then made for detection of the gonococcus.

Thayer and Martin medium contains antibiotics which suppress other organisms and allow the gonococcus to grow more rapidly.

Diagnosis is made on the following:

1. A history of infection.

2. The clinical findings.

3. The detection of Gram-negative intracellular diplococci in cultures.

4. The gonococcal complement fixation test of the blood is only reliable in certain cases.

Treatment

Penicillin is the antibiotic of choice. **Triplopen,** 1·25 mg., daily for two days. Many strains are now resistant to penicillin so erythromycin, 250 mg., four times daily is given for three to five days, and repeated if necessary. No local treatment is carried out other than swabbing the vulva to remove discharge. Vaginal tampons should not be used. **Advice is given regarding the means of preventing the spread of the disease.**

QUESTIONS FOR REVISION

DISEASES ASSOCIATED WITH PREGNANCY

CARDIAC DISEASE

Name the important points in the care of pregnant women with cardiac disease. IN WHAT POSITION is she delivered ? WHAT SIGNS should be reported to the doctor during labour ? **Why are the following drugs prescribed:** FRUSEMIDE, DIGOXIN ?

C.M.B.(Scot.) paper.—How does pregnancy affect a woman with mitral stenosis ? Describe the special care required during pregnancy, labour and the puerperium.

C.M.B.(Scot.) paper.—What are the risks to a patient with cardiac disease who becomes pregnant ? Describe the management during pregnancy and labour.

C.M.B.(N. Ireland) paper.—Give the nursing care of a patient in labour, who is known to have a moderate degree of cardiac disease.

ORAL QUESTIONS

Give 3 main causes of deterioration in pregnant cardiac patients

How would you manage each of the 3 stages of labour ?

Why is the lithotomy position not advisable ?

How would you cope with acute heart failure in the absence of medical assistance ?

DIABETES

What signs and symptoms would cause a midwife to suspect diabetes in pregnancy ? NAME THE CONDITIONS which may arise during pregnancy because of diabetes. DESCRIBE THE DUTIES of a midwife during labour, from the diabetic aspect.

C.M.B.(Scot.) paper.—In what way may diabetes in the mother complicate the pregnancy ? Outline the management of the case and immediate care of the baby.

C.M.B.(N. Ireland) paper.—What are the complications of diabetes in pregnancy? Describe the nursing care of the newborn baby of the diabetic mother.

C.M.B.(Scot.) paper.—Describe the methods used to reduce fetal loss in pregnancy complicated by diabetes.

Write not more than 10 lines on:
The effects of diabetes on childbearing. The management of the pregnant diabetic. The management of labour in diabetes.

Discuss in relation to diabetes: (a) hydramnios; (b) intra-uterine fetal death; (c the obstetric history.

ANÆMIA

Write not more than 10 lines on:

1. **The role of the midwife** in the prevention of anæmia.

2. **Causes of iron deficiency anæmia.**

3. **The effects of anæmia on child bearing.**

Underline the foods that are rich in iron: chocolate; wholemeal bread; green vegetables; milk; butter; oranges; liver; fish; treacle; prunes; eggs.

What is the connection between anæmia in pregnancy and the following: folic acid deficiency; hook worm infection; hyperchlorhydria; the sickle cell gene.

Why and how are the following substances administered: Imferon; ferrous fumerate; ascorbic acid; Alcopar; folic acid; packed red cells.

ORAL QUESTIONS

What advice would you give re administration of iron tablets ?

Describe foods rich in iron for each of the 3 main meals.

In which patients might hook worm infection be present ?

How frequently are hæmoglobin estimations made in pregnancy ?

C.M.B.(N. Ireland) paper.—Discuss the causes, prevention and treatment of anæmia in pregnancy.

C.M.B.(N. Ireland) paper.—Anæmia is noted at 34 weeks in a primigravida· Describe the possible dangers, investigation and treatment.

C.M.B.(Eng.) paper.—Anæmia still occurs during pregnancy. How may it be prevented and what are the dangers?

C.M.B.(Scot.) paper 1969.—What factors are responsible for the high incidence of anæmia in pregnancy? Describe the prevention and treatment of this condition.

C.M.B.(Scot.) paper 1970.—Give an account of anæmia in pregnancy.

TUBERCULOSIS

Write 10 lines on:
Pulmonary Tuberculosis as a social problem: the modern outlook regarding pulmonary tuberculosis and child-bearing.

C.M.B.(N. Ireland).—WHAT IS "B.C.G."? Which babies are especially likely to benefit from its use and what precautions must be observed?

RUBELLA

Rubella virus vaccine (1970) is recommended for girls before child-bearing age and not for pregnant women, or those liable to become pregnant within two months—why?

C.M.B.(Eng.) paper. 50 word question.—Rubella (German measles) in pregnancy.

PYELONEPHRITIS

Which is the most common INVADING ORGANISM? DESCRIBE THE SIGNS AND SYMPTOMS.

Write not more than 10 lines on: (a) asymptomatic bacteriuria; (b) factors that predispose to pyelonephritis; (c) nursing care in acute pyelonephritis.

The following drugs may be prescribed in pyelonephritis: state dose and purpose: Kanamycin, Cycloserine, Buscopan, sulphadimidine, papaveretum, ampicillin.

C.M.B.(Scot.) paper.—Describe the typical signs and symptoms of urinary tract infection in pregnancy and give the nursing treatment.

C.M.B.(N. Ireland) paper.—What is pyelonephritis? Describe the clinical features and nursing care of an acute case complicating pregnancy.

C.M.B.(Scot.) paper.—Describe the ætiology, diagnosis and treatment of pyelonephritis in pregnancy.

C.M.B.(N. Ireland) paper 1968.—Define Pyelonephritis. Give signs, symptoms and treatment of a moderately severe case.

C.M.B.(Scot.) paper 1969.—Give the signs and symptoms of pyelonephritis associated with pregnancy. Describe the nursing care of such a patient.

VENEREAL DISEASE

What signs of venereal disease may be evident on examination of the vulva?

State how you would (a) insert a penotrane vaginal pessary; (b) relieve vulval itching due to moniliasis; (c) recognize: (1) condylomata lata, (2) vulval warts.

Signs of congenital syphilis are rarely present prior to the .... month. Purulent blood stained nasal discharge is rarely evident before the .... month. Saddle nose becomes apparent after the .... month.

C.M.B.(Scot.) paper.—How may untreated venereal disease in a pregnant woman affect her baby? Describe in detail the conditions that may be found in the baby. How may they be prevented?

C.M.B.(N. Ireland) paper.—Describe the common venereal diseases. How may these complicate pregnancy, labour and the puerperium?

C.M.B.(Eng.) paper. 50 word question.—Why is the rise in incidence of gonorrhœa of concern to midwives?

C.M.B.(Scot.) paper.—Enumerate the possible ways in which the baby may be affected by the following maternal complications of pregnancy: (a) German measles. (b) Rhesus incompatibility. (c) Syphilis.

VAGINAL DISCHARGE

C.M.B.(Scot.) paper.—What are the causes of non-hæmorrhagic vaginal discharge in pregnancy? Give the usual treatment of one of the conditions you mention.

C.M.B.(Eng.) paper.—Describe the vagina and its anatomical relations. What are the causes of vaginal discharge during pregnancy?

C.M.B.(N. Ireland) paper.—Describe the vagina, mentioning its anatomical relations. What are the causes of vaginal discharge during pregnancy?

13

Antepartum Hæmorrhage

Although any vaginal bleeding prior to the birth of the baby might be considered to be antepartum, it is expedient to limit the source of bleeding to that from the placental site, and the time of occurrence to the period of fetal viability. (*Prior to the 28th week of pregnancy bleeding from the placental site would be a sign of abortion.*)

Some authorities include bleeding from other sources, such as lesions of the cervix (see p. 136) and vasa prævia (see p. 41). Bleeding from cervical lesions can be recognised by speculum examination.

Hæmorrhage from the placental site constitutes an urgent threat to mother and child which demands immediate admission to hospital for supervision and treatment. The midwife must appreciate the seriousness of placental site hæmorrhage.

DEFINITION

ANTEPARTUM HÆMORRHAGE

This is bleeding from the placental site due to premature separation of the placenta after the 28th week of pregnancy and prior to the birth of the baby (the first and second stages of labour are therefore included). Antepartum hæmorrhage is classified according to the situation of the placenta, *i.e.* whether it is implanted in the upper or lower uterine segment.

UNAVOIDABLE HÆMORRHAGE

Bleeding due to the premature separation of a placenta which is situated partly or wholly in the lower uterine segment, *i.e.* a placenta prævia.

ACCIDENTAL HÆMORRHAGE

Bleeding due to the premature separation of a normally situated placenta.

INCIDENTAL HÆMORRHAGE

Bleeding from other sources usually cervical.

ANTEPARTUM HÆMORRHAGE *(type undiagnosed)*

Patients with antepartum hæmorrhage have to be dealt with on district and in hospital before the hæmorrhage has been diagnosed as unavoidable or accidental. In both types the initial treatment is the same, but when, after admission to hospital, the diagnosis is made, the appropriate treatment is instituted.

To avoid unnecessary repetition *the initial treatment of antepartum hæmorrhage is not given when the management of unavoidable hæmorrhage and accidental hæmorrhage is described. Midwives must therefore when deliberating on the treatment of these refer back to initial treatment of antepartum hæmorrhage (type undiagnosed).*

MANAGEMENT

Hospitalization is imperative whether the bleeding is slight or severe. Every woman who bleeds *per vaginam* after the 28th week of pregnancy must be transferred to hospital as soon as possible. She is in danger of further and more serious hæmorrhage; intra-uterine death may occur, so all the facilities provided in a modern maternity hospital to preserve maternal and infant life and health should be made available.

Vaginal examination is dangerous. No attempt should be made on the district or anywhere outwith an operating theatre, to differentiate between unavoidable and accidental hæmorrhage by vaginal examination. Inserting a finger into the cervical canal or applying pressure through the vaginal fornices may induce profuse hæmorrhage, immediately or within a few hours, which may be almost uncontrollable.

TREATMENT BY MIDWIFE ON DISTRICT

1. **Prophylaxis is the midwife's first duty.** If the woman has been instructed to report any vaginal bleeding at once, is transferred to hospital promptly without vaginal or rectal examination, the prognosis is much better for mother and child, and the midwife is less likely to have to deal with severe hæmorrhage in the home.

2. **The woman is put to bed,** reassured, and kept flat.

3. **Medical aid is sent for without delay. If the doctor is not available and the situation is urgent,** e.g. severe bleeding, or shock and abdominal pain with or without slight bleeding, the midwife should summon the " flying squad " or communicate with a maternity hospital at once.

4. OBSERVATION

(a) **General condition.** Note pulse rate, pallor, blood pressure, œdema.

(b) **Blood loss.** The amount of blood should be assessed (pads and sheets set aside for inspection by the doctor). Enquiry is made as to previous bleeding and whether the onset of the present loss is related to undue physical exertion or emotional stress.

(c) **Abdominal examination** must be carried out with the greatest gentleness, noting pain, tenderness, uterine consistence, malpresentation, high head, fetal heart rate.

(d) **Recording.** A record is made of name, age, parity, week of gestation, blood loss, blood pressure; pulse every 5 to 15 minutes depending on the severity of the condition; amount of urine passed, fetal heart rate, drugs administered.

SEDATION AND TRANSFER TO HOSPITAL

The doctor will arrange for the woman to be transferred to hospital after a sedative such as pethidine, 100 or 200 mg., or papaveretum (Omnopon), 20 mg., or morphine, 15 mg. is administered. If the woman's condition does not warrant the journey the doctor will summon the " flying squad " who will give a blood transfusion before transferring her to hospital.

The midwife, taking with her the records she has kept, accompanies the woman, having applied two perineal pads and wrapped a linen and a plastic sheet round the woman's hips.

TREATMENT IN HOSPITAL
(*Type of Haemorrhage undiagnosed*)

Certain routine investigations are made on all patients when admitted to hospital with antepartum hæmorrhage, whether the bleeding is slight or severe. Booked patients will have had their blood examined previously, a procedure which saves valuable time when blood transfusion is urgently needed.

(A) PREPARATIONS TO BE MADE FOR INVESTIGATION AND TREATMENT

1. THE FOLLOWING EQUIPMENT MAY BE REQUIRED:

(a) **For ABO blood grouping and cross matching, hæmoglobin, Rh factor,** clotting time, plasma fibrinogen, and Wassermann reaction (if not already done).

(b) **For intravenous administration of blood,** dextrose, Ringer's lactate solution, oxytocin drip, fibrinogen.

(c) **For injection** of pethidine, papaveretum, atropine, nikethamide.

(d) **For shaving vulva.**

(e) **For urine analysis. Esbach's test.**

(f) **Baumanometer,** stethoscope, fetal stethoscope.

(g) **Cylinder of oxygen.** Polythene face mask.

2. PREPARE THE FOLLOWING CHARTS IN GRAPH FORM IF POSSIBLE.

(a) **Pulse,** 5 to 15 minutes.   (b) **Blood pressure,** 30 to 60 minutes.

(c) **Fetal heart,** 10 to 20 minutes.   (d) **Fluid balance.**

Have a " permission for operation and anæsthetic " form ready for signature.

(B) TREATMENT OF SLIGHT BLEEDING

(a) **The woman is put into a warmed bed** and not allowed to get up.

(b) **No vaginal or rectal examination is made.**

(c) OBSERVATION

Note blood loss, pallor, œdema.

Gentle abdominal examination, noting pain, tenderness, uterine consistence, high head, malpresentation, fetal heart.

(d) **Sedatives such as papaveretum, 20 mg. are administered** if necessary.

(e) **Blood is obtained for the necessary tests.**

(f) **Temperature, pulse and blood pressure** are recorded.

(g) **Routine vulval shaving and swabbing** are carried out.

(h) **A midstream specimen of urine** is obtained and examined for protein.

(i) **No routine enema on admission** (a small enema, Dulcolax suppository or mild laxative may be ordered after 48 hours).

(j) **Perineal pads are kept for inspection** by the doctor if the loss becomes more than slight.

(k) **Speculum examination.** This is made after two or three days to rule out cervical causes of bleeding. A Papanicolaou smear may be taken if the patient is unbooked.

(l) **Patient is allowed up after five days** if there is no bleeding during that time.

(*m*) **If after a further two days there is no bleeding, no pre-eclampsia, essential hypertension,** and no **placenta prævia** on X-ray or ultrasonic localization the woman may be permitted to go home, and told to return if bleeding occurs and for delivery.

(C) TREATMENT OF SEVERE BLEEDING

The woman will be in a dangerous state of collapse due to profuse or prolonged hæmorrhage.

Immediate resuscitation is imperative and no time should be lost in obtaining and administering blood.

1. **The woman is admitted to the special resuscitation unit.**

2. **The procedures as for slight bleeding are carried out.** See heading B (*a*) to (*h*) (p. 213).

3. **Maternal pulse and blood pressure** (see p. 213, A 2).

4. **Plasma fibrinogen and clot tests are made.**

5. **Sedatives are given** for apprehension, analgesics for pain.

6. **Dextrose 5 per cent and Ringer's lactate solution is given intravenously** while compatible blood is being procured.

7. **Blood transfusion is given.**

8. **The fetal heart is auscultated** every 10 or 15 minutes.

9. **Oxygen is administered** if necessary.

10. **Further treatment** will depend on whether the hæmorrhage continues, and if so a vaginal examination may be made, as outlined on page 218 (9) to determine if bleeding is due to placenta prævia. The appropriate treatment is then given.

UNAVOIDABLE HÆMORRHAGE

PLACENTA PRÆVIA

The premature separation of a placenta prævia is inevitable and bleeding unavoidable because when stretching of the lower uterine segment occurs during the latter weeks of pregnancy the anchoring chorionic villi are torn across, the venous sinuses in the placental site are exposed and blood escapes. **The initial bleeding may be very slight,** but, as further stretching of the lower segment proceeds, the bleeding recurs at intervals of hours or days.

When the placenta lies over the internal os the seriousness of the situation is intensified because massive separation with profuse hæmorrhage must occur while the cervix is being taken up and the os dilating.

CAUSES

The cause of low implantation of the placenta is not clearly understood.

1. **It occurs more commonly in multigravid women,** and may be due to some abnormal condition in the endometrium of the upper uterine segment which does not present a suitable nidus in which the ovum can embed.

2. The placenta may have developed from chorionic villi in the lower part of the decidua capsularis which should have atrophied before the decidua capsularis fused with the decidua vera at the 12th week; these villi then embed in the lower pole of the uterus.

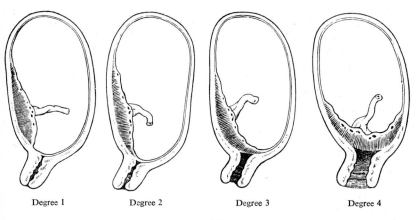

| Degree 1 | Degree 2 | Degree 3 | Degree 4 |

FIG. 139

DEGREES OF PLACENTA PRÆVIA.

1—The edge of the placenta dips into the lower segment.

2—The edge of the placenta is at the margin of the internal os.

3—The placenta lies completely over the os when closed and up to 4 cm. dilatation.

4—The centre of the placenta lies over the centre of the os.

Incidence

Placenta prævia is said to occur in about 1 in 200 cases.

At the Simpson Memorial Maternity Pavilion, Edinburgh, in 1969. *A total of 33 cases was admitted, 23 booked. Cæsarean section in 28 cases. Maternal mortality, nil. Perinatal mortality, 3 per cent.*

SIGNS AND DIAGNOSIS

The only sign is vaginal bleeding. A reliable method of diagnosis is by feeling the placenta through the cervical canal, but the risk of instigating massive hæmorrhage is so great that a vaginal examination is never made except when the patient is in the operating theatre set up in readiness for Cæsarean section.

Factors which are suggestive in making the diagnosis

1. TYPE OF BLEEDING.

Painless vaginal bleeding, for which no obvious cause is apparent; the bleeding often occurring during rest or sleep. The initial loss is usually slight and ceases spontaneously but may recur within hours or days and more rarely weeks; becoming more and more profuse. Occasionally the first bleeding is sudden and severe.

2. ABDOMINAL FINDINGS.

(*a*) **Transverse lie** occurs because the placenta encroaches on the lower pole of the uterus and prevents the fetus from adopting the longitudinal lie.

(*b*) **Malpresentation** particularly breech.

(*c*) **The head is high** and slips to one or other side when an attempt is made to make it enter the brim. (*The rare occasions when a central placenta prævia has permitted the head to enter the brim are of academic rather than practical interest.*)

(*d*) **The uterus is of normal consistence,** being neither hard nor tender on palpation.

(*e*) **No pain is experienced.**

3. LOCALIZATION OF PLACENTA.

(*a*) **Placentography. After the 33rd week the location of the placenta can be determined** on soft tissue X-ray (lateral view, woman erect, bladder empty). The junction of the upper and lower uterine segments is assumed to be on a level with the plane of the pelvic brim; the landmarks being the promontory of the sacrum and the symphysis pubis.

(*b*) **Arteriography** is used from the 28th to the 32nd week. After sedation and local anæsthesia Conray aqueous solution is injected via a catheter which is inserted into the femoral artery. In 6 seconds the X-ray will show the radio-opaque substance in the intervillous spaces.

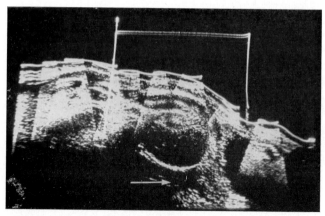

FIG. 140

ULTRASONOGRAM OF ANTERIOR PLACENTA PRAEVIA—DEGREE 3 (Arrow).

Partially filled bladder (black area on right) helps to delineate the position of the lower segment. The fetal head is moderately displaced upwards.

(*Queen Mother's Maternity Hospital, Glasgow*)

(*c*) **Radioactive isotopes** injected intravenously are used to locate the vascular placental site which has a high count rate.

(*d*) **Sonar (ultrasonic techniques)** are now being used with over 90 per cent accuracy. The level and margins of the placenta can be defined from the 26th week onward.

MANAGEMENT IN HOSPITAL

Initial treatment of antepartum haemorrhage is described on page 211

Treatment is aimed primarily at controlling hæmorrhage and saving infant life and will be active or expectant depending on (1) the amount of blood loss, (2) the week of gestation.

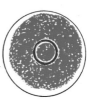

| Degree 1 | Degree 2 | Degree 3 | Degree 4 |

FIG. 141

FINDINGS ON VAGINAL EXAMINATION.

Membrane over os. Placenta may be felt on exploration of lower uterine segment.	Membrane over os. Placenta felt at margin of os.	Placenta may be felt over os until about 4 cm. dilatation.	Placenta lies over os until full dilatation.

Red line is margin of os.

ACTIVE TREATMENT

SEVERE BLEEDING.

(*a*) **Resuscitative measures** as for severe antepartum hæmorrhage (p. 214).

(*b*) **Preparations are made for Cæsarean section** which is performed immediately if, on admission or subsequently, bleeding is profuse.

MODERATE OR PERSISTENT BLEEDING.

If the woman is over 37 weeks pregnant, vaginal examination is carried out in the theatre set up for immediate operation. The treatment adopted (1) Puncture of membranes to induce labour, (2) Cæsarean section, will depend on the findings as in expectant treatment, (9 (*d*) to (*f*), see p. 218).

SLIGHT BLEEDING.

The treatment is expectant.

Expectant or Conservative Treatment

An attempt is made to prolong pregnancy until the fetus is sufficiently mature to have a reasonable chance of survival. Any interference which would be likely to incite the onset of labour, such as exploring the cervical canal or puncturing the membranes is postponed until the 38th week as recommended by Macafee of Belfast.

1. **The woman is kept in hospital, closely supervised** and usually confined to bed.

2. **Routine blood tests are made** (p. 213).

3. **Further bleeding** should be reported immediately: perineal pads kept for inspection if blood stained.

4. **A speculum examination is made** after two or three days to exclude cervical or vaginal lesions as sources of bleeding. (*A Papanicolaou smear is also taken.*)

15

5. **Blood transfusion is administered** if the hæmoglobin is low or further bleeding occurs.

6. **Food rich in iron,** as well as iron supplements, are given.

7. **The doctor is notified** if labour starts.

9. AT THE 38TH WEEK THE WOMAN IS TAKEN TO THE OPERATING THEATRE

(*a*) **All equipment is set out, patient's skin prepared, bladder emptied:** theatre staff " scrubbed up " in readiness for immediate Cæsarean section.

(*b*) **Cross-matched blood,** 1,200 ml. (at least), should be at hand, a saline drip set up, and facilities for resuscitation of collapsed patient ready.

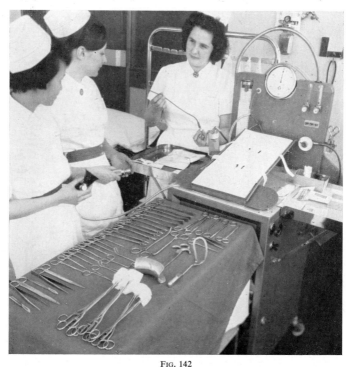

Fig. 142

CÆSAREAN SECTION FOR PLACENTA PRAEVIA.

Non-sterile " set up " for clinical instruction.

Sister, stressing the importance of clearing the airway prior to administration of oxygen, also demonstrating the use of the Resuscitaire. Student midwives holding baby laryngoscope and baby rebreathing bag.

(*County Maternity Hospital, Bellshill, Lanarkshire.*)

(*c*) A separate trolley is set up for puncture of membranes.

(*d*) **A vaginal examination may be made under general anæsthesia** by the obstetrician to determine the degree of placenta prævia. Two sterile gauze vaginal packs 1·82 m. × 10·2 cm. (2 yards × 4 inches) should always be in readiness to control the massive hæmorrhage which may occur. **When ultrasonic or radiological diagnosis of placental location is accepted,** exploration of the lower uterine segment and the hazard of (torrential) bleeding is avoided.

(*e*) CÆSAREAN SECTION IS PERFORMED—

(1) **If profuse hæmorrhage occurs.**

(2) **When placenta prævia degree 3 or 4 is diagnosed.**

(3) **If in degree 2 the placenta is situated posteriorly,** because it may prevent descent of the head and any bleeding would be difficult to control.

(4) **If the fetus lies transversely,** or the woman is an older primigravida.

(*f*) PUNCTURE OF MEMBRANES

(1) **This is done for degrees 1 and 2.** When labour ensues the woman usually delivers the baby spontaneously.

(2) **The baby's hæmoglobin level should be estimated** at birth because on occasions fetal blood is lost. If within four hours it is below 14·8 G. (100 per cent) a blood transfusion is given.

Student midwives should note that central placenta prævia does not obstruct labour. The reason why Cæsarean section is performed is to avoid massive hæmorrhage and so to save mother and baby.

TREATMENT FOR PLACENTA PRAEVIA
May be summarised as follows:

(*a*) PUNCTURE OF MEMBRANES FOR SLIGHT CASES

(*b*) CÆSAREAN SECTION FOR SEVERE CASES

Treatment rarely employed

Traction on the half breech or internal version and breech extraction is practically never employed because of the risk of extensive cervical lacerations and shock as well as increasing the stillbirth rate.

Vaginal packing is condemned.—When done without anæsthesia, shock is produced and the pack cannot be inserted efficiently. Further placental separation may result, and organisms may be introduced.

However, in remote areas or developing countries where no "flying squad" is available and the distance to hospital is too great for the patient's safe transportation, packing may be the only means of controlling torrential hæmorrhage and saving the woman's life. (For method see p. 142.)

The midwife is again reminded that serious bleeding is usually due to the unjustifiable digital exploration of the cervical canal or ill-advised attempts to puncture the membranes.

DANGERS OF PLACENTA PRÆVIA

1. **HÆMORRHAGE**

(*a*) **Antepartum,** particularly following vaginal examination.

(*b*) **Postpartum atonic** because the lower segment does not contract and retract efficiently.

2. **Stillbirth** occurs due to fetal anoxia; prematurity adds to the danger.

3. **Puerperal sepsis** is more liable to occur because of—

(*a*) loss of blood, (*b*) the proximity of the placental site to the vagina,

ACCIDENTAL HÆMORRHAGE

Abruptio Placentæ

This condition (defined on p. 211) **is not due to an injury as the name might imply.**
The term " accidental hæmorrhage " was first used by an obstetrician during the
18th century, meaning " by chance " in contradistinction to unavoidable hæmorrhage
due to placenta prævia, in which the reason for premature separation of the placenta
was obvious.

The term " **abruptio placentæ,**" means to tear asunder and is more descriptive.

CAUSES

SEVERE HYPERTENSION

Pre-eclampsia and essential hypertension are present in about 8 per cent of cases.

Any strenuous physical effort or acute emotional stress that temporarily raises the
blood pressure may precipitate the occurrence of accidental hæmorrhage.

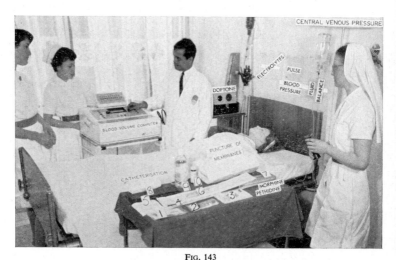

Fig. 143

Abruptio Placentae.

Obstetrician giving clinical instruction on equipment which may be used.

(1) **Plextrocan** intravenous cannula and needle. (2) **Syringe** 20 ml. (3) **Test tubes** for blood urea
and electrolytes, haemoglobin, serum fibrinogen Rh factor, group and cross matching. (4) **I.V. Cannula.**
(5) **Extension tube** 75 cm. (6) **Central venous pressure manometer** and stopcock. (7) **Giving set.** (8) **Arm
splint.** (9) **Intravenous fluid.** (10) **Uristix.** Packs: (*a*) Catheterization, (*b*) puncture of membranes.
Blood volume computer. Doptone. Drugs.

(*County Maternity Hospital, Bellshill, Lanarkshire.*)

HIGH PARITY

The condition is more common in multigravid patients and in those with poor nutritional status. (*Folic acid deficiency has been demonstrated in a series of cases.*)

TRAUMA

A fall or a blow on the abdomen, or traction on the cord, as might take place during
external version, is the cause in a minority of cases.

TYPES

1. EXTERNAL

Revealed accidental hæmorrhage in which blood escapes from the vagina.

2. COMBINED

The signs and symptoms of concealed and revealed hæmorrhage are both present, the hæmorrhage being primarily concealed.

3 CONCEALED

Accidental hæmorrhage, in which no vaginal bleeding is present. This is a very serious condition and fortunately much less common.

Incidence

The recorded incidence of accidental hæmorrhage has increased during recent years because more slight cases are being sent into hospital.

At the Simpson Memorial Maternity Pavilion in 1969. *A total of 336 cases was admitted, 281 cases were slight; Concealed, 8; Cæsarean section, 21; Maternal mortality, nil; Perinatal mortality 8 per cent. 88 were discharged after placentography or arteriogram or sonargram had excluded placenta praevia.*

1a. EXTERNAL ACCIDENTAL HÆMORRHAGE (SLIGHT)

This is the common type in which blood escapes through the cervix. Bleeding may however, become severe.

SIGNS AND SYMPTOMS

(*a*) **Vaginal bleeding.**

(*b*) **Abdominal pain** and tenderness may or may not be present.

(*c*) **Pre-eclampsia or essential hypertension** may be present in about 8 per cent of cases.

(*d*) **Normal presentation.** The head can usually be made to dip into the brim.

Treatment

On district and in hospital the initial treatment is that of antepartum hæmorrhage (type undiagnosed) (see p. 211).

1b. EXTERNAL ACCIDENTAL HÆMORRHAGE (SEVERE)

Treatment

(*a*) **As for severe antepartum hæmorrhage (type undiagnosed)** (p. 211).

(*b*) **Adequate blood transfusion.**—When the plasma fibrinogen is below normal, fresh rather than stored blood is used, because of its higher fibrinogen content.

(*c*) **A careful fluid balance record is kept.**

(*d*) **The woman should lie in the left lateral position until delivered** to facilitate more efficient kidney secretion. In the dorsal position shock may occur due to the supine hypotensive syndrome.

(*e*) **The membranes are punctured** and the liquor amnii drained off, as it is high in thromboplastin; the procedure being carried out in the theatre set up for Cæsarean section.

(*f*) **Cæsarean section is usually performed** when hæmorrhage persists, and in severe cases if the fetus is alive or if during labour fetal distress occurs.

(*g*) **An oxytocin drip is given by some authorities if labour does not commence** within a few hours and in cases where the fetus is dead. A syringe I.V. pump is used.

(*h*) **Urinary œstriol** assays are made in cases when bleeding has ceased and, if persistently low, Cæsarean section is considered.

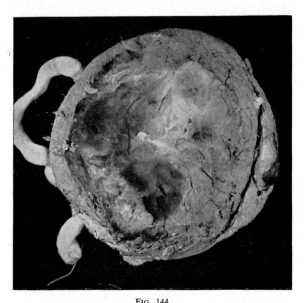

Fig. 144

Placenta with crater-like area on the maternal surface due to the pressure of old retroplacental blood clot. Infarction is also present.

2. COMBINED ACCIDENTAL HÆMORRHAGE

In this condition the hæmorrhage is primarily concealed, and then becomes revealed.

The patient exhibits a degree of shock, which is always greater than the blood loss warrants, and is usually associated with blood coagulation disorders and infiltration of the broad ligaments with blood as in concealed accidental hæmorrhage.

The uterus is tender, feels rigid but not necessarily board-like; abdominal pain is constant.

Signs of pre-eclampsia or essential hypertension may be present in about 8 per cent of cases.

TREATMENT is that of concealed accidental hæmorrhage.

3. CONCEALED ACCIDENTAL HÆMORRHAGE

This is a desperately serious condition with high maternal and fetal mortality rates. Fortunately it is the least common type of accidental hæmorrhage.

No vaginal bleeding occurs, but a retroplacental blood clot forms which may weigh as much as 1,588 G. (3½), lb. the placenta when expelled showing a crater-like area, or circumscribed depression on the maternal surface, containing dark old blood clot which may be adherent to it.

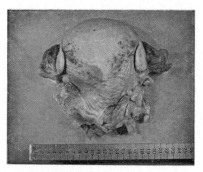

FIG. 145

CONCEALED ACCIDENTAL HÆMORRHAGE.
Uterus showing extensive discoloration due to extravasation of blood.

Blood coagulation disorders develop in many of these cases (see p. 224).

Folic acid deficiency has been found in some instances.

SIGNS AND SYMPTOMS

The following signs and symptoms are those of a severe case:—

1. **Shock is the outstanding feature** but the blood pressure may not fall to (90/60) in the hypertensive patient.

2. **The abdominal pain is excruciating and constant: never intermittent.**

3. **The uterus is exquisitely tender to touch,** hard and board-like.

4. **The pulse, which may be slow at first, becomes rapid and thready.**

5. **Very little urine is secreted.**

6. **The fetus cannot be palpated** because of uterine and abdominal wall rigidity; no fetal heart-beat is heard.

7. **Signs of pre-eclampsia or essential hypertension may be present** but protein always appears in the urine after concealed accidental hæmorrhage occurs and does not necessarily indicate the presence of pre-eclampsia.

Treatment on District

1. **Send for medical aid urgently;** if not available get the flying squad or communicate with a maternity hospital.

2. **Give pethidine, 100 mg.** (*The doctor may order morphine 15 mg. for severe pain.*)

3. **Keep a five-minute pulse chart.**

4. **Measure and save all urine passed.**

15 B

5. **In treating shock do not apply heat,** nor elevate the foot of the bed; removal of pillows is sufficient—the woman should lie on her side.

6. **The patient is transferred to hospital.**

Treatment in Hospital

1. **Measures to combat shock and blood loss** should be quickly initiated.

2. **Routine blood investigations are made** (see p. 213). **Plasma-fibrinogen and clotting-time tests** are performed. The Fi-test, Baxter-Hyland, for hypofibrinogenæmia is useful when laboratory facilities are not available. The Fibrindex thrombin test is made. **Expert hæmatological advice** is essential.

3. **Pethidine, 200 mg. or morphine 15 mg. may be given for pain.**

4. **Blood transfusion of at least one litre** fresh blood is administered rapidly, then more slowly, depending on the central venous pressure (normal being 8-12 cm. of water).

5. **Fibrinogen, 4 to 6 G.,** may be administered intravenously, followed by 1 G. at half-hourly intervals until the clotting mechanism is restored to normal.

6. **Triple or quadruple strength plasma is only given** if no fibrinogen is available.

7. **The membranes are punctured** to reduce retroplacental tension, prevent further absorption of thromboplastin and to induce labour.

8. **Oxygen is administered** if necessary.

9. **Each specimen of urine is examined for volume and protein.**

10. **Renal secretion is carefully observed** and ought to be at least 30 ml. per hour. **The fluid intake is recorded.**

11. **The pulse and blood pressure are taken every 15 and 30 minutes respectively,** and charted in graph form.

12. **An oxytocin drip may be administered** and kept running after delivery for 2 or 3 hours.

13. **Cæsarean section may be performed** (when the clotting defect is controlled).

14. **Postpartum hæmorrhage is a possible danger** if the uterus is atonic and any blood coagulation defect has not been corrected.

(*The weight of the retroplacental clot should be recorded.*)

THE PUERPERIUM

The hazard of acute renal failure is very great indeed so the woman must be observed carefully. The daily fluid intake should be restricted to 1,000 ml. for a few days and the diet low in protein, sodium and potassium. Blood urea estimations and potassium determinations are made for 3 days. An accurate fluid balance record is kept and signs of oliguria (less than 500 ml. urine daily) reported without delay. **Anæmia if present should be** treated and further blood transfusion may be indicated.

BLOOD COAGULATION DISORDERS IN OBSTETRICS

Serious hæmorrhage in obstetrics may be due to blood clotting failure.

(*a*) HYPOFIBRINOGENÆMIA, (*b*) EXCESSIVE FIBRINOLYTIC ACTIVITY or (*c*) A COMBINATION OF BOTH.

(*a*) **Hypofibrinogenæmia** is usually due to multiple micro-embolism and consumption of available maternal fibrinogen because of the abnormal entry of thromboplastin into the circulation (1) from the placental site in abruptio placentæ, (2) from amniotic fluid (which is rich in thromboplastin), (3) from tissue juice from a retained macerated fetus.

Tests.—The Fibrindex (Ortho) and the Baxter f i test are available for bedside diagnosis.

Expert hæmatological advice is needed in the differential diagnosis and treatment.

Treatment.—This includes giving intravenous human fibrinogen 4 G. to 6 G. with, in severe blood loss, adequate whole blood replacement. Dextran is definitely contra-indicated.

(*b*) **EXCESSIVE FIBRINOLYTIC ACTIVITY** can occur under the same conditions as (*a*) p. 224. It is due to excessive tissue plasminogen activator entering the maternal circulation and producing substances that inhibit normal blood coagulation. The maternal blood, in a test tube, may clot but rapid lysis follows at once.

Treatment.—**This may include the administration of a fibrinolytic inhibitor** such as epsilon-aminocaproic acid (EACA), intravenously, fibrinogen and/or whole blood as in (*a*), and heparin.

(*c*) **EXCESSIVE FIBRINOLYTIC ACTIVITY AND HYPOFIBRINOGEN-ÆMIA.** *Treatment includes fibrinogen, EACA, whole blood and heparin alone*, or in combination as individual circumstances indicate.

Fresh blood is a rich source of fibrinogen (about 3·3 G. in 1,800 ml.) as well as of fibrinolytic inhibitors and the successful outcome in many cases, where the more sophisticated products are not available, is often no doubt due to the prompt administration of adequate fresh blood.

Serious postpartum hæmorrhage may have to be dealt with should the uterus be atonic in the presence of blood coagulation disorders.

Couvelaire — blood in muscle of uterus causing labour.

QUESTIONS FOR REVISION

ANTEPARTUM HÆMORRHAGE

Define the following terms: (a) *Antepartum*; (b) *accidental*; (c) *unavoidable*.

What are the signs of concealed accidental hæmorrhage ?

Give a List of the Equipment you would have at hand for the reception of a patient with moderately severe antepartum hæmorrhage and for the investigations to be carried out in such a case.

ORAL QUESTIONS

How could you help to reduce the number of cases of serious ante-partum hæmorrhage ?

Why is bleeding from the placental site more serious than from other vaginal sources ?

Why must a vaginal examination not be made outwith a theatre equipped for a Cæsarean section ?

The active treatment of placenta prævia can be summarized for slight and severe cases as (a) . . . and (b) . . . Why is the woman required to lie on her side in cases of accidental hæmorrhage? **Why is Cæsarean section performed** in placenta prævia? **Why is vaginal packing not advocated** for placenta prævia?

What observation would you make in a case of antepartum hæmorrhage: (1) general condition; (2) history; (3) blood loss; (4) abdominal examination?

State 4 blood tests; 4 charts; 4 intravenous solutions; 4 methods of diagnosis that might be utilized.

Define the four degrees of placenta prævia.

Differentiate between: blood coagulation defect and **retroplacental clot; active** and **expectant treatment** of placenta prævia; **combined and concealed** accidental hæmorrhage.

C.M.B.(N. Ireland) paper.—What is placenta prævia ? When is this condition suspected ? What is meant by conservative treatment ?

C.M.B.(Eng.) paper.—Define antepartum hæmorrhage. Discuss the possible causes of such bleeding at the 34th week of pregnancy. What action should the midwife take in such cases ?

C.M.B.(Scot.) paper.—Describe the nursing care after delivery of a patient who has had concealed accidental hæmorrhage. What particular observations would you make ?

C.M.B.(Scot.) paper.—Describe the diagnosis and management of a case of concealed accidental hæmorrhage (*abruptio placentæ*).

C.M.B.(N. Ireland) paper.—What is Antepartum Hæmorrhage? Detail the nursing care of a patient with Antepartum Hæmorrhage at 32 weeks.

C.M.B.(Eng.) paper.—Give the possible causes of bleeding from the genital tract after the 28th week of pregnancy. How should this condition be investigated?

C.M.B.(N. Ireland) paper 1969.—Define accidental hæmorrhage. What are the symptoms and signs of concealed accidental hæmorrhage (abruptio placentæ) ? Describe the maternal complications which it may cause.

C.M.B.(Scot.) paper 1969.—What are the possible causes of slight vaginal bleeding at the 34th week ? Describe the management.

C.M.B.(Scot.) paper 1970.—What are the clinical features of a patient suffering from concealed accidental hæmorrhage? Describe the management.

14

Clinical Course: Physiological Changes: Mechanism of Normal Labour

THE CLINICAL COURSE OF LABOUR

Labour is described as the process by which the fetus, placenta and membranes are expelled through the birth canal. It involves more than the expulsive muscular effort of the uterus, being a strenuous ordeal in which the woman's whole body participates, and demanding physical stamina and emotional control. The term "labour" is used after the 28th week of gestation: before then the process is called "abortion."

NORMAL LABOUR *is known as* **EUTOCIA**

This has been described as one in which:

1. **The fetus is born at term and presents by the vertex.**

2. **The process is completed spontaneously** (*by the natural unaided efforts of the mother*).

3. **The time does not exceed 24 hours.** 4. **No complications arise.**

Difficult or Abnormal Labour is known as Dystocia

CAUSES OF THE ONSET OF LABOUR

The onset of labour appears to be the result of a combination of factors, hormonal, nervous and circulatory. It is possible that some signal is given from the feto-placental unit.

1. **Oxytocin from the posterior pituitary gland** and probably from the placenta has a stimulating action on the pregnant uterus which has been sensitized by some hormonal or other factor.

2. **Increased contractibility.**—As pregnancy advances, there is an increase in the contractibility of the uterus, which becomes more susceptible to stimulation as term approaches. Abdominal palpation will excite uterine contractions during the last month; drugs, such as oxytocin, will successfully induce labour in 50 per cent of women who are at term.

3. **The pressure of the presenting part on the nerve-endings in the cervix** is thought to stimulate a nerve plexus known as the cervical ganglion, and experience shows that labour is more likely to start on time when the head is engaged than when it is high.

4. **Overdistension of the uterus,** as occurs with twins or hydramnios, tends to induce premature labour, but high temperature, strong emotion, cyanosis and eclampsia have all been associated with the onset of premature labour.

THE PREMONITORY SIGNS OF LABOUR

During the three weeks previous to the onset of labour, certain changes take place which, when manifest, are useful to determine the approach of labour.

1. LIGHTENING.
2. FREQUENCY OF MICTURITION.
3. FALSE PAINS.
4. SLIGHT TAKING UP OF THE CERVIX.

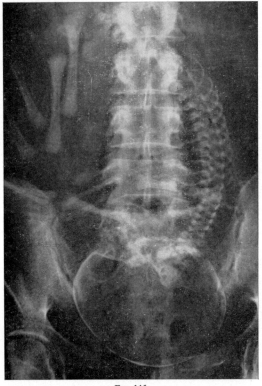

Fig. 146

X-ray photograph, showing vertex left occipito-anterior position.

(*Simpson Memorial Maternity Pavilion Edinburgh*)

1. LIGHTENING

This is the sinking of the uterus, which takes place about two or three weeks before term. Because the fundus no longer crowds the lungs, breathing is easier, the heart and stomach can function better and the relief of pressure experienced by the woman is described as lightening.

It occurs because:

(*a*) **The symphysis pubis widens.**

(*b*) **The softened, relaxed pelvic floor sags** by as much as 3·8 cm. (1½ inches) allowing the uterus to descend further into the true pelvis.

(*c*) **The lower segment stretches and the fetus sinks further down inside the uterus.**

The fundus is therefore at a lower level; the uterus becomes more prominent and if the abdominal muscles are in good tone, as is found in primigravid women, and no disproportion exists, *the head will enter the pelvic brim and become engaged.*

In multigravid women the bracing action of firm abdominal muscles may be absent, and the uterus will then sag further forwards, the abdomen becomes somewhat pendulous and the fetal head does not as a rule become engaged.

Walking is more difficult at this time, and the woman feels cumbersome and ungainly. Relaxation of the pelvic joints may give rise to backache or pain in the region of the symphysis pubis. Vague discomfort may be experienced in the lower abdomen, groins and thighs. The vaginal secretion becomes more profuse.

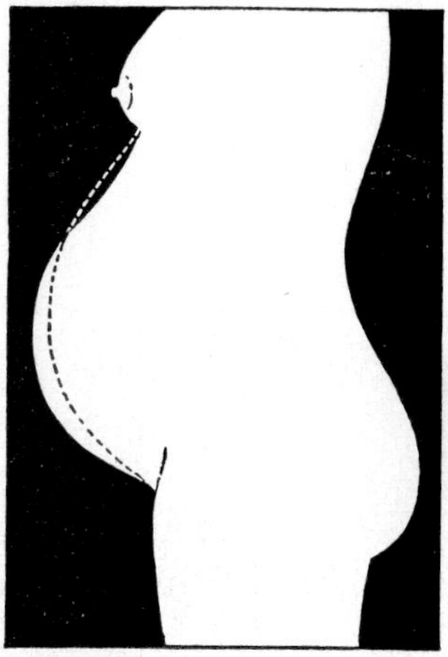

Fig. 147

LIGHTENING.

The dotted line shows the shape of the uterus prior to lightening.

2. FREQUENCY OF MICTURITION

This may be due to pressure of the fetal head on the bladder limiting its capacity and requiring it to be emptied more often. But sometimes there is a state of mild incontinence or poor control of the urethral sphincter, which may be accounted for by the lax condition of the softened pelvic floor at this time.

3. FALSE PAINS

These are erratic and irregular, causing the uterus to contract and relax, whereas in true labour the uterus contracts and retracts. They may be unduly troublesome and some consider this to be a mild form of inco-ordinate uterine action.

4. TAKING UP OF THE CERVIX

The cervix is somewhat shorter, because it is being drawn up and merged into the lower uterine segment. This sign is usually looked for, when, in the interest of mother or child, labour must be induced.

SIGNS OF TRUE LABOUR

1. PAINFUL, RHYTHMIC UTERINE   CONTRACTIONS.

2. DILATATION OF THE OS.

3. SHOW.

1. UTERINE CONTRACTIONS

These are now felt by the woman as tightening, discomfort or actual pain. During contraction the uterus feels hard to the touch.

Slight backache may also be present. These signs are explained in detail on page 267; and the diagnosis of true labour on page 269.

DILATATION OF THE OS

The physiology of this is explained on page 234 and diagnosis on page 274.

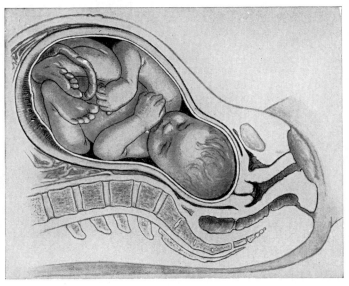

FIG. 148

Fetus *in utero* at beginning of labour.

3. SHOW

This is explained on page 234.

Rupture of the membranes cannot be accepted as a sign of true labour, as it sometimes occurs a few days before labour begins, or may not occur until the end of the second stage.

THE THREE STAGES OF LABOUR

THE FIRST STAGE

The first stage is that of dilatation of the os, and lasts from the onset of true labour to complete dilatation of the os.

THE SECOND STAGE

The second stage is that of expulsion of the fetus. It begins when the os is fully dilated and ends when the baby is born.

THE THIRD STAGE

The third stage is that of separation and expulsion of the placenta and membranes and is also concerned with the control of bleeding. It lasts from the birth of the baby to the expulsion of the placenta and membranes.

THE FOURTH STAGE

In order to stress the continued vigilance which is necessary because of the risk of postpartum hæmorrhage, **some authorities describe a fourth stage**—the period of six hours following the birth of the placenta.

THE DURATION OF LABOUR

There are wide variations in the duration of labour, depending on whether the woman is a primigravida or multigravida and on the time that has elapsed since the birth of her last child. The type of pelvis, size and presentation of the fetus and the strength and frequency of the uterine contractions, all influence the length of labour.

The greater part of labour is taken up with the first stage. Seldom is the second stage less than half an hour in a primigravida and the multigravid woman may have a second stage of 15 minutes or less. The duration of the third stage is usually between 5 and 20 minutes.

The consensus of opinion is that during the past 20 years the duration of labour has been shorter than previously, probably due to the greater use of relaxation, sedation and oxytocin. The figures given below could be considered fairly average to-day but experience proves that average figures can be misleading.

	First Stage	Second Stage	Third Stage	Total
PRIMIGRAVIDA	12½ hours	1 hour	½ hour	14 hours
MULTIGRAVIDA	7 hours	½ hour	½ hour	8 hours

A considerable number of primigravidæ have labours of under 12 hours, a number of multigravidæ have labours of six to eight hours and in many cases less than six hours.

THE PHYSIOLOGICAL CHANGES DURING LABOUR
First and Second Stages

It is advisable for the midwife to study the physiological changes that occur during labour, to enable her to interpret intelligently such observations as may be made and to appreciate deviations from the normal course.

PHYSIOLOGICAL CHANGES DURING THE FIRST STAGE

1. **CONTRACTION AND RETRACTION OF UTERINE MUSCLE.** *The primary powers*
2. **FORMATION OF THE UPPER AND LOWER UTERINE SEGMENTS.**
3. **DEVELOPMENT OF THE RETRACTION RING.**
4. **TAKING UP OF THE CERVIX.**
5. **DILATATION OF THE OS.**
6. **SHOW.**
7. **FORMATION OF THE BAG OF WATERS**
8. **RUPTURE OF THE MEMBRANES.**

1. CONTRACTION AND RETRACTION OF UTERINE MUSCLE

Uterine contractions (*sometimes known as the primary powers*) are **involuntary**: they are controlled by the nervous system and probably indirectly governed by endocrine influence.

Palpable contractions rarely last longer than 60 to 70 seconds, because, if prolonged, the compression of the blood sinuses in the uterine wall interferes with the oxygen supply to the fetus. They usually recur with rhythmic regularity, and the intervals between them gradually diminish from 15 minutes, more or less, at the beginning of the first stage, to two or three minutes at the end of the second stage.

Fundal dominance. Each contraction starts in the fundal region and spreads downwards, being stronger and persisting longer in the upper region. The fundus and mid-zone remain hard throughout the period of contraction, the transverse diameter decreases. On reaching the lower uterine segment the wave of contraction weakens considerably and this permits the cervix to dilate and the strongly contracting fundus to expel the fetus.

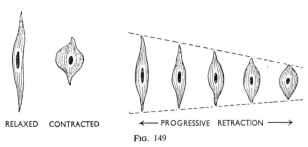

RELAXED   CONTRACTED   ⟵ PROGRESSIVE RETRACTION ⟶

Fig. 149

Diagrammatic representation of a uterine muscle fibre, showing how by retraction it retains some of the contraction and becomes shorter and thicker.

Polarity is the term used to describe the neuromuscular harmony that prevails between the two poles or segments of the uterus during labour. The nervous control of polarity is not understood and is the subject of much controversy.

During each uterine contraction these two poles act harmoniously; the upper pole contracting strongly and retracting to expel the fetus, the lower pole contracting slightly and dilating to allow it to be expelled.

If polarity is disorganized the progress of labour is inhibited.

RETRACTION

This is a special faculty of uterine muscle whereby the contraction does not pass off entirely; the muscle fibres retaining some of the contraction instead of becoming completely relaxed. Retraction assists in the progressive expulsion of the fetus; the upper segment of the uterus becomes shorter and thicker and its cavity diminishes.

2. FORMATION OF THE UPPER AND LOWER UTERINE SEGMENTS

At the end of pregnancy the uterus is divided functionally into two, the upper and the lower uterine segments. The upper segment is the thick muscular contractile part, and the lower segment is the thin distensible area, 7·5 or 10·2 cm. (3 or 4 inches) in length, which has developed from the isthmus of the uterus. When labour begins, the retracted longitudinal fibres in the upper segment pull on the lower segment, causing it to stretch: this is aided by the force applied by the descending head or breech. The thinned out area facilitates the expulsion of the fetus.

3. DEVELOPMENT OF THE RETRACTION RING

The ridge which forms at the lower border of the thick upper segment where it meets the thin lower segment is known as the retraction, or Bandl's ring. It is present in every labour and is perfectly normal so long as it is not marked enough to be visible above the symphysis pubis. In normal labour there is no need for the lower segment to become unduly distended, because the fetus is gradually being expelled through the dilating os.

In cases of obstructed labour, where the fetus cannot descend to pass through the os, the lower segment must stretch to accommodate it, because the fetus is being pushed out of the shortened upper segment. In such a case the retraction ring would be *palpable and visible as a depressed ridge* running transversely or slightly obliquely across the abdomen above the symphysis pubis. The greater the distension of the lower segment, the higher will the retraction ring rise and the more urgent is the danger of rupture of the uterus.

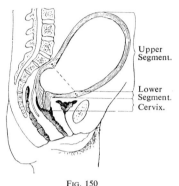

Upper Segment.

Lower Segment.
Cervix.

FIG. 150
Parturient canal before labour begins.

Although the terms " Bandl's ring " and " retraction ring " are synonymous, it is expedient for practical purposes to differentiate between the two. The term " Bandl's ring " is commonly applied to the retraction ring when it becomes visible and " retraction ring " to the normal invisible one.

4. TAKING UP OF THE CERVIX

Some shortening of the cervix has already taken place at the end of pregnancy, but when labour begins, the muscle fibres surrounding the internal os are drawn upwards by the retracted upper segment, and the cervix is shortened as it merges into and becomes part of the lower uterine segment. **The cervix is gradually effaced;** its canal widens from above to form a funnel, the external os being the narrowed portion. The process could in some measure be likened to the shortening of the neck of a toy balloon as the balloon is inflated.

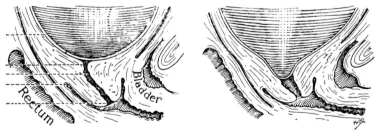

FIG. 151

Process of " taking up " of cervix by which its canal becomes continuous with the lower uterine segment.

N.B.—The **" taking up of the cervix "** should not be confused with **" no cervix felt "** on vaginal examination. which denotes complete dilatation of the os and signifies the end of the first stage.

16

5. DILATATION OF THE OS

This is the enlargement of the external os from a circular opening which would admit a uterine sound to one sufficiently large to permit passage of the fetal head. The mechanism of the process of dilatation is imperfectly understood but it is surmised that the upward traction, exerted by the retracted muscle fibres in the upper segment, exerts pull on the margin of the weakened area—the os—and makes it enlarge.

But without pressure applied from within the uterus, by a well-fitting presenting part, dilatation will not proceed normally. **The well-flexed head will, when closely applied to the cervix, aid dilatation.**

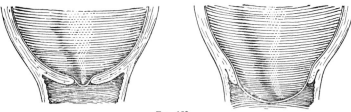

FIG. 152
Showing dilatation of the os, membranes intact.

Artificial rupture of membranes as a means of speeding up labour will only succeed if there is good application of head to cervix; weak uterine contractions or a high or badly-fitting presenting part invariably result in slow dilatation of the os.

In the primigravid woman the external os may be closed at the beginning of labour, or it may admit the tip of one finger, and does not dilate until the cervix has been taken up, but the internal os dilates during the process of taking up of the cervix.

In the multigravid woman the external os usually admits one finger prior to the onset of labour and the dilatation of the external and internal os proceeds simultaneously with taking up of the cervix.

6. SHOW

Show is the blood-stained mucoid discharge seen a few hours before, or within a few hours after, labour has started. The mucus is the thick, tenacious substance

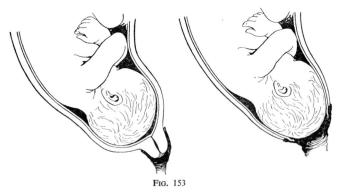

FIG. 153
The cervix at the beginning of labour.　　　　The os fully dilated.

which formed the cervical plug—**the operculum**—during pregnancy. The blood comes from the ruptured capillaries of the decidua vera where the chorion has become detached, and from the dilating cervix. Show resembles the beginning of a menstrual period.

7. FORMATION OF THE BAG OF WATERS

When the lower uterine segment stretches, the chorion becomes detached from it, and the increased intra-uterine pressure causes this loosened part of the sac of fluid to bulge downwards into the dilating internal os, to the depth of 6·2 mm. (¼ inch) or 12·4 mm. (½ inch).

The well-flexed head fits snugly into the cervix, so that the fluid in front of the head is cut off from the remainder of the amniotic fluid, and is known as the *fore-waters*; the remainder is known as the *hind-waters*. The purpose of cutting off the fore-waters is to prevent the pressure exerted on the hind-waters during uterine contractions from being applied to the fore-waters, and is Nature's method of keeping the membranes intact during the first stage.

General Fluid Pressure

While the membranes remain intact the pressure of the uterine contractions is exerted on the fluid, and as fluid is not compressible the pressure is equalized throughout the uterus and is known as **general fluid pressure.** When the membranes rupture and a quantity of fluid escapes, the placenta is compressed between the uterine wall and the fetus during contractions, and the oxygen supply to the fetus is thereby diminished.

With intact membranes there is less risk of fetal anoxia and uterine infection and it can be accepted as a good working rule that as long as the membranes are intact mother and fetus are relatively safe.

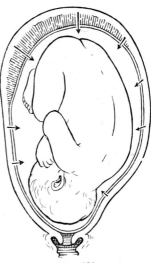

FIG. 154

GENERAL FLUID PRESSURE.

The pressure of the uterine contractions is exerted on the amniotic fluid and equalized. The placental circulation is only interfered with slightly.

8. RUPTURE OF THE MEMBRANES

The amniotic sac should remain intact until the os is fully dilated, but this by no means always happens. The membranes may rupture days before labour begins, or during the first or second stages, and in some instances not until the head is being born.

Towards the end of the first stage the bag of membranes receives very little support, because of the extensive dilatation of the os. It is also subjected to the increased force of the strong uterine contractions. If, for any reason, there is a badly fitting presenting part, the fore-waters are not cut off effectively and the membranes rupture early. but in some cases this happens for no apparent reason.

PHYSIOLOGICAL CHANGES DURING THE SECOND STAGE

1. THE CONTRACTIONS ARE STRONGER AND MORE FREQUENT.

2. THE SECONDARY POWERS ARE ACTIVE.

3. THE PELVIC FLOOR IS DISPLACED.

4. THE FETUS IS EXPELLED.

5. THE MECHANISM OF LABOUR PLAYS AN IMPORTANT ROLE IN THE SECOND STAGE OF LABOUR.

1. THE CONTRACTIONS ARE STRONGER

The uterus is irritated by being more closely applied to the fetus when some of the fluid escapes, so its contractile power is intensified. The vagina is being stretched by the fetus and this reflexly stimulates good uterine action

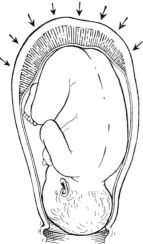

The upper uterine segment continues to become short and thick because of the retraction of the muscle fibres, and the placental circulation is interfered with to a greater extent than during the first stage. The fetus is gradually expelled.

The uterine contractions tend to straighten out the fetal spine and elongate the fetus, so the height of the fundus remains well above the umbilicus although the head is on the pelvic floor.

Fetal Axis Pressure

During each contraction the uterus rears forwards and the force of the contraction is transmitted via the long axis of the fetus and directs it through the birth canal. This is known as **fetal axis pressure** and differs from the general fluid pressure of the first stage.

FIG. 155

FETAL AXIS PRESSURE
(aids expulsion of the fetus).

The membranes have ruptured and much of the fluid has drained away. The pressure of the abdominal muscles and diaphragm is exerted on the buttocks and body of the fetus. The placental circulation is interfered with during contractions.

2. THE SECONDARY POWERS

The contractions of the abdominal muscles and diaphragm now come into play. Their expulsive action, known as " *bearing down* " or " *pushing*," is largely reflex at first and can be aided by voluntary effort, but when the presenting part reaches the pelvic floor and distends it this expulsive action becomes involuntary. The secondary powers are of tremendous assistance in overcoming the resistance encountered at the pelvic outlet.

As long as there is no obstruction to hinder the continued descent of the fetus the lower segment does not thin out to a dangerous degree.

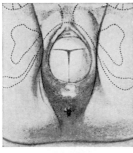

3. DISPLACEMENT OF THE PELVIC FLOOR

The fundus of the bladder rises into the abdomen where there is less risk of its being injured by the descending head, and at the same time more space is available in the pelvis for the passage of the fetus.

The advancing head dilates the vagina and may lacerate the mucosa, causing slight bleeding. The posterior segment of the pelvic floor is pushed downwards in front of the presenting part: the rectum is compressed by the advancing head, and any fæcal contents will be expelled.

FIG. 156

THE HEAD IS CROWNED.
The occipital prominence has escaped and the sinciput will now sweep the perineum.

The anus *pouts* and gradually gapes until the opening is 2·5 cm. (1 inch) in diameter, showing the anterior rectal wall.

The triangular perineal body is flattened out and instead of being 3·8 cm. by 3·8 cm. (1½ by 1½ inches) it becomes thin and almost transparent with a length of about 10·2 cm.

(4 inches). The thinned out perineum lengthens the posterior wall of the birth canal, causing the vaginal orifice to be directed upwards.

4. THE FETUS IS EXPELLED

The head is seen at the vulva, advancing with each contraction and receding between contractions, until crowning takes place, when the head is then born by extension.   The shoulders and body follow with the next contraction, along with the remainder of the amniotic fluid.   **The second stage culminates in the birth of the baby.**

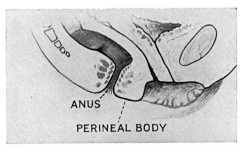

FIG. 157

Urethra, bladder, vagina, perineal body and rectum in the non-pregnant state. (*See Fig. 158 for comparison.*)

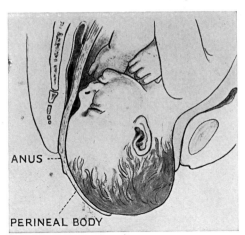

FIG. 158

Vagina distended, perineal body thinned out, rectum compressed, at the end of the second stage of labour.

5. THE MECHANISM OF LABOUR

The mechanism of labour is a series of passive movements of the fetus in its passage through the birth canal.   Such movements are essential, because the canal is cylindrical, with an inlet and outlet differing in size and shape and a forward curve at its lower end. The fetus is a flexible cylindrical body which, during the process of birth, is made to accommodate itself to the diameters and curve of the pelvic canal.

The skilful management of normal delivery is based on a knowledge of the mechanism of labour so it is imperative that these natural movements should be thoroughly understood. The student midwife must be taught the underlying principle of each movement; they are only of value when related to the management of labour.

Some authorities question the value of teaching the mechanisms of labour (admittedly they are valueless if learned by rote). But when each movement is understood this knowledge enables the midwife to observe the progress of normal and abnormal labour more intelligently. The successful conduct of delivery, whether vertex, breech or face, depends largely on facilitating Nature's method which is mechanism.

The terms—lie, presentation, position, etc., used in describing mechanisms, have been defined and explained on page 75.

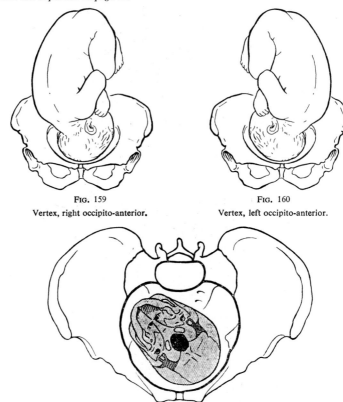

Fig. 159	Fig. 160
Vertex, right occipito-anterior.	Vertex, left occipito-anterior.

Fig. 161

Showing the advantage of an anterior position of the vertex. The wide biparietal diameter is in the roomy anterior part of the pelvic brim. The narrow bitemporal diameter lies in the sacro-cotyloid diameter of the pelvic brim.

MECHANISM OF VERTEX PRESENTATION
(Left Occipito-Anterior Position)

The lie, which is the relation of the long axis of the fetus to the long axis of the uterus, is longitudinal.

The attitude, which is the relation of the fetal limbs and head to its trunk, is one of flexion.

The presentation, which is the part lying at the pelvic brim, is the vertex.

The position, which is the relation of the part of the fetus, known as the denominator, to the six areas of the pelvic brim is the left occipito-anterior or L.O.A.   The occiput points to the left ilio-pectineal eminence, the sinciput to the right sacro-iliac joint.   The suboccipito-frontal diameter of the head is in the right oblique diameter of the pelvic brim.

The denominator is the occiput, and because it points to the ilio-pectineal eminence which is in the left anterior quadrant of the pelvis determines the position as left occipito-anterior (L.O.A.).

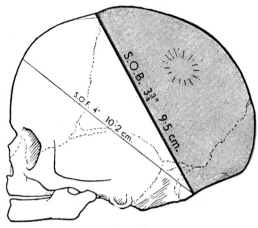

FIG. 162

Diagram of fetal skull showing the engaging diameters in a vertex L.O.A.   The S.O.F. diameter lies at the pelvic brim at the onset of labour.   With increase of flexion the S.O.B. diameter engages and passes through the birth canal.   The S.O.F. diameter sweeps the perineum.

The presenting part, which is the part of the presentation that lies over the os, is the posterior area of the right parietal bone.

The following movements take place during labour, as the result of the expulsive action of the uterine and abdominal muscles and diaphragm and the resistance offered by the pelvis, cervix and pelvic floor.

1. FLEXION OF THE HEAD
2. INTERNAL ROTATION OF THE HEAD
3. CROWNING OF THE HEAD
4. EXTENSION OF THE HEAD
5. RESTITUTION OF THE HEAD
6. INTERNAL ROTATION OF THE SHOULDERS
7. EXTERNAL ROTATION OF THE HEAD
8. LATERAL FLEXION OF THE BODY

Descent takes place throughout.

DESCENT

Descent begins in most primigravid patients two weeks before the onset of labour when engagement of the head occurs, unless disproportion between head and pelvis exists. Further descent takes place during the first stage, and is brought about by the

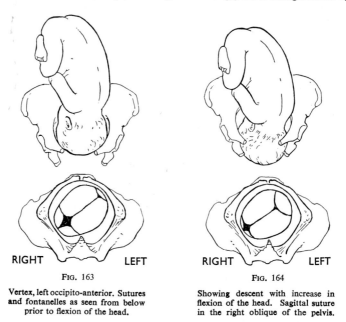

RIGHT   LEFT   RIGHT   LEFT

FIG. 163   FIG. 164

Vertex, left occipito-anterior. Sutures and fontanelles as seen from below prior to flexion of the head.

Showing descent with increase in flexion of the head. Sagittal suture in the right oblique of the pelvis.

force of the uterine contractions. When the head meets resistance, flexion is increased and the dilating os allows the flexed head to sink partly into it. During the second stage descent is more rapid because the abdominal muscles and diaphragm come into play and the fetus is being actively expelled.

1. FLEXION OF THE HEAD

The head is usually flexed at the beginning of labour, with the suboccipito-frontal diameter, 10·2 cm. (4 inches), lying at the pelvic brim, but when flexion is increased the suboccipito-bregmatic diameter, 9·5 cm. (3¾ inches), engages. This increased flexion facilitates descent.

Causes of Flexion

(*a*) **Exaggeration of an existing attitude.** The fetus *in utero* is already in an attitude of flexion; the uterine contractions will therefore tend to increase the existing attitude.

(*b*) **The lever theory.** When the head meets the resistance of the pelvis, cervix and pelvic floor, flexion is increased. This may be due to the fact that the fetal head articulates with the spine nearer the occiput than the sinciput, producing a lever with two arms of unequal length. Any force transmitted via the fetal spine causing fetal descent, *e.g.* fetal axis pressure, will exert greater pressure on the shorter arm of the lever and the occiput will descend (Fig. 165).

(*c*) **The wedge shape of the head.** When the head is partly flexed it forms a wedge one side of which, being short and steep, will meet less resistance and will, therefore, descend more rapidly (Fig. 166).

The result of increased flexion of the head is that the occiput becomes the leading part, and this influences the next movement—that of internal rotation.

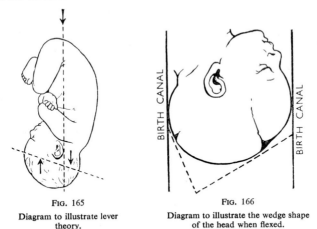

FIG. 165

Diagram to illustrate lever theory.

FIG. 166

Diagram to illustrate the wedge shape of the head when flexed.

2. INTERNAL ROTATION

Internal rotation is a turning forwards of whatever part of the fetus reaches one lateral half of the gutter-shaped pelvic floor first. *In an L.O.A. the occiput rotates forwards.* This movement makes the fetus conform to the lower curve of the birth canal, and

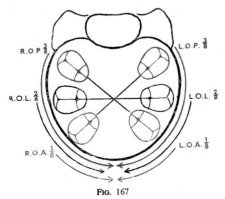

FIG. 167

Diagrammatic representation of internal rotation in anterior, lateral and posterior positions of the vertex presentation

causes the larger diameters of the head, shoulders and buttocks to emerge under the pubic arch in the antero-posterior, which is the largest diameter of the outlet.

The factors which bring about internal rotation are:

(a) **The passive recoil of one lateral half of the pelvic floor.** When the leading part reaches the level of the ischial spines it comes in contact with the left half of the pelvic floor. The force of the uterine contractions causes the occiput to stretch the left half of the pelvic floor and push it downwards and outwards; when the contraction passes off the pelvic floor recoils and because it slopes forwards the occiput glides along the left side of the pelvis. If the head is deflexed there is no leading part and the head comes in contact with both halves of the pelvic floor so rotation does not take place.

(*b*) **The gutter-shape of the pelvic floor.**—This tends to direct the leading part towards the front, where it passes through the weakened area of the pelvic floor and under the pubic arch.

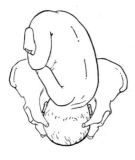

Fig. 168

Showing internal rotation of the head. The occiput lies behind the symphysis pubis, having rotated forwards one-eighth of a circle.

RIGHT   LEFT

The sagittal suture is in the antero-posterior diameter of the outlet.

(*c*) **The unequal flexibilities of the fetus.**—Because the head bends more readily in one direction than another (*nodding movement*), it conforms to the curve of the pelvic canal in much the same way in which the foot turns forwards if pushed sideways into a Wellington boot.

In an L.O.A. the occiput rotates forwards one-eighth of a circle, from the left ilio-pectineal eminence to the symphysis pubis, where it can escape under the pubic arch and allow the suboccipital region to pivot on the lower border of the symphysis pubis.

3. CROWNING OF THE HEAD

Crowning is the term used when the occipital prominence escapes under the symphysis pubis and the head no longer recedes between uterine contractions. (*The suboccipito-*

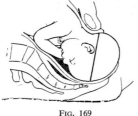

Fig. 169

Crowning of the head.

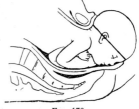

Fig. 170

Extension of the head

bregmatic diameter 9·5 cm. (3¾ inches), distends the vulval orifice instead of the larger suboccipito-frontal diameter, 10·2 cm. (4 inches).)

4. EXTENSION

Extension is a movement by which flexion of the head is undone. The nape of the neck pivots on the lower border of the symphysis pubis while the sinciput, face and chin pass over the thinned-out perineum. Extension results from the action of two forces; the uterine and abdominal muscles exert downward pressure; the pelvic floor and perineum resist this pressure and tend to push the head forwards and upwards through the weak area—the vaginal orifice. *The suboccipito-frontal diameter,* 10·2 *cm. (4 inches), sweeps the perineum.*

5. RESTITUTION

This is a turning of the head to undo the twist in the neck that took place during internal rotation of the head. In a vertex L.O.A. the occiput turns one-eighth of a circle to the left, back to where it was before internal rotation took place. (*This movement reveals whether the position is right or left, and when the midwife knows whether she is delivering an L.O.A. or an R.O.A. she is more likely to manage the birth of the shoulders without causing a perineal laceration.*)

6. INTERNAL ROTATION OF THE SHOULDERS

This is a movement similar to internal rotation of the head. The shoulders in an L.O.A. are in the left oblique diameter of the pelvic cavity. The anterior shoulder reaches the right side of the pelvic floor and rotates forwards bringing the shoulders

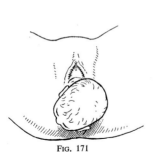

Fig. 171

Restitution of the head, occiput turns to left in an L.O.A.

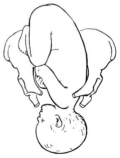

Fig. 172

Internal rotation of the shoulders. They are now in the antero-posterior diameter of the outlet. The head has also rotated externally.

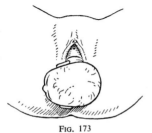

Fig. 173

External rotation of the head.

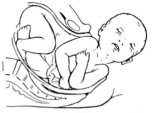

Fig. 174

Lateral flexion of the body.

into the antero-posterior diameter of the outlet. This should take place with the uterine contraction which occurs after the head has been born.

7. EXTERNAL ROTATION OF THE HEAD

This is a turning of the head which accompanies internal rotation of the shoulders. The occiput turns a further one-eighth of a circle; always in the same direction as in restitution. (*When the head has rotated externally, it indicates that the shoulders are now in the antero-posterior diameter of the pelvic outlet, in readiness for expulsion.*)

8. LATERAL FLEXION OF THE BODY

Lateral flexion is a sideways bending of the spine, which takes place while the body is being expelled, so that it conforms to the curve of the birth canal. The anterior shoulder escapes under the symphysis pubis; the posterior shoulder passes over the perineum, causing a smaller diameter to distend the vaginal orifice than if both shoulders were expelled simultaneously. (*The baby is carried forwards over the symphysis pubis towards the mother's abdomen to facilitate lateral flexion.*)

SUMMARY OF MECHANISM. VERTEX L.O.A.

1. **The lie is longitudinal.**
2. **The attitude is one of flexion.**
3. **The presentation is the vertex.**
4. **The position is the L.O.A.**
5. **The denominator is the occiput.**
6. **The presenting part is the posterior area of the right parietal bone.**

The head enters with the sagittal suture in the right oblique diameter of the pelvic brim.

Flexion.—Descent takes place with increasing flexion, the occiput becomes the leading part.

Internal rotation.—The occiput reaches the pelvic floor first and rotates one-eighth of a circle forwards, along the left side of the pelvis.

Crowning.—The occipital prominence escapes under the symphysis pubis and the head is crowned.

Extension.—The sinciput, face and chin sweep the perineum and the head is born by a movement of extension.

Restitution takes place and the occiput turns to the mother's left and the head rights itself with the shoulders.

Internal rotation of the shoulders.—The shoulders enter in the left oblique. The anterior shoulder reaches the pelvic floor first and rotates one-eighth of a circle forwards, along the right side of the pelvis.

External rotation of the head accompanies internal rotation of the shoulders. The occiput turns another one-eighth of a circle to the mother's left.

Lateral flexion.—The anterior shoulder escapes under the symphysis pubis, the posterior shoulder sweeps the perineum and the body is born by a movement of lateral flexion; the baby's back being towards the mother's left.

SUMMARY OF MECHANISM. VERTEX R.O.A.

The movements are identical to those in the left occipito-anterior, except that the word " *right* " is substituted for " *left* " and vice versa.

The head enters with the sagittal suture in the left oblique diameter of the brim.

The occiput points to the right ilio-pectineal eminence and the sinciput to the left sacro-iliac joint.

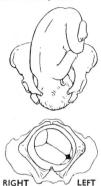

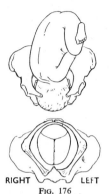

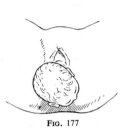

RIGHT	LEFT	RIGHT	LEFT	
Fig. 175		Fig. 176		Fig. 177

Right occipito-anterior. Head descending. Sagittal suture in the left oblique diameter of the pelvis.

Right occipito-anterior. Occiput has rotated one-eighth of a circle forwards. Sagittal suture in the antero-posterior diameter of the pelvic outlet.

Restitution, occiput turns to the right.

The occiput reaches the pelvic floor first and rotates one-eighth of a circle forwards along the right side of the pelvis, escapes and the head is crowned.

After extension, restitution takes place and the occiput turns one-eighth of a circle to the right; it then turns another eighth of a circle when the head rotates externally; the occiput being directed towards the mother's right thigh.

QUESTIONS FOR REVISION

ORAL QUESTIONS

What do you understand by normal labour ? Name 3 premonitory signs of labour ? 3 signs of true labour ?

What would you do if called out at night to a woman in false labour ? Which skull diameters engage in a well flexed head ?

How would you facilitate lateral flexion of the body during delivery ?

What do you understand by: polarity; show; bag of membranes.

Differentiate between: (*a*) contraction and retraction; (*b*) taking up of the cervix and no cervix felt; (*c*) false and true labour; (*d*) presentation and position; (*e*) restitution and external rotation; (*f*) upper and lower uterine segments; (*g*) retraction ring and Bandl's ring; (*h*) forewaters and hindwaters; (*i*) general fluid pressure and fetal axis pressure; (*j*) abortion and labour.

C.M.B.(Scot.) paper.—How do you recognize that labour has begun ? What changes take place in the uterus during the first stage of labour ?

C.M.B.(N. Ireland) paper.—Describe the normal action of the uterine muscle during labour. How may this be interfered with ?

C.M.B.(Eng.) paper.—Describe the second stage of normal labour, explaining (*a*) the action of the uterus; (*b*) the action of any other muscles which may help the movements of the fetal head.

17

C.M.B.(Scot.) paper.—Describe the course of normal labour.

C.M.B.(Eng.) paper.—Describe the mechanism of a vertex presentation, left occipito-anterior. In what way are these various movements of practical significance ?

C.M.B.(Eng.) paper.—Describe the changes that take place in the cervix during pregnancy and normal labour.

C.M.B.(N. Ireland) paper.—Describe the structure of the uterus. What changes take place in the cervix during the first stage of labour ?

C.M.B.(Scot.) paper, 1969.—Describe the physiology of the first stage of labour and state what may interfere with the normal process of the first stage.

C.M.B.(Scot.) paper, 1969.—Describe the uterus at term and enumerate the physiological changes which take place in the uterus during the first stage of labour.

C.M.B.(Scot.) paper, 1969.—The cervix. Describe its structure and the changes which take place in it during pregnancy and labour.

MECHANISM OF LABOUR

Arrange the following movements in correct sequence:

1. internal rotation of the head (2).
2. lateral flexion of the body (8).
3. flexion of the head (1).
4. restitution of the head (5).
5. crowning of the head (4).
6. internal rotation of the shoulders (3).
7. extension of the head (6).
8. external rotation of the head (7).

PRACTICAL APPLICATION

Explain how knowledge of the following are useful when delivering the baby: (*a*) external rotation; (*b*) crowning; (*c*) restitution; (*d*) flexion; (*e*) extension of the head; (*f*) position of the caput.

How would you recognize: (*a*) descent; (*b*) flexion of the head during labour.

Why should the midwife wait for external rotation of the head before delivering the shoulders ?

Lie is the relation of the......*foetus*.........**to the**....................**of the**....................

Position is the relation of the....................**to the**....................**of the**...................

Attitude is the relation of the.................**to the**....................

Name the denominators in the following } **Vertex ; Breech ; Face ; Shoulder.**
presentations.

occiput   Sacrum   mentum.

15

The Management of Normal Labour

BASIC PRINCIPLES, PSYCHOLOGY, RELIEF OF PAIN

BEFORE describing the various methods and techniques used in the management of labour, it should be understood that these are founded on certain basic principles. If the student midwife is aware of these she will readily grasp the numerous detailed procedures necessary in the conduct of labour.

The basic principles are as follows:

1. **TO UNDERSTAND AND MEET THE WOMAN'S PSYCHOLOGICAL NEEDS.**

2. **TO PROVIDE EFFICIENT BEDSIDE CARE.**

   A good midwife is essentially a good nurse, and will endeavour to:—

   (*a*) **Give comfort; relieve pain;** conserve strength; prevent exhaustion, injury and loss of blood.

   (*b*) **Maintain cleanliness, antisepsis and asepsis** throughout labour.

   (*c*) **Exercise vigilant observation.** This is an integral part of good nursing, and the midwife requires sufficient knowledge and experience to enable her to recognize normal progress and detect deviations from the natural course.

3. **TO REFRAIN FROM UNNECESSARY INTERFERENCE.**

   Nature is capable of performing her function without aid in most instances; meddlesome midwifery increases the hazards of birth.

4. **TO COPE WITH SUCH EMERGENCIES AS MAY ARISE.**

   Complications should be prevented where possible, recognized early and dealt with promptly and competently until the arrival of the doctor.

   These principles are not confined to labour only, for the management of labour begins during the prenatal period by:—

   (*a*) **Building up the woman's general health.**

   (*b*) **Gaining her confidence, promoting courage and serenity.**

   (*c*) **Giving expert supervision and advice.**

   (*d*) **Detecting abnormalities** which may adversely affect labour.

THE PSYCHOLOGY OF THE WOMAN IN LABOUR

It has been proved that the emotions of the woman in labour profoundly influence her reaction to discomfort and pain and are a contributory factor in determining the amount of physical and mental exhaustion she will experience.

THE FEAR OF LABOUR

The onset of labour gives rise to various emotions, particularly when it is the first baby. The woman is glad the long waiting period is over and pleased that labour has begun, for she is eagerly looking forward to seeing her infant. These emotions are pleasureable, but they are sometimes counterbalanced by emotions of the opposite type. She may be apprehensive about the process of labour and its possible outcome, and if the thought of the actual birth perturbs her such a state of uncertainty and anxiety culminates in fear.

A HOME-LIKE ATMOSPHERE

The hospital situation often suggests preparations for a surgical operation rather than a natural event in her life. If the woman is expected to relax, a well-sprung bed in which she can ease her cumbersome body should be provided. A low, broad, washable chair in which she can sew, read or listen to the radio will help to relieve the tedium of labour.

But the atmosphere created by the staff will overcome many furnishing defects, for a woman can be lonely and unhappy in perfect surroundings.

CHILDBIRTH A FAMILY OCCASION

It must never be forgotten that the birth of a baby is an important family affair, and the midwife should give adequate consideration to the relatives, for whom it may be a very trying ordeal. The fact that some relatives are troublesome is no reason why all women should be cut off from those who are so deeply concerned, particularly when labour is prolonged.

The husband should be permitted to remain with his wife, this gives comfort and happiness to both, and she needs the companionship, love and sympathy of those who are dear to her. Patients should always be told of telephone enquiries for them; it is only natural that a woman likes to know her relatives or friends are thinking of her, and it helps to keep up her morale.

When answering telephone calls from relatives during labour, the Sister or her deputy should dictate the reply. It is not sufficient to state that " Mrs . . . has not had her baby yet "; they should be told something simple and reassuring to allay their natural anxiety, by statements such as—" Had a good sleep during the night." " Quite comfortable, not in strong labour yet." " Enjoyed her lunch, everything is all right." " Her husband can see her to-night at visiting time." " Baby will be here soon: ring again in two hours." Otherwise they imagine the patient is writhing in agony and desperately ill. If the woman is not in hard labour and is reasonably comfortable, that information should be conveyed to her relatives.

THE INFLUENCE OF THE MIDWIFE

It has long been known that the personality and attitude of the midwife play an important part in influencing the behaviour of the woman in labour. If the midwife is endowed with a *calm, optimistic temperament* she is eminently suited from the psychological point of view for the work she is doing.

Her approach should always be friendly, and a kindly welcome makes all the difference to an apprehensive patient. The midwife needs sufficient imagination to appreciate what the woman is thinking and suffering, and although labour should be treated as a natural everyday occurrence, the midwife should not in any way belittle the fact that it is a strenuous, uncomfortable process and a momentous experience for the mother.

If the midwife conveys the impression that she is really interested and is doing her utmost to be helpful she will have a soothing influence. *The serene way* in which the midwife deals with her patients has a reassuring effect; there is no need for any display of authority or bristling competence; efficiency should always be tempered with mercy.

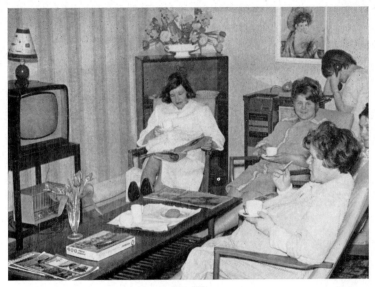

Fig. 178

Patients admitted prior to labour or during the early first stage relaxing in the labour ward sitting-room.

(*Simpson Memorial Maternity Pavilion, Edinburgh.*)

GOOD HUMAN RELATIONSHIPS

The successful midwife has the ability of understanding human nature and adapts her methods of approach to the needs of the different personalities. But the qualities that are acceptable to all women in labour, irrespective of temperament, intelligence, or social status, are *sympathetic understanding* and *patient kindliness*.

Women in labour are sometimes irritable. Some are poorly endowed to endure the discomfort of the first stage of labour, and much tact is needed in handling them.

Others are emotionally immature and unable to control their feelings, and in such cases the influence of a calm, patient midwife is invaluable. Although at times firmness must be exercised, this does not necessarily preclude kindness. Towards the end of labour the midwife may have to urge the patient to persevere, when her energy and her spirits tend to flag and she becomes disheartened and apprehensive. *A word of praise and encouragement will often stimulate the woman to renew her efforts.*

EMOTIONAL SUPPORT

This term is used to embrace the concept of meeting the emotional needs of the woman in labour as a feeling, suffering and probably apprehensive human being.

Building up the woman's confidence in the hospital, doctor and midwife, and providing competent physical care during labour, give the woman a feeling of safety that must not be underestimated as a valuable source of emotional support. But this is not enough.

Her emotional requirements must be met in order to prevent labour from becoming a nerve-wracking experience with emotionally traumatising effects. Obstetric care is neither completely effective nor wholly acceptable to the woman unless it is permeated with a sympathetic understanding of what she is feeling and suffering.

Not only must the midwife desire to give emotional support, she must at all times demonstrate this by her words and actions.

The woman must be helped to direct her energy into fruitful accomplishment rather than in wasteful emotional stress and tension.

COMPANIONSHIP IS NEEDED

Loneliness breeds fear, and fear is the arch enemy of the woman in labour who is going through one of life's most tremendous experiences, isolated from those to whom she would naturally look for solace. The comforting companionship of the midwife who will listen, explain, encourage and assure, or keep silent as required, is of inestimable value to the woman at this time.

When labour is well established the midwife should remain in constant attendance unless the woman is asleep under sedatives. In that case she should first be assured that baby's birth will not occur for some time, that she will be closely supervised while asleep, and her call-bell answered promptly when she awakes. When left for long periods the woman's confidence in her attendants and herself is shattered. The midwife should appreciate the expectant mother's fear that her baby will be born suddenly while she is alone.

ADEQUATE COMMUNICATION

It is essential for the peace of mind of most women that they be kept informed regarding the progress they are making. Women respond magnificently to a word of praise, and being given reasons or explanations, *e.g.* prior to vaginal examination the woman is told why this is being done and that if she relaxes the findings will be more complete: afterwards she is assured that all is well, and that the baby will, or will not, be born soon.

If the woman is made aware that she will never be expected to suffer more than she can stand, and that she will be given a sedative when she feels the need of it, she is less likely to clamour for relief too soon or to lose her nerve.

Women who scream during labour do so more from fear than from pain, and the midwife should communicate confidence by her calm, competent bearing and kindly actions. Telling the woman not to be frightened and not to worry suggests there is something to worry about.

THE WOMAN'S POINT OF VIEW

The woman desires and needs patient, almost maternal, care and companionship as well as the competent observation and obstetric skill she will undoubtedly receive. Soothing measures, such as rubbing the back, help to alleviate discomfort and the woman interprets this as an expression of solicitude.

She expects to practise what she has been taught and has rehearsed during pregnancy, *e.g.* relaxation and controlled breathing, and should be encouraged to do so.

Some women feel very deeply regarding being permitted to experience what is commonly known as " natural childbirth " with the profound joy in hearing their baby's first cry. Although the midwife may think it is more humane to administer inhalational analgesia she must respect and comply with the mother's wishes which, in this instance, will have no untoward effect on mother or child.

A PEACEFUL ATMOSPHERE

The atmosphere of the labour ward should be as quiet and tranquil as possible, and it is the midwife in charge who sets the tone. Nothing is more detrimental to the woman in labour than the irritable, impatient, apprehensive or indifferent midwife, and fortunately few of that type are attracted to the profession.

Student midwives may find the urgency of the situation overwhelming at times, but the impulse to rush about must be resisted as this produces an atmosphere of tension which is transmitted to the patients. The woman in labour should never be aware of any doubt or anxiety the student may experience such as inability to hear the fetal heart or that hæmorrhage is taking place. Great self-control is needed in maintaining an unperturbed demeanour in the presence of an emergency in which life is endangered and quick action required.

There should be no boisterous urging during the second stage; progress is just as rapid in the absence of excessive exhortation to push. Loud talking and noise create the impression of stress and strain which may leave the memory of terrific turmoil and difficulty when the labour was quite normal and straightforward. No conversation should take place between members of staff in the presence of the woman in labour other than is necessary for the conduct of labour.

An attitude of reverence should always prevail while in attendance on women during childbirth.

THE RELIEF OF PAIN IN LABOUR

Sir James Young Simpson will be remembered as one of the pioneers who attempted to alleviate the pains of childbirth. In the year 1847, while Professor of Midwifery in Edinburgh, he first used chloroform for this purpose; but strenuous objection from the clergy, the medical profession and the laity was encountered.

Six years later, chloroform was administered to Queen Victoria during the birth of her seventh child, and her enthusiastic appreciation of the drug did much to break down the opposition to its use. Chloroform tends to inhibit uterine contractions, so it has been superseded by substances which do not have its disadvantages and dangers.

Every woman in labour should be given the maximal relief from pain that is consistent with her own and her infant's safety; and drugs are not the only means whereby pain can be relieved. The midwife can, by creating a tranquil atmosphere and using suggestion combined with relaxation as well as distraction do much to alleviate pain.

An effort should be made during pregnancy to induce the proper attitude of mind in the woman and to build up confidence in herself and those who will attend to her.

Preparation for childbirth by midwives, which includes relief of pain and the various psychological methods employed, is described on p. 712. Included are hypnosis, relaxation, psychoprophylaxis, which utilize one or more of the following:— education, suggestion, assurance, concentration and distraction.

THE DETRIMENTAL EFFECT OF PAIN

Pain exhausts the woman physically and emotionally, so that her confidence is undermined and her courage dissipated. When in such a state the pain threshold is lowered and moderate pain becomes unbearable. Women vary in their ability to stand pain, and the sensitive or highly strung woman may interpret discomfort as pain.

SEDATIVE AND ANALGESIC DRUGS

The effect of pain-relieving drugs varies in different women. The dose is important, but the woman's temperament and the fact that she is amenable to suggestion and has been given instruction regarding labour and how to cope with it, influence the amount of relief obtained.

Drugs given by mouth are not so effective as by I.M. injection because the rate of gastric absorption is slow during labour.

The following rule of the Central Midwives Boards must be noted. " A practising midwife must not on her own responsibility use any drug, including an analgesic, unless in the course of her obstetric training, whether before or after enrolment she has been thoroughly instructed in its use and is familiar with its dosage and methods of administration or application." A midwife must observe the requirements of the Dangerous Drugs Regulations.

SEDATIVE DRUGS THAT MIDWIVES MAY GIVE

Pentazocine (Fortral), 30 to 60 mg.	**Pethidine,** 100 mg.
Welldorm tablets, 0·65 G. (gr. 10).	**Pethilorfan,** 2 ml.
Tricloryl tablets, 0·5 G. (dose 1 G.).	**Tricloryl syrup,** 5 ml.

PETHIDINE

Pethidine is rather similar to morphine and atropine in its chemical formula, but is not a derivative of opium; **it is habit forming and gives rise to drug addiction** of a very severe type. Pethidine, 100 mg., is about the equivalent of morphine, 10 mg. and comes under the **Dangerous Drugs Regulations:** midwives in domiciliary practice being required by law to keep records of the amount issued to and administered by them.

Pethidine relieves pain, is slightly sedative; its somewhat limited antispasmodic action relaxes plain muscle, including that of the lower uterine segment.

Dosage and Administration

Domiciliary midwives authorised by the Central Midwives Boards to administer pethidine or Pethilorfan to women in normal labour are required to comply with the Dangerous Drugs Regulations (see p. 670). The Central Midwives Board (Scotland) limit the total dose given by midwives to any one patient to 200 mg. If a further dose is necessary the doctor will prescribe it.

Midwives should remain with patients on district to whom they have given pethidine.

Pethidine, 100 mg., is not considered to be adequate, as an initial dose, by many labour ward sisters: 150 to 200 mg. has a deeper and more lasting effect: repeat doses of 100 mg. are given every two, three, or four hours, depending on the needs of the patient.

Pethilorfan, 2 ml., contains 100 mg. pethidine and 1·25 mg. levallorphan (Lorfan). The analgesic action of Pethilorfan is only 75 per cent of what is obtained from Pethidine. This drug should be reserved for the end of the first stage in cases of premature labour, and for the multigravid woman in quick labour. It is not repeated because of the depressant effect of too much Lorfan on the fetal respiratory centre.

The doctor sometimes prescribes 600 mg. of pethidine during a period of 24 hours; many give an initial dose of 150 or 200 mg.

ADVANTAGES OF PETHIDINE

Uterine contractions are not adversely affected.

The normal incidence of vomiting is not increased.

DISADVANTAGES

The depressing effect of pethidine on the fetal respiratory centre is intensified when given in conjunction with trichloroethylene. It is therefore essential that the effect of pethidine has practically worn off before giving trichloroethylene.

In cases of neonatal asphyxia due to morphine or pethidine excellent results have been obtained by injecting neonatal levallorphan (Lorfan), 0·05 mg. into the umbilical vein.

The action of pethidine is believed to be potentiated by the mono-amine oxidase inhibitors such as Nardil that are sometimes prescribed for mental depression. This combination of drugs may produce coma. Prior to giving pethidine the midwife ought to question the woman regarding drugs she may have been taking.

PENTAZOCINE (FORTRAL)

The Central Midwives Board (England) has sanctioned the use of this drug which can be obtained by midwives for use in their professional practice under section 20 (5) of the Pharmacy and Poisons Act 1933.

Pentazocine is a non-addictive analgesic drug which is not restricted under the Dangerous Drug Act. In analgesic properties 40 mg. is approximately equivalent to 100 mg. pethidine; giving slightly more pain relief during the first hour. Pentazocine is excreted more rapidly therefore its effect is of shorter duration than that of pethidine; less nausea and vomiting occurs.

The drug is available in ampoules 1 ml. 30 mg.: and should not be repeated within 3 hours. Two doses are usually sufficient. (*One hospital reports satisfactory results, giving a single dose of 60 mg. 2 ml.*)

Should neonatal respiratory depression occur, and this is rare, Ritalin, Vandid or nikethamide is administered. Nalorphine is not effective.

The tablets (25 mg.) are useful for pain in the post-natal period.

DRUGS WHICH MUST BE ORDERED BY THE DOCTOR

THE PHENOTHIAZINES

These include drugs such as promazine, and promethazine They reduce tension, relieve stress and induce a calm state of mind without clouding consciousness. They also potentiate some analgesic drugs.

Promazine (Sparine), 25 mg., is often given in combination with pethidine 100 mg. as an initial dose, and is particularly effective for the apprehensive woman and in cases of emotional instability. When nausea or vomiting is troublesome Sparine gives excellent results: it also potentiates the action of pethidine. The dose is usually limited to 25 mg. and is rarely repeated: rapid pulse and a fall in blood pressure may occur, particularly in patients who are dehydrated if larger doses are given.

Promethazine (Phenergan), 50 mg., one of the effective and long acting antihistamines, preferred by some in combination with pethidine, 100 mg., will provide three to four hours of analgesic detachment. *Fentazin is apt to produce agitation.*

OPIUM DERIVATIVES

Morphine, 15 mg., is popular in a number of centres, for primigravidæ, but is only given in very early labour; os 2 to 3 cm. dilated. It is not repeated because of its very depressant effect on the fetal respiratory centre; this is particularly important should Cæsarean section or forceps delivery be anticipated. (If, inadvertently, the baby is born in a state of asphyxia due to the effect of morphine, levallorphan (Lorfan), 0·05 mg., or neonatal nalorphine (Lethidrone), 0·5 mg., will counteract its depressant action.)

Morphine is extremely valuable when a long labour is anticipated, as in posterior vertex positions, because it relieves pain effectively and also induces sleep. To counteract the tendency of morphine to cause vomiting promazine (Sparine) or promethazine (Phenergan) can be given along with it.

Papaveretum (Omnopon), 20 mg., is frequently given in conjunction with promethazine, 25 to 50 mg., during early established labour and has a calming influence on the apprehensive woman.

THE BARBITURATES

These drugs are hypnotic and sedative with a very limited analgesic action some-times useful to induce sleep during the latent period following the induction of labour and in non-established labour: quinalbarbitone (Seconal); pentobarbitone Nembutal).

If given repeatedly throughout labour, the initiation of respiration in the infant may be slow and Lorfan and Lethidrone are not effective as antidotes.

TIME OF ADMINISTRATION

(a) NON-ESTABLISHED OR VERY EARLY LABOUR

Hypnotic and sedative drugs should be employed at this stage to induce sleep and to calm the apprehensive woman. They are ineffective when pain is present and may even increase sensitivity to pain. Suitable drugs would be dichloralphenazone (Welldorm), 1·3 G. (2 tablets), or amylobarbitone sodium (Sodium Amytal), 200 mg.

(b) ESTABLISHED LABOUR

This is commonly taken to be when the os is 2 to 3 cm. dilated with contractions lasting 30 seconds every five minutes. The woman's needs should be the factor indicating when analgesic drugs are necessary. Some require sedation earlier than others and it is better given too early than too late. **Definite discomfort** might be a good criterion. If the woman is allowed to become distressed it is much more difficult to achieve the maximal analgesic effect of the drug administered.

Suitable drugs are pethidine, papaveretum, morphine, pentazocine, promazine or promethazine (for dosage see pp. 252, 253).

Experience and judgment are of inestimable value when using the pharmacological method of pain relief. **If success is not achieved** the fault may be in (*a*) the choice of drug, (*b*) insufficient dosage, or (*c*) faulty timing.

(c) THE TRANSITION STAGE

This stage extends over the period during which the first stage ends and the second stage begins. It has been arbitrarily defined because this half-hour (more or less) is probably the most unpleasant part of labour for the woman and the most testing for the midwife.

Contractions are longer and stronger; cervical dilation is maximal (for the size of the baby); physical discomfort and emotional distress are more acute and particu-larly so when the woman's stamina is waning.

Although some have circumscribed the transition stage to within 7-9 cm. cervical dilatation this could only obtain with a baby weighing around 3,200 G.; feeling a " rim of cervix " might be a more accurate description.

Management

If the woman has been successfully managed and adequately sedated throughout labour she ought not to be unduly distressed.

Inhalational analgesia is usually administered at the transitional stage; drugs that would depress the fetal respiratory centre and delay the establishment of respiration at birth are not given within 3 hours of expected delivery.

Should the woman be admitted at this time acutely distressed with pain, pethidine, 50 mg., given intravenously by the doctor will give prompt relief.

PROTECTION OF THE PATIENT UNDER SEDATIVES

The dose must always be checked before being given. The midwife also has a duty to see that the woman comes to no harm because of her confused state of mind. Women have been known, when left unattended, to fall out of bed, to wander from the labour ward, or to drink antiseptic lotions. **Constant vigilance is necessary.**

When transferring a patient to hospital the domiciliary midwife should give a report of drugs, and the time they were administered, in writing.

PSYCHOLOGICAL METHODS OF PAIN RELIEF
(see also p. 712)

Many midwives have, by their sympathetic understanding manner, unknowingly used psychological methods of pain relief. They should now study the modern techniques and use them to supplement the pharmacological method.

The personality of the midwife is of paramount importance in handling women in labour. If her approach is kindly, her manner reassuring, and she exhibits by word and deed her interest in, and concern for, the woman in labour as an individual, she will provide the emotional support which is so essential at this time. If the woman has been instructed by the midwife during the prenatal period and is sustained emotionally during labour, the maximal analgesic effect of pain relieving drugs is more likely to be achieved.

The midwife can use suggestion as is done in hypnosis, relaxation as is practised in the Grantly D. Read method, and distraction and concentration as in psychoprophylaxis. These techniques help to raise the pain threshold. All methods need a basic educational foundation in order to give the woman some understanding of labour and the confidence and assurance to cope with it.

INHALATIONAL OBSTETRIC ANALGESIA

Inhalational analgesia is intended for the use of healthy women to relieve the pain of normal labour. The Central Midwives Boards permit midwives to administer, under certain conditions laid down by them, the following inhalational analgesics—

(1) **Premixed nitrous oxide,** 50 per cent, and oxygen, 50 per cent.

(2) **Trichloroethylene B.P.** Trilene, 0·35 to 0·5 per cent, and air.

(3) **Methoxyflurane** (Penthrane) 0·35 per cent in air.

(1) PREMIXED NITROUS OXIDE AND OXYGEN

The premixed gas is a definite advance over gas and air.

The apparatus consists of a cylinder of premixed gas under pressure (500 litres for domiciliary use : 2,000 litres for hospital use). The cylinder is fitted with a reducing valve that brings the pressure of the gas down to a level safe for inhalation : a pressure gauge provides an indication of the cylinder contents and the demand valve allows the premixed gas to be delivered only on inspiration by the woman inhaling it.

CONDITIONS OTHER THAN NORMAL IN WHICH PREMIXED GAS MAY BE USED

1. **Placental insufficiency.**	5. **Premature labour.**
2. **Post-maturity.**	6. **Severe anæmia.**
3. **Pre-eclampsia.**	7. **Diabetes.**
4. **Essential hypertension.**	8. **Mild fetal distress.**

The **Central Midwives Board have approved the Entonox apparatus** for use by midwives on their own responsibility provided they have been instructed in its use. Such instruction will include advice on the necessary precautions to be taken against the exposure of the cylinders of premixed gas to cold.

Because premixed gas contains a high percentage of oxygen—50 per cent—and because nitrous oxide is relatively non-cumulative it is safe to prolong its administration over a period of four or even more hours with little risk of fetal anoxia.

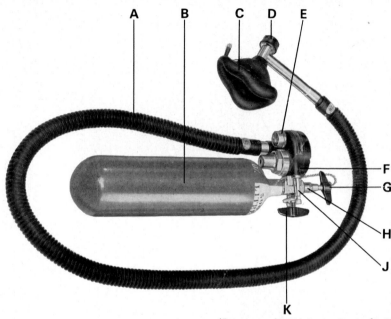

(By courtesy of British Oxygen Company Ltd.

Fig. 179

ENTONOX ANALGESIC APPARATUS, DOMICILIARY MODEL.

A, *Corrugated tube.*
B, *500 litre cylinder (50 per cent nitrous oxide/*
    50 per cent oxygen).   C, *Face mask.*
D, *Expiratory valve assembly.*

E, *Cylinder pressure gauge.*
F, *Demand regulator.*   G, *Cylinder valve key.*
H, *Non-interchangeable pin-index cylinder valve.*
J, *Cylinder yoke.*   K, *Cylinder yoke key.*

Precautions to be Observed

(A) CYLINDERS MUST NOT BE CHILLED

Cylinders of premixed gas must not be exposed to cold, *i.e.* temperature below freezing, 0° C. (32° F.). They should be stored at a temperature above 10° C. (50° F.).

If the cylinder is known to have been exposed to a low temperature 0° C. (32° F.) or shows ice or condensation on its surface, it should be placed in warm water not exceeding 35° C. (95° F.) for five minutes, avoiding water touching the valve, or placed in the delivery room for at least 2 hours. The cylinder should then be inverted three times to agitate its contents and remix the gases.

Oil or grease should never be applied to valves or fittings.

(2) TRICHLOROETHYLENE B.P. (Trilene)

Trilene is the trade name of the brand produced by Imperial Chemical (Pharmaceuticals) Ltd.

Trichloroethylene in concentrations over 0·5 per cent is an anæsthetic, but midwives are only permitted to use it as an analgesic in concentrations of 0·35 or 0·5 per cent. Two special thermostatically controlled machines have been designed for the use of midwives and approved by the Central Midwives Boards. These are the *Emotril Automatic* and the *Tecota Mark* 6. Both deliver trichloroethylene and air in the following mixtures:

MINIMUM OR WEAK CONCENTRATION, trichloroethylene 0·35 per cent.

MAXIMUM OR NORMAL CONCENTRATION, trichloroethylene 0·5 per cent.

A midwife must not on her own responsibility use any other machine or administer trichloroethylene unless she has complied with the requirements of the Central Midwives Boards Rules on the use of trichloroethylene.

Trichloroethylene is cumulative in effect. For that reason it is not given for prolonged periods, and is usually administered towards the end of the first stage. The fetal heart must be closely observed and a chart kept in graph form. If the woman is **excessively drowsy** the inhalation should be stopped temporarily and the concentration reduced to 0·35 per cent. **Slowing of the maternal pulse or rapid respirations, slowing of the fetal heart to below 120 are indications to cease administration.**

It passes the placental barrier and may produce fetal anoxia, when given in conjunction with pethidine within three hours of birth. Trichloroethylene should therefore not be administered until not less than two hours after the last dose of pethidine was given.

(3) METHOXYFLURANE (Penthrane)

The Central Midwives Board (Eng.) have approved (1970) the use of methoxyflurane B.P. 0·35 per cent administered with the approved Cardiff inhaler, by unsupervised midwives in accordance with Rule E5 of Statutory Instrument, 1955, No. 120.

The Cardiff inhaler must be tested when new and retested every 12 months according to British Standards Institution approved specification. Certificates will then be issued by the Board stating their fitness for use by unsupervised midwives.

Instruction on Penthrane, and a demonstration of its administration with the Cardiff inhaler should be given to student midwives in addition to instruction on the principles and practice of obstetric inhalational analgesia. (*Abbot Laboratories, Queensborough, Kent provide a suitable booklet.*)

Penthrane is administered intermittently to provide analgesia during labour and delivery. The effect of pethidine should have worn off before methoxyflurane (Penthrane) is given. The analgesic effect is good and is usually accompanied by physical and mental relaxation. Some patients object to the odour. Overdosage is manifest by excessive drowsiness.

The majority of babies have an Apgar score of 8 or more.

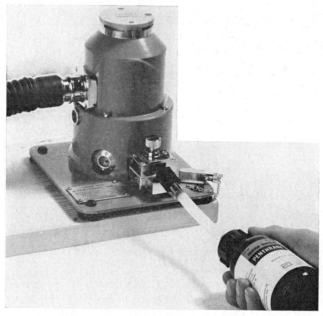

FIG. 180
CARDIFF INHALER FOR PENTHRANE.
(*Courtesy of Abbot Laboratories, Queensborough, Kent.*)

ADMINISTRATION OF INHALATIONAL ANALGESIA

ENTONOX   TRILENE   PENTHRANE

To be successful, instruction during the prenatal period is essential, for when feeling nervous on her admission to hospital, distracted with pain or stupefied by drugs the woman cannot comprehend the directions given her. Confidence in herself, and in the safety and efficiency of the apparatus are necessary; she should be shown how to relax and be proficient in using the face-mask. *These points are explained in a talk to mothers-to-be, page 728.*

TECHNIQUE OF ADMINISTRATION
DURING THE FIRST STAGE
(See also p. 728.)

Dentures are removed. The mask is applied closely to the face with the broad end resting on the chin, the narrow end on the bridge of the nose.

Analgesic gas is only administered during contractions.

Nitrous oxide and oxygen has to be inhaled for 20 seconds before having any analgesic effect, and it takes 45 seconds to obtain maximal relief, so inhalation must be started prior to the sensation of pain felt by the woman. **Trichloroethylene is slightly more rapid in action.**

By laying her hand on the fundus the midwife will feel the uterus contracting before the woman experiences pain; inhalation may be started then.

The midwife remains in the room, encouraging the woman and helping her to relax between contractions.

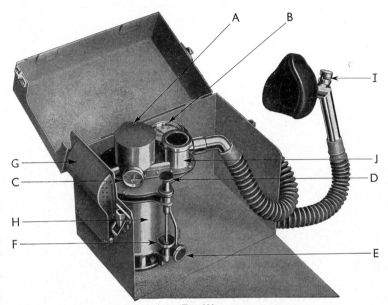

FIG. 181

THE EMOTRIL (AUTOMATIC). Trichloroethylene analgesia inhaler.

A, *Thermostat housing.*
B, *Thermometer dial.*
C, *Weak mixture control.*
D, *Filling control handle.*
E, *Trichloroethylene level gauge.*

F, *Filler and overflow.*
G, *Air inlets.*
H, *Vaporizing chamber.*
I, *Expiratory valve.*
J, *Valve to prevent rebreathing into vaporizing chamber.*

(*By courtesy of Medical and Industrial Equipment Ltd.*, 10 *New Cavendish Street, London, W.*1.)

When administering trichloroethylene the woman must not be left alone in case she extends the period of inhalation, becomes drowsy and rolls over on to her face. The potential dangers of this substance must always be kept in mind and constant vigilance maintained (see Disadvantages, p. 257).

It should be remembered that the effort of forced inhalation and of repeatedly applying the mask can be very tiring when continued for some time. The mouth becomes parched.

DURING THE SECOND STAGE

Inhalation of nitrous oxide and oxygen should be started 40 seconds prior to the uterine contraction: trichloroethylene 30 seconds, in order that as soon as the pain commences the woman can hold her breath and bear down. After doing so she takes one or two breaths of the analgesic gas and pushes again as long as the uterus is in a state of contraction. Timing the contractions is comparatively easy during the second stage as they are recurring at frequent intervals.

When the head is crowned an assistant holds the mask snugly in position, and the woman is told to take deliberate breaths to counteract the strong urge to push. During the few moments of the actual birth of the head gas is inhaled continuously.

Rubber masks should be thoroughly cleansed with soap and hot water, washed in Hibitane, 1-2,000, rinsed and dried, otherwise respiratory infections may be spread. *Unclean masks have an unpleasant odour.* Irritating antiseptics should not be used, because of the danger of eye and face burns.

RELIEF OF BACKACHE IN LABOUR

The need to make some positive effort in the alleviation of this distressing complaint is urgent. Many women assert that backache is the worst feature of labour, being even more painful than uterine contractions. The analgesic drugs that relieve

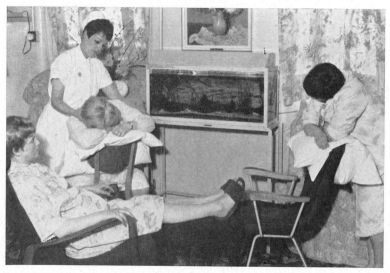

FIG. 182
DEMONSTRATION OF POSITIONS TO RELIEVE BACKACHE DURING LABOUR.
(*Gold fish tank a soothing distraction.*)
(*Royal Maternity Hospital, Rottenrow, Glasgow.*)

uterine pain do not always have a similar beneficent action on backache: analgesic gas helps some women but psychological methods of pain relief have little or no effect.

Low back pain may be present from the inception of labour; usually coinciding with the onset of cervical dilatation. The backache persists although it may be less severe during the second stage: while the uterus is contracting the pain is markedly intensified.

The pain is felt in the sacral rather than the lumbar region, sometimes radiating over the buttocks and occasionally down the thighs with a cramp-like sensation.

Causes

The backache of labour is a referred pain, probably due to a degree of resistance in the lower uterine segment and cervix.

The more severe forms are associated with—

1. DISORDERED UTERINE ACTION

(*a*) The upper and lower uterine segments are not functioning harmoniously.

(*b*) Hypertonus retards relaxation of the lower uterine segment.

(*c*) The rigid cervix.

2. **OCCIPITO-POSTERIOR POSITION OF THE VERTEX** is a well known cause of backache. The occiput, when posterior, may unduly compress the paracervical ganglia: inefficient uterine action and resistance to cervical dilatation are usually coexistent.

3. **A VERY LARGE BABY** causing excessive compression of the paracervical ganglia.

But many women who do not exhibit any of the causes mentioned suffer from backache, and a number of experienced midwives consider this condition to be more common and more severe than formerly (20 years ago). Postural backache should now be less frequent considering there are fewer multigravid women with flabby muscles, and greater opportunities to avoid or correct lordosis.

TREATMENT BY THE DOCTOR

PARACERVICAL NERVE BLOCK

This procedure has been used with success in cases of prolonged labour with backache especially in occipito-posterior position. It is employed during the second half of the first stage including just prior to full dilatation of the cervix. Unfortunately the relief from an injection only lasts for 1 to $1\frac{1}{2}$ hours (see p. 625).

EPIDURAL ANÆSTHESIA. This technique is employed in a number of centres (see p. 636). It may be given throughout labour and has been used in cases of severe backache associated with high tone in the lower uterine segment. Complete relief is obtained.

MANAGEMENT BY MIDWIVES

During pregnancy the midwife should—

(*a*) **advise re posture and correct this when faulty,**

(*b*) **direct exercises to maintain good muscle tone.**

During labour—

(*a*) **The woman should not be recumbent too soon** unless tired.

(*b*) **Effective analgesic drugs should be administered.**

(*c*) **During contractions the woman should be advised to curve her back forwards.** She may stand behind a chair on the top of which is placed a pillow on which she rests her arms and head.

(*d*) **Between contractions she may sit astride the seat of a chair,** arms and head resting on a pillow placed over the top of the chair-back.

(*e*) **Squatting, crosslegged, may help** some, others find relief by flexing the legs at hip and knee joints.

BACK MASSAGE

Back rubbing is the most effective means of providing relief employed by midwives and approximately 70 per cent of women obtain some easement from this. How massage helps is not perfectly understood. By improving the subcutaneous circulation, tissue fluid tension in the deeper structures is reduced.

Method

With the woman lying on her left side, the midwife, facing the patient's back, uses her left hand. Power is directed from the shoulder with a relaxed elbow and hand.

Deep circular massage is applied mainly over the sacral region. Pressure should be firm but not excessive; the palm being used to a greater extent than the fingers. There should be no friction between the woman's back and the midwife's hand which should adhere to the skin and move the subcutaneous tissues: brisk superficial rubbing is not effective and will only irritate the skin.

As an additional measure in refractory cases, both hands can be used; the woman sitting up with her back towards the midwife.

(*a*) **Starting at the upper outer border of the sacrum** the hands are firmly stroked along the iliac crests.

(*b*) **The buttocks are massaged** with curving strokes radiating laterally from the sacrum.

(*c*) **Stroking the sacrum vertically from the tip upwards** with the palmar surface of the fingers.

As a soothing measure massage of the lumbar region and thighs would be appreciated between uterine contractions.

QUESTIONS FOR REVISION

Write not more than 10 lines on each of the following statements:
1. Childbirth is a family occasion.
2. The midwife should provide emotional support to the woman in labour.
3. Pain exhausts the woman physically and emotionally.
4. The effect of pain relieving drugs varies in different women.

ORAL QUESTIONS

How would you prevent or deal with screaming by a woman in labour ?

How would you deal with severe pain during the transitional stage ?

Why is pethidine controlled by the D.D.A. ?

Name 3 drugs to relieve pain that a midwife is permitted to administer ?

How would you deal with neonatal asphyxia when pethidine had been administered one hour before delivery ?

How would you deal with a cylinder of mixed nitrous oxide and oxygen that had been chilled ?

Name 3 drugs prescribed by the doctor that are given in conjunction with pethidine ?

Compare the effects and advantages of pethidine and pentazocine (Fortral).

RELIEF OF PAIN

Give reasons (*in five lines*) **why and when during labour** you would as a midwife administer each of the following: (1) Entonox; (2) pethidine 100 mg.; (3) Tricloryl tablets 1 G.; (4) Pethilorfan 2 ml.; (5) Trilene 0.35 per cent; (6) pentazocine 60 mg.

C.M.B.(Eng.) paper.—Which drugs are commonly used for the relief of pain in labour? Briefly explain their value.

C.M.B.(Eng.) paper.—What measures can a midwife take to reduce discomfort and pain in labour ?

C.M.B.(N. Ireland) paper.—What methods are available to the midwife for the relief of pain in labour ?

C.M.B.(Eng.) paper.—How may a midwife alleviate pain in labour ? What regulations must she observe in the use of drugs for this purpose ?

C.M.B.(Eng.) paper. 100 word question.—(*a*) The Entonox analgesia apparatus. (*b*) Pethidine.

C.M.B.(Eng.) paper, 1969.—Describe the ways in which a midwife can relieve discomfort and pain during labour.

Enumerate other methods which are available to a doctor.

C.M.B.(Eng.) paper, 1970.—50 word question.—What are the rules concerning the administration of inhalational analgesics by a midwife?

16

The Management of Normal Labour (contd.)

OBSTETRICAL NURSING CARE DURING THE FIRST STAGE OF LABOUR

1. CLEANLINESS, ANTISEPSIS, ASEPSIS.   3. TAKING THE HISTORY OF LABOUR
2. ADMISSION OF THE WOMAN.   4. EXAMINATION OF THE WOMAN.
5. PREPARATION OF THE WOMAN.

1. CLEANLINESS, ANTISEPSIS AND ASEPSIS DURING LABOUR

LABOUR should be conducted with the same antiseptic and aseptic precautions that would be employed in a surgical theatre, for the woman must be protected by every available means from infection, which may cause ill-health and loss of life.

The woman is vulnerable to infection for the following reasons:

   (*a*) **Lacerations in her perineum,** vulva, vagina and cervix permit organisms to enter.

   (*b*) **Harmless organisms that live in the vagina become pathogenic** when tissue is bruised, and bruised tissue readily becomes infected.

   (*c*) **The large placental site is a raw area** through which organisms can readily gain entrance to the blood stream.

   (*d*) **The uterus immediately after labour provides an excellent medium for the growth of organisms.**

   (*e*) **Her general resistance may be lowered** because of exhaustion and loss of blood.

THE PATIENT AS A SOURCE OF INFECTION

The patient herself can be a source of infection directly and indirectly. She should be free from any focus of infection, such as a septic finger, discharging ear or boils. **The rectum,** vulva and skin of the patient are teeming with organisms, so the giving of an enema or suppository and bath, shaving and swabbing the pubes and vulva, are carried out for antiseptic reasons.

The patient's hands should be clean, her finger nails short and she should be instructed not to touch her vulva.

Paper handkerchiefs should be supplied in labour wards, used once and discarded, and when the patient has a cold, extra hand-washing should be practised. It is doubtful whether mask-wearing by the woman in labour, who has a respiratory infection, is as important as the use of paper handkerchiefs and frequent hand-washing.

All patients who are potentially or actually infected on admission should be isolated and it is a wise precaution when taking the history of the labour to make sure that the woman has not been in recent contact with an infectious disease.

THE MIDWIFE AS A SOURCE OF INFECTION

If the midwife has a cold, sore throat, or other focus of infection, or if she has been nursing a patient suffering from an infectious condition, **she should not be in attendance on the woman in labour.** The use of paper handkerchiefs, followed by hand-washing is an excellent hygienic practice.

The midwife is responsible for carrying out a technique whereby neither she herself, the patient, nor the environment will be a source of infection. But in our zeal for asepsis **we must never underestimate the value of soap and water.**

Good wholesome cleanliness is the first prerequisite in midwifery and is as important as an impeccable aseptic and antiseptic technique. Throughout labour the midwife should wear a clean dress; during delivery a sterile gown. Her nails should be short and clean; rings should not be worn when hands require to be obstetrically clean. Gloves are worn for vaginal examinations and during the delivery of the patient.

Mask Wearing

Unless a mask is worn intelligently, it simply becomes an additional source of infection. The mask should be applied with clean, but not necessarily sterile, hands and should always be worn while " scrubbing up " to prevent the hands from being contaminated with the spray of saliva while talking.

Masks need only be worn **when the vulva or sterile equipment is exposed:** if worn constantly, the mouth becomes an incubator for organisms.

The mask should never be touched, once it has been applied, because it is infected, and by contaminating the hands infection is spread; nor should one mask be worn for longer than two hours.

On removing the mask, it ought to be handled by the tapes and destroyed if disposable or dropped into a covered container of antiseptic, washed later, dried and autoclaved to destroy the organisms of the wearer. If masks are not well washed, they have an objectionable odour *A mask must never hang around the neck or be carried in the pocket.* To do so shows disregard or ignorance of the technique of mask-wearing.

Disposable paper masks for short periods of use are admirable

THE ENVIRONMENT AS A SOURCE OF INFECTION

The risk of cross-infection is very great in hospital because of the large number and close proximity of patients, and on that account special precautions must be taken. Every woman in labour should, if possible, be bathed and dressed in clean clothing before being admitted to the labour ward proper. Her own clothing, which is usually soiled, should be sent home with relatives.

Single labour and delivery rooms are ideal in limiting infection, and should be well aired, as well as being scrupulously clean.

Domestic Cleanliness

Daily dusting should be carried out with clean damp cloths. Thorough scrubbing of the labour ward bed, furniture and floor should follow each delivery, and the mop used for removing blood from the floor should be thoroughly washed after use and kept in a bucket of disinfectant.

EQUIPMENT FOR LABOUR IN HOSPITAL

The amount of equipment used for a normal confinement varies in different hospitals, and it is not feasible to state requirements that would meet with universal approval.

Adequate equipment.—Disposable or metal ware should be in good supply, and an ample amount of linen is necessary. Labour ward blankets should be of cellular cotton. Bed-pans must be disinfected, and common lavatory seats should never be used in a labour ward because of the risk of infection. A (metal) commode, in which a bed-pan can be placed, could be provided.

(*Photographs of pack contents and lists of equipment are given, throughout the text, for the guidance of midwives not accustomed to making such preparations.*)

The trolleys are washed with soap and water, then wiped with Hibitane, 1 in 2,000. Instruments, linen and dressings for each trolley are wrapped in double heavy sheeting, and when the pack is unpinned the wrapper acts as a table-cover.

Trolleys on which patients are transferred to the puerperal wards can be a source of infection and should be washed daily. If clean sheets for the trolley are not available for each patient, it is better to use the plastic and linen sheets off her labour ward bed.

Perspex cots with hinged lids and control valve for oxygen-air mixture are excellent for labour ward use. The baby is under constant vision.

2. ADMISSION OF THE WOMAN IN LABOUR

When the patient arrives in hospital she should be welcomed in a friendly manner and made to feel that she is expected. The midwife notes whether delivery is imminent, and, if so, makes immediate preparations to cope with it. While helping the woman to undress, enquiry is made as to whether this is her first baby, and as to the expected date of confinement.

A decision must be made as to whether the woman is in true labour or not, and this is done by taking a short history of her labour and by examination and observation of the patient. The midwife must also try to decide how far labour has advanced, before giving an enema and carrying out the full admission procedure.

If the type of contractions is taken into consideration and how much has been accomplished since the onset of labour, it may be possible to estimate, within limits, whether labour will be long or short. The length of previous labours also gives some idea as to what may be expected, and if the youngest child is under 15 months a more rapid labour can be anticipated.

The majority of booked patients coming to hospital in labour are normal; abnormal booked cases are usually admitted for rest and observation previous to the onset of labour. Many of the unbooked patients are sent to hospital because some complication has arisen; *it is commendable that in many hospitals the domiciliary midwife is permitted to remain with her patient until she is delivered if she wishes to.*

The patient's religion and the address of her nearest relative must always be recorded.

Relatives ought to be treated with consideration and courtesy, any anxiety allayed and told when to enquire again.

CONSENT FOR OPERATION AND ANÆSTHETIC

It is customary and expedient for midwives to request women admitted in labour to sign a **permission slip** for the surgeon-in-charge to carry out any treatment or operation which may be considered necessary, including an anæsthetic.

This is a wise precaution, particularly at the present time when unscrupulous persons may initiate litigation against medical staff or Hospital Boards. It would even be prudent

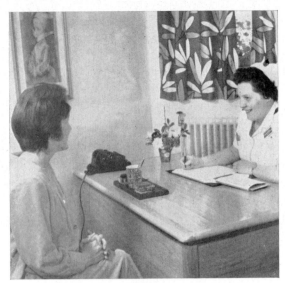

FIG. 183
Sister taking history of labour
(*Aberdeen Maternity Hospital*)

to include treatment and operative procedures that may be carried out on the fetus and newborn baby.

Those who consider the signing of forms on admission in labour to be at an inappropriate time could obtain the signature at the prenatal clinic. The form should be read to the patient so that she knows the purpose of her signature.

The age of consent is now 16 years.

Prior to sterilization a special consent form signed by husband and wife is essential.

3. TAKING THE HISTORY OF LABOUR

The history of labour is taken under four headings, and the midwife notes whether her own observations coincide with the woman's statements. Questions are asked regarding:

(*a*) THE UTERINE CONTRACTIONS. (*c*) RUPTURE OF THE MEMBRANES.
(*b*) SHOW. (*d*) SLEEP: REST: FOOD.

(*a*) UTERINE CONTRACTIONS

The woman is asked when regular contractions (*pains*) **began,** how often they are coming and if she has had backache. At the beginning of labour, backache may be the only symptom. Later, discomfort or pain is experienced in the lower abdomen, and when the first stage is more advanced the pain may resemble intestinal colic. Backache may persist throughout labour (see p. 260).

The woman's statement regarding the length, strength, severity or expulsive character of the contractions should be corroborated by observation, and a certain amount of discrimination used in assessing the history given, for many women in false labour are under the impression, because they have had occasional pain, that they have been in true labour for one or more days. **False labour should never be included in the recorded time of true labour.**

(b) SHOW

The woman is asked if she has seen any show (*blood and mucus*) and her under garments examined for staining. Show may appear a few hours before or after the commencement of labour, and the multigravid patient has less than the primigravid one because of her gaping cervix. Patients sometimes give a history of bleeding, which on investigation is found to be only show.

(c) THE MEMBRANES

The patient may not be sure whether her " waters " have broken or not; they may have ruptured in the bath or toilet, unknown to her. She should be asked if she has noticed a gush or trickling of water. Frequency or slight incontinence, due to the laxity of the pelvic floor and the pressure of the uterus on the bladder, may be mistaken for the draining of liquor amnii. Without having actual proof that the membranes have ruptured, " patient's statement " should be added when reporting or recording the fact. The use of litmus paper may be helpful, as liquor amnii is alkaline and urine is commonly acid.

(d) SLEEP: REST: FOOD

Enquiry should be made as to whether the patient has been deprived of sleep. Many women are kept awake for nights with false, niggling pains, and in such a case it would be advisable to give a sedative to ensure a good rest before the contractions become severe.

The patient should be asked if she has had food recently, for when admitted a night she may feel hungry. If labour is not well established a light meal should be served.

HISTORY OF PREVIOUS LABOURS

From her prenatal record, certain important facts regarding previous labours will be noted; but if she is not booked, enquiries will have to be made in regard to them. The weights of her babies delivered spontaneously give a clue to pelvic capacity, particularly if they were 3,630 G. (8 lb.) or over. Previous instrumental delivery, Cæsarean section or stillbirth should be reported to the doctor.

HISTORY OF THE PRESENT PREGNANCY

The prenatal record will state whether cephalo-pelvic disproportion exists. Her age, if over 30, is significant should this be her first baby or if she has no living children. Any abnormal condition existing during pregnancy will also have been recorded, such as **pre-eclampsia, anæmia, diabetes,** or **cardiac disease.**

In patients whose Rhesus factor is negative, a history of babies with icterus neonatorum, or of stillbirth is of serious import, and if antibodies are present in her blood the fact should be reported to the doctor at once, so that the pædiatrician can be notified and arrangements made for the provision of suitable blood for mother and baby should the need arise.

4. EXAMINATION OF THE WOMAN IN LABOUR

(a) HAS LABOUR BEGUN ?	(d) VULVAL EXAMINATION.
(b) GENERAL EXAMINATION.	(e) VAGINAL EXAMINATION.
(c) ABDOMINAL EXAMINATION.	(f) RECTAL EXAMINATION.

(a) HAS LABOUR BEGUN ?

When labour has really started, little difficulty is experienced in making the diagnosis, but it sometimes takes a number of hours before labour is properly established. At the onset, it is not always easy to decide whether the woman is in false labour or in poorly established true labour.

False or True Labour ?

False labour is far more common in multigravid women and is frequently troublesome at night. The contractions tend to be erratic and irregular; they often last longer than one minute and are not usually felt in the back. An enema will generally disperse them, whereas it will stimulate true contractions—no show is present.

If true labour has begun, the midwife may detect on vaginal or rectal examination the shortened cervix, and during a contraction the tense bag of waters is felt over the os if the membranes have not already ruptured. The diagnosis is more difficult in the multiparous woman who has a patulous cervix and in whom dilatation of the external os is commonly present during the later weeks of pregnancy, but regular contractions and progressive dilatation of the os are the best guides in such cases.

When a woman is near term and has been admitted during the night or from a distance in false labour, it is a good plan to administer a sedative to ensure sleep, *e.g.* dichloralphenazone (Welldorm) tablets, 1·3 G. If labour does not start during the ensuing 24 hours, the woman may be discharged after the situation has been assessed unless over 40 weeks gestation.

TO INITIATE OR ACCELERATE LABOUR

If the woman is admitted not in labour and the membranes have ruptured, labour would be induced by the I.V. or buccal administration of oxytocin.

If the woman appears to be in labour but contractions are weak or infrequent, the os dilating slowly, the membranes would be punctured and an oxytocin I.V. drip started with 0·5 unit Syntocinin in 540 ml. dextrose or Buccal Pitocin may be administered (see p. 610).

THE UTERINE CONTRACTIONS

TRUE LABOUR	FALSE LABOUR
(1) Are always present.	(1) Are not always present.
(2) Are accompanied by abdominal tightening, discomfort or pain.	(2) Are not always painful.
(3) Rarely exceed 60 seconds.	(3) May last three to four minutes.
(4) Recur with rhythmic regularity.	(4) Are erratic and irregular.
(5) Are often accompanied by backache.	(5) Are not accompanied by backache.

THE CERVIX

TRUE LABOUR	FALSE LABOUR
(1) The cervix is shortened.	(1) The cervix is not shortened.
(2) The os is dilating.	(2) The os is not dilating.
(3) The membranes feel tense during a contraction.	(3) The membranes do not become tense.
(4) Show is usually present.	(4) There is no show.

(b) GENERAL EXAMINATION

1. BUILD AND STATURE.   4. ŒDEMA.
2. APPEARANCE.   5. URINE ANALYSIS.
3. TEMPERATURE AND PULSE.   6. BLOOD PRESSURE.

1. BUILD AND STATURE

Particular attention is paid to the build and stature of the woman, and especially when she is less than 1·6 m. (5 feet 3 inches) in height, or if there is evidence of limp or deformity. The doctor should be notified of such cases.

2. APPEARANCE

The woman's general appearance will convey an impression of her health and nutrition, and the midwife must be on the alert for conditions that would in any way affect the course of labour.

Pallor might be due to anæmia and would be marked in patients admitted because of severe antepartum hæmorrhage, but more frequently it is nutritional in origin. *Breathlessness* would suggest a cardiac condition and when accompanied by cyanosis it is of serious import. Patients with *respiratory infections* should be nursed under barrier precautions because of the danger of infecting others.

If the woman is suffering from a condition that is contagious, e.g. untreated *venereal disease* or scabies, she should be seen by the doctor so that isolation and treatment can be carried out.

3. TEMPERATURE AND PULSE

The temperature is taken and, if elevated, the cause should be sought and the patient isolated or nursed under barrier precautions. The **pulse** is counted, but not during a uterine contraction, as both pulse and respirations are slightly increased then. Temperature, pulse and respirations do not rise during a normal labour, so any elevation or increase is significant.

4. ŒDEMA

Œdema may be due to pre-eclampsia, and if so will be accompanied by raised blood pressure and probably proteinuria. A tight wedding ring or puffiness of the face denotes a marked degree of œdema which is serious. Œdema of the vulva is shown on page 169.

5. URINE ANALYSIS

The urine is examined for protein and ketones, the specimen being obtained when the vulva is clean, e.g. after shaving, but before enema and bath, which are likely to cause involuntary micturition. A trace of protein in a voided specimen after the membranes have ruptured has no significance. In some hospitals the urine is examined for glucose.

The urine is tested for protein and ketones every four hours; after 12 hours every specimen is tested.

6. BLOOD PRESSURE

The blood pressure of every woman admitted in labour is taken. Cases are known where no pre-eclampsia was present during pregnancy and the woman showed no protein in her urine on admission, yet eclamptic convulsions occurred during labour. **If the blood pressure is over 130/80, the doctor should be notified so that sedatives can be prescribed.** The blood pressure rises about 10 mm. during normal labour, but this is most evident towards the end of the first and during the second stage.

(c) ABDOMINAL EXAMINATION

Abdominal examination should be carried out systematically by inspection, palpation and auscultation, as described on page 107, to determine the period of gestation, lie, presentation, position; whether the head is engaged and the presence of disproportion, if any. It is essential to listen to the fetal heart, not only as an aid to diagnosis of presentation and position but to find out if the fetus is alive and vigorous. The uterine contractions and the descent of the fetus will be noted abdominally and are described under Observation (p. 287).

(d) VULVAL EXAMINATION

If the woman is in strong labour on admission, the vulva may be inspected without actually touching it; and any gaping of the vaginal orifice or anus and bulging of the perineum are suggestive signs of the second stage of labour.

The colour and odour of the liquor amnii are noted. If the odour is *offensive* it usually means that the liquor is infected, and this is most likely when the membranes have ruptured early. **Green liquor** would necessitate listening to the fetal heart, as the presence of meconium may be due to fetal distress.

Any bleeding other than a mere show should be reported and the possibility of antepartum hæmorrhage considered.

Profuse or purulent vaginal discharge should have been dealt with during the prenatal period, but, if present, special precautions should be taken to avoid ophthalmia neonatorum.

Œdema of the vulva can assume large proportions; on occasions the labia being the size of the closed fists. This is as a rule due to pre-eclampsia. Reducing the œdema by multiple incisions is recommended by some authorities, but such treatment is seldom necessary as gross œdema of the labia will not appreciably delay the birth of the head but may predispose to labial or perineal laceration. *Sores and warts of the vulva are considered under Venereal Disease* (p. 205).

(e) VAGINAL EXAMINATION

A vaginal examination should not be necessary during every labour and should always be preceded by abdominal examination. The presentation, position and descent of the fetus can be ascertained by abdominal palpation during the first stage of labour, but there are occasions when it is imperative that a vaginal examination be made. **It is the only certain method of determining the degree of dilatation of the os,** which is one of the criteria by which progress during labour is assessed. When in doubt, the midwife should not hesitate to examine the woman vaginally, for failure to confirm the suspicion of some abnormality may have serious consequences.

INDICATIONS FOR VAGINAL EXAMINATION

(1) **To decide whether the woman is in labour.**

(2) **When there is doubt** regarding the presentation, as may arise in a primigravid patient with rigid abdominal walls.

(3) **In an obese patient,** to determine whether the head is engaged or not.

(4) **In district practice,** where the midwife has other patients to visit, in order to decide whether the patient can be safely left.

(5) **Before giving an enema** to a multiparous patient having strong contractions in case she is nearing the second stage.

(6) **When in doubt as to whether the second stage has begun,** *e.g.* persistent pushing at end of first stage.

(7) **In cases of prolonged labour,** to determine the cause of delay and to report such facts as the level of the presenting part, size of the caput and the degree of moulding to the doctor.

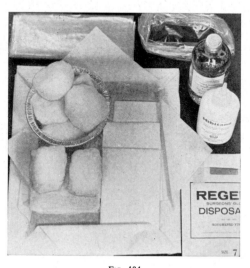

Fig. 184

VAGINAL EXAMINATION REQUIREMENTS.

1 solution bowl. 12 wool balls. gloves. perineal pad. 1 sheet steri paper.	180 ml. Savlon. Hibitane cream. 2 paper towels. 1 polythene sheet. 1 polythene bag for soiled swabs.

(*Aberdeen Maternity Hospital.*)

(8) **When prolapse of cord is likely to occur:**

    (*a*) After the membranes have ruptured in hydramnios.

    (*b*)   ,,   ,,   ,,   in breech or face presentation.

    (*c*)   ,,   .,   ,,   in a multiparous patient when the head is not engaged.

(9) **If prolapse of cord is suspected** because of fetal distress.

(10) **If there is doubt regarding the lie** of the second twin, or in order to puncture the second bag of membranes when contractions have not recommenced after five minutes.

(11) **When some abnormality** of the fetus is suspected, *e.g. anencephaly or hydrocephaly.*

N.B.—**In cases of antepartum hæmorrhage,** vaginal examination should **never** be made outwith the operating theatre because of the danger of producing serious hæmorrhage, and also because of the risk of infection.

METHOD

Need for Asepsis.—The introduction of the fingers into the vagina gives rise to the **danger** of exogenous infection (*introduced from outside the vulva*). **The greatest risk lies in the introduction of organisms by the attendant,** but intelligent mask-wearing, the conscientious preparation of hands and vulva and wearing of sterile gloves will greatly minimize the risk of sepsis.

The woman should be told what is about to be done, and if she is assured that the procedure will not be painful she is more likely to relax, and the examination will be easier to do and the findings more complete. It is a matter of personal preference whether the midwife examines the patient in the dorsal or left lateral position, but it is generally agreed that the examination can be more comprehensive when the woman lies on her back; when lying on her side, she feels less exposed and less draping is needed. **The bladder should be empty.**

The midwife, wearing a mask, prepares her hands and the patient's thighs and vulva prior to swabbing with the left hand. She puts on a gown, and drapes the patient with towels. **The first two fingers** of the right hand, wearing a disposable plastic glove, are dipped into antiseptic cream and gently inserted into the vagina, while the labia are held apart by the thumb and first finger of the left hand.

Care should be taken not to touch the labia, and the fingers to be introduced are held on a higher level than the vaginal orifice, during their insertion, to avoid contact with the anus. The fingers are directed along the anterior vaginal wall, and should not be withdrawn until the required information has been obtained, for a perfunctory examination will have to be repeated and the risk of infection is in the insertion of the fingers.

While turning the hand to explore the vagina, the thumb must not be brought into contact with the anus and then with the vaginal orifice.

FINDINGS ON VAGINAL EXAMINATION

THE CONDITION OF THE VAGINA.	PRESENTATION.
THE CERVIX AND OS.	POSITION.
THE BAG OF WATERS.	DEGREE OF MOULDING.
LEVEL OF THE PRESENTING PART.	ABNORMALITIES.

THE CONDITION OF THE VAGINA

The vaginal walls should feel soft and dilatable; when firm and rigid a longer labour can be anticipated. The presence of scar tissue in the lower vagina, following a previous perineal laceration or episiotomy, may, because of lack of elasticity, cause delay during the perineal phase of the second stage of labour, and the perineum is also more liable to rupture. *A cystocele* may be felt in the multigravid woman. A loaded rectum could resemble a tumour, but its putty-like consistency is diagnostic of fæces.

THE CERVIX

If the cervix is found to be 2·5 cm. long and the os closed, it can usually be concluded that labour is not likely to commence for some time. At the beginning of labour the cervix can be readily felt, although somewhat shortened, but by the time labour is established the cervical canal is completely taken up or effaced and the cervix is often closely applied to the fetal head. A thin, effaced cervix may be difficult to detect, and in primigravid patients it may not lie directly below what is presenting, so the examining fingers should be directed backwards and upwards.

If the cervix feels rigid and unyielding, whether it is thick or thin, dilatation is likely to be slow.

Towards the end of the first stage, an *œdematous anterior lip of cervix* may be present (see p. 398).

DILATATION OF THE OS

This is determined by encircling the circumference of the cervix with the fingers and forming a mental image of its size. This is described according to the measurement of the diameter of the os in centimetres. Recording dilatation in graph form focuses attention on slow progress.

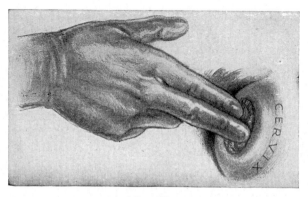

FIG. 185
Os 4 cm. dilated.

Centimetres			Approx. fingers	Centimetres		
1	.	.	. tip	4·5 .	.	half dilated
2	.	.	. 1 large	6		
3	.	.	. 2	7 .	.	three-quarters
4	.	.	. 3	8 .	.	rim of cervix

When fully dilated no cervix is felt

The figures given above would only obtain when the baby weighs about 3·1 kg. (7 lb.). With a 1·3 kg. (3 lb.) baby full dilatation might be imminent when the diameter of the os is 6 cm. It may take three hours for the os of the primigravid woman to reach 3 cm. dilatation and two hours for the multiparous os to reach 4 cm.

Rim of cervix. This term is used when the width of the cervical tissue surrounding the os is 0·5 or 1 cm. This indicates, that, no matter what the measurement of the dilated os, the stage of full dilatation is imminent. With a baby of 1·3 kg. (3 lb.) the os might be 6 cm. dilated when it was approaching full dilatation.

An important point to be grasped is that **when no cervix is felt** it has slipped up over the fetal head, **the os is fully dilated** and the second stage of labour has begun.

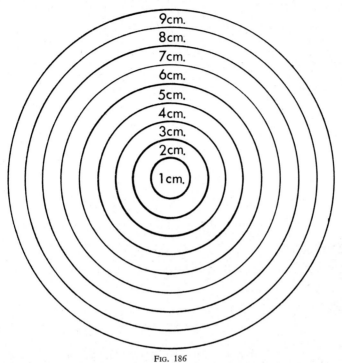

FIG. 186
DIAGRAMMATIC REPRESENTATION OF DILATATION OF THE OS IN CENTIMETRES TO SCALE.

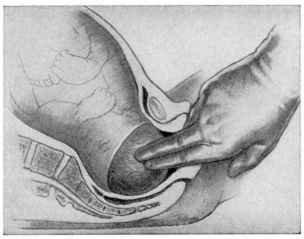

FIG. 187
Os almost fully dilated.

THE BAG OF WATERS

When the membranes are intact and the amount of fore-waters is scanty (6·2 mm. (¼ inch) or less in depth) the bag of waters may be difficult to detect on vaginal examination if the membranes lie in close contact with the fetal head. The scalp when covered with mucus has the same smooth slippery feeling that the bag of waters has, but during a uterine contraction the **membranes become tense** and can then be felt with the hard head lying immediately behind them and fluid between.

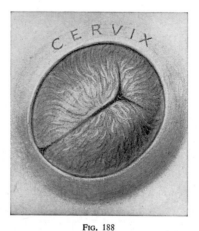

FIG. 188

Vertex L.O.A., os three-quarters (7 cm) dilated.

Usually the fore-waters are found by the examining finger to be shaped like a watch-glass but, if the "fit" between the presenting part and the lower segment is not good, some of the liquor from the hind-waters is forced into the fore-waters, causing the membranes to protrude through the cervix like a glove finger. The intra-uterine pressure exerted on these bulging fore-waters causes them to rupture early, so they are not often found on examination.

When there is doubt as to whether the membranes have ruptured, upward pressure on the head will allow amniotic fluid to escape.

Occasionally, in cases where there has been an escape of liquor amnii and the membranes are believed to have ruptured, the fore-waters are found on vaginal examination to be intact. The possible explanation is that there may have been a slight rupture of the hind-waters and when the head was forced into the lower segment by good uterine contractions further escape of fluid was prevented.

Avoidance of artificial rupture of membranes —As a general rule, the membranes should not be punctured by the midwife during the first stage of labour. Occasionally, in cases when contractions are poor and a well-flexed head presents, it has been found that by puncturing the membranes the head sinks down on to the cervical nerve endings and stimulates uterine action. The inexperienced midwife would be well advised not to meddle, and to look upon intact membranes as a protection for mother and baby.

LEVEL OF THE PRESENTING PART

If the head is deeply engaged it can be felt low in the pelvic cavity, at the level of the ischial spines. The caput may, however, be below that level. If the head is just engaged it can be touched or tipped, but when the head is above the brim it cannot be reached vaginally.

DIAGNOSIS OF PRESENTATION

In 95 per cent of cases the vertex presents and is recognized by feeling the hard skull bones, the fontanelles and sutures.

The diagnosis of malpresentations is described under their respective headings.

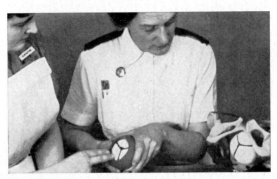

Fig. 189

Demonstration of dilatation of os and position of the vertex.
Note.—Halves of a series of rubber balls used to denote the dilating cervix.
(*Aberdeen Maternity Hospital.*)

DIAGNOSIS OF POSITION

In the vertex presentation, position is determined by recognizing which fontanelle lies anteriorly, *i.e.* the posterior fontanelle in anterior positions, the anterior fontanelle in posterior positions and whether it is to the left or right side of the pelvis.

DEGREE OF MOULDING

This can be judged by feeling the amount of overlapping of the skull bones, and, when excessive, it indicates that *intracranial injury* is likely to have taken place.

ABNORMALITIES

Prolapse or presentation of cord, anencephaly, hydrocephaly and compound presentation can be diagnosed vaginally.

N.B.—Student midwives should note that P.V. stands for "*per vaginam,*" and not "*per vagina.*"

(*f*) RECTAL EXAMINATION

There is much controversy regarding the making of rectal examinations during labour and many authorities condemn the procedure. It is true that when the finger in the rectum presses the lower vaginal wall up into the os, organisms could be transferred upwards, but the source of infection during labour is from outside the vulva rather than from the vagina. *That some make too many rectal examinations is not a justifiable censure on the procedure but on the persons.*

18

One practical advantage is the time factor. Vaginal examination entails scrubbing the hands and swabbing the vulva, which takes at least seven minutes. Rectal examination requires clean, but not surgically clean, hands.

A rectal examination should always be preceded by an abdominal examination to get a more complete assessment of the situation.

Seldom is it necessary to make more than two rectal examinations during a normal labour, and if labour is advancing quickly none is required.

Method

The patient lies on her back or on her left side at the edge of the bed, with knees drawn up. If she is told what is about to be done and asked to relax and to breathe deeply, the procedure causes little discomfort.

A mask is worn, and the hands should be washed for at least one minute and a plastic disposable glove worn. The thumb is held across the palm of the hand under the middle finger to avoid its touching the vulva, and the lubricated forefinger is slowly introduced through the anal sphincter and directed upwards and inwards.

Care must be taken to avoid bruising the rectal mucosa or causing anal fissures. On withdrawing the finger, precautions should be taken to avoid contaminating the vulva with fæces, but the risk of contamination is probably less when the woman lies in the left lateral position. The anus should be wiped clean with wool swabs, as there is usually soiling with lubricant if not with fæces.

The findings will be similar to those on vaginal examination, but not quite so well defined. If the head is in mid-cavity, it will be reached when the finger is inserted to the middle joint: when in high cavity the head can just be tipped and when at or above the brim it cannot be reached.

While the membranes are intact the cervix can be recognized as a circular ridge surrounding a depressed centre. After the membranes have ruptured, the caput may be felt in the os as a boggy wrinkled mass which may on occasions obliterate fontanelles or sutures.

An inexperienced person may mistake the thin cervix that is taken up and 2 or 3 cm. dilated, for one that is fully dilated, but the short contractions and absence of other signs of the second stage should prevent such an error from being made. As an aid to learning, it is a good plan for beginners to make a rectal examination immediately after having made a vaginal examination, when the findings are then known to be correct.

PREPARATION OF THE WOMAN IN LABOUR

1. SHAVING.
2. EVACUATION OF LOWER BOWEL.
3. BATH OR SHOWER.
4. ATTENTION TO HAIR AND NAILS.
5. VULVAL SWABBING.

1. SHAVING

The pubic hair is usually shaved or clipped because otherwise it is difficult to keep the vulva clean throughout labour or during the puerperal period. *In some centres neither shaving nor clipping is practised; the majority of midwives prefer shaving to be done and many think patients' objections to this have been exaggerated.*

The razor blade should be sharp, the pubic hair well lathered with green soap and the shaving strokes made in a downward direction to avoid unnecessary pain. Before using the razor, the strong antiseptic should be thoroughly rinsed off.

Disposable razors are on the market.

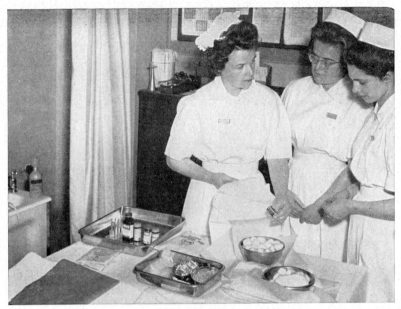

Fig. 190
Labour ward admission room. Sister showing pre-packed equipment for shaving.
(*Simpson Memorial Maternity Pavilion, Edinburgh.*)

2. EVACUATION OF LOWER BOWEL

N.B.—If the woman is suffering from eclampsia or antepartum hæmorrhage an enema or suppository is not given.

It is advisable that every woman should have her lower bowel emptied at the beginning of labour. (*Some prefer suppositories, Beogex or Dulcolax, but they are slow in action and do not empty the bowel as effectively as a plain water enema does; soiling tends to occur during the second stage.*)

(*a*) It stimulates uterine action. There is some connection between the nerve supply to the uterus and bowel, so that stimulation of the bowel appears to excite better uterine contractions.

This fact should be kept in mind, lest the baby be born during the expulsion of an enema given inadvisedly to a woman in strong labour. Judgment is needed in deciding when it is safe to give an enema. Although there would be no risk in giving one to a primigravid woman whose os was 6 cm. dilated, it would not be wise to give an enema to a multiparous patient at that stage, because in her case the second half of the first stage is so rapid. There is less soiling from a firm stool than the fluid returned from an enema.

When in doubt, it is advisable to make a vaginal or rectal examination to ascertain the degree of dilatation of the os, but the strength of the uterine contractions and what has been accomplished since the onset of labour should also be taken into consideration.

(b) **An empty rectum allows more room for the descent of the fetus.** The colon and rectum lie in the pelvic canal, and a loaded rectum occupies space that is needed for the passage of the fetus.

(c) **It ensures a clean field during delivery.** If the lower bowel is not emptied, the descending head will cause fæces to be expelled immediately before, and during the birth of the baby.

3. BATH OR SHOWER

This is given following shaving and enema, and thorough cleansing of the vulva and pubic region with Phisohex is recommended; a shower with a mobile hand-spray is excellent. If there is not time for a complete bath an effort should be made to wash the woman from the umbilicus to the knees at least.

If the patient kneels in a bath which is one-third full, it is doubtful whether bath water does enter the vagina. From the practical point of view there is much to commend a shower or tub bath; otherwise it is difficult to remove all the short cut hair after shaving.

A clean nightdress, cotton stockings and a washable dressing-gown are then worn.

4. HAIR AND NAILS

The hair is combed, inspected for pediculi in hospital and subsequently treated if necessary. **Long nails harbour organisms** and may infect the woman's vulva during labour. No person can handle a baby safely with long sharp nails.

It is equally important that *nail-paint, rouge and lip-stick* should be removed during labour, and if the woman is told that her natural colour is the best guide as to how she is faring she will usually co-operate. The use of cosmetics may keep up her morale, but **obstetric precautions must be observed.**

5. VULVAL SWABBING

The principle of swabbing technique is to cleanse the vulva of secretions and organisms without contaminating the birth canal. There is no " *best* " swabbing technique. It is **the conscientious thorough application of any satisfactory method,** rather than the method *per se*, that constitutes good technique. The equipment used and the method employed may vary slightly from hospital to hospital, mainly depending on whether (a) sterile gloves, or (b) the non-touch technique, or (c) disposable equipment is used.

Swabbing is done as much for the comfort of the woman as for its aseptic value and merely cleansing the labia is not enough. In all cases swabbing should be preceded by washing the pubes, groins, inner thighs and buttocks with soap and water unless a bath has been recently given.

The vulva is swabbed on admission and at six-hourly intervals during labour, as well as immediately preceding *vaginal examination and delivery.*

QUESTIONS FOR REVISION

ASEPSIS: ANTISEPSIS

C.M.B.(Eng.) paper.—What precautions can a midwife take during labour and the puerperium to prevent the occurrence of puerperal sepsis ?

C.M.B.(Eng.) paper.—Give the reasons for the measures which are adopted to avoid infection in a maternity unit.

C.M.B.(Eng.) paper.—Describe the measures you take to prevent infection during labour and the puerperium.

ADMISSION OF THE WOMAN IN LABOUR

What questions regarding her labour would you ask?

Under what circumstances should a vaginal examination not be made by the midwife?

Give reasons why the woman in labour should be given an enema.

CLINICAL APPLICATION

Give examples as to how domestic cleanliness can prevent infection in the labour ward. In what way is the history of labour significant ? How would a woman, 24 hours after admission in false labour, be dealt with ?

State whether labour is true or false in the following circumstances:

Contractions (a) painful ....; (b) lasting 2 minutes ....; (c) erratic ......; **on vaginal examination** (a) cervix is shortened ....; (b) os not dilating .... (c) membranes tense ....; (d) no show ....

The urine is examined every .... hours.

Blood pressure is taken every .... hours.

Discuss (a) vaginal versus rectal examination; (b) shaving versus non-shaving; (c) water enema versus suppository.

Differentiate between (a) urine and amniotic fluid; (b) the vulva of a primigravid and a multigravid woman; (c) thin cervix 2 cm. dilated and one that is fully dilated; (d) an L.O.A. and an R.O.P. vaginally; (e) intact and ruptured membranes P.V.

C.M.B.(N. Ireland) paper.—What examination of a patient would you make at the beginning of labour ? How would you decide that labour was likely to be normal ?

C.M.B.(N. Ireland) paper.—What are the indications for vaginal examination during labour ? Indicate how the findings might influence the conduct of labour.

C.M.B.(Eng.) paper.—You are called to attend a woman who has just started labour. Give the reasons for the examinations you would make.

C.M.B.(Eng.) paper.—When should a midwife make a vaginal examination during labour ? What information could she obtain ?

C.M.B.(N. Ireland) paper.—An unbooked multiparous patient is admitted in early labour. What would make you think the labour should proceed normally ?

C.M.B.(Eng.) paper.—Describe the anatomy of the vagina. What information may be obtained from a vaginal examination in labour?

17

The Management of Normal Labour (contd.)

OBSTETRICAL NURSING CARE DURING THE FIRST STAGE OF LABOUR

1. POSTURE OF THE WOMAN IN LABOUR.
2. DIET OF THE WOMAN IN LABOUR.
3. ATTENTION TO BLADDER AND BOWEL.
4. REST AND SLEEP.
5. COMFORT AND ASSISTANCE.
6. OBSERVATION AND RECORDING

1. POSTURE OF THE WOMAN IN LABOUR

No hard and fast rule can be laid down regarding the posture to be adopted by the woman in labour If a multgravid woman goes into labour during the evening, being a busy housewife she will be tired and should be advised to lie down, and snatch such sleep as she can, while there is a reasonable interval between contractions.

The rested woman can be encouraged to continue with her household duties or to walk about the room in hospital. It is a good working rule to *rest the tired woman* and stimulate the rested one, but a certain amount of judgment must be used, for labours vary in length and women have different degrees of physical stamina. Labour always seems longer and more painful to the woman who goes to bed and stays there as soon as contractions begin, waiting apprehensively for each pain.

The Upright Position

There is a distinct advantage in the assumption of the upright position; the fetus sinks into the lower pole of the uterus and by pressing on the cervical nerve endings stimulates good uterine action. It also facilitates dilatation of the os. In the erect position the antero-posterior diameter of the pelvic brim is enlarged because a certain degree of movement takes place at the sacro-iliac joints.

Very often the woman instinctively adopts postures that are advantageous, such as standing on tip-toe during a contraction with her back bent and her abdominal muscles drawn inwards and upwards. She rests her hands or elbows on the bed and her tense abdominal muscles act as a brace which helps to direct the fetus into the pelvic canal. A similar advantage can be obtained by sitting in a low chair, or in bed, leaning forwards during a contraction.

The Recumbent Position

When the intensity of the contractions gives rise to suffering, the woman should of course be in bed so that she can relax and conserve her strength and in order that analgesics may be given to relieve the pain. The woman in hard labour should certainly be in bed and when the uterus is overdistended with fluid or twins she needs extra rest because of the heavy load she is carrying.

Where there is a badly fitting presenting part and the membranes are liable to rupture early, some authorities keep the woman in bed because they believe the cord is more likely to prolapse when she is on her feet.

When much liquor is draining, the recumbent position should be adopted to prevent undue loss of liquor which might cause fetal distress. (Posture during the second stage is considered on p. 296.)

2. DIET DURING LABOUR

This subject presents great difficulties; both the nutritional requirements of the woman in labour and the grave risk of anæsthetic deaths must be given due consideration. The modern tendency is to withhold food when labour is well established and to give glucose intravenously if needed.

The Need for Glucose

Glucose is essential for efficient functioning of the uterine and cardiac muscles during labour. A tremendous amount of energy is expended in combating the stress of the first stage as well as in the expulsion of the baby during the second stage.

Deprivation of glucose leads to ketosis which produces vomiting, extreme exhaustion and a predisposition to shock, so the urine is examined for ketones every 4 hours (each specimen after 12 hours). When ketones are present or sooner an intravenous drip of 10 per cent dextrose is set up.

But even when no food has been partaken for hours during labour, inhalation by the unconscious woman of the acid gastric juice may produce broncho-spasm, cyanosis, pulmonary œdema and, in some cases, death may ensue. To counteract the acidity of the gastric contents some obstetricians prescribe Aludrox or magnesium trisilicate 10 ml. two hourly throughout labour.

Pain and nervous tension inhibit appetite and retard the absorption of food. The woman may not bother to chew her food properly so it should be sieved. Undigested food may be vomited 6-8 hours after it is partaken.

EARLY LABOUR

During early labour small light meals should be served such as tea and toast; strained non-greasy soups; sieved chicken; fruit jellies; cornflour pudding; ice-cream. The glucose in digestible carbohydrate foods is less irritating to the stomach than concentrated glucose solutions which if vomited and inhaled are bronchial irritants.

When in strong labour food should be withheld and fluid only (weak tea, water) given. Dehydration must be avoided so it is prudent to keep a fluid balance chart in every labour. Copious aerated fruit juices may cause nausea, vomiting and dehydration as well as gaseous distension of the stomach and intestine.

PROLONGED LABOUR

Although this is now rarely permitted to occur, it presents a serious problem for the midwife. If food is withheld for many hours until the woman is profoundly dehydrated and suffering from ketosis **she is a very grave risk** when operative measures under general anæsthesia are undertaken. **A dextrose drip 10 per cent should be given** as soon as oral feeding is precluded and always prior to operative procedures.

POSSIBLE ANÆSTHETIC DIFFICULTIES

The question as to whether an anæsthetic will be necessary should be kept in mind, and the woman ought not to be given food or copious fluids within three hours of delivery. Many obstetricians are using pudendal nerve block in preference to a general anæsthetic for forceps delivery.

A plastic oesophageal tube No. 18 E.G. should be passed before a general anæsthetic is administered to the woman in labour.

3. ATTENTION TO THE BLADDER

It is the duty of the midwife to see that the woman empties her bladder (every two hours) throughout labour. A bladder containing 90 or 120 ml. of urine will be seen and felt, well above the symphysis pubis during labour, and it will have a soft fluctuating consistency. When overdistended, it forms a smooth round tense swelling and above its upper margin a very definite depression is evident. This dip is sometimes mistaken for **Bandl's ring** (see p. 233).

Disadvantages of an Overdistended Bladder

A full bladder may prevent the head from entering the brim, and this is most frequently seen in the multigravid woman. It may retard descent of the fetus, so in all cases of delay the bladder should be palpated and percussed.

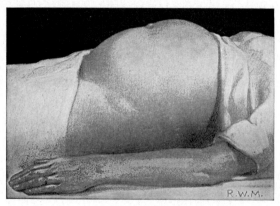

Fig. 191
Distended bladder during labour

It will cause much unnecessary pain during labour, and by interfering with the tone of the bladder may predispose to retention of urine after delivery.

Poor uterine contractions are often associated with a full bladder, and in such cases an improvement in uterine action is usually apparent as soon as the bladder is emptied.

During prolonged labour, and particularly when minor cephalo-pelvic disproportion exists, the **bladder may be nipped** between the fetal skull and pelvis, but this is most likely to happen when the bladder is not emptied regularly. The bruised area may slough during the puerperium, giving rise to a **vesico-vaginal fistula.**

RETENTION OF URINE

This frequently occurs during labour, for the following reasons:

(*a*) **The bladder may lack tone,** especially when hypotonic uterine action is present, (*b*) **Using the bedpan is an uncomfortable procedure** for the cumbersome woman in labour. (It should be placed on a low stool beside the bed, or better still, in a sani-chair, which gives firm support to her arms and buttocks and allows better relaxation of the pelvic floor muscles.)

(*c*) **Pressure on the urethra.**—Inability to void during the latter part of the first stage is usually due to pressure of the fetal head on the neck of the bladder, and in such circumstances posture and suggestion are of no value. **If the woman has not passed urine for six hours, the bladder is visibly distended and the woman unable to void, a catheter ought to be passed.** Medical permission should first be obtained.

CATHETERIZATION

Every effort must be made to encourage micturition during labour to obviate the necessity for catheterization.

Plastic disposable catheters are commonly used.

Need for asepsis.—It may be unnecessary to stress the need for aseptic technique in catheterization, as most nurses are aware of this, but the conditions existing during labour enhance the risk of infection, *e.g.* trauma and over-distension of the bladder, retention and stasis of urine.

If difficulty is encountered while introducing the catheter, the sterile gloved fore-finger of the left hand should be inserted into the vagina and placed along its anterior wall. The tip of the catheter can then be felt, and if it is directed parallel with the finger in the vagina, the catheter will enter the bladder without injury to the urethra. If the catheter is obstructed by the fetal head, upward pressure on the head by the finger in the vagina will permit passage of the catheter.

INSTILLATION OF CHLORHEXIDINE

The instillation of 60 ml. of chlorhexidine aqueous solution 1 in 5,000 into the bladder, before withdrawing the catheter, is recommended to reduce the risk of infection.

Indications for Catheterization

In all cases where medical aid is summoned during labour, the patient should be encouraged to empty her bladder. Many obstetricians are now reluctant to pass a catheter unless the bladder is distended and the woman unable to void. Others consider that damage to the bladder can be more dangerous than urinary tract infection and that catheterization should be performed prior to vaginal operative manipulations during labour.

ATTENTION TO THE BOWEL

An enema should never be given at the end of the first stage, because during its expulsion it is usual for the action of the uterus to be intensified, and further descent of the fetal head may prevent the complete return of the fluid, so that with each subsequent contraction there will be spluttering of liquid fæces.

Gaseous distension of the bowel can be exceedingly troublesome and is most likely to occur when the uterus is inert. The drinking of copious cold sweet fluids seems to favour its occurrence.

It is not commendable to permit patients to use " the toilet " throughout labour. *They are unable to differentiate between the desire to defæcate and the similar sensation preceding expulsion of the baby's head. When a bedpan is used and the midwife empties it, the amount of urine can be measured and any abnormal vaginal discharge noted.*

4. REST AND SLEEP

The need for **adequate rest and sleep during labour cannot be over emphasized;** for discomfort, pain and anxiety are each exhausting and the woman in labour may experience all three. She needs sleep, not only to give respite from these, but also to refresh her weary body and to maintain her mental equilibrium.

If the woman is tired her uterus also becomes tired and does not function well; labour is prolonged, with all its attendant hazards. When worn out from lack of sleep the *pain threshold is lowered,* the woman lacks energy to co-operate by pushing during the second stage, and the need for operative interference is therefore increased.

Night is the best time for sleep, and unless nearing the end of labour an effort should be made for the woman to rest and sleep at this time.

The usual nursing procedures to induce sleep should be employed :

(*a*) **The bladder is emptied;** (*b*) a nourishing drink given; (*c*) the bed ought to be comfortable; (*d*) **the room darkened;** (*e*) an effort is made to ensure **quietness.**

If the woman is assured that " all is well," told that the midwife is near, given a suitable sedative and tucked up in a kindly manner, she will almost certainly relax and sleep.

5. COMFORT AND ASSISTANCE

Personal toilet.—The midwife can add greatly to the comfort of the woman in labour by attending to her personal toilet. Pain is very demoralizing and she may lose interest in her appearance and feel disinclined for the effort such care entails. The midwife should wash her patient's face and hands and help to dress her hair. The buttocks and thighs should be washed and the vulva swabbed six-hourly for the woman's comfort, even by those who do not consider it to have any antiseptic value.

Clean clothing is most refreshing.—Soiled bed-linen is unhygienic as well as uncomfortable, and when liquor amnii is draining freely, "under" pads can be placed beneath the buttocks. The term, **dry labour,** is used by the laity to describe a labour when the membranes have ruptured early, but for the patient it is very wet indeed.

Cramp in the leg may be very distressing, and one way of obtaining quick relief is to extend the leg and dorsiflex the foot. (*The toes of the straightened leg are brought towards the knee.*)

Backache (*see* p. 260).

Bearing down should be forbidden during the first stage of labour, because, when the os is not fully dilated, the woman pushes her uterus downwards and puts such great strain on the transverse cervical ligaments and the para-cervical tissue, that subsequent uterine prolapse is likely.

Premature pushing causes the cervix to be compressed between the fetal head and the symphysis pubis, making the anterior lip of cervix become œdematous and hard, thereby increasing the pain and delaying labour. It is possible that if the head is forced through an os which is almost but not quite fully dilated, the cervix might be lacerated. The increased intra-uterine pressure may cause premature rupture of the membranes as well as fetal distress.

The patient who bears down too soon must be asked to stop, turned on her side and shown how to refrain by breathing deliberately, accentuating inspiration rather than expiration during contractions. Raising the foot of the bed may help. If inhalational analgesia is administered, the woman can co-operate more readily. It is essential that a midwife remain with the woman.

6. OBSERVATION OF THE WOMAN IN LABOUR

This is an integral part of good obstetrical nursing care, and, although the majority of labours are normal, the midwife must never lower the high standard of conscientious observation needed for the safety of the two lives in her care.

Observation can be considered under the following headings:

(*a*) UTERINE ACTION.

(*b*) DILATATION OF THE OS.

(*c*) DESCENT OF THE PRESENTING PART.

(*d*) DISCHARGE FROM THE VAGINA

(*e*) THE FETAL CONDITION.

(*f*) THE MATERNAL CONDITION.

(*g*) COMPLICATIONS.

(*a*) UTERINE ACTION

The frequency, length and strength of the contractions should be noted: four-hourly when the woman is up and about in early labour; every hour when labour is established and then every half hour. At the beginning of labour, pain is often felt in the sacral region, and some women complain of pain in the groins and thighs. It may, however, be some hours before rhythmic regular contractions are evident and labour is properly established.

The strength of a contraction cannot be judged by the reaction of the woman, but always by laying the hand on the uterus and noting the degree of hardness during the contraction and by timing its length. Some women appear to experience great pain and yet the contractions may be neither long nor strong and very little is accomplished; other women appear to suffer very little, yet good progress is made.

When a uterine contraction begins, it is painless for a number of seconds and painless again at the end, so the midwife is aware of the approach of a contraction before the patient feels it, and this knowledge can be utilized when giving inhalational analgesia. The uterus should always relax between contractions. Should the contractions be unduly long or very strong and rapid, concern would be felt in case fetal anoxia develops.

(*b*) DILATATION OF THE OS

Until the os begins to dilate, the woman is not considered to be in true labour but when it is 4 cm. dilated and accompanied by regular contractions, labour is said to be well established. The progress of labour is usually assessed by the degree of dilatation of the os.

In cases where the doctor wishes to be present for the delivery it is usual to call him when the os is fully dilated in a primigravida and when three-quarters dilated (7 cm.) in a multigravid woman, but other factors, such as the strength and frequency of the contractions and the rate of advance, must be taken into consideration when predicting the probable time of delivery.

(*c*) DESCENT OF THE PRESENTING PART

During the first stage this can be noted almost entirely by abdominal palpation but when doubt exists a vaginal or rectal examination is made.

In the primigravid woman the fetal head is commonly engaged before labour begins and its continued descent can be followed by abdominal palpation. Should the head be above the brim in a primigravida, close watch must be kept by frequent palpation to find out whether with good contractions the head enters the brim.

When the head is engaged the occiput has descended into the pelvic cavity and can only be felt with difficulty from above. The sinciput may still be palpable above the brim because of the increased flexion of the head until the occiput reaches the pelvic floor.

In a multigravid patient the head may not descend appreciably until labour is well established and sometimes not until the membranes rupture.

A full bladder may prevent descent.

The descent of the presenting part can also be detected from below by vaginal or rectal examination and in cases where there is excessive moulding and a large caput, a misleading impression of advance can be gained, as it is possible for a caput to be showing inside the vulva while the head is actually above the ischial spines and the os not fully dilated.

(d) DISCHARGE FROM THE VAGINA

Show is the blood-stained mucus seen early in labour. Towards the end of the first stage a trickle of blood may appear, due to the slight laceration of the cervix which usually takes place when it is dilated to its maximum. This is sometimes called " a bright red show," but it is not " show " in the real sense of the word.

Liquor amnii may be seen trickling from the vagina after the membranes have ruptured, and is a pale odourless fluid, but if doubt exists as to whether it is urine or liquor, its alkaline reaction, obtained by the use of litmus paper, will help to settle the question.

The presence of meconium in the liquor suggests fetal distress, except during the second stage in cases of breech presentation. **If the liquor looks milky** or contains white specks, this is only due to vernix caseosa and has no significance.

Golden liquor is seen in some cases when the fetus is suffering from Rh hæmolytic disease.

EARLY RUPTURE OF THE MEMBRANES

If the membranes have been ruptured for 24 hours or more, the liquor may become infected and will have an offensive odour. This is dangerous, because the fetus may inhale some of the liquor, with resultant pneumonia. Infection of the birth canal may also occur. The doctor should be notified; an antibiotic, such as ampicillin, 500 mg. followed by 250 mg., 6 hourly, is usually prescribed.

(e) THE FETAL CONDITION

THE FETAL HEART IS THE BEST GUIDE AS TO HOW THE FETUS IS FARING

The heart beat should be carefully counted at the beginning of labour, so that the average rate for this particular fetus is known. The normal rate ranges from 120 to 140 beats per minute, and it is a good plan **to record it in graph form** so that any upward or downward trend will be detected. *The normal rhythm* is that of a double beat, with a short first sound and a long second sound.

Rate, volume and rhythm should be noted.

The fetal heart is not usually taken during the height of a uterine contraction. The mother ought not to be disturbed while she is suffering pain, and any changes in rate at that time would not be a true reading. Towards the end of the first stage, when the contractions are long, strong and frequent, the interference with the placental circulation causes a slight increase or decrease in the fetal heart-rate, but this usually disappears towards the end of the contraction or within a few seconds after the contraction has ceased. If not, and marked slowing occurs, fetal anoxia may be present.

Frequency of Auscultation

No hard and fast rule can be laid down as to how often the fetal heart should be listened to during the first stage of labour. Patients who are up and about, with intact membranes and not in strong labour, could have the fetal heart taken every half-hour. Some authorities would consider this to be unnecessary, others would want it done every 15 minutes.   If the woman is asleep, she ought not to be disturbed.

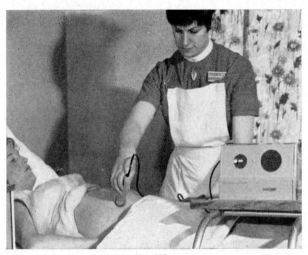

FIG. 192
THE DOPTONE ULTRASONIC FETAL BLOOD FLOW DETECTOR.
Used by the midwife to clarify indistinct fetal heart sounds.
(*Aberdeen Maternity Hospital.*)

The fetal heart should always be checked when the membranes rupture and particularly when there is a badly fitting presenting part, in case the cord has prolapsed.   More frequent auscultation is needed when the membranes are no longer intact.

Towards the end of the first stage, when the woman is in strong labour, it would be advisable to listen to the fetal heart every five minutes.

FETAL DISTRESS

The danger of fetal distress occurring during the first stage is not great, unless some complication is present such as disproportion, or during a prolonged first stage with early rupture of membranes.

Anoxia is the commonest cause of fetal distress, and the likelihood of prolapse of cord should always be kept in mind.   Oxygen lack may cause stillbirth: in less severe cases the baby may be born asphyxiated: anoxia may also cause brain damage resulting in cerebral palsy.

Some carry out fetal blood sampling (see p. 414) when fetal distress is anticipated, as in placental dysfunction or Rh incompatibility.

Continuous electronic fetal heart monitoring is now being employed in high risk cases.

THE SIGNS OF FETAL DISTRESS ARE AS FOLLOWS :

Meconium-stained liquor amnii.

Fetal heart that is slow or rapid.

Fetal heart that is irregular, intermittent or weak.

Excessive fetal movements may occur when death is imminent, but this sign is not reliable.

Fetal distress is discussed in detail under prolonged labour (p. 413).

(f) THE MATERNAL CONDITION

During normal labour there is rarely any need for anxiety regarding the woman's general condition. If given light nourishing food early in labour to maintain her strength and analgesic drugs for the relief of pain and to ensure adequate rest and sleep, the average woman remains in good physical condition throughout labour.

Pulse and temperature are useful guides as to how she is standing up to labour, and on that account both should be taken on admission and at **four-hourly intervals** throughout the first stage. The pulse is taken every one or two hours when in strong labour.

Blood pressure should be estimated four-hourly, some do so two-hourly.

A fluid balance chart is kept.

The urine should be examined for protein and ketones four-hourly: after 12 hours every specimen is examined.

EMOTIONAL DISTRESS

The woman may exhibit a certain amount of emotional or psychological fatigue when labour lasts longer than 18 hours. She is more discouraged than exhausted, and the student midwife must learn to differentiate between such a condition and actual physical exhaustion, which is commonly known as **maternal distress.** The emotionally tired woman shows no physical signs of exhaustion, such as rising pulse and temperature. She is disheartened owing to the length of labour and because she may feel that very little progress is being made.

Many women in this state say " *they cannot stand it any longer,*" but that is not a real indication of maternal distress. Much encouragement is needed to tide them over this difficult period, and drugs such as pethidine are invaluable. In such cases, as soon as labour is over the woman recovers quickly, she is interested in her baby and ready for food.

MATERNAL DISTRESS

Maternal distress is serious, and should not arise in good midwifery practice. It does not happen like a " *bolt from the blue,*" for it is usually associated with obstructed labour, the cause of which the midwife should have diagnosed earlier. Maternal distress may occur in an unduly prolonged labour, without obstruction, particularly when dehydration and ketosis have been allowed to develop and the woman has lost much sleep. This is unlikely to occur today.

The good midwife forestalls such a situation by competent obstetrical nursing. She does not wait for signs of maternal distress to be established before sending for medical assistance: experience has taught her how much the average woman can be expected to endure; she anticipates that the woman is reaching a state of exhaustion.

SIGNS OF MATERNAL DISTRESS (*Ketosis*)

1. RISING PULSE RATE.
2. INCREASE IN TEMPERATURE.
3. PINCHED, ANXIOUS EXPRESSION.
4. THE WOMAN FEELS ILL.
5. MARKED RESTLESSNESS.
6. DARK VOMITUS.

Maternal distress is considered under prolonged labour (p. 411).

(g) COMPLICATIONS

Conditions present during pregnancy such as eclampsia or antepartum hæmorrhage may persist during labour, but the commonest complications during the first stage are due to factors which give rise to delay, *e.g.*

Disordered uterine action.   Big baby: malpresentation: malposition.
Contracted pelvis: rigid cervix.

Such complications should be prevented when possible, recognized early and **medical aid summoned.** (*They are considered elsewhere under their respective headings.*)

The midwife should always refrain from unnecessary interference during normal labour, for meddlesome midwifery increases the dangers to mother and child. **Emergencies** must, however, be dealt with proficiently until the arrival of the doctor.

QUESTIONS FOR REVISION

OBSTETRICAL NURSING CARE IN NORMAL LABOUR

ORAL QUESTIONS

What are the advantages of a woman continuing with household duties in early labour ? How can the history of labour influence your management ?

Describe suitable food for a woman in early labour.

Why is Aludrox or magnesium trisilicate sometimes given during labour ?

What can you learn from abdominal examination during labour ?

What can you learn from inspecting the vulva during labour ?

What are the signs that labour is established ?

Write not more than 10 lines on: (a) attention to the bladder in labour; (b) attention to the bowel in labour; (c) comfort and assistance in labour; (d) early rupture of the membranes; (e) findings on vaginal examination in labour; (f) intelligent mask-wearing.

Differentiate between: (a) physical and emotional distress; (b) the cervix of a primigravid and a multigravid woman; (c) true and false labour.

What could be done for the following conditions: Backache, cramp in the leg, premature bearing down ?

Give five signs of fetal distress. Give five signs of maternal distress.

C.M.B.(Eng.) paper.—Describe the anatomy and relations of the bladder. Why is it important to keep the bladder as empty as possible during labour ?

C.M.B.(N. Ireland) paper.—Describe your care of a primigravida from the time she is admitted to the labour ward until she is ready for delivery 24 hours later.

C.M.B.(Scot.) paper.—How can a midwife assess whether labour is progressing normally ? Explain briefly what may interfere with the normal progress.

C.M.B.(Eng.) paper.—What do you understand by early rupture of the membranes ? Discuss the causes and management thereof.

C.M.B.(Scot.) paper.—Describe the care of a patient in the first stage of labour under the following headings: 1. Relief of pain. 2. Diet. 3. Observation. 4. Asepsis.

C.M.B.(N. Ireland) paper.—What would lead you to suspect that labour was not proceeding normally ? What examinations would you carry out to determine the cause ?

C.M.B.(N. Ireland) paper.—What are the possible causes and complications of early rupture of the membranes ? Describe the admission of a patient in early labour whose membranes have ruptured.

C.M.B.(N. Ireland) paper.—What information can be obtained from auscultation of the fetal heart during labour and how does this influence your care of the patient ?

C.M.B.(N. Ireland) paper.—Describe in detail your care of a primigravida during the first stage of labour.

C.M.B.(Eng.) paper.—Describe the management and nursing care of a primigravida during the first stage of labour.

C.M.B.(Scot.) paper.—What information can be obtained from a vaginal examination carried out during labour ? How might the findings influence the conduct of labour ?

18

The Management of Normal Labour (contd.)

THE SECOND STAGE

During the second stage of labour mother and fetus require unremitting supervision, for both are subjected to trauma and other dangers which do not arise during the first stage. The midwife must now remain in constant attendance; indeed, the woman in her own home should not be left from the time the os is three-quarters dilated.

C.M.B.(Scot.) Rule. (Eng.) Code of Practice.—*When in charge of a case of labour, a practising midwife* must not leave the patient without giving an address *by which she can be found without delay.* After the beginning of the second stage she must stay with the patient *until the expulsion of the placenta and membranes, and as long as may be necessary (Scotland, at least one hour).*

SIGNS OF THE SECOND STAGE

The transition from the first to the second stage is not always clearly defined clinically. **There is only one positive sign,** which involves making a vaginal examination, and it is neither desirable nor necessary to make repeated vaginal examinations for this purpose. There are a number of probable signs and an aggregation of these can be accepted with a fair degree of reliance, but no one probable sign is infallible.

POSITIVE SIGN

No cervix felt on vaginal examination

PROBABLE SIGNS

1. NO CERVIX FELT RECTALLY.
2. EXPULSIVE UTERINE CONTRACTIONS.
3. TRICKLING OF BLOOD.
4. RUPTURE OF MEMBRANES.
5. ANUS POUTING AND GAPING.
6. TENSENESS BETWEEN COCCYX AND ANUS.
7. VULVA GAPING.
8. PRESENTING PART APPEARING.
9. BULGING OF PERINEUM.

1. NO CERVIX FELT ON RECTAL EXAMINATION

Rectal examinations are not conclusive, for it is not always possible to palpate the whole circumference of a cervix that is almost fully dilated. Mistakes are sometimes made by inexperienced midwives when making a rectal examination on a primigravida. When the os is only 3 cm. dilated, the cervix, if closely applied to the head, may not be recognized and a wrong diagnosis of full dilatation made.

2. THE EXPULSIVE TYPE OF CONTRACTION

This is fairly diagnostic, but when the head is deeply engaged, the rectum loaded or the occiput posterior, the woman may have a strong inclination to bear down during the latter part of the first stage.

3. A TRICKLE OF BLOOD

This may come from slight lacerations of the cervix when it is stretched to nearly full dilatation, but with a large head the cervix may sustain slight laceration when the os is only three-quarters dilated. There may, of course, be no bleeding although the os is fully dilated. Later, when the head descends into the vagina, lacerations of the vaginal mucosa may cause slight bleeding.

4. RUPTURE OF THE MEMBRANES

They may rupture before labour begins or at any time up until the birth of the head: a most uncertain sign.

5. ANUS POUTING AND GAPING

When the head has reached the pelvic floor, the anus pouts and then gapes, but this can occur during the last phase of the first stage if the head is engaged deeply in a multipara with a lax pelvic floor. When the anus gapes and fæces are expelled the os is usually fully dilated. If a woman in labour, particularly a multigravid patient, asks urgently for a bed-pan because she thinks her bowels are about to move, the student midwife should first look at the vulva: the head will probably be showing.

6. TENSENESS BETWEEN ANUS AND COCCYX

This is a very useful test that can be made by pressing the middle finger deeply between the anus and coccyx. Before the head is low enough to be felt, there is a tenseness of the tissues that is probably due to the pressure exerted by the descending head on the rectum and pelvic floor. When the head descends further, its hard consistency can be recognized by this method.

7. GAPING OF THE VULVA

This is a more valuable sign in the primigravida, for the vulva of the multigravid woman will gape if she resorts to premature bearing down.

8. THE PRESENTING PART APPEARING

This is usually accepted as being an almost positive sign, and in the majority of instances it is so; but in the case of a footling breech presentation, the os would not necessarily be fully dilated although a foot appeared at the vulva.

On rare occasions, when there is excessive moulding of the head, a large caput may be visible inside the vagina during a contraction, although the head may be above the ischial spines and the os only three-quarters dilated.

9. BULGING OF THE PERINEUM

This is one of the good later signs and usually means that delivery is imminent.

DURATION OF THE SECOND STAGE

The second stage is relatively short, but its length is vitally important, for, if unduly prolonged, it is fraught with danger to mother and child. For that reason it is essential that the midwife should recognize its onset.

A primigravid patient may be half an hour or more in the second stage before the presenting part appears at the vulva so the commencement of the second stage should not be calculated from the time of the appearance of the head.

It has been usual to regard two hours in a primigravida and one hour in a multi-gravida as the limit of normal length as a good working rule for the inexperienced midwife. Many obstetricians consider this to be too long and would advocate making an episiotomy. In some hospitals the application of forceps is considered when the head is seen and not advancing satisfactorily in 30 minutes.

Time may be a convenient means of assessment for the novice, but with greater knowledge and additional experience the midwife develops judgment and will take the strength and frequency of the contractions and the condition of mother and fetus into consideration.

Many multigravid patients have a second stage of 15 minutes or less, but it would probably be safer to allow a primigravida, who always has a strong uterine wall, to go one hour, than to permit a woman who has had more than four children to go much longer than half an hour.

TWO PHASES OF THE SECOND STAGE

It is expedient to divide the second stage into two phases:

1. THE STAGE OF DESCENT. 2. THE PERINEAL PHASE.

1. The stage of descent lasts for only a few moments in the majority of multigravid women, the head descending to the perineum almost immediately after full dilatation of the os. In a primigravida the head is usually showing within 30 minutes, and if it does not appear then, a vaginal examination should be made to determine the cause of delay.

2. The perineal phase.—From the time that the head appears it is generally agreed that it should be born within three-quarters of an hour. Some authorities believe that half an hour is sufficient, but the strength and rate of the contractions and the maternal and fetal conditions have also to be considered.

Advance should take place with each contraction and some obstetricians wish to be summoned if no advance occurs with good contractions during a period of 15 minutes.

OBSERVATION

THE FETAL CONDITION

The fetal heart is listened to assiduously, for the risk of anoxia and intracranial injury is infinitely greater during the second stage. The fetal heart should be auscultated after every contraction.

The point of maximal intensity moves downwards and towards the midline of the mother's abdomen as the second stage advances, and when the head is on the perineum the fetal stethoscope should be placed just above the symphysis pubis.

THE MATERNAL CONDITION

This must be noted, and the pulse taken every 10 minutes, or more often if the second stage is prolonged.

Uterine action requires particular attention; the strength and frequency of the contractions and whether the uterus is relaxed between them must be closely watched

Although tonic contractions rarely occur and Bandl's ring is seldom seen, such possibilities must always be kept in mind, particularly in the multigravid woman, for the possibility of rupture of the uterus is much more likely during the second stage.

For signs of maternal distress see page 411.

ADVANCE OF THE PRESENTING PART

It is imperative that descent should proceed steadily even if slowly, and this can be seen from below. But only because of the delay that may occur before vulval signs of advance are manifest, should it be necessary to resort to vaginal or rectal examination.

GENERAL CARE AND ASSISTANCE

Because of the danger of inhaling vomited fluid under general anæsthesia, nothing more than a mere sip should be taken during the second stage of labour. When inhaling analgesic gas, the mouth becomes very dry: the woman is warm, perspiring and thirsty when pushing, especially in a hot climate.

A soft towel should be available to dry the woman's face if she is perspiring, and she will appreciate having her face and hands sponged with cool water.

THE BLADDER

A full bladder should be recognized and emptied at the end of the first or the beginning of the second stage. If the woman is unable to void at this time, the fetal head is no doubt compressing the urethra or the neck of the bladder. Catheterization will be necessary if the woman has not passed urine for six hours and the bladder is visibly distended.

On no account should a woman be permitted to enter the third stage with a full bladder, for this may interfere with the process of separation and expulsion of the placenta. Because a distended bladder can inhibit good uterine contractions during and after the third stage, postpartum hæmorrhage is likely to ensue, a catastrophe every midwife will endeavour to prevent.

PUNCTURE OF MEMBRANES

The membranes should have ruptured by the end of the first stage, their function is finished and they are only a hindrance during the second stage. The descent of the fetus will be retarded if it is still contained within the intact sac of fluid, the sac being attached to the uterus by the placenta. The membranes should be punctured, when tense during a contraction, by using a pair of artery forceps.

Should the intact membranes appear at the vulva they ought to be punctured at once. The baby's head will then appear and be born with the next contraction or within a few minutes. If the membranes are not punctured there will be more delay and the baby's head may be born covered with amnion (a **caul** or cap) which must be removed from the face immediately to allow the infant to breathe.

The explanation of how the membranes can remain intact and appear at the vulva is that the chorion lying over the os ruptures and the amnion remains intact. The amnion becomes detached from the chorion right up to the umbilical cord and can therefore descend to the vulva.

POSITION OF THE PATIENT

At the commencement of the second stage, positions such as squatting, kneeling or lying on the side with rounded back can be tried if progress is slow, but the woman should not be made to adopt attitudes that are contrary to her wishes.

ADVANTAGES OF THE DORSAL POSITION

1. **The woman can push more effectively.**

She can rest and relax between contractions and will often doze for short periods.

2. **Observation of her abdomen** can be more readily carried out, and at this stage intensive vigilance is necessary.

3. **The fetal heart can be listened to more readily** and more frequently.

(When the woman lies on her side, she becomes annoyed when she has to turn on to her back every few minutes for auscultation of the fetal heart.)

4. **The woman's face is in full view the whole time.**

A close check can be kept on her general condition, and early signs of distress detected.

5. **Cardiac patients and cases of multiple pregnancy** are more comfortable in the dorsal position.

The Exaggerated Lithotomy Position

Should there be delay during the perineal phase of the second stage of labour and no doctor available in some remote area, the exaggerated lithotomy position can be used during each contraction. The flexed legs, with knees well apart, are drawn up until the thighs are in contact with the abdomen, to act as a brace for her abdominal muscles and aid her expulsive efforts. During the manœuvre the woman's back is rounded and the attitude adopted is similar to squatting; the antero-posterior diameter of the outlet is enlarged and this may facilitate advance of the head.

The patient at this stage is usually tired, so she should be helped to raise her legs, and the midwife could augment the woman's efforts by applying judicious pressure on her thighs, the woman grasping her legs, either under or in front of her knees.

This procedure should not be continued too long; if progress is not evident after 15 minutes it should be discontinued.

Fundal pressure is sometimes applied in similar circumstances, but is **not** recommended. It impedes the placental circulation: bruises the uterine and abdominal walls and the bladder may also be subjected to trauma, besides causing intense pain to the woman.

WHEN TO BEAR DOWN

The woman may be told to " push " when the presenting part appears at the vulva; to do so before then incurs the risk of the os not being fully dilated.

The natural urge to " bear down " is experienced by the woman when the presenting part reaches the pelvic floor, so then would seem to be the proper time for her to be encouraged to do so. If she is told to " push " as soon as the os is fully dilated and the head has not descended to the pelvic floor, she fritters away her energy and will have no strength left to push properly when the need arises to overcome the resistance of the perineum.

(*Some authorities do not approve of encouraging the woman to make any expulsive effort and do not find undue prolongation of the second stage because of this.*)

How to " Bear Down "

The woman takes a deep breath, while the uterus is contracting, closes her lips (and glottis) and " bears down " (*a long sustained push is more efficacious than a series of short ones*).

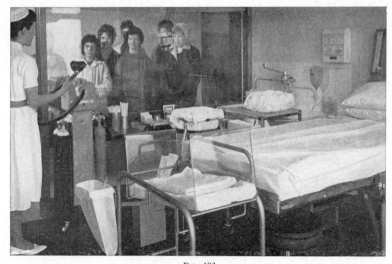

Fig. 193

Single Labour and Delivery Room.

Relaxation class having a preview.

(Photographed at County Maternity Hospital, Bellshill, Lanarkshire.

At the onset of each contraction she should plant her feet firmly on the bed and grasp her thighs under the flexed knees which are wide apart. She should be told not to tighten her pelvic floor muscles while bearing down, but to relax them to allow the baby to escape.

She must not cry out or make any sound, because much of the expulsive force will be wasted. It may be helpful to administer some analgesic gas with each contraction, for when the acuteness of the pain is reduced the woman can often be persuaded to push more vigorously.

Pushing can be maintained after the pain has gone, so long as the uterus is still in a state of contraction, but the woman must not be encouraged or permitted to push between contractions, or she will overstretch the transverse cervical ligaments and predispose to uterine prolapse.

Between contractions her legs should be flat so that she can relax and rest.

Encouragement should be given, and a word of commendation after each effort is opportune, for praise is a good stimulus to continued endeavour. As a rule, women complain less of pain at this stage, no doubt because they are taking an active part in the proceedings and are conscious that progress is being made and that labour is nearly over.

PREPARATION FOR DELIVERY

About one hour prior to the expected time of delivery and before the head is showing the woman ought to be encouraged to empty her bladder If she fails to do so and the bladder is distended catheterization is indicated.

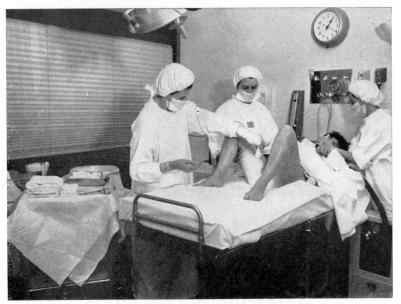

FIG. 194
DELIVERY TAKING PLACE IN ROOM SHOWN IN FIGURE 193.
Note blind drawn in window to corridor. Inner pack wrapping is now the trolley cover.
(*County Maternity Hospital, Bellshill, Lanarkshire.*)

NORMAL DELIVERY PACK

LINEN: DRESSINGS

1 Gown. 1 Draping sheet.
1 Waterproof paper sheet 100 × 100 cm. (40 × 40 inches).
Cord ligatures. 1 Baby wrap.
Wool swabs. 2 Perineal pads.

INSTRUMENTS

1 Mucus extractor.
2 17·8 cm. (Seven-inch) Spencer Wells forceps.
1 Disposable scissors.
1 Triangular placenta basin.

PACKED SEPARATELY

Caps and masks.
Gloves and hand towel.
Catheter and disposable dish.
Mucus extractors.
Episiotomy scissors.

BOWL PACK

2 Hand lotion polypropylene bowls. One used before, one after delivery.
2 Swabbing lotion polypropylene bowls. One used before, one after delivery.
1 Litre measuring jug.

Tray with syringes and drugs at hand.

The **pubic region**, thighs and buttocks should be washed with soap and water, using a sterile perineal pad. A clean short gown and white stockings are put on.

The baby's cot and cellular cotton blanket must be warm.

The delivery pack, basins and floor bucket are placed in position.

The hypodermic tray is in readiness for immediate use.

WHEN TO "SCRUB UP"

It is not possible to state the exact time at which the midwife should start scrubbing her hands in readiness for delivery: it depends on the rate of advance and whether the woman is a multipara or primipara.

In the multiparous woman who is progressing rapidly, towards the end of the first stage would be appropriate.

In the primigravida, a reasonable time would be when a diameter of about 5 cm (2 inches) of head is showing at the vulva during contractions. Experience is the best

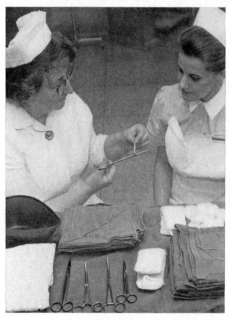

FIG. 195

LABOUR WARD SUPERINTENDENT giving non-sterile demonstration on normal delivery: pre-packed tray: showing student midwife rubber band for cord ligation.

LINEN AND DRESSINGS

1 gown. 2 draping sheets.
2 dressing towels.
10 wool swabs.
1 baby wrap.

INSTRUMENTS

2 Mayo forceps.
1 Mayo scissors (15 cm.).
1 Mayo scissors. (20 cm)
1 Spencer Wells forceps to apply cord rubber band.
1 polypropylene receiver for placenta.
1 hand lotion and
1 swabbing bowl.

LOWER SHELF

Pre-packed gloves and hand towel, catheter, mucus extractors, cord ligatures, syringes, needles, baby identification bands, jug to measure blood loss.

DRUG TRAY

Syntometrine, ergometrine, Syntocinon, neonatal nalorphine (Lethidrone), levallorphan (Lorfan), lignocaine 1 per cent.

REQUIREMENTS FOR RESUSCITATION OF INFANT

Laryngoscope, mechanical suction, endotracheal tubes, ampoules of sodium bicarbonate.

(Simpson Memorial Maternity Pavilion, Edinburgh.)

teacher. The midwife should not be scrubbed up too soon, or she is liable to become contaminated and the woman may disarrange the sterile drapes.

Method

The midwife, with clean hands, puts on a plastic apron, clean cap and mask; prepares hand and swabbing lotions; opens packs; places the patient in the correct position for swabbing and delivery.

Hands and arms are scrubbed with a soft brush in running water for five minutes.

It is a good plan to swab the vulva with the scrubbed hands before wearing gloves in order to avoid contaminating them. Sterile forceps can be used for this purpose and also to apply antiseptic cream.

The only areas which should be considered sterile are: The equipment on the trolley; swabbing lotion; the inner surface of the vulva and the baby's head. Drapes and gown soon become contaminated when in contact with the patient and the bed, and should be touched with the gloved hands as little as possible.

Methods of Delivering the Baby

The technique used in delivering the baby varies in different countries and different hospitals, but the basic principles are the same; in all cases an endeavour is made to deliver an uninjured child with minimal trauma to the mother. Where doctors and trained midwives are in attendance and when analgesics and anæsthetics are administered the dorsal or left lateral position is employed but a squatting attitude is the one adopted by primitive tribes.

DELIVERY IN THE DORSAL POSITION

The woman lies on her back with knees flexed and widely separated. The midwife stands on the right side of the bed, facing towards the woman's feet. She places the palm of her left hand on the advancing head, with fingers pointing to the sinciput. Some midwives alter their grip as in the left lateral position (Fig. 198,E), so that the parietal eminences are grasped, to assist in completing extension of the head.

Advantages of the Dorsal Position

1. **It is less tiring for the woman than the left lateral position** in which the right leg has to be held up by an assistant or the patient herself.

2. **When a midwife is delivering a woman alone, it is easier for both.**

3. **There is less opportunity or temptation to interfere prematurely** with the natural process of extension of the head, and so perineal trauma is minimized.

4. **One particular advantage in using the dorsal position is that the woman does not have to be turned on her side previous to crowning, nor on to her back again for the conduct of the third stage.**

DELIVERY IN THE LEFT LATERAL POSITION (No. 1)

The woman lies on her left side, buttocks at the edge of the bed and legs slightly flexed.

When the head is almost ready for crowning **the midwife stands behind the woman's buttocks, facing her feet,** and an assistant on the right or left side of the bed raises the right leg sufficiently to take its weight off the midwife's hand.

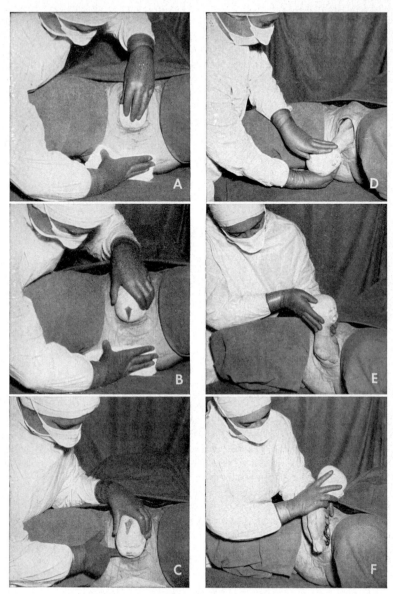

FIG. 196
Demonstrating delivery in the dorsal position.
(*Simpson Memorial Maternity Pavilion, Edinburgh.*

By passing her left arm over the patient's abdomen the midwife brings her hand between the thighs and down to the vulva where the fingers rest lightly on the baby's head, poised in readiness to retard any sudden expulsive movement.

LEFT LATERAL POSITION (No. 2)

The woman lies on her left side, as for position number 1. **The midwife sits or stands facing the vulva,** and when the baby's head is almost ready for crowning she places her right hand on it with the fingertips on the occiput. The palm rather than the thumb should be used, if necessary, to restrain any sudden advance (Fig. 198, C).

After crowning has taken place the position of the right hand is changed and the fingers are placed on the head parallel with the sagittal suture, finger tips pointing towards the sinciput.

Another grip can be used after the sinciput is born, and is useful to aid extension. The finger tips are moved on to the right parietal bone, with the thumb on the left,

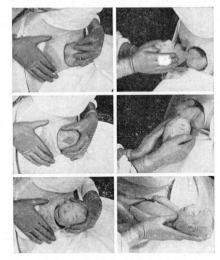

Fig. 197

Demonstrating delivery in left lateral position (No. 1).

(*Simpson Memorial Maternity Pavilion, Edinburgh*)

and the parietal eminences are grasped so that good control of the head is obtained.

Advantages of the Left Lateral Position

1. **More assistance can be given in aiding extension** of the head in cases where the woman is anæsthetized.

2. It is claimed by some that **fewer perineal lacerations occur.**

3. **When difficulty is encountered with the shoulders of a large baby,** the necessary manipulation is more easily carried out.

DELIVERY OF THE HEAD

The majority of midwives agree that not until the occipital prominence is free (*the head crowned*) should active extension be permitted to take place.

When the stage of crowning approaches, the woman is asked to stop pushing; she continues to inhale whatever analgesic gas is being administered.

During and after crowning the fingers are spread equally over the vertex, (to avoid depressing one of the skull bones,) with their tips pointing towards the bregma, in order to resist any sudden expulsive effort.

The sinciput is allowed to glide slowly over the perineum at the end of a contraction and during this time the woman is inhaling analgesic gas with deliberate breaths to avoid pushing. A certain amount of restraint may have to be applied to the baby's head during the height of this contraction, and such pressure should be evenly distributed to avoid intracranial injury.

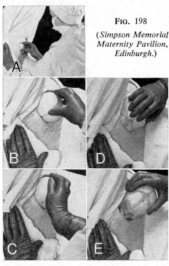

FIG. 198

(*Simpson Memorial Maternity Pavilion, Edinburgh.*)

A, Demonstrating delivery of head in left lateral position (No. 2).

B, Hand poised lightly maintaining flexion.

C, Restraining extension of head until end of the contraction.

D, Allowing head to extend slowly.

E, Using " horse shoe " grip to extend head.

Whether forward pressure applied with a pad on the area between the coccyx and anus is necessary to aid extension appears to be a controversial point, but the modern tendency is to allow the head to extend naturally.

Some aid extension of the head. A pad held in the palm of the right hand is placed over the anus and when crowning has taken place the midwife exerts steady forward pressure with the heel of her right hand on the area between anus and coccyx, while with her left hand she retards any sudden expulsive movement.

" Stripping " the perineum.—A few midwives draw the perineum down over the baby's face after the most prominent part of the sinciput has escaped. Such a manœuvre is probably traditional rather than necessary and if the thumb and middle fingers are placed on the outer lateral borders of the perineum and brought slightly towards the midline, tension on the perineum is diminished while it is being wiped down over the face.

The chin is freed, if necessary, by slipping the index finger under the side of the jaw and sweeping it below the chin and out at the other side.

ATTENTION TO THE CORD AROUND THE NECK

In about 40 per cent of cases the umbilical cord is looped round the baby's neck usually once but sometimes two or three times. Unwinding these loops seldom cause difficulty, but the novice tends to be over-anxious and is inclined to premature clamping and cutting of the cord, when it is not necessary.

Cord manipulation may induce spasm of the umbilical vessels and cause anoxia but the baby usually recovers quickly from the short period of oxygen deprivation at this stage of labour.

In a case at the Simpson Maternity Pavilion a 106·7 cm. (42-inch) cord, looped five times around the neck, was slipped over the head without clamping.

The fingers of the clean hand (*not the hand that was used to hold the pad over the anus*) should be inserted into the vagina to feel if the umbilical cord is round the baby's neck. The finger tips should be placed down the baby's back to shoulder level and drawn up towards the neck, where they will find the coil of cord which should be gently taken over the baby's head.

Strong traction must not be used in case a thin cord should break, but if the cord will not come over the head two Mayo forceps should be applied and the cord cut between them. *This should never be done without due cause*, as the baby's oxygen supply is now cut off, and if there is delay in the delivery of the shoulders, or if the baby is anoxic, his chances of survival are reduced.

Should the shoulders appear before there is time to deal with the loop of cord, an attempt should be made to slip it over the anterior shoulder and to deliver the baby through the loop.

ATTENTION TO NOSE AND MOUTH

While waiting for the shoulders to rotate internally, an opportunity is provided to wipe any mucus from the mouth and nostrils with a gauze swab.

DELIVERY OF THE SHOULDERS AND BODY

In a natural birth the shoulders are born during the contraction following the birth of the head. This contraction causes the anterior shoulder to rotate forwards so that the shoulders are in the antero-posterior diameter of the outlet. This will be evident by seeing **external rotation of the head.**

The tendency to hurry this phase of the delivery should be resisted. The baby's face will certainly look reddish blue, but such congestion is a necessary stimulus to respiration. Many experienced midwives practise slow delivery of the body and do not drag the baby out.

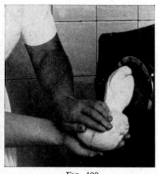

FIG. 199

DELIVERY OF THE SHOULDERS.

Labour ward sister demonstrating on model how downward traction is applied after shoulders have been rotated into the antero-posterior diameter of the outlet.

(*Aberdeen Maternity Hospital.*)

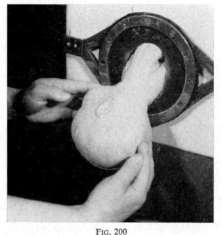

FIG. 200

Some prefer to grasp the head by the mentum and occiput.

If, however, the blue colour becomes dark the uterus ought to be stimulated to contract by massaging it, fundal pressure applied, or the woman asked to push to expel the baby.

Syntometrine, 1 ml., is given when the anterior shoulder appears, remembering the danger should there be a second fetus in utero. If the baby is large this is the ideal time to give Syntometrine.

To facilitate expulsion of the anterior shoulder the head may be gently depressed towards the anus but no attempt made to get the anterior arm out. If the anterior arm comes of its own accord it is not likely to be harmed, but if it is deliberately brought down under the pubic arch the risk of fracturing the humerus is intensified.

The important point is that **traction exerted should be minimal** and ought not to make the neck twist or bend sideways because of the risk of injury to the brachial plexus, causing paralysis of the baby's upper arm. (Erb's paralysis.)

When the anterior shoulder is free, the head is guided in an upward direction towards the mother's abdomen so that the posterior shoulder can escape over the perineum. This should take place slowly and smoothly; the contraction of the uterus being sufficient to accomplish the expulsion of the body.

As soon as the baby is born the midwife looks at the clock, which should be at the correct time, so that the exact moment of birth can be recorded on the birth certificate.

Some prefer to give Syntometrine, 1 ml., at this stage.

DELAY WITH THE SHOULDERS

The conscious woman can be asked to bear down or an assistant, if present, may apply fundal pressure.

Delay at this stage is usually due to incomplete internal rotation of the shoulders, so with a finger hooked into the anterior axilla forward rotation followed by downward traction is usually successful but care must be exercised (see shoulder dystocia, p. 615).

ATTENTION TO THE EYES

Each eyelid should be wiped with separate swabs of dry, sterilized cotton wool to remove secretions containing organisms from the birth-canal. *Some authorities do not approve of wiping the eyelids.*

The midwife's hands should be clean when dealing with the eyes, and dipping them into weak antiseptic solution is not an efficient method of cleansing them.

Wool swabs if used should be the size of a golf ball, so that antiseptic lotion and organisms from badly fitting or contaminated gloves will not come in contact with the baby's eyes.

PERINEAL LACERATIONS

CAUSES: SIGNS: PREVENTION

Perineal lacerations cannot always be avoided, but the extent of the damage can often be minimized by skilful manipulation.

The principles of management are:

1. That the smallest possible diameters of head and shoulders should be permitted to emerge and distend the vulval orifice.

2. That the actual birth of the head should take place slowly and without expulsive force.

The various methods of delivery have been devised with the intention of giving maximal control during the expulsion of the infant. The midwife ought to know which measurements of the skull are involved in the various presentations and whether, by assisting flexion or extension of the baby's head, the smallest possible diameters can be made to distend the vulval orifice. Certain conditions other than faulty management by the midwife predispose to perineal lacerations and they are usually due to disproportion between the fetal head and the outlet of the birth canal.

CAUSES OF A THIRD DEGREE TEAR

A large baby; vertex face to pubes; face presentation; the aftercoming head in a breech presentation.

A rigid perineum, and particularly when scar tissue from a previous laceration or episiotomy is present.

The android type of pelvis which causes the head to be forced backwards on to the perineum.

SIGNS THAT THE PERINEUM IS LIABLE TO TEAR

1. **A perineum that resists the pressure** of the descending head and is not stretching

2. **A long perineum,** particularly if it lacks elasticity or is œdematous.

3. **Trickling of blood** from the vagina when the head is on the perineum is usually due to laceration of the vaginal mucosa on the inner surface of the perineum, which tears as a rule before the perineal skin.

4. **When the perineum has a bluish appearance** in the midline, which later becomes white, shiny and transparent.

5. **If the fourchette begins to tear before the head is crowned,** an extensive laceration can be anticipated.

On rare occasions a perineal laceration may start in the centre of the perineum, the so-called " button-hole " or central tear.

Prevention

Undue prolongation of the perineal phase of the second stage is now condemned as a cause of fetal anoxia and intracranial injury, as well as damaging the pelvic floor.

Obstetricians consider it is better that an episiotomy should be made and subsequently repaired in an efficient manner, than to have an overstretched, although intact, perineum which is too lax to provide adequate support to the pelvic organs.

MEANS OF LESSENING THE RISK OF PERINEAL LACERATION

1. **Obtaining the woman's co operation.**—If the woman is conscious during delivery, her co-operation is necessary. She should have been told, prior to, or at the beginning of labour what she is expected to do. When distracted with pain or stupefied by analgesic drugs, the woman is incapable of comprehending instruction.

The art of relaxation should have been practised and the use of the face mask rehearsed, for the calm relaxed woman is more likely to be co-operative. The woman who is frightened is liable to become hysterical and unmanageable.

The only satisfactory method of inhibiting the desire to push, which is involuntary and overwhelmingly strong when the head is distending the perineum, is for the woman to take deliberate breaths through her mouth without accentuating expiration.

It is imperative that, from the time of crowning, the woman should only push when instructed to do so. Uterine contraction alone is sufficient at this stage, and while the head is actually being born the woman must desist from any expulsive effort.

2. **Having control of the advancing head.**—The midwife must scrub up in time, so that she is ready to retard any sudden advance of the head. The woman may push, cough or move *suddenly*, and the midwife must always anticipate such a possibility by having her finger tips on or near the head, poised ready to restrain it.

The midwife should watch the head during each contraction, and when crowning has taken place, absolute concentration is needed; her eyes and hands must not leave the baby's head for one instant.

3. **Getting small diameters to distend the vaginal orifice.**—By maintaining flexion and controlling too rapid extension of the head in vertex presentations.

4. **Preventing " active " extension before crowning.**—The sinciput should not be permitted to glide over the perineum, until the occipital prominence, and, if possible, the parietal eminences have been born.

5. Keeping the hands off the perineum.—Supporting, or what is commonly called " guarding," the perineum will not prevent lacerations. Any pressure applied by the fingers thins the perineum still further or causes bruising which favours tearing. The perineum should not be puckered in an attempt to prevent laceration, nor should descent of the head be retarded by pressure applied over the perineum.

Placing the palm of the hand posterior to the anus, with finger and thumb on the lateral boundaries of the perineum, and bringing the connective tissue forwards will provide greater laxity of the perineum.

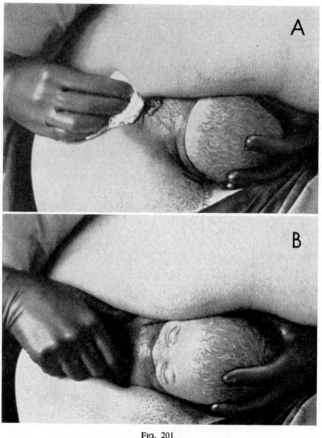

FIG. 201

The head is allowed to extend slowly to prevent perineal laceration.

(*Simpson Memorial Maternity Pavilion, Edinburgh.*)

6. Giving the perineum time to stretch.—The head should not be allowed to advance too quickly. The woman in such a case should stop pushing and breathe steadily, concentrating more on inspiration than expiration.

7. Delivering the head at the end of or between contractions.—If the head is born during a uterine contraction, too much force is exerted by the primary and probably by the secondary powers. The perineum is more tense then and will rupture more readily.

When the height of the contraction has passed or, alternatively, when the contraction has ceased, the head should be permitted to escape. If the patient is under a general anæsthetic it may be necessary to assist the delivery of the head by applying pressure behind the anus as described under " delivery of the head " (p. 304).

8. **Allowing the woman to " breathe the head out."**—This midwife's phrase lucidly explains a manœuvre whereby the actual extension of the head takes place with a slow gliding movement. During this time the woman breathes in a deliberate way to avoid pushing while the sinciput and face emerge from under the perineum.

9. **Avoiding too wide separation of the legs.**—If an assistant is supporting the woman's right leg, while she is in the left lateral position, it should not be lifted up too high.

10. **Taking care in delivering shoulders and body.**—If the shoulders are dragged or pushed out before they have rotated internally, they will rotate while passing through the vulva and the strain on the perineum is liable to result in a perineal tear. Not all lacerations of the perineum occur during the birth of the head. Very often a slight nick is extended into a gash during the birth of the shoulders.

The occurrence of restitution is not an indication to deliver the shoulders. External rotation of the head must take place as this indicates that the shoulders have rotated into the antero-posterior diameter.

By permitting the anterior shoulder to escape first a smaller diameter emerges, and when the baby is carried upwards over the mother's abdomen its weight is taken off the perineum. As the baby is being born its arms should be grasped alongside the body. If the midwife grasps the body under the arms their outward thrust puts additional strain on the perineum.

(For repair of perineal lacerations see page 621.)

PRECIPITATE LABOUR

Precipitate labour is one in which the fetus is expelled after three or four painful uterine contractions. The condition is rare, and the term should not be applied when early signs of labour have been overlooked. It is probable that the woman has had a **painless first stage** and that the cervix and vagina are unusually soft and dilatable.

The risks are greatest when the birth occurs in some inconvenient place, such as the " toilet " or the street. The baby may suffer from **intracranial injury** or cephal-hæmatoma, due to rapid expulsion; he might fall to the ground and be injured; the cord may rupture, but bleeding does not occur to the same extent as when the cord has been cut.

The mother may sustain a perineal laceration; inversion of the uterus, due to cord traction, is not likely to occur, because the uterus will be contracting strongly.

When a woman has had one precipitate labour, she should be admitted to hospital prior to her next confinement to avoid such consequences as those mentioned above.

Immediate Care of the Baby
CLEARING THE AIR PASSAGES

This is an urgent duty that must be performed without delay, for, if the baby inhales into its bronchi the mucus and liquor amnii which may be present in the pharynx, atelectasis or pneumonia may ensue.

If the baby cries immediately there should be no need to use any means of clearing the airway, but the trachea of the asphyxiated baby is often blocked with thick mucus which may be tinged with blood from the vagina, or meconium that has been passed by the distressed fetus. It is imperative that this material be removed without delay.

19

Some hold the baby upside down, with the head slightly extended for a few seconds before laying him on the bed, to allow any fluid in the trachea to drain out. This should be done with due care, and, to avoid letting the baby slip, the forefinger of the hand grasping the ankles should be placed between them.

The infant cannot breathe if the airway is plugged with mucus, and if inhaled into the lungs its tenacious consistency prevents the alveoli from becoming inflated and its irritant propensity is likely to cause pneumonia. Thick mucus will not drain out when the infant is held upside down.

THE USE OF SUCTION

Various mechanical devices for applying suction are used in hospital, *e.g.* via the water tap, a cylinder of oxygen, or electric apparatus, but all must be used with gentleness and caution. A rubber mucus extractor with a glass trap can be employed. Disposable extractors are on the market.

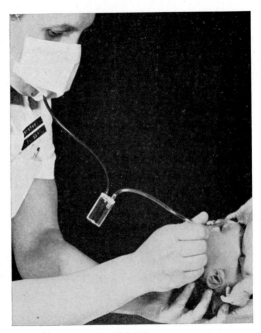

Fig. 202
USING DISPOSABLE MUCUS EXTRACTOR.
(*Aberdeen Maternity Hospital.*)

The tubing must be fine with a lumen of 2 or 3 mm. and the end bevelled like a rectal tube. In an emergency, a rubber catheter, No. 10 (Eng. gauge), a gauze swab, or the finger can be used to remove mucus.

In using a mucus extractor it should be directed over the dorsum of the tongue into the pharynx, not more than 5·1 cm. (2 inches) of tubing being inside the baby's lower gum.

A word of warning is necessary in regard to the excessive use of suction, for, if continued after the airway is clear, the baby is deprived of oxygen. Inexperienced midwives can produce fetal shock by this means.

The mucus extractor is a life-saving device when used judiciously.

APGAR SCORING

This is a means of standardizing the method of evaluating and recording the condition of the baby, in numerical terms at one minute after birth and if necessary at 5 minutes.

Signs	SCORE		
	0	1	2
Colour	blue-pale	body pink, limbs blue	completely pink
Respiratory effort	absent	slow, irregular weak cry	strong cry
Heart rate	absent	slow, less than 100	over 100
Muscle tone	limp	some flexion of limbs	active movement
Reflex response to flicking foot	absent	facial grimace	cry

Five vital signs are each given a score of 0, 1 or 2 points, i.e. colour, respiratory effort, heart rate, muscle tone, reflex response.

One minute score

Severe 0—2   moderate 3—4   mild 5—7   no asphyxia 8—10

The pædiatrician is notified if the score is 3 or under at 1 minute.

Five minute score

The score at 5 minutes gives a more accurate prediction regarding survival: a low score at 5 minutes being more serious than a low score at one minute.

The pædiatrician is notified if the score is 6 or under at 5 minutes.

Gastric Suction

In some hospitals mucus is extracted from every baby's stomach. This procedure is believed to reduce the incidence of vomiting and mucus gastritis. When the amount of gastric contents is excessive (over 10 ml.) the possibility of high intestinal obstruction is considered.

EXAMINATION OF THE BABY

Particular attention is paid to the baby's respirations and colour: a vigorous cry usually denotes satisfactory respiratory effort.

The presence of pallor or cyanosis is noted, the baby treated if necessary and closely observed for improvement. Muscle tone should be good.

Serious illness or gross malformation are readily detected (*medical aid is summoned*); a detailed examination is carried out later, usually prior to bathing.

More than a cursory glance at the genital organs is needed before recording the sex of the infant.   When doubt exists expert investigations are made.

THE NEED FOR WARMTH

While the baby is being attended to, he must not be allowed to become chilled. The thermal centre does not function well at birth, and the baby loses much heat by evaporation from his wet skin (see neonatal hypothermia, p. 560).

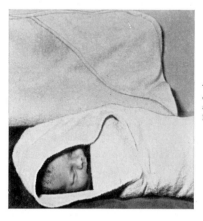

FIG. 203
Baby wrap and head cover to prevent hypothermia.
This turkish towelling 91·4 cm. (1 yd.) square is designed to envelop the body and head when applied cornerwise. Note the additional triangular piece stitched on one corner is flat to facilitate laundering.
(*Aberdeen Maternity Hospital.*)

The room in which the baby is born should be 21·1° C. (70° F.); the baby should be dried and received into a warm sterile towel and two warm cellular cotton blankets, one of which is wrapped over his head.   The baby can lose a lot of heat from his exposed wet head which is one quarter of the area of the baby.

DANGER OF BURNING

Hot-water bottles are potentially dangerous in a busy unit, where inexperienced staff may use water that is too hot or neglect to apply adequate covering to the bottles.

The newborn baby's skin is extremely sensitive and will blister very readily.   If as is the practice in some hospitals, the baby is wrapped in a 91·4 cm. (36-inch) cotton cellular blanket lined with a sterile towel it can wriggle until it comes in contact with the hot-water bottle.   Blankets should be adequate in size to envelop the baby properly and so avoid exposure due to limb movements.   **Electric blankets are not without risk.**

MEANS OF IDENTIFICATION

Before cutting the cord, whatever means of identification is used should be applied to the infant.   The system of checking the name and verifying the sex should be fool-proof.   It entails grave responsibility, and the danger of mixing babies in hospital must constantly be kept in mind.

The different methods are:—

1. **Wrist name tape.** (*These should be checked daily and a record kept of this.*)

2. **A string of lettered china beads** that are clamped with a lead seal around the neck or wrist before the cord is cut.

3. **Footprints are a positive means of identification** if they are clear enough to make the fine ridge detail on the baby's skin legible. A high standard of legibility is not readily attained by finger-print experts much less the nursing staff in a busy labour ward.

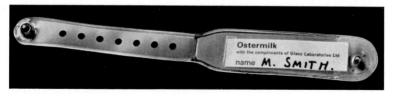

Fig. 204

IDENTIFICATION BRACELET.

(*Courtesy of Glaxo Laboratories Ltd.*)

Footprints must always be read by a finger-print expert so they are not as useful as beads and name-tapes for the daily routine identification of babies in maternity hospitals.

ATTENTION TO THE UMBILICAL CORD

There is a difference of opinion as to whether to tie the cord immediately or to wait for pulsation in the cord vessels to cease. It has been stated that the infant obtains 40 to 60 ml. of extra blood from the placenta if the cord is not tied until pulsations cease. Others believe that the baby obtains the full complement of placental blood within 20 seconds of birth.

By tying the cord at once, excessive exposure and chilling of the wet infant is avoided.

TYING AND CUTTING THE CORD

Plastic clamps, rubber bands, linen or tape ligatures are applied to the umbilical cord to act as a hæmostat to the umbilical blood vessels.

If the mother is Rh isoimmunized or diabetic or if the baby weighs less than 2,000 G. umbilical catheterization may be necessary. In such cases the cord should be ligated not closer than 4 cm. from the umbilicus.

A ligature that is too fine, even although strong, might sever the cord, so traction on the ligature should be exerted slowly, without jerking, and the knot should be of the reef or other variety that will not slip.

The first ligature may be placed about 2·5 cm. (one inch) from the umbilicus. Another ligature is applied 5·1 cm. (2 inches) on the outer side of the first one, but some midwives place it near the vulva as a means of detecting lengthening of the cord during the third stage. This other ligature is only necessary as a precautionary measure in case the placenta *in utero* is being shared by another baby, a monozygotic twin.

The scissors used to cut the cord should be blunt-pointed and sterile, and those previously used for episiotomy are no longer sterile. While cutting the cord it should be placed in the palm of the hand and the points of the scissors directed into the partly closed fist to avoid injuring the kicking infant. *Many now examine the cut end of cord; the absence of one artery occurs in 1-200 babies and suggests the presence of congenital abnormalities.*

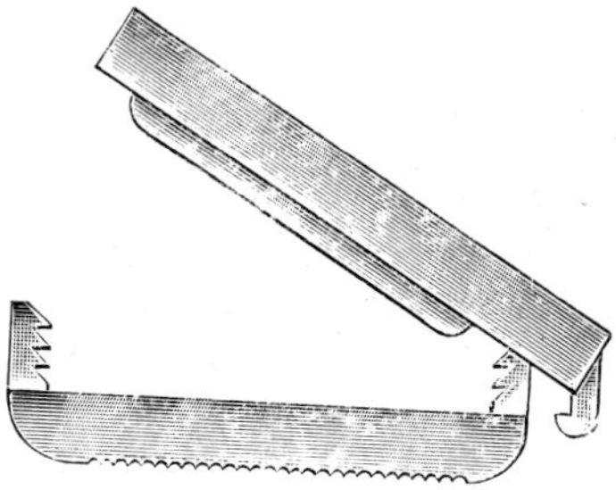

Nobecutane varnish or Octaflex may be applied to the cut end of the cord; the umbilicus is dredged with Ster Zac powder (hexachlorophane).

When the baby goes to the ward a second ligature is applied, after bathing, about 2·5 cm. (1 inch) from the umbilicus.

FIG. 205

Stericlam disposable cord clamp made in polyamide.

(*Obtainable from Down Bros. and Mayer & Phelps Ltd.*)

PLASTIC CLAMPS

Disposable plastic cord clamps are applied about one centimetre from the umbilical skin and closed by finger pressure. The cord is cut 1 cm. beyond the clamp to prevent it from slipping off the cut end of the cord. The clamp should be removed after 48 hours, but some prefer to leave it until the cord separates. Plastic clamps are effective but expensive.

RUBBER BANDS—COMPRESSION LATEX TUBING

(a) **Rubber bands,** 3·5 cm. long by 2 mm. wide, are wound four times around an average size cord: **they are considered to be more efficient than tape** which may allow leakage: elastic bands may cut through a thick cord.

(b) **Pieces of compression tubing** (*not ordinary rubber tubing*) 4 mm. wide are most effective. Umbilical cord-tape 15·2 cm. (6 inches) long is threaded through the lumen of the tubing and knotted.

Method.—Through the lumen of the tube a pair of sterile 17·8 cm. (7 inch) Spencer Wells forceps is passed to just beyond the joint. With these forceps the cord is clamped 5·1 cm. (two inches) from the umbilicus; another pair of forceps is applied 2·5 cm. (one inch) from the first pair on the placental side of the cord. The cord is cut between the two pairs of forceps. The umbilical cord tape is used to draw the latex tubing off the Spencer Wells forceps, which is clamping the cord, on to the cord stump; the tubing is positioned 2·5 cm. (one inch) from the skin edge. Forceps and tape are then removed. The tubing is more easily applied when wet.

These bands provide continued pressure as the cord shrinks.

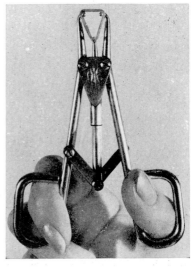

FIG. 206

INSTRUMENT TO APPLY CORD BAND TUBING.

(*Courtesy of National Woman's Hospital, Auckland New Zealand.*)

Octoflex or Nubecutane is applied to the cut end of the cord and Ster Zac powder applied to the umbilical area.

The midwife must look repeatedly at the cord during the first six hours to make sure there is no bleeding. **Fatal hæmorrhage** can occur, for the loss of 30 ml. of blood to the newborn is equivalent to the loss of 600 ml. to an adult. Artery forceps should be sterilized pending the doctor's arrival and applied if medical aid is not available.

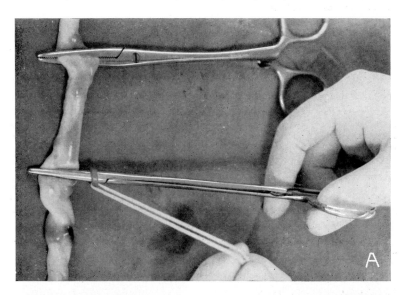

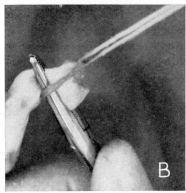 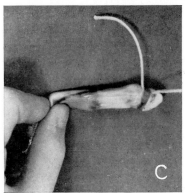

FIG. 207

APPLICATION OF LATEX COMPRESSION TUBING.

A, Spencer Wells forceps, with latex tubing, applied 5·1 cm from umbilicus.
B, After cutting umbilical cord between the two Spencer Wells forceps, the tape is used to pull the latex band on to the stump of cord.
C, Tape being withdrawn.

N.B.—This demonstration was not carried out on a baby.

(*County Maternity Hospital, Bellshill, Lanarkshire.*)

CARE OF THE EYES

No longer is the routine instillation of silver nitrate or argyrol in the eyes of the newborn advocated. It is believed that silver nitrate, 1 per cent, produces a mild chemical burn which lowers the resistance of the conjunctiva to organisms and may predispose to conjunctivitis neonatorum.

REST AFTER THE TRAUMA OF BIRTH

The baby should be placed in a warmed cot and allowed to recover from the strenuous experience of birth. Routine lowering of babies' heads is not now advocated.

The baby's colour should be noted.

Any mucus ought to be removed from the nose and mouth.

There should be no routine time, such as one hour after birth, for giving the first bath: the correct time is when the baby is pink, warm and vigorous. Bathing is not an essential procedure. A clear airway and warmth are the baby's immediate needs; bathing and food are secondary during the first 24 hours of life.

TELEPHONE INQUIRIES

Student midwives should be meticulously careful when receiving inquiries and giving information over the telephone regarding the birth of a baby, for much dissatisfaction is caused to relatives when erroneous statements are made.

The name should be clearly identified and repeated, for more than one patient may have the same surname. The use of the words " boy " and " girl " are less likely to be confused than " male " and " female ".

The Sister will always confirm name and sex from the chart, and will answer the call herself if the baby is stillborn.

MOTHER AND BABY

The question as to when a mother should be shown her baby, and given it to cuddle, is a moot one. Some authorities think the mother should see her infant immediately it is born, and before the umbilical cord is severed, believing that the emotional stimulus will cause the uterus to contract strongly.

The wishes of the mother should be ascertained and respected. In hospital, women are usually shown their babies in the labour ward before they are taken to the nursery. After the baby is dressed and the mother's toilet completed, would seem to be an appropriate time for her to have her baby to cuddle.

Midwives should remember that they are accustomed to the appearance of newborn babies, but an inexperienced mother seeing her own infant for the first time, unwashed, may experience a feeling of disappointment that she may later regret ever having entertained towards her child. The first glimpse of her baby is a momentous occasion and should be treated with due regard to its importance. The main thing is that the mother's feelings are considered and everything done to foster her appreciation of the beauty and sanctity of motherhood.

MANAGEMENT OF SECOND STAGE OF LABOUR

ORAL QUESTIONS

Name 6 probable signs of the second stage. How do you know when the cervix is fully dilated ? How often do you auscultate the fetal heart during the second stage ? Why is the fetus in greater danger during the second stage ?

How would you deal with the following: (*a*) membranes at the vulva intact; (*b*) cord around the baby's neck; (*c*) delay with the shoulders; (*d*) Apgar score of 6 at 5 minutes; (*e*) bleeding from the umbilical cord.

Write not more than 10 lines on: (*a*) the bladder during the second stage; (*b*) teaching the mother how to bear down; (*c*) avoiding perineal laceration.

What assistance can the midwife give to a woman during the second stage of labour ? **State the length of time** you would consider as safe for the second stage. What are your duties when it is unduly prolonged ?

C.M.B.(Scot.) paper.—How may perineal laceration during delivery be avoided ? What are its dangers and possible complications ?

C.M.B.(Scot.) paper.—What maternal structures may be damaged during labour and how is this damage caused ? What are the signs and symptoms of this damage afterwards ?

C.M.B.(Scot.) paper.—What observations should be made during the second stage of labour ? How do they affect the management of labour ?

C.M.B.(Eng.) paper.—What do you understand by delay in the second stage of labour ? What are the possible causes and how may the condition be relieved ?

C.M.B.(N. Ireland) paper.—Describe in detail your treatment of the umbilical cord at birth and subsequently. What possible complications may arise and how would you avoid them ?

C.M.B.(Eng.) paper.—What indications would lead you to send for a doctor during the second stage of labour ?

C.M.B.(Scot.) paper.—How would you know that a patient was established in labour? Describe the management of a normal second stage.

C.M.B.(N. Ireland) paper, 1969.—What would make you suspect that a patient was in the second stage of labour? How could you satisfy yourself that the second stage was progressing normally? What would you regard as undue delay?

C.M.B.(Scot.) paper, 1969.—Discuss the causes of delay in the second stage of labour. Enumerate the procedures which may be adopted to effect delivery.

C.M.B.(Eng.) paper, 1969.—Outline your management of the second stage of labour in a primigravida. What are the causes of delay in this stage of labour?

19

The Third Stage of Labour

PHYSIOLOGICAL CHANGES: MANAGEMENT

THE third stage is that of the separation and expulsion of the placenta, which lasts from the birth of the baby until the placenta is expelled. **The usual length is 5 to 15 minutes,** but any period up to one hour may be considered normal.

The administration of oxytocic drugs with the anterior shoulder or birth of the head shortens the third stage and some authorities are of the opinion that 30 *minutes should now be considered the limit of normal.*

MECHANISM OF PLACENTAL SEPARATION

Separation of the placenta is brought about by the contraction and retraction of the uterine muscle, which thicken the wall and reduce the capacity of the upper uterine segment so that the area of the placental site is diminished.

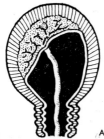 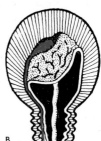

A Fig. 208 B

DIAGRAMMATIC REPRESENTATION OF PLACENTAL SEPARATION.
A, Uterine wall partly contracted but not sufficient to cause separation of placenta.
B, Further contractions and retraction thicken uterine wall, reduce the size of the area of the placental site, and cause the placenta to become detached.
Note.—The thin lower uterine segment has collapsed like a concertina following the birth of the baby.

The placenta has no power of contraction, but it does become thicker and more compact when its cotyledons are crowded more closely together. This can be proved when handling the placenta; it can be spread out on the outstretched hands, and the cotyledons can be bunched together in the cupped hands.

Before the end of the second stage the area of the placental site is somewhat diminished, and it is surmised that it must be reduced by half before placental separation begins. There is a marked reduction in the size of the placental site **during the contraction that expels the baby's body;** after the birth of the baby further contractions and retraction of the uterine muscle continue the process of separation: the more powerful the contractions the sooner will the placenta be detached, probably within five minutes.

318

Separation usually begins in the centre of the placenta, but may begin at the lower edge, and at the level of the deep spongy layer of the decidua, but if the ovum has embedded too deeply separation will not readily take place. The process has been likened to the detachment of postage stamps at the perforations between them. At the area of separation the blood sinuses are torn across, causing 30 to 60 ml. of blood to collect between the maternal surface of the placenta and the decidua basalis—**the retroplacental clot or hæmatoma.**

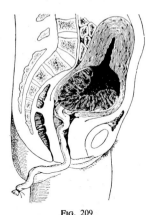

Subsequent uterine contractions completely detach the uterus from the placenta which is then forced out of the upper segment into the lower uterine segment or the vagina. The lower segment, which had collapsed like a concertina as the baby was born, becomes distended with the placenta. The empty upper uterine segment contracts effectively, forming a hard round mass, which is pushed upwards and perched on top of the placenta which is now lying in the lower uterine segment.

Fig. 209

THIRD STAGE.

Placenta in lower uterine segment

The membranes do not separate as readily as the placenta, for they tend to wrinkle, thus accommodating themselves to the diminished area of the uterus. The traction of the descending placenta slowly peels them off the decidua, but the membrane attached to the area round the cervix may remain adherent until the placenta is actually being expelled outside the vulva.

CONTROL OF BLEEDING

If Nature did not make some provision whereby bleeding from the large torn placental sinuses could be controlled, the woman would bleed to death in a matter of minutes. The contraction and retraction of the uterine muscle fibres that bring about separation of the placenta also act as " **living ligatures** " by compressing the blood vessels and controlling the bleeding.

Clotting of blood plays little part during this phase, but a few hours later, when the uterine contractions are less vigorous, bleeding is prevented by the blood clot which has formed in the sinuses. The presence of clots in the cavity of the uterus does not prevent hæmorrhage, in fact, by inhibiting uterine contractions, they might be a cause of hæmorrhage.

Recent research has shown a transitory activation of the coagulation and fibrinolytic mechanism in the uterine blood circulation during and immediately following placental separation. This beneficial clotting occurs in the uterine blood vessels and sinuses at the placental site.

N.B.—The presence of clots in the uterine cavity would inhibit uterine contractions and predispose to haemorrhage.

Nature's Method of Expulsion of the Placenta

Nature has two methods of expelling the placenta, which have been described by Schultze and Matthews Duncan. These methods are not under the control of the attendant.

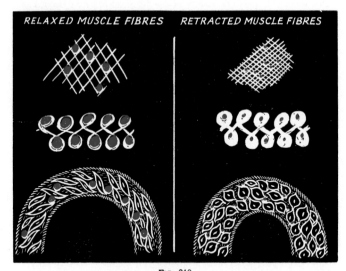

FIG. 210

Diagrammatic representation of the action of the uterine muscle fibres in the control of postpartum bleeding from the placental site.

The Schultze method is usually said to be the more common. The placenta slips down into the vagina through the hole in the amniotic sac; the fetal surface appears at the vulva with the membranes trailing behind like an inverted umbrella as they are peeled off the uterine wall. The maternal surface of the placenta is not seen, and any blood clot is inside the inverted sac.

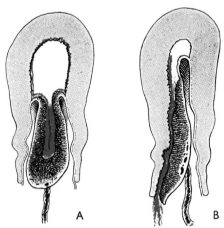

FIG. 211

EXPULSION OF THE PLACENTA.
A, The Schultez method.   B, The Matthews Duncan method.

The Matthews Duncan method.—The placenta slides down sideways and comes through the vulva with the lateral border first, like a button through a buttonhole. The maternal surface is seen, and the blood escapes as it is not inside the sac. There is more likelihood of ragged membranes with the Matthews Duncan method, as they are not peeled off as completely as in the Schultze method.

MANAGEMENT OF THE THIRD STAGE OF LABOUR

PROPHYLAXIS

Good management of the third stage begins during the prenatal period, for the woman should be brought into labour in excellent physical condition, so that the uterus will have the power to contract and retract, and in order that normal blood loss will not produce collapse. Such management should continue during the first and second stages of labour, when the midwife prevents conditions arising that would exhaust the woman and seeks medical assistance for the treatment of complications that interfere with good uterine action.

Many experienced midwives believe that slow delivery of the baby's body lessens the incidence of postpartum hæmorrhage.

The administration of oxytocic drugs, e.g. Syntometrine 1 ml. with the birth of the anterior shoulder shortens the third stage, reduces blood loss and **the incidence of hæmorrhage.**

IMMEDIATE CARE OF THE BABY

Although the care of the baby is not an integral part of the third stage, it is carried out while the third stage is in progress, and must therefore be mentioned under management.

The airway is cleared, the cord clamped and cut. Apgar score made and recorded. If any abnormal condition is present, medical aid should be summoned, but a more detailed examination of the baby is carried out later, usually prior to bathing.

The baby is dried and warmly wrapped, placed in a safe, warm place; plastic cots are excellent for supervision of babies in the labour ward. The immediate care of the baby is described on page 309.

ASEPSIS AND ANTISEPSIS

The need for asepsis is greater now than in the preceding stages of labour, for the mother's resistance, both general and local, is diminished. **Laceration and bruising devitalize the tissues** of the vulva and vagina, and render them prone to invasion by organisms. In the raw placental site and the alkaline lochia, organisms find an ideal nidus in which to flourish.

An aseptic technique must be rigorously observed.—The wearing of masks is essential. Hands should be rescrubbed and lotions changed before swabbing, and as the introitus is gaping, care must be taken that no swabbing lotion gains entrance to the vagina.

POSITION OF THE PATIENT

The dorsal position has numerous advantages:

1. **The uterus can be observed better.**   2. **The uterus remains in the midline.**

3. **It is more comfortable for the woman.**   4. **Her face is in full view.**

5. **Assistance in expelling the placenta can be given.**

6. **There is said to be less danger of an air embolism,** because, when lying in the left lateral position, air may enter the vagina and reach the blood sinuses in the placental site.

WARMTH

The need for warmth at this time should be appreciated, for the woman has undergone strenuous physical exercise which has made her perspire, and she has lost much heat from her body in the baby and liquor. If exposed, an attack of shivering is likely to occur, which is not a true rigor, but often alarms the woman and can be prevented by the avoidance of chilling. **The room should be warm: any soiled wet linen should be removed from under the patient:** if necessary, warm cellular cotton blankets are tucked over her arms and chest and around her legs.

OBSERVATION DURING THE THIRD STAGE

1. FOR PERINEAL LACERATION

When the woman is delivered in the left lateral position, the perineum can be examined before she is turned on her back, and if two wool swabs are used to separate the labia, the perineum and posterior vaginal wall can be inspected quite easily. The hands should, of course, be scrubbed and the vulva gently swabbed to remove blood. **Medical assistance should be obtained to suture all lacerations other than a mere nick.**

2. GENERAL CONDITION

In the majority of cases, the woman's general condition is good; she may feel rather tired, but not ill; she is happy that " all is well," and interested in her baby. In the case of twins, or after the birth of a very large baby, the woman may feel limp, although not actually shocked, because of the great reduction in abdominal pressure.

But after a long, exhausting labour, an instrumental delivery, or when there has been much bruising or laceration of the birth canal, the woman may suffer from shock.

THE PULSE

The pulse is the best guide as to the woman's condition, so the midwife should keep her finger on the pulse throughout the third stage. The rate should range between 60 and 70, as it is usually slightly slower than normal at this time. If the pulse is rising, and particularly when it reaches 90, the question of hæmorrhage or shock must be considered. The skin should feel warm and dry.

Pallor, which is a very serious sign, is caused by severe exhaustion, shock, hæmorrhage, or cardiac failure.

Blood pressure should be taken and recorded; The systolic should be over 110 mm.

3. THE UTERUS

(a) Size and Consistency

After the birth of the baby, the upper border of the fundus is about 2·5 cm. (1 inch) below the level of the umbilicus (15·2 cm. (6 inches) above the symphysis pubis) and in shape the uterus is broader laterally than antero-posteriorly.

The consistency is that of a firm sorbo-rubber or tennis ball. Every two or three minutes when a contraction occurs, the uterus will feel like a cricket ball, for about 30 seconds, and the woman may have slight pain or discomfort. But the student midwife must not expect the cricket ball consistency of the strongly contracting uterus to be constantly maintained. Between contractions, the firm distinct outline of the uterus should be clearly defined ; it should not feel soft and flabby.

FUNDUS ABOVE UMBILICUS

If, after the birth of the baby, the fundus is more than 2·5 cm. (1 inch) above the umbilicus, four causes must be considered.

(1) There is another baby *in utero.*—Palpate for fetal parts and listen for the fetal heart.

(2) The placenta is unduly big.—This will be present in the case of twins and where the baby is suffering from hydrops fetalis.

(3) Blood clot present.—The uterus will feel boggy; the mother's pulse will be rapid; blood may or may not be seen at the vulva.

(4) A full bladder.—This would only occur if the woman has not been under competent supervision throughout labour.

(b) SIGNS THAT THE PLACENTA HAS LEFT THE UPPER UTERINE SEGMENT

When controlled cord traction is used signs of placental descent are not waited for.

(1) THE FUNDUS FEELS HARD AND ROUND.

(2) THE FUNDUS RISES TO THE UMBILICUS AND TO THE SURFACE.

(3) THE UTERUS IS MOBILE.

(4) THE CORD LENGTHENS.

(5) THE PLACENTA IS SEEN AT THE VULVA.

The small gush of blood, 30 to 60 ml., is merely a sign that separation of the placenta has begun.

A combination of these signs is usually accepted as evidence that the placenta has separated and left the upper uterine segment.

(1) THE FUNDUS FEELS HARD

In shape it is round or globular, instead of having the broad flattened contour of the upper segment that contains a placenta, as previously described.

(2) THE FUNDUS RISES TO THE UMBILICUS

In thin patients it can be seen as a prominence at the umbilicus (17·8 *cm.* (7 *inches*) *above the symphysis pubis*), and in all patients the fundus can be palpated as a hard round mass, just under the abdominal wall, sometimes slightly above the umbilicus.

Occasionally a slight bulge may be apparent immediately above the symphysis pubis, produced by the placenta when it is lying in the lower uterine segment, but this is not always noticeable. If the placenta has descended into the vagina, no bulge will be visible.

(3) THE UTERUS IS MOBILE

The fundus, having been pushed upwards, is no longer restrained by the pelvic brim. Only two fingers should be used in testing the mobility of the uterus, the middle finger of each hand or the middle finger and thumb of one hand. Great gentleness should be exercised as the uterus is very tender. If the midwife is doubtful as to whether the uterus is freely movable, she should consider doubt to be a negative sign. On occasions, when the mother is lying on her left side, while the midwife attends to an asphyxiated baby, she may find the fundus has fallen over to that side. This is a sign of mobility and denotes that the placenta has left the upper segment.

(4) THE CORD LENGTHENS AT THE VULVA

This occurs when the placenta slides down into the lower segment or vagina.

The cord can sometimes be seen slipping out of the vulva, and if a ligature or clamp is placed on the cord near the vulva, its descent will be obvious.

The kinks in the cord are straightened by slight traction and then, when the uterus is firmly contracted, gentle downward fundal pressure is applied. If the placenta is in the lower segment the extra length of cord that appears at the vulva **will not recede,** but if the placenta is still in the upper segment the cord will recede when pressure on the fundus is released.

Alternatively, the fingers dipped down behind the pubic bone will produce a similar result. These methods, however, cannot be recommended, as the receding cord may carry organisms from the vulva back into the vagina.

(5) THE PLACENTA IS SEEN AT THE VULVA

This is a very good sign, but it is possible that part of the placenta may still be adherent to the lower uterine wall. If the fetal surface is visible, the placenta is usually completely separated.

No one sign is absolute

A combination of signs is usually accepted as being reliable. Although separation of the placenta begins during the contraction which expels the baby's body, it may be five minutes before the placenta leaves the upper uterine segment and what are usually known as " signs of separation and descent " become evident.

In some cases it may be 20 minutes: but, as long as there is no separation of placenta there can be no bleeding.

4. AMOUNT OF BLOOD LOSS

The average amount of blood lost during and immediately after the third stage is 120 to 240 ml., but, as there is usually some liquor amnii in the blood, such an amount is not serious.

Blood is a very precious fluid, and the midwife ought to take pride in conducting the third stage with the minimal loss. It is an excellent plan to measure the blood, adding clots from the placenta and estimating what is spilt on the bed.

The vulva is always exposed during the third stage, so that undue blood loss will be detected immediately, for the possibility of hæmorrhage must constantly be kept in mind.

A midwife ought to take action to control excessive bleeding even although the loss is not sufficient to be classified as postpartum hæmorrhage.

GUARDING THE UTERUS

This term is used to describe the " manual " method of observing the uterus during the third stage of labour. With the use of oxytocic drugs the period of guarding is shorter; some would say, unnecessary.

The midwife watches for :

1. **Signs that the placenta has left the upper uterine segment.**

2. **Signs of hæmorrhage.** *Pallor is a late* sign and it may be more than one minute after hæmorrhage has begun before the pulse quickens. There may be 300 ml. of blood, or more, *in utero* before it escapes from the vagina.

3. **Any change in the size and consistency of the uterus.**

This can be readily detected by the sense of touch, so the slightly cupped left hand is laid lightly on the fundus to note:

(*a*) **Its height in relationship to the umbilicus.**   (*b*) **Its size or bulk.**

(*c*) **Whether it feels firm or flabby.** *The hand is kept perfectly still.*

The aortic pulse can be felt by dipping the little finger of the left hand down behind the fundus.

The uterus cannot contract properly with a partially separated placenta *in situ.*

The student midwife ought to be aware that kneading and squeezing the uterus prevents and disturbs the clotting of blood that should be taking place in the uterine sinuses. The idea that squeezing the uterus or pushing it down into the pelvis prevents it from filling up with blood is quite erroneous, and the practice is harmful. It is primarily the contraction and retraction of the muscle fibres acting as " living ligatures " that control blood loss.

EXPULSION OF THE PLACENTA

The expulsion of the placenta was probably intended by Nature to be accomplished by the force of gravity, with the mother in the squatting attitude, as adopted for defæcation; but when the third stage is conducted in the dorsal position, the midwife's help is usually necessary.

The woman lies with her knees drawn up and well separated. She is told that the after-birth has to come away, and that the process may be uncomfortable but not painful.

(1) CONTROLLED CORD TRACTION

Delivering the placenta by controlled cord traction following the administration of Syntometrine 1 ml. provides a safe and successful means of reducing blood loss and shortening the third stage of labour. By this regime normal blood loss has been diminished by 30 to 60 ml.; the incidence of post-partum hæmorrhage lowered from 7 to 3 per cent.

Successful results depend upon (1) understanding the pharmacological action of Syntometrine; (2) timing the procedure properly; (3) being alert to the possibility of twins *in utero.*

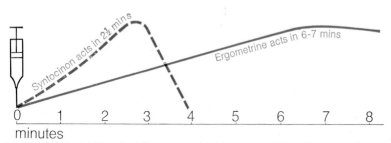

TO SHOW RAPID ACTION OF SYNTOCINON IN COMPARISON WITH ERGOMETRINE

Fig. 212

(*Courtesy of Sandoz Products Ltd.*)

Syntometrine 1 ml. consists of 5 units of oxytocin (Syntocinon) and 0·5 mg. ergometrine maleate B.P. When administered intramuscularly Syntocinon acts within 2½ minutes and ergometrine within 6 to 7 minutes. Ergometrine tends to cause spasm of the lower uterine segment so the placenta should be delivered before the ergometrine acts; (when ergometrine is given intravenously its rapid action within 1 to 2 minutes may cause trapping of the placenta as well as hypertensive episodes).

Syntometrine must not be used after the expiry date, **i.e. nine months after manufacture.**

TIMING THE ADMINISTRATION OF SYNTOMETRINE

Giving Syntometrine when the anterior shoulder appears has certain advantages; the length of time between administration of the drug and delivery of the placenta can be accurately controlled. If given with crowning of the head Syntometrine may be administered too soon, for the act of crowning is not always properly understood or recognized; the placenta is not then delivered within 4 minutes and is liable to be trapped.

Some administer Syntometrine when the head is born, others think that shoulder dystocia is less likely to occur if it is given when the anterior shoulder appears.

TIMING OF CONTROLLED CORD TRACTION

The placenta should be extracted with the first uterine contraction after the birth of the baby usually between 2 to 4 minutes. (Some do not wait for this, but attending to the baby occupies two or three minutes.)

(*Waiting for separation and descent of the placenta has been traditional teaching for midwives, but this cherished idea should be abandoned.*)

While waiting for signs of placental separation and descent more than seven minutes may elapse; the ergometrine comes into action and the placenta may be trapped.

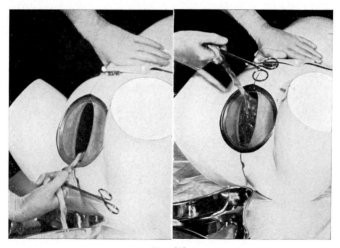

FIG. 213

CLASSROOM DEMONSTRATION OF CONTROLLED CORD TRACTION
Note left hand bracing back the uterus.
(*Aberdeen Maternity Hospital.*)

Method

The bladder should have been emptied prior to delivery of the baby.

Apply Kocher's artery forceps to the cord near the vulva. This provides a better hold for traction and reinforces the sensation of placental descent to a greater degree than when the cord is wound around the fingers.

Wait until the uterus contracts strongly, usually about 2-4 minutes after delivery.

Place the left hand on the lower abdomen, the palmar surface bracing back the upper uterine segment, the fingers stretching the lower uterine segment upwards towards the umbilicus to prevent inversion of uterus.

Traction on the umbilical cord should begin gently, and be continued steadily, without jerking to avoid breaking the cord. Should the uterus relax, traction is stopped temporarily. The hand on the abdomen can, with practice, detect that the uterus is not being pulled downwards as would occur if the placenta were still adherent to it. If after 20 to 30 seconds of traction the placenta does not descend, the attempt should be abandoned for one or two minutes when it can again be resumed.

The direction of pull should first be downwards then outwards as the placenta descends and upwards when it appears at the vulva, following the axis of the birth canal. The safety of the procedure, in avoiding inversion of the uterus, lies in bracing back the uterus while cord traction is applied.

Fundal pressure and cord traction must never be combined as this would be very liable to cause inversion of the uterus.

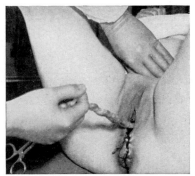

FIG. 214
CONTROLLED CORD TRACTION.
The left hand braces the contracted uterus upwards.
(*Photographed at Simpson Memorial Maternity Pavilion, Edinburgh.*)

Hypertensive episodes. With Syntometrine these are slight, transient and less frequent than with ergometrine given intravenously. Pre-eclamptic patients and those with essential hypertension are given Syntocinon 5 units in preference to Syntometrine or ergometrine. Syntometrine does not cause hypertensive episodes in normotensive women.

BREAKING OF THE CORD

Cord traction should not be applied when the fetus is macerated, or if the baby is premature: in both instances the tensile strength of the cord is much reduced. Fundal pressure would be preferable if the woman cannot expel the placenta by her expulsive effort.

If the cord should snap, the sterile gloved hand is introduced into the vagina and the placenta grasped and extracted.

(2) BRANDT-ANDREWS MANŒUVRE

Brandt, during 1930, and Andrew, during 1940, modified Aristotle's method of delivering the placenta by cord traction. They recommended applying tension, but not traction, to the umbilical cord with one hand; the other hand on the abdomen pushing the uterus upwards off the placenta, which in most cases was partially, if not completely, separated.

(3) THE WOMAN'S BEARING DOWN EFFORT

When the uterus contracts she is instructed to hold her breath and bear down as she did for the birth of the baby.

Some multigravid women have lax abdominal muscles which cannot be effectively used in bearing down. The midwife could assist in such cases by laying both her hands, palms downwards, across the woman's abdomen below the umbilicus to provide a brace against which the woman can push.

The primigravida often has a rigid pelvic floor, and assistance may be required to overcome its resistance, unless an episiotomy has been made, or an extensive perineal laceration is present.

If the woman fails to expel the placenta by pushing, assistance must be given.

(4) USING THE FUNDUS AS A PISTON *(rarely used in Britain)*

The firmly contracted fundus is used as a piston to push the placenta out, in the same way that the piston is used to push fluid out of the barrel of a syringe.

(*a*) **The uterus must be in a state of contraction** (of cricket ball consistency). (*b*) **The bladder ought not to be distended.** (*c*) **Only one hand should be used.** (*d*) **No undue force should be exerted.**

The woman is asked to open her mouth and to breathe through it slowly and quietly, for the abdominal muscles must be relaxed. (*It is difficult for the midwife to expel the placenta by using the fundus as a piston if the woman is bearing down at the same time.*) The midwife stands on the woman's right and uses her left hand to grasp the fundus, during a contraction, with her fingers behind the uterus and her thumb on the anterior surface.

Pressure is applied with the palm of the hand in the axis of the pelvic inlet, then in a downward and backward direction. If too much force is used, the transverse cervical ligaments are strained and this may predispose to uterine prolapse.

The causes of failure are usually due to pushing in the wrong direction, so that the placenta is jammed against the pubic bones. A full bladder makes the procedure very difficult indeed.

The right hand receives the placenta at the vulva, but when it is almost completely expelled both hands should be used, as it is too big and slippery for a midwife to hold with one hand, and if it should drop into the basin any adherent membrane will be torn and retained.

The membranes usually slip out with the placenta, but, if not, they may be still attached to the decidua in the area of the lower uterine segment near the cervix. It is believed that the detachment of the chorion is completed by the weight of the descending placenta stripping the chorion off the decidua, and it should take place slowly.

Summary of Fundal Heights during Third Stage

FUNDAL HEIGHT RELATIVE TO	UMBILICUS	SYMPHYSIS PUBIS
A, At the beginning of the third stage	2·5 cm. below (1 inch)	15·2 cm. above (6 inches)
B, Placenta in lower segment (separated)	1·3 cm. above (½ inch)	19 cm. above (7½ inches)
C, End of third stage (placenta expelled)	3·8 cm. below (1½ inches)	14 cm. above (5½ inches)

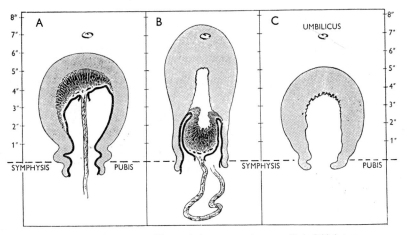

Beginning of third stage.   Placenta in lower segment.   End of third stage.

Fig. 215

The Fourth Stage of Labour

The first hour after expulsion of the placenta is sometimes designated the fourth stage of labour, in order to stress the fact that vigilance is still necessary in case hæmorrhage should occur.

The empty uterus should now be firmly contracted.

If an oxytocic drug has not already been given the midwife should now administer an ergot preparation, such as ergometrine, 0·5 mg., or Syntometrine, 1 ml.

Any blood clot present should be expelled while the uterus is in a state of contraction by gently squeezing and cautiously pressing the uterus in a downward and backward direction with due regard to the danger of predisposing to uterine prolapse. Routine massage of the uterus at this period, when it is contracting satisfactorily, is to be deprecated.

ADHERENT MEMBRANES

In an attempt to detach adherent membranes the placenta can be turned around to make a complete circle which will twist the membranes into a rope and strengthen them. If twisted too much, the membranes may tear off at the edge of the placenta and be retained. The usual method employed is to apply a pair of artery forceps to the membranes and to exert gentle traction in an up and down, sideways and circular manner, in an endeavour to coax the membranes out. If the chorion still remains adherent, the placenta is laid aside and the artery forceps left attached to the membrane at the vulva, so that it cannot slip back into the vagina. The chorion usually comes away within a few hours.

EXAMINATION OF THE PLACENTA

Management of the third stage is not complete until the placenta has been examined to make sure that no part of it has been retained, and this must be done in a careful systematic manner. It is advisable to examine the membranes first, as they are apt to become torn while inspecting the maternal surface of the placenta.

INSPECTION OF THE MEMBRANES

The amount of chorion should be sufficient to have contained the fetus and amniotic fluid and, if not complete, an effort must be made to assess the amount of membrane that is missing. *In utero* the chorion is adherent to the decidua, and pieces of chorion may remain attached to it after the placenta is expelled.

The amnion ought to be peeled from the chorion right up to the umbilical cord, for it is not possible to determine that the chorion is complete until the amnion has been detached from it. Filling the amniotic sac with water as a means of testing for complete membranes is valueless, as the amnion is practically always complete.

Meconium staining.—When the membranes are stained with meconium it is possible that the baby may have inhaled meconium stained liquor and develop pulmonary complications. Antibiotics may be prescribed by the doctor as a prophylactic measure.

BLOOD VESSELS IN THE MEMBRANE
They may denote a Succenturiate Lobe

Blood vessels in the membrane should be traced from source to destination. **They may run from the main placenta to a succenturiate lobe situated in the membrane,** and when such a lobe is present (*visibly*) there is no cause for concern, but if the lobe has been retained, the vessels will be seen running to the hole in the membrane where the lobe had been.

There will, of course, be a large hole in the membrane through which the baby has come, and there may be a hole due to the retention of a piece of membrane; but in neither instance will there be any blood vessels going to these holes. **The vessels may run to a velamentous insertion of cord,** or they may return to the placenta again— the so-called aberrant vessels which are of no significance.

Incomplete Membranes

The state of the membranes must be recorded on the chart, *e.g.* " complete," " half retained," and if the membranes are torn but appear to be complete the term " ragged membranes " is used.

When the membranes are incomplete, the midwife in remote areas may give one of the ergot preparations, b.i.d. for two or three days; and inspect all lochial discharge until the membrane is passed.

The danger of hæmorrhage must be kept in mind and the doctor summoned if the membrane is not passed within 48 hours, if the lochia are persistently red, or if postpartum or puerperal hæmorrhage occurs.

INSPECTION OF THE MATERNAL AND FETAL SURFACES

Blood clot should be removed from the maternal surface and placed in the jug used for measuring blood loss. The placenta should be dark bluish-red in colour and of firm consistency. An unhealthy placenta is soft and mushy, and when hydrops fetalis is present the placenta is large, pale and œdematous, with water oozing from it. (Other abnormalities are considered on page 35.)

All the cotyledons should be present, and, if the placenta is laid flat, the cotyledons will fit together if the placenta is intact.

The placenta is inspected for infarcts, which are whitish areas usually about 2·5 cm. (1 inch) or more in diameter. *The position of the insertion of the cord is noted*, its length measured and the number of arteries scrutinized. *The placenta is weighed*, and pertinent facts regarding it are recorded on the chart.

The examination of the placenta is a most important duty, and because of the grave danger of a cotyledon (*or a succenturiate lobe*) being left behind, the Central Midwives Board for Scotland rules state that the placenta and membranes must be examined before they are destroyed. If the placenta is normal and the doctor has not requested that it should be kept for his inspection, it is disposed of by burning if possible.

DANGERS OF RETAINED LOBE OF PLACENTA

Serious postpartum or puerperal hæmorrhage may occur when a lobe of placenta is left behind and no steps are taken to promote its expulsion. It is also a predisposing cause of puerperal sepsis. Retained placenta is more dangerous than retained membrane, because it is deeply embedded and when it sloughs off may open up large uterine vessels. This hæmorrhage may occur after the woman has been discharged, and can be fatal. To avoid such a catastrophe the obstetrician will explore the uterus under a general anæsthetic in the operating theatre and remove the lobe. Blood should be available for transfusion.

In district practice medical assistance must be obtained when the placenta is not complete, and it is likely that the woman will be transferred to hospital. If the retained piece of placenta is very small, ergometrine, 0·5 mg., or other ergot preparation will be ordered and given b.i.d.

Continued red lochial discharge is a warning sign, which should be reported at once and preparations made for exploration of the uterus.

NURSING CARE DURING THE FOURTH STAGE

The vulva is swabbed and a sterile pad placed in position, buttocks dried and any wet linen removed, so that the woman will be warm and comfortable. A sterile towel is laid over the lower abdomen and thighs and the woman covered with warm cellular cotton blankets.

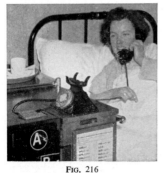

Fig. 216

PORTABLE TROLLEY TELEPHONE.

Newly delivered mother talking to her husband.

(*Simpson Memorial Maternity Pavilion, Edinburgh.*)

The midwife remains at the bedside, noting the woman's pulse and colour. At frequent intervals she palpates the uterus to make sure it is not filling up with blood, and looks at the pad to ensure that the blood loss is not excessive.

The pulse rate should be between 60 and 70, but if it is over 90 investigation and continued supervision are necessary. The temperature is taken, and may be subnormal because of loss of body heat, but occasionally it is 37·2° C. (99° F.), due to reaction following a difficult labour.

The blood pressure is taken during the first half hour after delivery; 118 mm. is the average. The systolic pressure should be above 110, but, if less, and especially if accompanied by a pulse of over 100, it is usually due to collapse from hæmorrhage or shock. If the blood pressure is higher than anticipated it is taken every half hour.

The woman will appreciate a cup of tea and toast, and there is no reason why she should not have a light meal if she desires it. Half an hour should elapse before the woman is bathed; she needs that period of rest, quiet and warmth.

The woman is encouraged to pass urine before being left in her home or transferred to the puerperal ward in hospital, but if she has emptied her bladder prior to delivery she may have no desire to urinate.

Swabbing is repeated, and a large perineal pad placed on the vulva.

Rest and sleep should be encouraged.—After seeing her husband and one other near relative, the room should be darkened and quietness assured. Even although the mother may feel elated and not inclined for sleep, it is sound practice to give a sedative at this time.

C.M.B.(Scot.) Rule.—*The midwife must not leave her patient until at least one hour after the birth of the placenta, and only then if:*

VAGINAL BLOOD LOSS IS NORMAL.   PULSE BELOW 90.

FUNDUS FIRM.   SYSTOLIC BLOOD PRESSURE 110 mm./hg. OR OVER.

BABY'S CONDITION GOOD.

The more common reasons for obtaining medical assistance during the third stage are: Hæmorrhage, adherent and retained placenta. These and the other complications are discussed on page 428.

RECORD KEEPING

It is the duty of the midwife, whether in hospital or domiciliary practice, to record her observations during labour. The two best aids to good record keeping are :

1. **A plan of work** that ensures the carrying out of every essential treatment and examination at stated times throughout labour.

2. **Suitable charts** that are designed for the recording of all necessary observations and treatment at specific intervals. Such charts serve as a reminder for making observations and giving treatments and help the midwife to organize the nursing care of the woman in labour.

There are differences of opinion as to which observations are absolutely necessary and how frequently they should be made. There should be no slavish adherence to the making of any observation merely to fill the blank spaces in a chart. The midwife in charge uses her discretion, allowing the woman to rest and sleep when necessary. Although there may be educational value in requiring the student midwife to keep detailed records, *e.g.* the time, length and severity of each contraction, this may divert her attention from the suffering human being.

Time is sometimes spent in writing reports that should be devoted to giving emotional and physical support to the woman.

PROMPT RECORDING SHOULD BE THE RULE

The filling up of charts, long after the findings were made, is most unreliable. If facts are recorded at once, the progress of labour can be assessed by any member of the staff, in the absence of the person who made the examination.

Charts should, if possible, be completed as soon as labour is over, so that they can be sent to the puerperal ward along with the patient. The sister will, of course, make her own observations of mother and baby as soon as they are admitted to her ward; but she should be given certain information regarding the type of delivery and what the condition of mother and baby has been during the postpartum hour. The puerperal ward sister will note *the following facts, which should have been recorded so that any necessary precautions and treatment can be instituted.*

1. **Delivery:** Spontaneous; malpresentation; forceps.

2. **Anæsthetic:** General; epidural; local.

3. **Blood loss:** Amount.

4. **Placenta and membranes:** Complete; incomplete.

5. **Perineum:** Laceration; episiotomy; number of non-absorbable sutures.

6. **Drugs given to mother:** *e.g.* oxytocic preparations; sedatives.

7. **Baby:** Prematurity ? Dysmaturity. Condition at birth. Apgar score. Rhesus incompatibility ? Drugs given, *e.g.* Konakion (vitamin K); levallorphan.

Legibility is essential and the dosage of drugs given ought to be clearly printed. *Abbreviations* should be avoided, except for those which are universally employed, such as, L.O.A., P.V.

ACCURACY IS IMPERATIVE

The chart should present a clear, concise, reliable record so that when reviewing the case at the end of labour, or prior to a subsequent delivery, the pertinent facts are available. Records are sometimes utilized for statistical purposes and for obstetrical research, so facts and figures must be correct.

The legal aspect of record keeping is also important during labour.

The date and hour of birth, sex of the child, and whether alive or stillborn, are required for the registration and the notification of births.

The length and weight at birth might be needed as evidence of the period of gestation in cases when the paternity of the child is under question.

QUESTIONS FOR REVISION

THE THIRD STAGE OF LABOUR

ORAL QUESTIONS

What does the midwife observe during the third stage ? Why is it important to take the pulse during the third stage ? Why might the uterus be unduly large during the third stage ? How could you help a woman to expel her placenta ? When should you not apply cord traction ? What would you do if the cord broke ? What is the normal amount of blood loss ?

The patient's condition should be satisfactory when left one hour after the placenta has been expelled. Explain what you mean by " **satisfactory** " under three headings.

Write not more than 10 lines: (*a*) controlled cord traction; (*b*) examination of the placenta; (*c*) retained lobe of placenta; (*d*) nursing care during the fourth stage.

Differentiate between: (*a*) the Schultze and Matthews Duncan method; (*b*) Brandt-Andrews method and controlled cord traction; (*c*) adherent and retained placenta; (*d*) Syntometrine and Syntocinon.

C.M.B.(Scot.) paper.—What are the signs that the placenta has left the uterus in the third stage of labour, and what errors in the management of this stage may lead to a dangerous condition of the mother ?

C.M.B.(Scot.) paper.—Describe briefly how you would examine the placenta, and state what complications may occur if the placenta or membranes are found to be deficient.

C.M.B.(Eng.) paper.—Draw a diagram showing the arrangement of the muscle fibres in the uterine wall. Describe the process of separation of the placenta and the natural arrest of hæmorrhage on completion of labour.

C.M.B.(N. Ireland) paper.—Discuss the conduct of the third stage of labour in a patient with a history of postpartum hæmorrhage at an earlier confinement.

C.M.B.(N. Ireland) paper—Describe the placenta at term. Why is it necessary to examine the placenta and membranes after delivery ?

C.M.B.(Eng.) paper.—Describe the mechanism of the third stage of labour. How do you conduct this stage in practice ?

C.M.B.(N. Ireland) paper.—Describe the physiology of the third stage of labour and state how a normal third stage should be managed.

C.M.B.(Eng.) paper, 1969.—Describe the management of the third stage of labour. In what circumstances should the midwife send for a doctor during this stage?

C.M.B.(N. Ireland) paper, 1969.—Describe the placenta at term. Why is it important to make a careful examination of it immediately the third stage is completed?

C.M.B.(N. Ireland) paper, 1969.—Describe the management of the third stage of labour.

20

Occipito-posterior Positions of the Vertex

Although the vertex is a normal presentation, the course of labour can border on the abnormal when the occiput occupies a posterior instead of an anterior part of the pelvis.

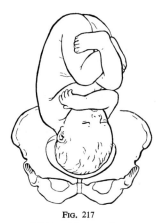

FIG. 217
Right occipito-posterior.

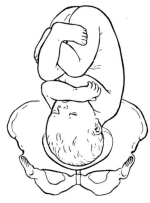

FIG. 218
Left occipito-posterior.

VERTEX PRESENTATION.

In about one-fifth of posterior vertex positions labour will be prolonged, and in no instance is the presence of a patient, competent midwife so valuable as in tedious labours due to this cause.

FREQUENCY

The vertex presents in 96 per cent of cases and authorities are not in agreement as to what proportion are posterior. Ten per cent might be considered a fair average. Right occipito-posterior is three times more common than left occipito-posterior, for the same reason that L.O.A. is more common than R.O.A.

CAUSE

There is no satisfactory explanation why the occiput should be posterior. It has been said that in as many as 60 per cent of vertex presentations the fetal head lies at the pelvic brim in the transverse diameter and that it is just a matter of chance whether the head will enter the brim with the occiput slightly anterior or posterior.

335

DIAGNOSIS

RIGHT OCCIPITO-POSTERIOR

ABDOMINAL EXAMINATION

INSPECTION

There is a saucer-shaped depression at or immediately below the umbilicus, because when the back is not in front, there is a " dip " between the upper and lower poles of the fetus. The high head with the depression above it looks rather like a full bladder.

2. PALPATION

(*a*) THE HEAD IS HIGH

The commonest cause of a high head in a primigravida during the last two weeks of pregnancy is posterior position. This is because the large engaging diameter O.F. 11.4 cm. (4½ inches) will not enter the brim until labour begins and flexion takes place.

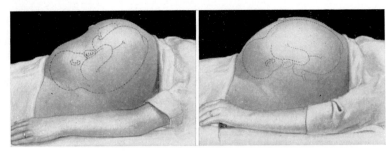

Posterior.   Anterior.

FIG. 219

Comparison of abdominal contour in posterior and anterior positions of vertex presentation.

(*b*) THE HEAD FEELS UNDULY LARGE

This is also due to the larger circumference of the deflexed head.

(*c*) THE OCCIPUT AND SINCIPUT ARE ON THE SAME LEVEL

(It will be remembered that in palpating anterior positions the occiput will be lower than the sinciput because the head is flexed.) The sinciput is in closer proximity to the abdominal wall than the occiput.

(*d*) THE BACK IS DIFFICULT TO PALPATE

It is found well out on the right side. The anterior shoulder will be 7·6 to 10·2 cm. (3 to 4 inches) from the midline, and because the head is high, the shoulder will be about 12·7 cm. (5 inches) above the symphysis pubis.

(*e*) LIMBS ARE FELT ON BOTH SIDES OF THE MIDLINE

In anterior positions they are only felt on one side.

3. AUSCULTATION

The fetal heart-beat will be located in the right flank and it will be somewhat muffled as the muscles there are thick. It may also be heard in the midline near the umbilicus or slightly to the left, because when the back is not well flexed the fetal heart is heard through the fetal chest which is thrown forwards.

DIAGNOSIS DURING LABOUR

Posterior position should be suspected where there is no disproportion and a vertex presentation is held up at the brim in spite of good uterine action.

The vaginal findings will depend on the degree of flexion of the head, and locating the anterior fontanelle to the left anterior is diagnostic of an R.O.P. **The sagittal suture will be in the right oblique diameter of the pelvis.** Very occasionally in an

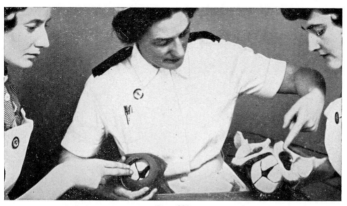

Fig. 220

Labour ward superintendent demonstrating vaginal findings in vertex right occipito-posterior. Note half of rubber ball used to denote the cervix.
(*Aberdeen Maternity Hospital.*)

R.O.P. with a well flexed head, the posterior fontanelle is felt in the right posterior quadrant, but with fingers of average length it is most unlikely that it could be reached.

During the second stage of labour a vaginal examination is often necessary because of delay. The large caput may make identification of sutures and fontanelles difficult and in such cases the doctor usually inserts his hand so that an accurate diagnosis and assessment of the situation can be made.

MECHANISM OF VERTEX PRESENTATION

Right Occipito-posterior Position

The lie is longitudinal.
The attitude is that of flexion.
The presentation is the vertex.
The position is the R.O.P.

The denominator is the occiput.
The presenting part is the middle or anterior area of the left parietal bone.

The occipito-frontal diameter, 11·4 cm. (4½ inches), lies in the right oblique diameter of the pelvic brim. The occiput points to the right sacro-iliac joint, the sinciput to the left ilio-pectineal eminence.

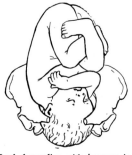

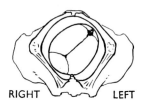

Head descending with increase in
flexion.

Sagittal suture in the right oblique
diameter of the pelvis.

Fig. 221

RIGHT OCCIPITO-POSTERIOR.

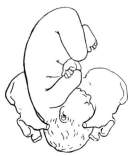

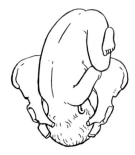

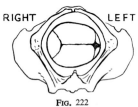

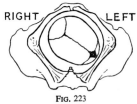

Fig. 222

Fig. 223

The occiput and the shoulders
have rotated one-eighth of a circle
forwards. The sagittal suture is
in the transverse diameter of the
pelvis.

The occiput and shoulders have
rotated two-eighths of a circle
forwards, now being similar to
an R.O.A. The sagittal suture is
in the left oblique diameter of the
pelvis.

Flexion.—Descent takes place with increasing flexion. The occiput becomes the leading part.

Internal rotation of the head.—The occiput reaches the pelvic floor first and rotates three-eighths of a circle forwards along the right side of the pelvis. The shoulders turn two-eighths of a circle with the head from the left to the right oblique. (*This is not internal rotation of the shoulders as they have not yet reached the pelvic floor.*)

Crowning.—The occiput escapes under the symphysis pubis and the head is crowned.

Extension.—Sinciput, face and chin sweep the perineum and the head is born by a movement of extension.

Restitution takes place and the occiput turns one-eighth of a circle to the right and the head rights itself with the shoulders.

Internal rotation of the shoulders.—The shoulders enter in the right oblique of the pelvis the anterior shoulder reaches the pelvic floor first and rotates one-eighth of a circle forwards, along the left side of the pelvis.

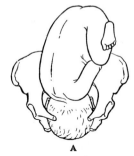

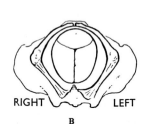

A   Fig. 224   **B**

Occiput has rotated three-eighths of a circle forwards.   Note twist in neck.

The sagittal suture is in the antero-posterior diameter of the pelvic outlet.

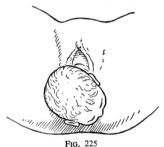

Fig. 225

RESTITUTION.

The occiput turns one-eighth of a circle
to the right.

External rotation of head.—The occiput turns a further one-eighth of a circle to the right.

Lateral flexion.—The anterior shoulder escapes under the symphysis pubis, the posterior shoulder sweeps the perineum and the body is born by a movement of lateral flexion.

THE PROBABLE COURSE OF LABOUR

1. **Long internal rotation of the head commonly takes place.**—Good uterine contractions produce flexion and descent of the head so that in 90 per cent of cases the occiput rotates forwards three-eighths as described above.   The long rotation does not necessarily take a long time as the head rotates quite rapidly once it reaches the pelvic floor.

2. **Short internal rotation of the head takes place in 10 per cent of posterior position** because flexion of the head does not occur.   The sinciput reaches the pelvic floor first rotates forwards and the baby is born face to pubes.

CLINICAL FEATURES

1. **Labour may be prolonged,** for the following reasons:

(*a*) **Larger diameters of the skull** present, and the suboccipito-frontal diameter 10·2 cm. (4 inches) instead of the suboccipito-bregmatic diameter 9·5 cm. (3¾ inches) will have to pass through the pelvis.

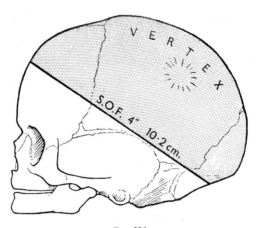

FIG. 226

The suboccipito-frontal diameter of the skull passes through
the birth canal in posterior vertex positions.

(*b*) **The os will have to dilate to a greater extent** to allow passage of the larger circumference of the head.

(*c*) **The anterior lip of cervix may be nipped** between the head and the pubic bone.

(*d*) **Weak uterine contractions are sometimes associated with occipito-posterior positions,** because the deflexed head does not fit snugly into the lower uterine segment and stimulate the cervical nerve endings.

(*e*) **The deflexed head does not dilate the cervix effectively.**

(*f*) **The head may be arrested in the transverse diameter of the pelvic cavity.**

(*g*) **The head may be born face to pubes.**

2. **The necessity for interference is greater.**—More vaginal examinations are needed because of delay in progress. **Paracervical nerve block or epidural analgesia** may be used for backache during the last hours of the first stage. Rotation of the head may have to be assisted manually or by forceps; application of forceps is frequently required because of delay in the second stage, or on account of fetal or maternal distress.

Traction by the Malmstrom extractor (ventouse) facilitates internal rotation and descent of the head.

3. **The fetal mortality and morbidity rates are higher** because of intracranial injury and anoxia.

SUMMARY OF CLINICAL FEATURES

The head descends slowly, even when there are good contractions.

The uterine contractions are sometimes weak.

Dilatation of the os is retarded.

The membranes usually rupture early.

Backache is frequently complained of.

Difficulty in micturition is common and may necessitate catheterization.

The urge to bear down at the end of the first stage is especially great, probably because the occiput is pressing on the rectum.

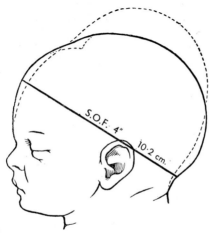

Fig. 227

Moulding of the head in an occipito-posterior position of the vertex. Shown by dotted line.

NURSING CARE

Although only 20 per cent of these patients will have a prolonged or difficult labour, such a possibility should be anticipated in every case so that further complications can be averted. Additional nursing care, including observation of the maternal and fetal conditions, **as described for prolonged labour (p. 410), will be** necessary.

DEEP TRANSVERSE ARREST

Transverse arrest of the head may be associated with occipito-posterior positions of the vertex, but it occurs more frequently in cases in which the occiput is lateral, *i.e.* L.O.L. or R.O.L. when flexion does not take place at pelvic floor level.

21

The head is arrested deep in the pelvic cavity, with the sagittal suture in the transverse diameter of the pelvis. Arrest may be due to weak contractions.

It is sometimes associated with the type of pelvis with a straight sacrum, or with one that is narrowed at the bispinous diameter of the outlet, and the occiput is prevented from rotating forwards.

Unless the head becomes flexed no rotation can take place because there is no leading part.

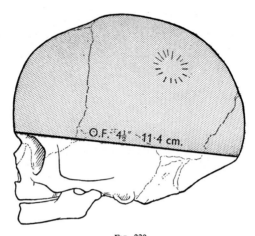

Fig. 228

Diameter engaging in face to pubes position.
Occipito-frontal 11·4 cm. (4½ inches).

DIAGNOSIS

Deep transverse arrest would be suspected when, after half an hour (or less) of second stage contractions, the head is not visible at the vulva.

On vaginal examination the sagittal suture will be felt in the transverse with a fontanelle at either end. The head will be at the level of the ischial spines, although the caput may be below this.

Treatment

Medical assistance should be obtained, and pending the doctor's arrival the woman could be given an inhalational analgesic. Perineal infiltration or pudendal nerve block should be anticipated and preparations made for catheterization, episiotomy, forceps delivery, the reception of an anoxic baby and perineal suturing.

The doctor will attempt to increase flexion by pushing up the sinciput and with his whole hand in the vagina will rotate the head. The midwife may be asked to push the anterior shoulder forwards and hold it there while the doctor applies forceps. Obstetricians frequently rotate the head with Kielland's forceps.

UNREDUCED OCCIPITO-POSTERIOR

When the occiput fails to rotate forward in an R.O.P., it is known as a right unreduced occipito-posterior or R.U.O.P. The occiput goes into the hollow of the sacrum and the term " *persistent occipito-posterior* " is sometimes applied. The baby is born face to pubes.

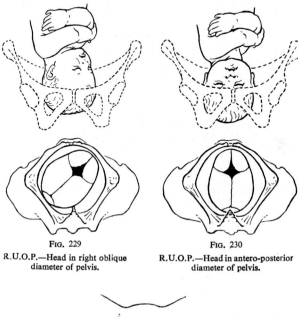

FIG. 229

R.U.O.P.—Head in right oblique
diameter of pelvis.

FIG. 230

R.U.O.P.—Head in antero-posterior
diameter of pelvis.

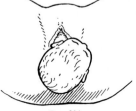

FIG. 231

Restitution.—Sinciput turns to
the left.

CAUSES

1. **Deficient flexion of the head and spine.**—In posterior positions the fetus tends to adopt the military attitude and the occipito-frontal diameter, 11·4 cm. (4½ inches), presents in the right oblique diameter of the pelvic brim. The wide biparietal diameter being posterior is liable to be caught in the sacro-cotyloid diameter, 8·9 cm. (3½ inches). (*If the head becomes flexed, the parietal eminences are brought forwards and clear the sacro-cotyloid diameter.*)   Descent of the occiput is retarded, and if the sinciput becomes the leading part it reaches the pelvic floor first and rotates forwards.

2. Small head or large pelvis.—If the head is small in relation to the pelvis, it need not flex before descent can take place and in that case the sinciput might reach the pelvic floor first and rotate forwards.

The occipito-frontal diameter of the head engages with the sagittal suture in the right oblique diameter of the pelvic brim.

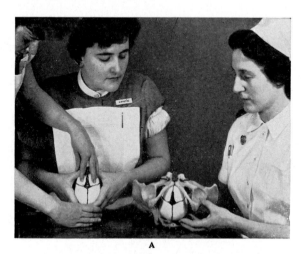

A, Holding sinciput back until occiput sweeps the perineum.

B, Bringing the face down from under the symphysis pubis by a slight movement of extension.

A

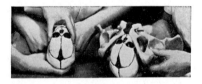

Labour ward superintendent demonstrates. Note hands being used as vulva.

B

Fig. 232

DELIVERY FACE TO PUBES IN THE DORSAL POSITION.
(*Aberdeen Maternity Hospital.*)

SUMMARY OF MECHANISM
VERTEX. RIGHT UNREDUCED OCCIPITO-POSTERIOR POSITION

The **lie** is longitudinal.	The **denominator** is the occiput.
The **attitude** is " military."	The **presenting part** is the anterior area of the left parietal bone.
The **presentation** is the vertex.	
The **position** is the R.U.O.P.	The **leading part** is the sinciput.

Descent takes place with deficient flexion. The biparietal diameter is held up in the sacro-cotyloid diameter. The sinciput becomes the leading part.

Internal rotation.—The sinciput reaches the pelvic floor first, rotates one-eighth of a circle forwards along the left side of the pelvis, and impinges on the under surface of the symphysis pubis.

Flexion and extension.—The occiput sweeps the perineum and the head is born by a movement of flexion, followed by a slight movement of extension which brings the face down from under the symphysis pubis.

Restitution takes place. The sinciput turns to the left and the head rights itself with the shoulders.

Internal rotation of the shoulders.—The shoulders enter in the left oblique diameter of the pelvis. The anterior shoulder reaches the pelvic floor first and rotates one-eighth of a circle forwards along the right side of the pelvis.

External rotation of the head.—The head rotates a further one-eighth of a circle, sinciput to left.

Lateral flexion.—The anterior shoulder escapes under the symphysis pubis, the posterior shoulder sweeps the perineum and the body is born by a movement of lateral flexion.

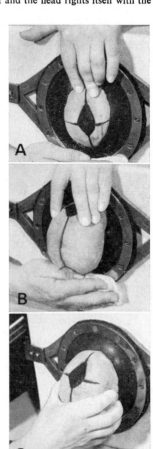

DIAGNOSIS OF FACE TO PUBES POSITION

During labour the head is slow to engage, and the usual degree of flexion does not take place. The fetal heart may be heard clearly in the midline at about umbilical level, because the chest of the fetus is in close proximity to the abdominal wall.

Delay in the second stage should arouse suspicion and a vaginal examination would reveal the anterior fontanelle behind the symphysis pubis. Sometimes the fontanelle is obliterated by a large caput and in that case the doctor will feel for the pinna of the ear which if directed towards the sacrum will determine that the occiput is posterior.

Excessive bulging of the perineum and gaping of the anus are sometimes evident because the broad biparietal diameter instead of the bitemporal is distending the perineum. In this case the head will be showing and the anterior fontanelle can be felt just below the symphysis pubis.

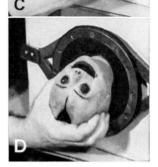

Fig. 233

Demonstrating delivery of vertex face to pubes in the dorsal position.

A, Holding the sinciput back until the occiput sweeps the perineum.

B, The occiput is born by a movement of flexion.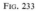

C, Grasping the head to bring the face down from under the symphysis pubis.

D, The movement is now one of extension.

(*Aberdeen Maternity Hospital.*)

Management

An episiotomy will facilitate delivery and avoid serious perineal trauma.

The midwife will maintain flexion by holding the sinciput back under the symphysis pubis so that the area anterior to the bregma will be the point which pivots under the symphysis pubis. After the occiput comes over the perineum, the midwife grasps the vertex and brings the face down from under the symphysis pubis.

UNDIAGNOSED FACE TO PUBES POSITION

The forehead is seen slipping down under the symphysis pubis, the head pivots on the glabella and the occipito-frontal diameter distends the vulval orifice. Because the biparietal diameter is also stretching the perineum, a third-degree tear is likely.

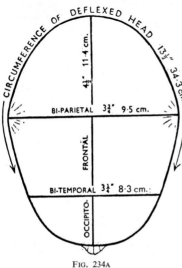

FIG. 234A

A circumference of 34·3 cm. (13½ inches) will distend the vulval orifice if flexion is not maintained. This occurs in undiagnosed cases.

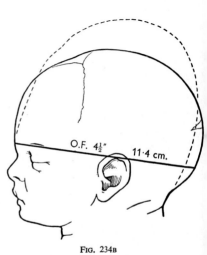

FIG. 234B

Moulding in vertex, face to pubes, shown by dotted line. Note the " sugar loaf " head.

The moulding of the head in these babies is typical, with the caput on the anterior part of the parietal bone, giving what is known as the " *sugar-loaf* " head. Because the vault of the skull is raised, intracranial injury and hæmorrhage may occur.

N.B.—It should be noted that transverse arrest never occurs in an unreduced occipito-posterior position, because the head is never in the transverse diameter of the pelvic canal.

Multiple Pregnancy

When there is more than one fetus *in utero* the term " plural " or " multiple " pregnancy is applied. Twins occur approximately once in about every 80 pregnancies, and the tendency is manifest in certain families. Triplets occur once in about every 7,000 pregnancies, quadruplets once in 500,000, but quintuplets are very rare indeed.

TWO TYPES OF TWINS

1. MONOZYGOTIC (UNIOVULAR)

Monozygotic or single ovum twins are known as **identical twins** because their physical and mental characteristics are so similar. They develop from one ovum which has been fertilized by one spermatozoon and are always of the same sex. They are definitely uniovular if they share one placenta and one chorion; a few have two chorions. There is a connection between the circulation of blood in the two babies.

DIZYGOTIC OR BINOVULAR

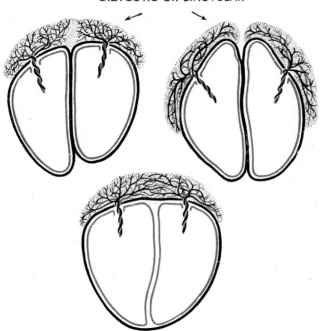

MONOZYGOTIC OR UNIOVULAR

FIG. 235

TWIN PLACENTÆ.

Dizygotic twins have two placentæ which may fuse, and two chorions. Monozygotic twins have one placenta; if they have one chorion they are definitely uniovular, but some have two chorions.

MONOZYGOTIC	DIZYGOTIC
Uniovular	*Binovular*
ONE OVUM.	TWO OVA.
ONE SPERMATOZOON.	TWO SPERMATOZOA.
ONE PLACENTA.	TWO PLACENTÆ *(may fuse)*.
ONE CHORION *(a few have two)*.	TWO CHORIONS.
TWO AMNIONS.	TWO AMNIONS.
ONE SEX.	ONE OR TWO SEXES.

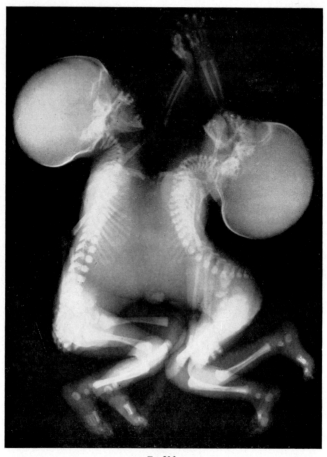

FIG 236

X-ray of conjoined twins delivered by Cæsarean section at onset of labour at 35th week of pregnancy. (Note extension of heads and spines.)

Errors in development are more likely in monozygotic twins, so abnormal fetuses are more common; conjoined twins, usually known as Siamese, are uniovular in type. The fetal mortality rate is much higher.

2. DIZYGOTIC (BINOVULAR)

Dizygotic or double ovum twins, which are five times more common than uniovular twins, develop from the fertilization of two ova and two spermatozoa.

The babies may or may not be of the same sex and their physical and mental characteristics can be as different as in any two members of one family. Dizygotic twin bearing is hereditary either through the mother or father, but probably mainly *via* the mother.

They each have a separate placenta and chorion, but, although the placentæ may fuse, the fetal circulations do not mix. The differentiation between monozygotic and dizygotic twins at birth is not always easy, because some monozygotic twins have two chorions.

If the babies are of different sexes or have two separate placentæ, they are definitely dizygotic. But sometimes the two ova embed close to each other so that the placentæ fuse and appear to the naked eye to be one single placenta. In that case, if the sex of the babies is the same, the diagnosis is made by examination of the membranes of the fetal sac, and in dizygotic twins two chorions are present.

Although twin babies are as a rule small and often premature, ranging from 2,268 G. to 2,722 G. (5 to 6 lb.), normal weights are not uncommon; the author having seen twins weighing 4,054 G. and 3,969 G. (8 lb. 15 oz. and 8 lb. 12 oz.); 4,337 G. and 4,309 G. (9 lb. 9 oz. and 9 lb. 8 oz.).

Very occasionally one fetus may die and be retained *in utero* until term when it will be expelled with the placenta as a flattened paper-like fetus—**a fetus papyraceous.**

DIAGNOSIS OF TWINS

The diagnosis of twins is not always easy in primigravid women with firm abdominal walls, or in obese women, and experienced doctors and midwives may not always detect them. The period of gestation is also difficult to assess.

ON INSPECTION

Suspicion is aroused when the uterus is unduly large for the period of gestation after the 20th week. The uterus looks round or broad and fetal movement may be seen over a wide area, but this is not diagnostic. At term, a woman of average build has an abdominal girth of about 101·6 cm. (40 inches). The possibility of hydramnios must be considered, and it can be present in conjunction with or independent of twins, but palpation should help to clinch the diagnosis.

ON PALPATION

Finding two heads is diagnostic.—When one head lies in the fundus and one in the lower pole, they are more readily palpated; but in 40 per cent of cases both fetuses present by the vertex, and the second head may be palpated in the iliac fossa. If one fetus lies in front of the other, it may not be easy to detect two heads or two backs.

Should the fetal head seem small in comparison with the size of the uterus this rather suggests the presence of two fetuses.

Excessive fetal parts might make one surmise that twins were present.

AUSCULTATION

Hearing two fetal hearts is not a reliable method of diagnosis because with a large, vigorous fetus, the fetal heart can sometimes be heard over a wide area.

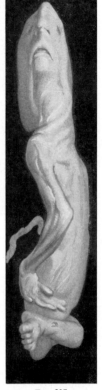

FIG. 237

FETUS PAPYRACEOUS.

Drawing of a specimen in the classroom for student midwives at the Simpson Memorial Maternity Pavilion, Edinburgh.

Ultrasonics will demonstrate two heads at mid-term. Two gestational sacs have been seen at eight weeks.

X-RAYS MAY BE USED AFTER THE 30th WEEK

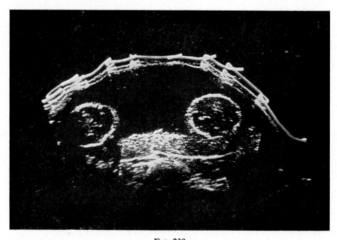

Fig. 238.
ULTRASONOGRAM.

Twins at 21½ weeks gestation demonstrated by both heads seen in oblique section.
Note placenta (speckled area situated posteriorly near the bottom of the picture.)
(*Courtesy of Queen Mother's Maternity Hospital, Glasgow*).

UNSUSPECTED TWINS

These may first be diagnosed by finding the uterus large and the fundus well above the umbilicus after the birth of the first baby. The presence of fetal parts and hearing the fetal heart will confirm the diagnosis.

THE EFFECT OF TWINS ON PREGNANCY

1. **Pre-eclampsia** is more common than in single pregnancies.

2. **Hydramnios** occurs with twins and adds to the woman's discomfort. Acute hydramnios is almost invariably associated with twins: the usual outcome being abortion.

3. **Anæmia** develops because of the increased fetal demands for iron : the incidence of megaloblastic anæmia is increased and may be suspected by a sudden fall in hæmoglobin.

4. **Pressure symptoms** due to the weight and size of the uterus may be troublesome. (*a*) The tendency to œdema of the ankles and varicose veins is increased because of pressure on the veins returning blood from the lower limbs. (*b*) Dyspnœa, bladder irritability, constipation and indigestion are more marked.

5. **The minor disorders and general discomforts of pregnancy are more pronounced:** morning sickness, nausea and heartburn are more persistent. General ungainliness, œdema, varicose veins and backache are common complaints.

MANAGEMENT OF PREGNANCY

NUTRITION

As soon as twins are diagnosed a close check should be kept on the mother's **hæmoglobin** and advice given regarding foods rich in iron. Ferrous preparations are usually prescribed and vitamin supplements are essential. Most obstetricians give a preparation of folic acid *e.g.* Fefol, 0·5 mg., daily and until four weeks after delivery.

The woman should drink at least 1,200 ml. (2 pints) of milk daily to prevent her calcium reserves from being depleted. Her protein intake must be adequate, a moderate salt diet should be advocated.

In order to detect pre-eclampsia which is three times more common in multiple pregnancy, the woman is seen weekly from the time twins are diagnosed, *i.e.* the 20th week.

To relieve the discomfort of a heavy uterus, a good supporting maternity belt will be appreciated. A "roll-on" worn at night in the later weeks gives abdominal support, and extra pillows are needed for sleep, as the woman feels more comfortable when propped up. When lying on her side a small pillow tucked under her abdomen will ease any dragging sensation. **Vague pains due to overstretched muscles and ligaments,** as well as the excessive fetal movements, tend to disturb sleep and in some cases a mild sedative is necessary.

Adequate rest is essential during the last 12 weeks to increase uterine blood flow.

The woman should be admitted to hospital from the 30th to the 36th week to avoid premature labour by providing rest, and to improve her nutrition. This measure will, it is hoped, reduce the high perinatal mortality rate in twins.

She should not be permitted to go beyond term but the majority start labour prior to then.

THE EFFECT OF TWINS ON LABOUR

Although multiple pregnancy may not be regarded as abnormal in itself, many complications that endanger fetal and maternal life do arise (see p. 353).

Labour is often premature: the babies tend to be immature even when at term, especially if the mother is suffering from pre-eclampsia. The smaller baby may be dysmature so the blood glucose should be assessed (see p. 547).

The perinatal mortality rate is about 10 per cent, as against less than 3 per cent in single births.

The mortality rate of the second twin is twice that of the first, and this may be due to reduction in the placental circulation and partial separation of placenta following the birth of the first twin.

For these reasons hospitalization for delivery is advocated.

THE MANAGEMENT OF LABOUR

Heavy sedation should be avoided.

If delay occurs due to hypotonic uterine action an oxytocin drip may be given after puncture of the membranes and kept running until both babies and placentæ are delivered.

PREPARATIONS SHOULD BE MADE FOR:

1. **The reception of two immature babies,** who may show signs of asphyxia or intracranial injury. Additional swabs, cord clamps, ligatures, scissors and mucus

extractors and baby blankets should be set out. Two incubators or cots should be in readiness.

2. The treatment of shock and hæmorrhage.

The room ought to be warm, and extra cotton blankets should be available for the slight degree of shock that often follows delivery because of marked reduction in abdominal pressure.

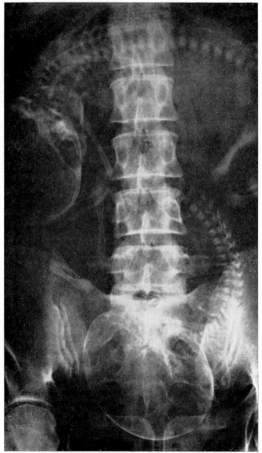

FIG. 239

Twins. One is presenting by the vertex; the other is lying transversely in the fundus

(*Simpson Memorial Maternity Pavilion, Edinburgh*)

Ergometrine 0·5 mg. or Syntometrine 1 ml. should be drawn up in readiness to be given as soon as the placentæ are born, or during the third stage if hæmorrhage occurs. It is a wise precaution to have 600 ml. of compatible blood available.

Active Treatment

The woman will be more comfortable if delivered in the dorsal position with additional pillows if necessary.

Perineal infiltration or pudendal nerve block is commonly employed.

An episiotomy is made *in an endeavour to lower the high perinatal mortality rate.*

The airway of the first baby is cleared.

The cord should be ligatured in two places, for although the placental end of the cord is tied or clamped at every delivery, it is because of the possibility of undiagnosed monozygotic twins that this is done.

The first baby, after being marked No. 1, is laid in a warm cot and the midwife keeps her " *ear and eye on it.* "

The abdomen is palpated without delay to ensure that the lie of the second twin is longitudinal. Presentation and position are diagnosed, but are of less importance: **the fetal heart is listened to.** After swabbing the vulva, clean drapes are applied and the limbs and chest covered with warm cellular cotton blankets.

The midwife stands by. She will closely observe the uterus, probably keeping her hand lightly on it to detect uterine contractions.

The fetal heart should be checked frequently.

With three or four good contractions and the woman pushing effectively the second baby ought to be born. But if, when 5 minutes have elapsed, contractions have not recommenced, the midwife should scrub up and after making sure that the head or the breech is presenting she should puncture the bag of membranes and massage the uterus to stimulate uterine action.

The second baby should be born within 20 minutes after the first baby.

(Doctors in hospital frequently deliver the second baby within a few minutes.)

Ergometrine, 0·5 mg., or Syntometrine, 1 ml., should be given intramuscularly as soon as the placentæ are born to prevent postpartum hæmorrhage. Warm cotton blankets are used if necessary. The woman should not be left until at least two hours after the birth of the placentæ, and to ensure sleep a sedative is given.

COMPLICATIONS AND INDICATIONS FOR MEDICAL ASSISTANCE

1. **TRANSVERSE LIE OF THE SECOND TWIN.**

2. **DELAY IN THE BIRTH OF THE SECOND TWIN.**

3. **PROLAPSE OF CORD** because of malpresentation and hydramnios (see p. 421).

4. **THE EXPULSION OF A PLACENTA OR BLEEDING BEFORE THE BIRTH OF THE SECOND TWIN.**

5. **POSTPARTUM HÆMORRHAGE** is said to occur due to the overdistended uterus and large placental site from which an atonic uterus can bleed, but this is not usually excessive.

6 **LOCKED TWINS.**

1. TRANSVERSE LIE OF THE SECOND TWIN

If, after the birth of the first baby, the second baby is found to be presenting by the shoulder, the midwife should send for the doctor, but she must act pending his arrival because of the risk that the second bag of membranes will rupture and the arm prolapse.

The midwife ought to attempt external version between contractions: this should not be unduly difficult, if the membranes are intact (see p. 612).

The doctor will probably perform internal version for transverse lie of the second twin and do a breech extraction. In very remote areas, with no medical help available, the midwife should do likewise if external version has not been successful.

2. DELAY IN THE BIRTH OF THE SECOND TWIN

Should contractions not recommence within half an hour after having punctured the membranes medical assistance must be sought. Cases are known in which two or three days have elapsed between the births of the first and second babies: this should not be permitted to occur.

The disadvantages of such delay are:

(a) The fetus *in utero* may die of anoxia should the placentæ separate.

(b) The risk of sepsis is increased when the cord is lying outside the vulva.

(c) The os closes to a certain extent and will have to dilate again.

Having ensured that the lie is longitudinal, the doctor will probably puncture the membranes, and give an oxytocin drip, then when the uterus begins to contract he may apply forceps or use the Malmstrom extractor.

4. The expulsion of a placenta or bleeding before the birth of the second twin gives warning that the placenta still *in utero* may also be separating and causing anoxia of the unborn twin; in which case, the midwife should massage the uterus and expel the second twin as soon as possible by using fundal pressure. (The usual sequence of events is for both babies to be born and then the placentæ.)

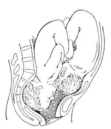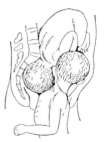

Fig. 240
Two varieties of locked twins.

5. Postpartum hæmorrhage (see p. 428).

6. Locked twins are very rare indeed, and the most serious variety occurs when the first fetus is presenting by the breech and the head of the second fetus which is presenting by the vertex gets in front of the aftercoming head of the first baby. The heads become impacted and decapitation of the head of the first baby is usually necessary.

MANAGEMENT OF THE PUERPERIUM

Involution of the uterus may be slow; afterpains are more troublesome. The care of the babies is a most urgent problem, as the number of twin babies who die is alarmingly high, the smaller one may be dysmature (small for dates) (see p. 546).

The mother will need help and advice in regard to feeding, and should not be discharged from hospital until the babies are gaining weight satisfactorily.

OCCIPITO-POSTERIOR POSITION OF THE VERTEX
ORAL QUESTIONS

Why does a high head occur in posterior positions of the vertex ? How would you diagnose posterior position on (*a*) inspection; (*b*) palpation; (*c*) auscultation.

Describe on vaginal examination: R.O.P.; deep transverse arrest.

Describe head moulding in face to pubes. How would you diagnose face to pubes when the head is on the perineum ?

Write not more than 10 lines on: (*a*) diagnosis of R.O.P. during labour; (*b*) clinical features of labour in R.O.P.; (*c*) management of transverse arrest; (*d*) delivery of baby face to pubes.

C.M.B.(Scot.) paper.—Describe how posterior position of the occiput may influence the course of labour.

C.M.B.(Scot.) paper.—What do you understand by the term " persistent occipito-posterior " ? How would you recognize that delay in labour was due to this cause?

C.M.B.(N. Ireland) paper.—How would you diagnose an occipito-posterior position in labour ? How may this position affect the course of the second stage ?

C.M.B.(Eng.) paper. 1969.—Discuss the course of labour in an occipito-posterior position and mention the common complications.

C.M.B.(Eng.) paper, 1969.—How would you diagnose an occipito-posterior position during labour? Describe the midwife's care of a young primigravida with an occipito-posterior during the first stage of labour.

C.M.B.(N. Ireland) paper, 1969.—Describe the diagnosis of an occipito-posterior position in labour. How does the degree of flexion affect the course of labour?

MULTIPLE PREGNANCY
ORAL QUESTIONS

Why is it advisable for twins to be born in hospital ? What procedures, normally outside her province, might a midwife have to perform during delivery of twins ?

Give another name for: (*a*) conjoined twins; (*b*) monozygotic twins; (*c*) fetus papyraceous. Why does the woman pregnant with twins become anæmic ? Why is folic acid always prescribed ? What advice could you give to relieve pressure symptoms ? What is the danger of giving Syntometrine in a twin labour ? How would you do external version for the second twin ? The smaller of twin babies may be dysmature; what will the midwife be required to do in such a case ?

Differentiate between: (*a*) uniovular and binovular twins; (*b*) twins and hydramnios: (*c*) multiple pregnancy and multiparity.

Write not more than 10 lines on: (*a*) the effect of twins on pregnancy; (*b*) nutrition of the pregnant woman with twins; (*c*) the effect of twins on labour; (*d*) the management of labour in twins; (*e*) delay in the birth of the second twin.

What type of twins would you diagnose if the findings were as follows:	
Type or Types	Type or Types
ONE SEX TWO CHORIONS ONE PLACENTA TWO SEXES	TWO AMNIONS TWO PLACENTÆ ONE CHORION

C.M.B.(N. Ireland) paper.—You are unexpectedly faced with the delivery of twins and the first baby has been born. Describe the subsequent conduct of the case.

C.M.B.(Scot.) paper.—What would make you suspect the presence of twins ? What complications may arise in (*a*) the ante-natal period, and (*b*) labour ?

C.M.B.(N. Ireland) paper.—How is a twin pregnancy diagnosed ? Describe the conduct of delivery from the time the first twin is born until the end of the third stage.

C.M.B.(Scot.) paper.—Describe the investigation of a patient with excessive abdominal enlargement at the 30th week of pregnancy.

C.M.B.(N. Ireland) paper, 1969.—Describe the conduct of a twin *delivery*.

C.M.B. (Scot.) paper, 1969.—Describe the management of labour in a multiple pregnancy. What complications may arise?

C.M.B. (Scot.) paper, 1969.—Describe the management of labour in a twin pregnancy.

21

Malpresentations

BREECH PRESENTATION

IN breech or pelvic presentation, the fetus lies with its buttocks in the lower pole of the uterus.

VARIETIES

1. COMPLETE BREECH

The fetal attitude is one of complete flexion, thighs and legs both flexed.

2. INCOMPLETE BREECH

(*a*) **Breech with extended legs (frank breech).** The legs are extended on the abdomen thighs flexed.

(*b*) **Footling presentation** (*rare*). One or both feet present because neither thighs nor legs are fully flexed.

(*c*) **Knee presentation** (*rarer still*). Thighs are extended, one or both legs are flexed

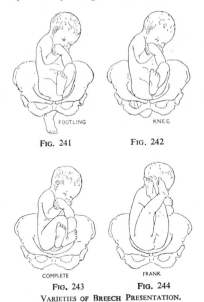

FIG. 241   FIG. 242

FIG. 243   FIG. 244

VARIETIES OF BREECH PRESENTATION.

POSITIONS

There are six positions, the denominator being the sacrum.

Right sacro-posterior	R.S.P.	Left sacro-posterior	L.S.P.
,, ,, lateral	R.S.I.	,, ,, lateral	L.S.L.
,, ,, anterior	R.S.A.	,, ,, anterior	L.S.A.

FREQUENCY

Breech presentation occurs in about 3·3 per cent of cases after the 34th week of pregnancy. During mid-term the frequency is higher because the greater ratio of liquor facilitates spontaneous version of the fetus.

CAUSES

In the majority of cases there is no obvious reason why the fetus presents by the breech at term, for the ovoid shape of the uterine cavity and greater breadth in the fundus is conducive to cephalic presentation:—

1. EXTENDED LEGS.   3. PREMATURITY.   5. HYDRAMNIOS
2. MULTIPLE PREGNANCY.   4. MULTIPARITY.   6. HYDROCEPHALY.

Extended legs occur in over 60 per cent of cases commonly in **primigravid women** with high uterine muscle tone and this inhibits the free turning of the fetus which usually occurs at mid-term.

The cavity of the uterus may be round because of excessive liquor as in hydramnios; or because the uterine muscle is lax as in multiparity, or a combination of both as in multiple pregnancy. Movement of the fetus is thereby facilitated at the time when the presentation should be stable. Prior to the 34th week the ratio of liquor is greater.

The fetal head may be proportionately large as in hydrocephaly or to some extent in the premature baby and can be more readily accommodated in the fundus.

PRENATAL DIAGNOSIS

This may not be easy in the primigravid woman who has firm abdominal muscles. (The figures of undiagnosed breech presentation range from 10 to 15 per cent, depending on the skill of the person who is palpating.)

ABDOMINAL EXAMINATION

INSPECTION

The abdominal contour of the complete breech is not different from that of the vertex presentation.

PALPATION

1. **At the pelvic brim a large, soft, indefinite mass is felt.**

2. **In the fundus, at one or other side, a round, hard mass may be detected,** and by ballotting this mass with one or both hands it can be made to move independently of the back (nodding of the head). To identify the head, the fetal back is grasped between the palms of both hands and an attempt made to ballott with the fingers what is thought to be the head.

If the breech is anterior and the fetus well flexed it may be difficult to locate the head. In that case the woman should be turned on her side and if the under-surface of the uterus is palpated and percussed deeply the hard head may then be detected. If doubt still exists, the combined grip is useful (p. 116).

AUSCULTATION

The fetal heart is heard at or above the level of the umbilicus in a complete breech, because (1) the presenting part is high; and (2) the fetal heart is further from the buttocks than from the head.

PRENATAL TREATMENT

If the midwife suspects or detects a breech presentation on or after the 32nd week she should arrange for her patient to see a doctor or attend a prenatal clinic.

X-rays are not employed as frequently as formerly, because of radiation hazards, except in cases of failed version.

The following points are noted on X-ray :

1. The size and shape of the pelvis.
2. Size of the fetus.
3. Whether the legs are extended.
4. Fetal abnormalities, *e.g.* hydrocephaly.

External Version

External version is usually attempted (if no contraindications exist) for two reasons:

1. Cephalo-pelvic disproportion cannot be detected unless the head is at the pelvic brim.

2. To avoid the dangers to the fetus of breech delivery.

The optimal time for performing version is between the 32nd and 36th week: but some authorities do so earlier. If external version fails a careful assessment of the pelvis is made.

Spontaneous cephalic version may take place up to the 34th week (*rarely later*). The risks of external version are rupture of membranes and placental separation due to traction on the cord, but these are less frequent than the actual dangers of breech delivery. The midwife's duties during external version are described on page 614.

Contraindications

The doctor is likely to decide against external version if there is antepartum hæmorrhage or if a Cæsarean section has previously been performed.

If the fetus is hydrocephalic, breech presentation is an advantage, as it may be possible after the buttocks are born to drain off the cerebro-spinal fluid *via* the spinal canal.

MECHANISM OF LABOUR

LEFT SACRO-ANTERIOR, L.S.A.

Lie, longitudinal.

Attitude, complete flexion.

Presentation, breech.

Position, left sacro-anterior.

Denominator, sacrum.

Presenting part, anterior buttock.

The bitrochanteric diameter, 10·2 cm. (4 inches), enters in the left oblique diameter of the pelvic brim. The sacrum points to the left ilio-pectineal eminence.

Descent takes place with increasing compaction, due to increased flexion of limbs.

Internal rotation of the buttocks.—The anterior buttock reaches the pelvic floor first and rotates one-eighth of a circle forwards along the right side of the pelvis. The bitrochanteric diameter is now in the antero-posterior diameter of the outlet.

Lateral flexion of the body.—The anterior buttock escapes under the symphysis pubis, the posterior buttock sweeps the perineum and the buttocks are born by a movement of lateral flexion.

Restitution of the buttocks.—The anterior buttock turns slightly to the patient's right side.

Internal rotation of the shoulders.—The shoulders enter in the same oblique of the brim as the buttocks—the left oblique. The anterior shoulder rotates forwards one-eighth of a circle along the right side of the pelvis and escapes under the symphysis pubis, the posterior shoulder sweeps the perineum and the shoulders are born.

Internal rotation of the head.—The head enters in the transverse diameter of the pelvic brim. The occiput rotates forwards along the left side, and the sub-occipital region (*nape of the neck*) impinges on the under surface of the symphysis pubis.

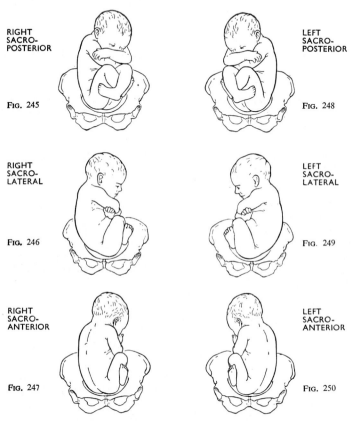

RIGHT
SACRO-
POSTERIOR

FIG. 245

LEFT
SACRO-
POSTERIOR

FIG. 248

RIGHT
SACRO-
LATERAL

FIG. 246

LEFT
SACRO-
LATERAL

FIG. 249

RIGHT
SACRO-
ANTERIOR

FIG. 247

LEFT
SACRO-
ANTERIOR

FIG. 250

SIX POSITIONS IN BREECH PRESENTATION.

External rotation of the body.—The body turns so that the back is uppermost, a movement which accompanies internal rotation of the head.

Birth of the head.—The chin, face and sinciput sweep the perineum and the head is born in a flexed attitude.

RIGHT SACRO-ANTERIOR

The mechanism of the right sacro-anterior, R.S.A., is the same as in the L.S.A. except that " right " is substituted for " left "

SACRO-POSTERIOR

The mechanism of the right sacro-posterior, R.S.P., is the same as in the L.S.A. There is no three-eighths rotation forwards as in a posterior vertex, because the leading part is the anterior buttock and no matter whether the sacrum is anterior or posterior one buttock will be in the anterior part of the pelvis. One-eighth rotation forwards is all that is necessary.

The mechanism of the left sacro-posterior, L.S.P., is the same regarding rotation as in the R.S.P. except that " left " is substituted for " right."

DANGERS OF BREECH PRESENTATION

MATERNAL

The hazards to the mother are increased because of the conditions giving rise to breech presentation, *e.g.* hydrocephaly. Cephalo-pelvic disproportion may not be apparent until the baby is born as far as the umbilicus, and the necessary interference in dealing with the obstruction causes tissue trauma.

DANGERS TO THE BABY

The dangers to the baby are very great indeed and except in the hands of experts the perinatal mortality rate is 20 per cent. It has been proved that fetal loss in multigravid women is equal to that in primigravidæ, probably because the delivery is often conducted by less experienced persons.

Some induce labour at 38 weeks if the fetus is large.

(1) PREMATURITY

Prematurity, particularly if the baby weighs under 1,814 G. (4 lb.) intensifies all the other dangers and 50 per cent of breech stillbirths are premature. The skull bones are soft and the brain is easily damaged. The relatively large head may be " held up " by a cervix which has allowed extended legs to pass, causing dangerous delay and anoxia. (*The complete breech dilates the cervix to a greater extent.*)

(2) INTRACRANIAL HÆMORRHAGE

This is due to the rapid compression of the aftercoming head which has not had the opportunity of slow moulding as when the vertex presents.

The severe compression of the head on the pelvic floor and its sudden release when extracted quickly (like a cork out of a bottle) also produce intracranial trauma.

To avoid this an episiotomy is made.

(3) ANOXIA

This may be due to the following causes:

(A) *Interference with the Utero-placental Circulation*

(*a*) By the application of fundal pressure (*inadvisedly*).

(*b*) When the placenta separates while the head is still in the vagina.

(*c*) By marked retraction of the placental site before birth of the head.

(B) *Interference with the Cord Circulation*

(*a*) Cord compression. This is inevitable with a large baby and when the legs are extended, because the cord becomes nipped when the fetal head enters the pelvic brim. (The head does not enter the brim until the baby presenting by the breech is born as far as the umbilicus.)

(*b*) **Prolapse of cord.** This occurs because the complete breech is a badly fitting presenting part and also because the umbilicus is so near the buttocks.

(C) *Premature Inspiration*

If the oxygen supply is diminished because of the preceding causes the fetus will be stimulated to breathe and will inhale liquor or mucus which may prevent expansion of the lungs at birth and may cause pneumonia.

4. INJURIES

The fetus is usually injured because of rough or wrong handling. Patience and gentleness are needed, but when interference becomes imperative the midwife must know how to avoid injuries to the baby such as:

(*a*) **Fractures of humerus** or clavicle when dealing with extended arms.

(*b*) **Damage to the brachial plexus** by twisting the neck, causing Erb's paralysis.

(*c*) **Ruptured liver,** produced by grasping the abdomen.

(*d*) **Damage to adrenals** by grasping the baby's body at kidney level.

(*e*) **Crushing the spinal cord** or fracturing the neck by bending the body backwards over the symphysis pubis while delivering the head.

Bruising and congestion of the external genitalia may occur, especially when the legs are extended.

MANAGEMENT OF LABOUR

Because of the risks to the fetus, multigravidæ as well as primigravidæ should be delivered in hospital where expert assistance is available. The woman should not be allowed to go beyond her dates; labour is induced. Cæsarean section may be necessary when complications other than breech presentation exist, *i.e.* infertility, older primigravida, bad obstetric history.

THE PRINCIPLES OF TREATMENT ARE:

1. **Patience and the avoidance of unnecessary interference.**

2. **Prompt intelligent action,** carried out with manual dexterity when assistance is needed.

3. **The avoidance of fetal injury and anoxia.**

THE FIRST STAGE OF LABOUR

Labour is conducted in the same manner as in vertex presentation. An enema should be given, and if the breech is engaged the woman ought to be allowed up until the need for analgesia arises. (Early rupture of membranes cannot be avoided by keeping the woman in the recumbent position, and it is also doubtful whether prolapse of cord can be prevented by that means.)

The passage of meconium during the first stage should be considered a sign of fetal distress.

VAGINAL EXAMINATION

A vaginal examination is always made in breech presentation, immediately after the membranes rupture, for the following reasons:

1. **To find out whether the cord has prolapsed.**

2. **To ascertain whether the breech is complete or incomplete.**

3. **To determine the dilatation of the os.**

1. **Prolapse of cord** is probably the cardinal indication for making the vaginal examination and is a serious complication.

2. **Complete breech.**—A high, soft, irregular mass presents, with feet lying alongside the buttocks: sacrum and coccyx are recognizable. The anal sphincter will grip the examining finger. (Meconium on the examining finger is diagnostic of breech presentation.)

Incomplete breech.—If the legs are extended, no feet are felt. The external genitalia are very evident.

In a footling presentation doubt may arise as to whether the prolapsed limb is a hand or a foot. Toes are all the same length; they are shorter than fingers and the great toe cannot be abducted. The foot is at right angles to the leg and the os calcis (heel bone) has no equivalent on the hand.

3. **Dilatation of the os.**—This ought to be carefully assessed, because it is important that the midwife should be aware when the first stage is completed.

SEDATION

Dichloralphenazone (Welldorm) tablets may be prescribed and followed later, if necessary, by two doses of pethidine, 100 mg., to ensure rest, so that the woman will have energy to co-operate by pushing during the second stage.

THE AVOIDANCE OF PREMATURE PUSHING

No pushing should be permitted until the buttocks are bulging at the vulva.

In a footling presentation the os may be only half dilated when the foot appears at the vulva. (It is possible that with extended legs the os may not be fully dilated although the buttocks are visible on separating the labia.) If the buttocks are forced through an imperfectly dilated cervix, the birth of the head may be delayed at the critical moment after the shoulders are born.

The head of the premature baby, being proportionately large, is liable to be held up by the cervix which has not been fully dilated by the smaller buttock mass.

THE SECOND STAGE

When the buttocks are bulging at the vulva, the woman should be lying on her back, with two pillows under her head, and encouraged to bear down. The temptation to assist, by using fundal pressure, must be resisted in case the placental circulation is impeded, oxygen supply reduced and the fetus stimulated to breathe *in utero*.

Using traction is much more liable to cause extension of arms and head than the mother's expulsive efforts so she must be encouraged to push.

PREPARATIONS FOR DELIVERY

The room should be warm and the cot ready to receive an anoxic baby. Mucus extractors may be needed.

The bladder should be empty so that supra-pubic pressure will be effective and bladder injury avoided.

Syringes, a local analgesic, requirements for pudendal nerve block, scissors and suturing requirements ought to be set out for a large episiotomy.

Some obstetricians prefer that an anaesthetist be present at every breech delivery.

Forceps for the aftercoming head should always be in readiness, for, if required, there must be no delay. This is a routine procedure in some centres, to give adequate control of the head.

The paediatrician is present in a number of hospitals to take charge of the baby.

POSITION FOR DELIVERY

In undiagnosed cases delivered at home the woman lies in the cross bed position, with each foot on a chair. With the buttocks at the edge of the bed it is possible to allow the baby to hang and to apply supra-pubic pressure to the head if required.

The midwife would be justified in making an episiotomy, *e.g.* a primigravid woman, or a multigravida with a small or very large baby.

The fetal heart is checked after every contraction, but, unless the placental circulation is being interfered with, the fetal heart should remain good. Cord compression does not occur until the head enters the brim, *i.e.* the baby is born as far as the umbilicus.

(It is essential that a doctor or senior midwife, who is competent and thoroughly experienced in breech deliveries, should be scrubbed up in readiness to assist the novice should the need arise.)

The administration of Syntometrine is delayed until the baby is born.

BIRTH OF THE BABY

The buttocks should be expelled by the unaided, bearing-down efforts of the mother and it is therefore an advantage to have a conscious patient so that she can co-operate.

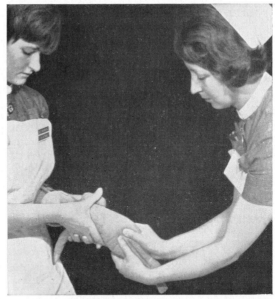

Fig. 251

STUDENT MIDWIVES PRACTISING DELIVERY OF BREECH.

Grasping iliac crests: 2 thumbs on sacrum to avoid compression of adrenals: using downward traction to deliver anterior shoulder.

(*Aberdeen Maternity Hospital classroom*)

" **Hands off the breech** " is a good motto at this stage for the midwife, who should exhort the woman to push. The buttocks curve upwards, the feet become disengaged at the vulva, and with the same contraction the baby is born as far as the umbilicus. *Doctors in hospital tend to do an " episiotomy and assisted breech delivery"; some give a pudendal nerve block.*

A loop of cord is pulled down, mainly to avoid traction on the umbilicus. The cord should be handled gently to avoid inducing spasm of the cord vessels; traction on the cord occurs if it is not pulled down and this will also induce spasm. If the cord is being nipped under the pubic arch it should be moved down to the perineum.

The cord pulsations at this stage are almost certain to be slow, but the midwife should not become agitated, because, if the delivery is hurried, intracranial hæmorrhage will probably occur and the baby be less likely to survive. The fetus will stand 8 to 10 minutes of cord compression and more babies die of intracranial damage, due to rapid extraction, than of anoxia because of cord compression.

Feel if the elbows are on the chest: they usually are. Wait calmly for the next contraction. Do not hurry the birth of the baby.

DELIVERY OF THE SHOULDERS

The weight of the buttocks will bring the shoulders down on to the pelvic floor, where they will rotate into the antero-posterior diameter of the outlet.

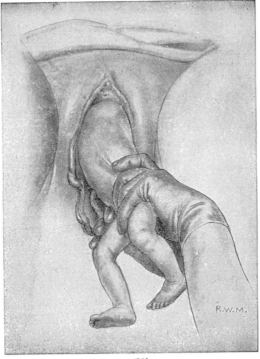

FIG. 252
Delivery of the anterior shoulder.

The midwife can assist the expulsion of the shoulders by using downward traction while the uterus is contracting and the woman pushing.

The baby should be grasped by the iliac crests (*with thumbs on the sacrum and not high enough to compress the adrenals*). A towel may be wrapped round the baby's hips as it is slippery to hold but this should not interfere with the necessary manipulation.

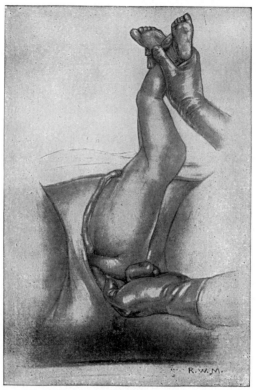

FIG. 253
Delivery of the posterior shoulder.

When the anterior shoulder escapes, the buttocks are elevated to allow the posterior shoulder and arm to pass over the perineum.

The back must not be turned uppermost until the shoulders have been born, in order that the head will descend through the transverse diameter of the pelvis. If the back is turned up before the shoulders are born, the head will enter the antero-posterior diameter of the brim and become extended; the shoulders may then become impacted at the outlet and the extended head may cause difficulty.

DELIVERY OF THE HEAD

The Burns Marshall Method

As soon as the shoulders are born, the infant is allowed to hang by its own weight, which brings the head down to the pelvic floor on which the occiput rotates forwards.

If the occiput fails to rotate forwards two fingers should be placed on the malar bones and the head rotated.

The back is now uppermost.—Gradually the neck elongates, the hair-line appears and the sub-occipital region can be felt. The baby can be allowed to hang for one or two minutes.

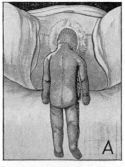
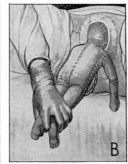

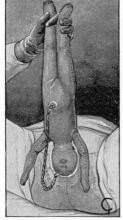

(A) Baby hangs for one or two minutes until the hair-line appears.

(B) Baby grasped by the feet and held on the stretch.

(C) Mouth and nose are free. The vault of the head is delivered slowly.

Fig. 254

THE BURNS MARSHALL METHOD OF DELIVERY.

The baby is grasped by the feet and held on the stretch; sufficient traction being applied to prevent the baby's neck from bending backwards and being fractured. The sub-occipital region, and not the neck, should pivot under the apex of the pubic arch, or the spinal cord may be crushed.

The feet are taken up through an arc of 180 degrees until the mouth and nose are free at the vulva.

The baby is now being held upside down and any mucus or liquor can drain from the lungs and trachea. Mechanical suction or mucus extractors may be used. The nose and mouth are wiped with gauze swabs. If the airway is clear the baby will breathe because lungs, trachea, nose and mouth are free. Two or three minutes should elapse to allow the vault of the head to be expelled, and this is best accomplished when the mother takes deliberate regular breaths—" **breathing the head out.**"

The use of the Burns-Marshall manœuvre has reduced the perinatal mortality rate, because the unhurried gentle delivery of a well-flexed head prevents intracranial injury. This method can be recommended to midwives, but the hair-line must be visible and the body and neck kept on the stretch. **Suprapubic pressure may be required** to aid expulsion of the head.

BREECH WITH EXTENDED LEGS

The frank breech occurs in about 60 per cent of breech presentations and is commonly found in primigravid women, probably because firm uterine walls and strong abdominal muscles predispose to a more rigid attitude of the fetus.

DIAGNOSIS

ON INSPECTION
The uterus looks long and narrow.

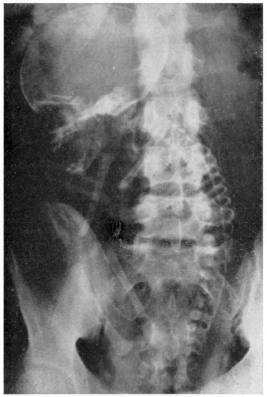

Fig. 255
X-ray of frank breech.
Simpson Memorial Maternity Pavilion, Edinburgh.)

ON PALPATION

The frank breech forms a snug, firm mass that may engage before labour begins and may easily be mistaken for the head. If the breech does not engage, the straight spine may cause the head to be pushed under the costal margin where it is not readily palpated. (The woman complains of pain in that region when she is sitting.) The nodding movement of the head is not manifest if the head is caught between the feet; the knobbly feet and knees are not palpable.

Failed external version is suggestive of extended legs.

ON AUSCULTATION

The fetal heart will be heard below the umbilicus when the frank breech is engaged, and this adds to the likelihood of the diagnosis of vertex, L.O.A., head engaged—instead of breech, L.S.A.

PER VAGINAM

If, after the os is four fingers dilated, no feet can be felt, the legs are extended. The buttocks are firm to the touch, round and smooth because the presenting mass is more compact. The external genitalia are more evident.

MANAGEMENT OF EXTENDED LEGS

The frank breech is a better fitting presenting part than the complete breech, so it descends more rapidly during the first stage. The os dilates more quickly and the risk of cord compression is greater but prolapse of cord is less likely. Some delay may occur at the outlet (p. 373).

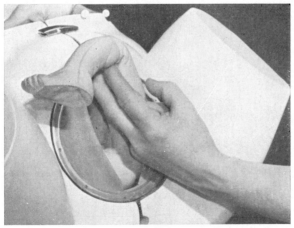

FIG. 256

CLASSROOM DEMONSTRATION OF ASSISTING DELIVERY OF EXTENDED LEGS AT
THE VULVAL ORIFICE
Pressure on popliteal space. Splinting and abduction of femur.
Flexion of knee joint. Extraction of foot.
(*Aberdeen Maternity Hospital.*)

The baby can be born with its legs extended, but some assistance is usually required. When the popliteal fossæ appear at the vulva pressure on the fossa of the most accessible leg combined with abduction of the thigh will flex the knee and aid extraction of the foot from the vagina.

THE LØVSET MANŒUVRE

This manœuvre is a combination of rotation and downward traction, that can be used successfully **whether the arms are extended, flexed, or round the nape of the neck.** It makes delivery of inaccessible extended arms possible, and is efficacious in cases when, because of a large baby, there is no room in the vagina for manipulation in bringing arms down.

Procedure (L.S.A.)

When the umbilicus is born and the shoulders are in the antero-posterior diameter, traction is applied until the axilla is visible, the midwife grasping the baby by the iliac crests with thumbs on the sacrum. While doing so the body is raised to allow the posterior shoulder to descend.

The body is rotated half a circle, 180 degrees (when starting rotation the back must be turned **uppermost** in order that the shoulders may enter the transverse of the pelvic brim). The posterior arm is now anterior and is delivered from under the pubic arch by splinting the humerus or drawing down the elbow if the arm is not born without aid.

Steady downward traction must be maintained throughout the manœuvre or it will not succeed.

The body is then rotated back half a circle in the opposite direction, bringing the back uppermost: the arm lying posteriorly is now anterior and is delivered by splinting, if necessary.

SUMMARY OF LEFT SACRO-ANTERIOR

Turn the body anti-clockwise, half a circle (to the left), deliver the arm which is under the pubic arch. **Turn the body clockwise half a circle (to the right) and deliver the other arm** from under the pubic arch.

N.B.—**The direction of rotation, in each instance, must bring the back uppermost.**

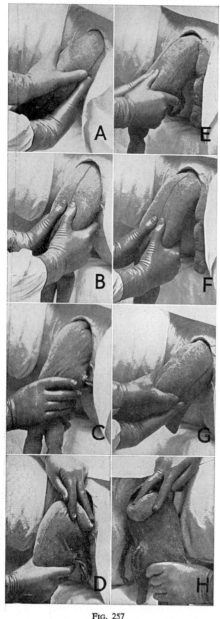

Fig. 257

The Løvset Manœuvre, L.S.A.
Simpson Memorial Maternity Pavilion, Edinburgh.)

The knee is a hinge joint that bends only in one direction so traction must not be exerted on the anterior surface of the knee. Severe injury to the knee joint can occur from doing so.

EXTENDED ARMS

Extended arms are diagnosed when the elbows are not felt on the chest after the umbilicus is born or if there is no advance then, with good contractions.

The district midwife must act or the baby may be stillborn: she must know what to do and how to do it; for unless the manipulation is carried out competently, fracture or paralysis of the arms may result.

The Løvset manœuvre is so successful in the bringing down of extended arms that it is now used in preference to the classical method.

(A)

Midwife's left hand supports the buttocks. Posterior arm brought down first, using hand corresponding to the baby's back. Index and middle fingers splint the humerus to avoid fracturing it. Baby's forearm is flexed over his face like a " cat washing its face." The wrist is grasped and the hand brought out.

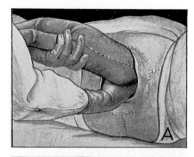

(B)

The hands splint the body while rotating it in the same direction as the hand that is out is pointing (otherwise the arm in the vagina will be displaced behind the baby's neck in the nuchal position, a serious complication which can be avoided or rectified by the Løvset manœuvre).

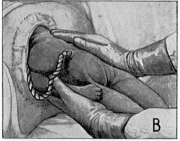

(C)

Midwife's right hand supports the buttocks and with her left hand the posterior arm is brought down as in (A)

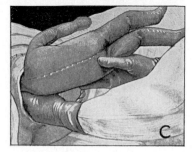

FIG. 258

THE CLASSICAL METHOD OF BRINGING DOWN EXTENDED ARMS.

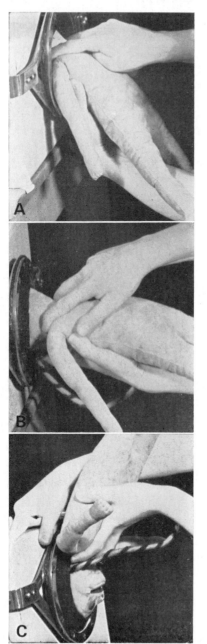

EXTENDED HEAD

If, when the body has been allowed to hang, the neck and hair-line are not visible, it is probable that the head is extended.

MANAGEMENT

The doctor will apply forceps: the midwife uses the Mauriceau-Smellie-Veit manœuvre.

MAURICEAU-SMELLIE-VEIT MANŒUVRE

A moderate degree of suprapubic pressure is used in a downward, backward direction to increase flexion and descent of the head. (To avoid injury to the bladder, while using suprapubic pressure, the bladder is always emptied during preparation for delivery of breech presentation.)

(A)

Baby astride left arm with palm supporting chest.

First and third fingers of left hand on malar bones to flex head. (Some place the middle finger in the mouth (well back) to aid flexion.)

First two fingers of right hand hooked over shoulders, pull in a downward direction.

(B)

Traction is exerted in an outward rather than downward direction as the head descends in the curved birth canal.

(C)

Traction exerted in an upward direction to expedite birth of the head. Nose and mouth are free so the air-way is cleared. The vault is delivered slowly.

FIG. 259
MAURICEAU-SMELLIE-VEIT MANŒUVRE.

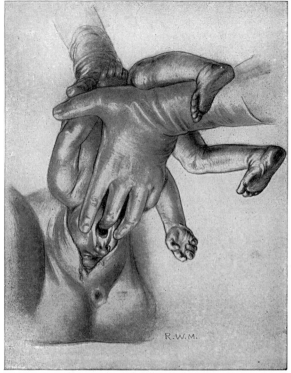

FIG. 260

EXTRACTION OF THE HEAD BY MAURICEAU-SMELLIE-VEIT GRIP.
Middle finger in mouth, first and third fingers on malar bones to aid flexion.

Posterior rotation of the Occiput

This malrotation of the head is rare and is usually the result of mismanagement, for the back should always be turned upwards after the shoulders are born.

To deliver the head, face to pubes, the chin and face are permitted to escape under the symphysis pubis as far as the root of the nose; the occiput then sweeps the perineum. The application of forceps may be necessary.

CAUSES AND TREATMENT OF DELAY IN BREECH PRESENTATION

DELAY IN THE FIRST STAGE

This may be caused by impaction due to a large baby or small pelvis or to weak contractions. Medical aid is necessary.

DELAY DURING THE SECOND STAGE

This is usually caused by extended legs and in such a case the midwife should not interfere until the buttocks are showing at the outlet. If the doctor is not available and fetal or maternal distress is manifest, a medio-lateral episiotomy ought to be made then steady traction should be used with two fingers in the groins, pulling mainly in the posterior groin, in an outward upward direction, to aid lateral flexion.

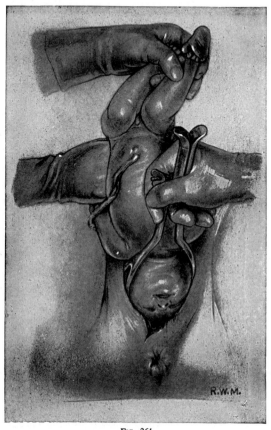

FIG. 261
Application of forceps to the aftercoming head.

DELAY IN THE BIRTH OF THE HEAD

A footling presentation does not dilate the cervix adequately to allow passage of the head.

The head of a premature baby is large in proportion to the breech and is held up.

If the midwife is unable to extract the head and the baby is making gasping movements, she should mop the vaginal wall in contact with the baby's face and by inserting two fingers make a channel through which air can reach the baby.

If the head is arrested high in the pelvic cavity disproportion may exist; suprapubic pressure may help but the application of forceps will likely be necessary. Should the baby be small the possibility of a hydrocephalic head must be considered. Perforation of the skull will be required (see p. 649).

The baby should be admitted to the intensive care unit for the first few days.

Face Presentation

When the attitude of the head at the pelvic brim is one of complete extension, with the occiput in contact with the spine, the face will present at the pelvic brim.

The frequency is about 1 in 500 cases and the majority develop from vertex to face after the onset of labour, *i.e.* secondary face presentation. When the face presents before labour, the term " primary face presentation " is used, and the anencephalic fetus is the main example.

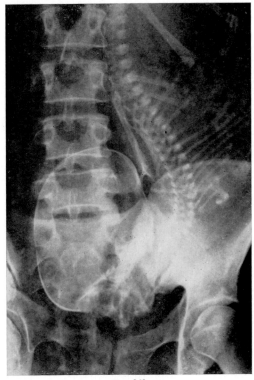

FIG 262

X-ray of face presentation. Left mento-posterior. Note extension of the spine.

POSITIONS

There are six positions in face presentation: denominator the mentum.

RIGHT	MENTO-POSTERIOR		R.M.P.	LEFT	MENTO-POSTERIOR		L.M.P.
,,	,,	LATERAL	R.M.L.	,,	,,	LATERAL	L.M.L.
,,	,,	ANTERIOR	R.M.A.	,,	,,	ANTERIOR	L.M.A.

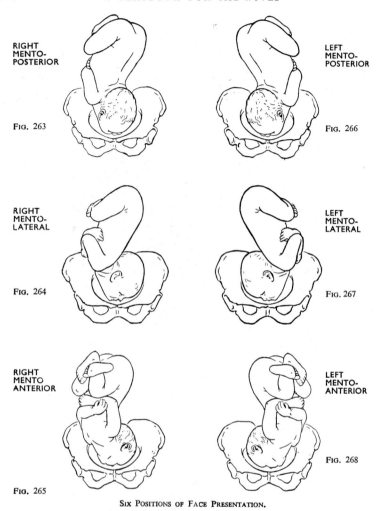

RIGHT
MENTO-
POSTERIOR

FIG. 263

LEFT
MENTO-
POSTERIOR

FIG. 266

RIGHT
MENTO-
LATERAL

FIG. 264

LEFT
MENTO-
LATERAL

FIG. 267

RIGHT
MENTO
ANTERIOR

FIG. 265

LEFT
MENTO-
ANTERIOR

FIG. 268

SIX POSITIONS OF FACE PRESENTATION.

CAUSES

MATERNAL	FETAL
ANTERIOR UTERINE OBLIQUITY.	ANENCEPHALY.
CONTRACTED PELVIS.	SPASM OF MUSCLES OF NECK.
HYDRAMNIOS.	TUMOURS OF NECK (RARE).

ANTERIOR UTERINE OBLIQUITY

This is the commonest maternal cause. When the fetus presents as a posterior vertex, the pendulous abdomen causes the fetal buttocks to lean forwards and the force of the uterine contractions is exerted in a line directed to the chin rather than to the occiput, causing the head to extend.

CONTRACTED PELVIS

In the flat pelvis, the head enters in the transverse of the brim and the parietal eminences may be held up in the obstetrical conjugate, the head becomes extended and face presentation develops. Or, if the head in the posterior position (vertex presenting) remains deflexed, the parietal eminences may be caught in the sacro-cotyloid diameter, the occiput does not descend, the head becomes extended, and face presentation results.

HYDRAMNIOS

If the vertex is presenting and the membranes rupture spontaneously, the head may extend with the rush of fluid.

ANENCEPHALY

This is a common fetal cause because the vertex is absent, and if the head lies in the lower pole of the uterus when labour starts the face enters the pelvic brim.

Increased tone of neck muscles and tumours of the neck are two rare causes of extension of the head.

DIAGNOSIS

ABDOMINAL EXAMINATION

ON INSPECTION:

There is nothing diagnostic.

ON PALPATION:

Face presentation may not be detected. (If the doll is placed in the pelvis as a right mento-posterior, the prominent occiput can be seen in the left anterior quadrant of the pelvis with a furrow between the occiput and the extended back, but in practice the prominent occiput may be mistaken for the sinciput and an erroneous diagnosis of vertex (R.O.A.) made.)

In mento-anterior positions the limbs are readily palpated being in close proximity to the abdominal wall.

AUSCULTATION

When the chin is anterior the fetal heart is heard distinctly because the fetal chest is in contact with the mother's abdominal wall.

When the chin is posterior the fetal heart is not easily heard because the fetal thorax is not in contact with the mother's abdominal wall.

VAGINAL EXAMINATION

The presenting part is high, soft and irregular.

A malpresentation is suspected when the smooth, hard vertex is not felt and sutures and fontanelles are absent.

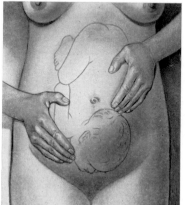

FIG. 269
PALPATION OF HEAD IN FACE PRESENTATION.
Right mento-posterior.

Gums are diagnostic. Confusion between mouth and anus could arise, but the mouth is open, whereas the anus grips the examining finger and stains it with meconium.

To determine position the chin should be located and, if it is posterior, the midwife should decide whether it is lower than the sinciput; if so, it will rotate forwards.

In an R.M.P. the orbital ridges will be felt in the left oblique diameter of the pelvis.

Care must be taken neither to injure nor infect the eyes with the examining finger.

MECHANISM OF LABOUR

The mechanism is fundamentally similar to that in a vertex presentation, except that, instead of an increase in flexion, there is increased extension, and the chin, instead of the occiput, becomes the leading part and rotates forwards. The head is born by flexion instead of extension.

LEFT MENTO-ANTERIOR

LIE, longitudinal.

ATTITUDE, extension of head and back.

PRESENTATION, face.

POSITION, L.M.A.

DENOMINATOR, mentum.

PRESENTING PART, left malar bone.

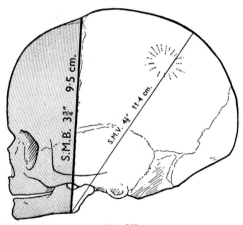

FIG. 270

ENGAGING DIAMETERS

The submento-bregmatic diameter, 9·5 cm. (3¾ inches) presents at the brim and appears at the vulva. The submento-vertical diameter 11·4 cm (4½ inches) sweeps the perineum.

Descent takes place with increasing extension.

Internal rotation occurs when the chin reaches the pelvic floor and rotates forwards one-eighth of a circle. The chin escapes under the symphysis pubis.

Flexion takes place when the sinciput, vertex and occiput sweep the perineum; the head is born.

Restitution occurs when the chin turns one-eighth of a circle to the patient's left.

The shoulders enter in the left oblique and the anterior shoulder rotates one-eighth of a circle forwards along the right side of the pelvis, **accompanied by external rotation of the head. (*The shoulders are born as in a vertex presentation.*)**

Right Mento-posterior

The chin rotates forwards three-eighths of a circle along the right side of the pelvis, and the shoulders turn two-eighths of a circle with the head. The remainder of the mechanism is similar to that in an R.M.A.

PROGNOSIS AND COURSE OF LABOUR

If the chin is anterior, less difficulty is encountered; if posterior and the head is well extended and contractions are effective, the chin will rotate forwards and the face will be born as in the anterior position.

1. DELAY IN LABOUR IS COMMON

For the following reasons:

(*a*) **The face is a badly fitting presenting part** and does not stimulate good uterine contractions.

(*b*) **The face is a poor cervical dilator.**

(*c*) **The face bones do not mould.**

(*d*) **The face is shallow** and to enable the chin to reach the pelvic floor the shoulders must also enter the pelvic cavity.

(*e*) **There is misdirected force,** because the fetal axis pressure is directed to the chin, and the head is almost at right angles to the spine.

(*f*) **Internal rotation may be arrested** when the chin is posterior.

(*g*) **The face becomes impacted** when persistent mento-posterior occurs.

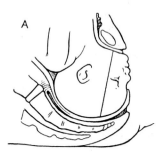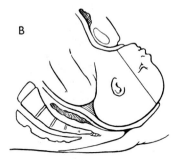

Fig. 271

MECHANISM OF BIRTH OF HEAD IN MENTO-ANTERIOR POSITION.

A. Submento-bregmatic diameter at outlet, chin escapes under symphysis pubis.

B, Head is born by movement of flexion; the submento-vertical diameter will sweep the perineum.

2. THE CORD MAY PROLAPSE

3. PERINEAL LACERATION OCCURS

Because the submento-vertical diameter, 11·4 cm. (4½ inches), sweeps the perineum, which is also distended by the biparietal diameter.

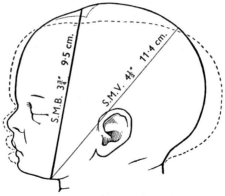

FIG. 272

Typical moulding in a face presentation, shown by dotted line.

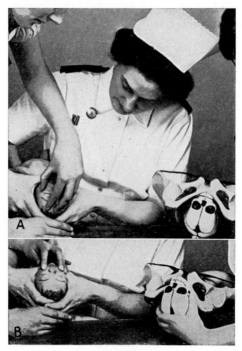

FIG. 273

DELIVERY OF FACE PRESENTATION IN DORSAL POSITION.
Labour ward superintendent demonstrates with doll:
hands used as vulva.

A, Keeping sinciput back until chin is delivered.
B, Pressure on malar bones to deliver face by flexion.
(*Aberdeen Maternity Hospital.*)

4.MANAGEMENT OF LABOUR

(a) **The midwife must notify the doctor,** but in 75 per cent of cases the babies are born spontaneously.

(b) **A vaginal examination is made when the membranes rupture,** to find out whether the cord has prolapsed; taking care neither to infect nor injure the eyes.

(c) **The fetal heart requires careful observation.**

(d) **In mento-posterior cases** the midwife must observe closely that the chin is the lowest point and that rotation and descent are taking place. If the head remains high in spite of good contractions Cæsarean section should be anticipated.

(e) DELIVERY OF THE BABY

The important point is to get the chin out before the head flexes, so, when the face appears at the vulva, extension should be maintained by holding back the sinciput to permit the chin to escape under the symphysis pubis before the occiput is allowed to sweep the perineum. In this way the submento-vertical diameter, 11·4 cm. (4½ inches), distends the vaginal orifice instead of the mento-vertical diameter, 13·3 cm. (5¼ inches)

(f) **An episiotomy and delivery by forceps may be necessary.**

(g) **The baby should be cot-nursed and kept quiet for a few days.**

Head retraction persists for some days; the face is congested and bruised, the eyelids and lips œdematous, but this is less marked when the patient is multiparous. The babies stand labour remarkably well, however, considering the stretching to which the blood vessels and nerves in the neck are subjected. *If the blue discoloration and the disfiguring œdema are excessive the mother should not see her baby until they have subsided.*

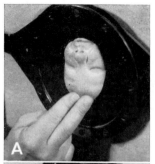
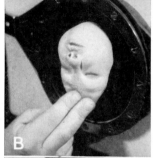
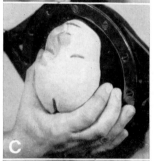
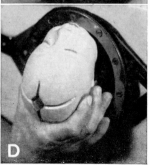

DELIVERY OF FACE PRESENTATION
FIG. 274

A, Holding back sinciput to increase extension of the head until the chin is born.

B, Chin is born, the head can now be flexed by the mother ' breathing the head out '.

C, Bringing the occiput over the perineum.

D, Flexion completed—head born.

(Aberdeen Maternity Hospital classroom).

PERSISTENT MENTO-POSTERIOR

In this case the head is incompletely extended and the sinciput reaches the pelvic floor first and rotates forwards one-eighth of a circle: the chin passes into the hollow of the sacrum.

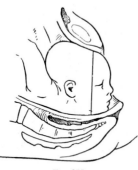

There is no further mechanism: the face becomes impacted because the head and neck are completely extended and cannot negotiate the posterior wall of the pelvis. **(Whatever lies in the hollow of the sacrum must sweep the perineum to be born.)** In a persistent mento-posterior this is not possible because the fully extended neck lies in the hollow of the sacrum and the head cannot extend further.

Management

Cæsarean section is now frequently performed.

The midwife must get medical aid at once and prepare for Cæsarean section or pudendal block, episiotomy, forceps delivery and an asphyxiated baby.

The doctor may attempt to increase extension of the head by pushing up the sinciput; he will then manually rotate the head and apply forceps.

Fig. 275

PERSISTENT MENTO-POSTERIOR POSITION.

Head cannot extend further to sweep the perineum, so becomes impacted.

In a neglected case when the face is impacted and the baby dead, craniotomy through the orbit will be necessary.

Brow Presentation

The fetus presents by the brow when the area of the skull bounded by the orbital ridges and the anterior fontanelle lies at the brim of the pelvis. The attitude of the head is midway between that of a vertex and a face presentation; in fact, during the process of a vertex developing into a face presentation, the brow will present temporarily, and in 1 in 1,000 cases brow presentation will persist.

The maternal causes are similar to those of face presentation (see p. 376).

It is not necessary to consider the positions in brow presentation because only on rare occasions is any mechanism of labour possible. Commonly, the head attempts to enter the pelvis with the mento-vertical diameter 13·3 cm. (5¼ inches) in the transverse diameter of the brim.

DIAGNOSIS

Brow presentation is seldom diagnosed before the onset of labour.

On abdominal examination the head is high, seems to be unduly big, and in spite of good uterine contractions does not enter the pelvic brim.

On vaginal examination the presenting part cannot be reached, but as labour proceeds the anterior fontanelle may be felt at one side of the pelvis and the orbital ridges at the other; neither vertex nor face can be felt.

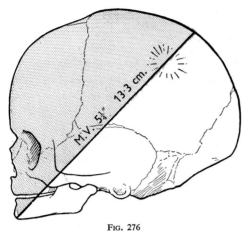

FIG. 276

BROW PRESENTATION.

The mento-vertical diameter, 13·3 cm. (5¼ inches), lies at the pelvic brim.

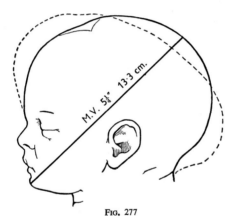

FIG. 277

Typical moulding in a brow presentation
shown by dotted line.

PROBABLE COURSE OF LABOUR

It is possible that with a large pelvis in a multiparous woman, a small baby could be born with the aid of forceps. The brow reaches the pelvic floor, rotates forwards and is born by a mechanism rather similar to that of a vertex face to pubes.

The midwife should never anticipate such a favourable outcome, as the majority of brow presentations give rise to obstructed labour.

Management

When the back is anterior and the condition is diagnosed early, before the membranes rupture, the doctor may, by combined abdominal and vaginal manipulation, attempt to increase flexion of the head and convert the brow into a vertex. **Cæsarean section is usually resorted to.**

When the back is posterior, the doctor may attempt to increase extension and convert the brow into a face presentation, because an anterior face might be more favourable than a posterior vertex, but **Cæsarean section is often necessary.**

The moulding of the head is typical, with a large caput on the brow.

In cases of neglected brow presentation when the head is wedged into the pelvic brim, or when labour has been in progress for some time and the uterus is moulded round the fetus, it may be necessary to perform craniotomy to avoid rupture of the uterus.

The midwife must always view brow presentation with concern and immediately send for medical assistance. The doctor will transfer the patient to hospital without delay.

Shoulder Presentation

When the fetus lies with its long axis across the long axis of the uterus (*transverse lie*)

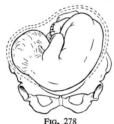

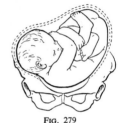

Fig. 278
Shoulder presentation,
dorso-anterior.

Fig. 279
Shoulder presentation,
dorso-posterior.

the shoulder is most likely to present. Occasionally the lie is oblique, but this does not persist, as the uterine contractions during labour make it longitudinal or transverse.

Two positions are commonly described.

1. DORSO-ANTERIOR

The fetal back is in front, conforming to the mother's abdominal wall: the acromion process (*and, of course, the head*) could be to the right or the left.

2. DORSO-POSTERIOR

The fetal back is behind, directed towards the mother's spine, the acromion process and head are to the left or right.

Frequency

Shoulder presentation occurs in 1 in 250 cases near term and the incidence is five times greater in multigravidæ than in primigravidæ.

CAUSES

Any condition that increases the mobility of the fetus *in utero* or which prevents the head from entering the brim will produce any malpresentation, including shoulder.

MATERNAL

1. **Anterior obliquity of the uterus.**—When the abdominal muscles are lax, the uterus leans forwards and the fetus does not maintain the longitudinal lie.

2. **Multiparity.**—If the uterine walls have been frequently stretched, due to repeated childbearing, the snug ovoid shape of the uterus is absent.

3. **Hydramnios.**—Because the uterus is globular, the fetus can move freely in the excess fluid.

4. **Bicornuate uterus.**—When the septum extends part way down into the uterine cavity, the fetal head may be in one horn, the breech in the other: **external version fails.**

5. **Contracted pelvis**
6. **Placenta prævia** }prevent the head from entering the pelvic brim.
7. **Fibroid tumours** (low)

FETAL

1. **Twins,** especially the second twin.

2. **Prematurity.**—Because the amount of liquor is relatively greater, the fetus is mobile.

3. **Macerated fetus.**—Lack of muscle tone causes the fetus to slump down into the lower pole of the uterus.

DIAGNOSIS

Every qualified midwife should be competent to diagnose shoulder presentation during pregnancy and early labour; (traditional birth attendants should also be taught this).

It is reprehensible when the condition is not recognized until labour is well advanced. The results can be disastrous, *i.e.* obstructed labour, rupture of uterus, maternal and fetal death.

1. DURING PREGNANCY

ABDOMINAL EXAMINATION

(*a*) **Inspection.**—The fundus is low, sometimes being higher at one side than the other; the uterus is wide.

(*b*) **Palpation.**—On pelvic and fundal palpation, neither head nor breech is felt. The mobile head is located in the iliac fossa, the breech on the opposite side, slightly higher.

(*c*) **Auscultation.**—The fetal heart is heard below the umbilicus but this is not diagnostic.

2. DURING LABOUR

When the membranes have ruptured the **irregular outline of the uterus is more marked.** If the uterus is contracting strongly and becomes moulded round the fetus, palpation is very difficult; the pelvis is no longer empty, the shoulder being wedged into it.

PER VAGINAM

Early in labour the presenting part is so high that it is beyond the reach of the midwife's fingers and this should immediately arouse suspicion. The membranes have usually ruptured because of the badly fitting presenting part.

Later, the shoulder is felt as a soft irregular mass and if the fetus is small the ribs may be palpated; their gridiron conformation is diagnostic. When the shoulder enters the brim, prolapse of an arm is liable to occur.

A hand can be differentiated from a foot *as follows:*

The elbow feels sharper than the knee.	**The thumb** can be abducted.
The fingers are longer than the toes.	**The palm** is shorter than the sole.
The fingers are of unequal length.	**No os calcis** can be felt.

The hand is not at right angles to the arm.

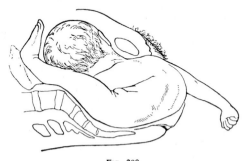

Fig. 280

Spontaneous evolution.

THERE IS NO MECHANISM FOR A SHOULDER PRESENTATION

The rare processes by which a macerated, premature fetus may be expelled in a doubled-up manner are only of academic interest to midwives. These are: (1) **Spontaneous evolution.** (2) **Spontaneous expulsion** (see Glossary).

The likelihood of the lie becoming longitudinal by the occurrence of **spontaneous version** or **spontaneous rectification** at the beginning of labour, is so remote that the midwife should never even entertain the idea of such a possibility.

In all cases of transverse lie the midwife must get medical assistance.

TREATMENT

The main treatment is prophylactic and where adequate prenatal care is practised a shoulder presentation ought to be diagnosed, the cause investigated, and the condition rectified or appropriate treatment arranged for prior to labour.

External version is performed when the lie is transverse after the 32nd week of pregnancy. If unsuccessful or if the lie is again transverse when seen within a few days the woman is admitted to hospital where a full investigation is made to determine the cause.

Contracted pelvis in the primigravid woman and the possibility of **placenta prævia** will be considered; in both instances Cæsarean section would be performed at term.

1. **At the beginning of labour** if the membranes are intact, the doctor may do **external cephalic version,** followed by puncture of membranes; close supervision is essential to ensure that the longitudinal lie is maintained.

2. **Cæsarean section is the method of choice** (*a*) when attempts to correct shoulder presentation have failed; (*b*) when the membranes are ruptured; (*c*) if the cord prolapses; (*d*) if labour has been in progress for some hours; the outcome being more favourable for mother and child.

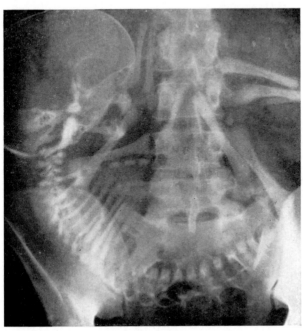

FIG. 281

X-ray of shoulder presentation.

3. BI-POLAR VERSION

This procedure, which is hazardous for both mother and fetus, is rarely employed and often condemned but may be useful in remote areas where facilities for Cæsarean section are not readily available.

When the os is two fingers dilated, membranes intact or recently ruptured, a general anæsthetic is administered and bi-polar podalic version carried out while the uterus is relaxed between contractions (p. 614).

4. INTERNAL PODALIC VERSION

The danger of internal version is very great: the thinned out lower uterine segment is very easily ruptured (particularly in the multigravid woman); the stillbirth rate is high. Some authorities condemn the practice with a mature live baby, or at all.

In remote areas where facilities for Cæsarean section are not available internal podalic version may be done under a general anæsthetic. When the os is sufficiently dilated to admit the whole hand a leg is grasped and brought down to prevent the fetus from reverting to the transverse lie.

PROLAPSE OF CORD

This is a possible complication, so a vaginal examination is made immediately the membranes rupture. Cæsarean section is a recognized method of treating prolapse of cord as well as of shoulder presentation.

NEGLECTED SHOULDER PRESENTATION

In this condition, the shoulder becomes impacted. It is forced down and wedged into the pelvic brim; the membranes will have ruptured and if the arm has prolapsed it becomes swollen and blue.

The uterus goes into a state of tonic contraction, the over-stretched lower segment is tender to touch, the fetal heart fails and all the maternal signs of obstructed labour are manifest. The outcome is that of **obstructed labour,** with **rupture of uterus and stillbirth.**

TREATMENT

A general anæsthetic is given immediately, to stop the contractions, in an endeavour to avert uterine rupture, and preparations made for Cæsarean section.

Some obstetricians consider the risk of uterine rupture to be so great that they perform a Cæsarean section even if the fetus is dead.

Internal version is dangerous and may rupture the uterus.

In remote areas it may be necessary to decapitate the fetus (see p. 649): evisceration may be needed if the neck is not accessible.

With adequate prenatal care and competent supervision during labour, impacted shoulder presentation should never occur. The midwife must always treat shoulder presentation during labour as a dangerous emergency which demands immediate action by the doctor.

UNSTABLE LIE

This term is applied when after the 36th week of pregnancy the lie, which should at this time be stable as longitudinal, is found to vary (breech, vertex, or shoulder presenting), from one examination to another.

Causes

Any condition in late pregnancy that increases the mobility of the fetus in utero, *e.g.*

(*a*) lax uterine muscles as in multiparity

(*b*) hydramnios.

MANAGEMENT OF UNSTABLE LIE

1. **The woman is admitted to hospital** at the 37th-38th week of pregnancy and remains there until she is delivered,

   (*a*) to avoid the unsupervised onset of labour with a transverse lie.

   (*b*) to receive the essential expert supervision necessary prior to and throughout labour.

2. **Further attempts to correct the abnormal presentation by external version are made.**

3. **Some authorities puncture the membranes at the 38th week,** having first corrected transverse lie, to ensure that the woman goes into labour with the vertex presenting: others do so when labour starts. A number of obstetricians do not approve of puncturing the membranes because of the risk of prolapse of cord.

4. **An intravenous oxytocin drip** is usually given; extreme caution being exercised if the woman is a grande multipara.

5. **Cæsarean section will be considered if the transverse lie is uncorrected** at term.

6. **Vigilant supervision is mandatory throughout labour** to ensure that:—

(*a*) **the longitudinal lie is maintained**: a meticulous abdominal examination being made at the onset of labour, and repeated at intervals even although the membranes are ruptured.

(*b*) **prolapse of cord is recognised** and treated without delay: the fetal heart must be auscultated more frequently than is usual.

7. **The bladder should be emptied every two hours** (the rectum having been evacuated at the onset of labour) to facilitate preservation of the longitudinal lie.

COMPOUND OR COMPLEX PRESENTATION

When a hand, or occasionally, a foot, lies alongside the head, the presentation is said to be compound. This tends to occur with a small fetus or roomy pelvis and seldom is difficulty encountered except in cases where it is associated with a flat pelvis. On rare occasions, **head, hand** and **foot** are felt in the vagina; a serious situation which usually occurs with a dead fetus.

If diagnosed during the first stage of labour, medical aid must be sought. An attempt could be made to push the arm upwards over the baby's face.

During the second stage if the midwife sees a hand presenting alongside the vertex at the vulva, she could try to hold the hand back, directing it over the face. The author saw a case in which both feet were showing at the vulva with the head (*following external version in a frank breech*); the feet were held back, and with no delay the baby was delivered spontaneously.

———————

QUESTIONS FOR REVISION

MALPRESENTATIONS

BREECH

Fill in the following facts.—The percentage of breech presentations at term..................
The perinatal mortality rate......................... How many minutes will a fetus stand cord compression ?.................. Main cause of fetal death...................

How would you diagnose a frank breech on inspection—palpation—auscultation—vaginal **examination.**

Give three maternal and three fetal causes of breech presentation.

Give two reasons why external version should be performed during pregnancy.

Write 10 lines on the following procedures: (*a*) Burns-Marshall method; (*b*) Løvset manœuvre; (*c*) Mauriceau Smellie Veit manœuvre.

How would you differentiate P.V. between: (*a*) complete and frank breech; (*b*) knee and elbow; (*c*) hand and foot.

Why is it advisable that breech presentations should be delivered in hospital ? Give two reasons why the cord is liable to prolapse.

Explain how the following are produced: anoxia; intracranial injury; rupture of liver; fracture of humerus; fracture of neck; Erb's paralysis.

Why should the following procedures be avoided ? (*a*) fundal pressure; (*b*) traction on the breech; (*c*) turning the back up prior to birth of the shoulders; (*d*) pulling the head out quickly.

The following colloquial terms are useful reminders—explain them. " Hands off the breech," " like a cat washing its face," " not like a cork out of a bottle," " breathing the head out."

C.M.B.(Scot.) paper.—Describe the management of a breech delivery in a multiparous woman. What dangers to mother and child does this complication involve ?

24

C.M.B.(Scot.) paper.—Describe the management of a breech delivery where the legs are extended.

C.M.B.(Eng.) paper.—How is a breech presentation diagnosed ? Discuss the investigations which would be made and what treatment would be carried out during the antenatal period.

C.M.B.(Scot.) paper.—Describe the management of a multiparous breech delivery. What are the increased dangers to the child associated with this malpresentation ?

C.M.B.(N. Ireland) paper.—What are the principal dangers of breech delivery ? What can be done to avoid them ?

FACE PRESENTATION

Give three maternal and three fetal causes of face presentation. In making a vaginal examination, what is the diagnostic landmark ? Why must you avoid the eyes ?

WRITE 10 LINES ON

(*a*) The management of labour in face presentation; (*b*) persistent mento-posterior.

Why is labour long ? Which diameters of the skull (*a*) engage ; (*b*) appear at the vulva ; (*c*) sweep the perineum ? How will you ensure that the chin is born first ?

C.M.B.(Eng.) paper.—How would you diagnose a face presentation during labour ? Briefly describe the conduct of labour in such a case.

C.M.B.(Scot.) paper.—Describe the course of labour in a face presentation and indicate briefly the treatment of any difficulties which may arise.

BROW PRESENTATION

How would you (*a*) suspect a brow presentation, on abdominal examination ; (*b*) diagnose it on vaginal examination ? What would you do in such circumstances ? What treatment might be carried out ?

SHOULDER PRESENTATION

Give three fetal and three maternal causes of shoulder presentation and explain why they produce a transverse lie. Place the doll in the dorso-anterior position and explain what the findings would be on abdominal examination.

What would you do if the shoulder was presenting in the following circumstances :

In the overseas service, with the doctor ten hours' journey distant : (*a*) woman at beginning of labour ? (*b*) os half dilated ? (6 cm.)

WRITE 10 LINES ON

(*a*) The outcome of an undiagnosed shoulder presentation. (*b*) **Unstable lie.**

(*c*) The dangers of internal version during labour for shoulder presentation.

C.M.B.(Scot.) paper.—Discuss the diagnosis of transverse lie, both by abdominal and vaginal examination. If the membranes are unruptured, how may it be corrected ? What is the risk of leaving it alone ?

C.M.B.(Scot.) paper.—What are the complications and dangers of transverse lie at full term ? How may they be avoided ? In what type of patient are you likely to find a transverse lie ?

C.M.B.(N. Ireland) paper.—What are the dangers of a transverse lie of the fetus near term ? How would you diagnose this condition, and what steps are usually taken to deal with it ?

C.M.B.(Scot.) paper.—What are the possible causes of a transverse lie ? How is this diagnosed ? What may be the treatment in such a case ? What are the risks to mother and baby ?

C.M.B.(Scot.) paper.—How would you recognize a transverse (or oblique) lie ? Describe the management before and during labour.

C.M.B. (Eng) paper, 1970.—50 word question.—Unstable lie at 36th week of pregnancy.

22

Disordered Uterine Action.   Contracted Pelvis.
Trial Labour.   Obstructed Labour

There is no absolute pattern among different women in the length, strength and frequency of uterine contractions during normal labour. Uterine action has been studied by using an instrument—the tocograph—that records the degree of uterine

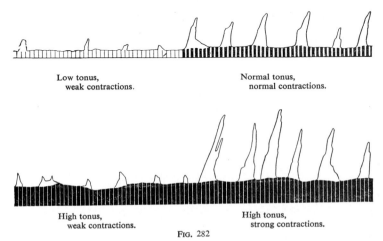

Low tonus,
weak contractions.

Normal tonus,
normal contractions.

High tonus,
weak contractions.

High tonus,
strong contractions.

FIG. 282

DIAGRAMMATIC REPRESENTATION OF UTERINE TONUS AND CONTRACTIONS.

tonus, which may be low, normal or high, and also the length and strength of each uterine contraction. By this means a better comprehension of disordered uterine action has been attained.

DISORDERED UTERINE ACTION

Many theories have been propounded regarding the causation of disordered uterine action, **but none provides a satisfactory solution.**

A state of uterine neuro-muscular disharmony exists.

The following clinical conditions are believed to be predisposing factors:

1. **Parity.**—Disordered uterine action is much more common in primigravidæ.

2. **A badly fitting presenting part,** *e.g.* disproportion, malpresentation, posterior positions of the vertex prevent the head from exerting pressure on the cervical nerve endings. **Post-maturity** may be associated with failure of the lower uterine segment to dilate and accommodate the fetal head.

The following terms are applied to disordered uterine action:
1. HYPOTONIC UTERINE INERTIA
2. INCO-ORDINATE UTERINE ACTION
3. CERVICAL DYSTOCIA

HYPOTONIC UTERINE INERTIA

The term **uterine inertia** is usually applied when labour in the absence of disproportion is prolonged over 24 hours but the condition can be diagnosed before that time, *e.g.* with weak contractions and slow dilatation of the os.

In this condition the tone of the uterus is poor; on palpation the normal degree of firmness is absent; **contractions are weak, short, of low amplitude and do not give rise to much pain.** They may also be irregular and infrequent, sometimes going off for a number of hours.

This state of affairs may exist from the onset of labour and it is sometimes difficult to differentiate between false labour and hypotonic inertia.

Preventive Treatment

When progress in established labour is slow, uterine action is stimulated after 6 hours by some authorities without waiting for prolonged labour to develop (*disproportion is of course ruled out*).

Puncture of membranes is carried out and if labour is not accelerated an I.V. oxytocin infusion is given (see below).

EFFECT ON LABOUR

Dilatation of the os is slow.

When labour lasts over 24 hours the perinatal mortality is increased.

ACTIVE TREATMENT

Admit to hospital when in labour for 18 hours, or earlier.

Hypnotic drugs such as dichloralphenazone (Welldorm), 1·3 G., or Trichloryl, 1 G., are useful for the apprehensive woman.

Sleep is induced by papaveretum 20 mg.

Biochemical control and electrolyte replacement are instituted.

Dextrose 5 per cent is administered intravenously before dehydration or ketosis develops.

Oxytocin drip, 0·5 units Syntocinon in 540 ml. of 5 per cent Dextrose (*some add* 150 *mg. Pethidine*), may be ordered by the doctor, if no contra-indications to oxytocin drip are present (see p. 609). Increase to 1 unit in half an hour and gradually up to 2·5 units if the maternal and fetal conditions are satisfactory. It is continued for one hour after completion of the third stage to prevent postpartum hæmorrhage.

Vigilant supervision is necessary. Continuous monitoring of the fetal heart may be done by cardiotocograph.

A high vaginal swab is taken after 24 hours.

Much encouragement should be given. The nursing care is similar to that which is described for prolonged labour (p. 410).

The possibility of postpartum hæmorrhage ought to be kept in mind, and Syntometrine, 1 ml., given as soon as the anterior shoulder appears, if an oxytocin drip is not being administered.

OBSERVATION

1. THE MATERNAL CONDITION

(a) ABDOMINAL EXAMINATION

Note frequency, length and strength of the uterine contractions; descent of the presenting part.

(b) VAGINAL OR RECTAL EXAMINATION

Note dilatation of the os and descent of the presenting part. The precise time when the membranes rupture should be recorded.

(c) GENERAL CONDITION

Note and record temperature, pulse and blood pressure every four hours: record amount of food and sleep.

(d) FLUID BALANCE CHART

A record should be kept of fluid intake and kidney output.

(e) URINE ANALYSIS

The urine should be examined for ketones, chlorides and protein every four hours, and every specimen after 12 hours.

(f) SIGNS OF DISTRESS

These are not usual if the membranes are intact and the amount of sleep, nutriment and fluid are adequate. (For signs see p. 411).

2. THE FETAL CONDITION

The fetal heart should be auscultated every 15 minutes, towards the end of the first stage every five minutes, and recorded in graph form. When the membranes rupture signs of fetal distress are watched for assiduously. Saling's method of fetal blood sampling is sometimes carried out to determine the pH of the blood (see p. 414).

Operative Measures

Puncture of membranes in conjunction with oxytocin drip.

Cæsarean section is being performed with greater frequency for this condition.

The vacuum extractor (Malmstrom) is sometimes employed (see p. 629) when the os is half-dilated (6 cm.) and the head below mid-cavity.

Forceps delivery is often necessary because the woman is tired after the prolonged first stage and does not push effectively.

Pudendal nerve block is employed in preference to general anæsthesia in order to lessen the risk of fetal anoxia.

INCO-ORDINATE UTERINE ACTION

HYPERTONIC UTERINE ACTION

This state of dysfunction is manifest when the progress of labour is very slow in spite of apparently strong painful uterine contractions.

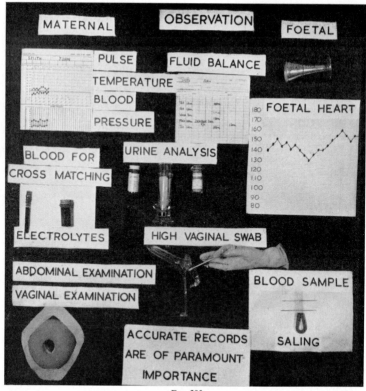

FIG. 283

REPRESENTATION OF REQUIREMENTS FOR OBSERVATION (FETAL AND MATERNAL) IN CASE OF DISORDERED UTERINE ACTION.
(*Bellshill Maternity Hospital classroom.*)

EFFECT ON LABOUR

THE UTERUS

(*a*) **Uterine tone is high.** At the height of a contraction the wall of the uterus is tender to touch and cannot be indented by the finger tips. High tone persists after the contraction subsides.

(*b*) **The contractions may be frequent but ineffective;** they are extremely painful, sometimes irregular and erratic. The woman feels pain at the beginning and end of each contraction, periods that should be painless.

(*c*) **The lower uterine segment is also hypertonic** and its resistance impedes descent of the head and gives rise to persistent low abdominal pain and severe backache.

(*d*) **Colicky uterus occurs** when the two poles of the uterus are not acting rhythmically as a whole. The upper segment contracts strongly but spasmodically, with intense cramp-like pain but little expulsive power, and **pain is felt at the onset and termination of each contraction.** Uterine tenderness and severe backache are present.

(*e*) **The os dilates slowly** because of the uterine dysfunction. The cervix may be thick or thin but feels tight **and unyielding.**

EFFECT ON THE WOMAN

(1) EXHAUSTION DUE TO

    (*a*) **Constant severe pain.**   (*b*) **Lack of rest and sleep.**

    (*c*) **Ketosis (causing weakness, apathy, lethargy).**   (*d*) **Diminished morale.**

(2) KETOSIS

The metabolic disturbance gives rise to signs formerly known as those of maternal distress. It is due to deficient intake of carbohydrates interfering with the metabolic breakdown of fats. Ketone bodies appear in the urine.

Ketosis usually occurs after 18 hours in labour and dehydration and lack of food accentuate the condition. This in turn contributes to uterine dysfunction and if neglected the maternal and fetal conditions deteriorate.

Electrolytes—particularly potassium—are depleted.

(3) DILATATION OF (*a*) STOMACH, (*b*) COLON, (*c*) BLADDER

The relaxation of involuntary muscle may be due to ketosis and potassium depletion.

    (*a*) **Overdistension of the stomach delays the digestion and absorption of food.** Fluid accumulates, vomiting occurs and dehydration ensues.

    (*b*) **Gaseous distension of the colon reduces peristalsis** and gives rise to pain and discomfort that add to the woman's misery.

    (*c*) **Inability to empty the bladder is a troublesome accompaniment of uterine dysfunction** and if overdistension is manifest catheterization (and instillation of chlorhexidine) may have to be resorted to.

EFFECT ON THE FETUS

Hypertonic uterine action is extremely dangerous for the fetus even when the membranes are intact. Ketosis adds to the hazards.

(1) ANOXIA

The fetus is deprived of oxygen because the utero-placental circulation is diminished by the hypertonic state of the uterus. Fetal anoxia is a constant threat that becomes more serious in ratio to the length of time the membranes have been ruptured and labour has lasted.

(2) STILLBIRTH

The fetal mortality rate is doubled in such cases after 36 hours.

(3) RESPIRATORY INFECTIONS

Pneumonia is common in cases when the membranes have been ruptured for 24 hours.

MANAGEMENT

One very important point is that oxytocic drugs, *i.e.* Pitocin or Syntocinon drip are not given in cases of hypertonic uterine action.

Maternal and fetal condition is observed. (As on p. 393.)

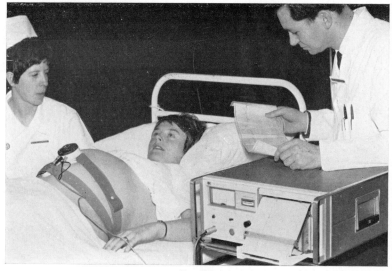

FIG. 285

THE HEWLETT-PACKARD CARDIOTOCOGRAPH SYSTEM.

This apparatus simultaneously measures and records uterine activity and fetal heart frequency. The outputs of the transducers are fed to two distinct channels in the cardiotocograph, where they are processed to give a direct reading of fetal heart frequency and relative uterine activity. These readings are indicated by meters on the front panel of the instrument and simultaneously by the recorder.

(*Simpson Memorial Maternity Pavilion, Edinburgh.*)

TO RELIEVE UTERINE SPASM

Pethidine is invaluable for this purpose and an intravenous drip with 1,000 ml. Dextrose (5 per cent) and 400 mg. Pethidine may be given over a period of 24 hours.

TO RELIEVE PAIN AND ENSURE SLEEP

Analgesics, sedatives and narcotics are prescribed, *e.g.* morphine, 15 mg., or papaveretum, 20 mg.

Trichloryl, 1 G., will soothe the apprehensive woman. Pethidine, 150 mg., with promazine, 25 mg., may be ordered (if not being given by intravenous drip) if pain or backache is severe.

Paracervical nerve block may be given during the latter part of the first stage (see p. 625).   Epidural anæsthesia is advocated.

Biochemical Control and Electrolyte Replacement

This should be instituted in all labours lasting over 18 hours.

DEXTROSE IS GIVEN INTRAVENOUSLY

(*a*) **Where ketonuria is present.**   (*b*) **If vomiting or distension of colon occurs.**

(*c*) **Before signs of dehydration or ketosis are evident.**

TREATMENT OF VOMITING

Oral fluids are stopped: the intravenous route is utilized.

HIGH VAGINAL SWAB

If the membranes have been ruptured 24 hours a bacterial culture is made and an antibiotic administered, *e.g.* ampicillin, 500 mg., followed by 250 mg. 6 hourly.

Operative Procedures

CÆSAREAN SECTION

The termination of labour by lower segment Cæsarean section is employed earlier and more frequently than formerly; the possibility being considered for fetal distress or after 18 hours with ruptured membranes or 24 hours with membranes intact and the os not more than 5 cm. dilated. The midwife should always anticipate Cæsarean section and make tentative preparations: speed is vital in such cases and the pre-pack system facilitates this.

FORCEPS DELIVERY

Episiotomy and application of forceps under pudendal nerve block are commonly necessary to shorten the second stage. Following a long first stage neither mother nor fetus will stand up to a prolonged second stage.

NURSING CARE

The following points are made in addition to what is given under normal and prolonged labour :

Good nursing which includes intelligent observation (based on knowledge and experience) is essential during this difficult labour, the course and outcome of which are often unpredictable.

The competent midwife does not allow dehydration or ketosis to develop, she anticipates them. The experienced midwife knows how much or how little mother and fetus can endure and seeks medical aid before flags of distress are exhibited. She also provides the necessary physical and emotional support.

CONSTRICTION RING DYSTOCIA

This localized spasm of a ring of circular muscle fibres, a condition occurring in about 1 in 1,000 labours, is due to disorganized uterine action. It may occur in the upper or lower segment, commonly near the junction of both, and usually embraces a narrow part of the fetus, *e.g.* the neck.

The constriction ring may form during the first or second stage and when present during the third stage is known as an **hour-glass contraction.**

CAUSES

The spasm may arise in such circumstances as:

(*a*) When the uterus is hypertonic.

(*b*) When the membranes rupture early and the uterus becomes irritated by being moulded round the fetus.

(*c*) Following intra-uterine manipulation, *e.g.* internal version.

Signs

There is no advance of the presenting part. The upper segment feels tender to touch.

The constriction ring is diagnosed vaginally, during the investigation of delay or prior to and during operative delivery. It must not be confused with Bandl's retraction ring.

Treatment

Papaveretum or pethidine is used as in cases of hypertonic uterine action. It may be necessary to achieve immediate relaxation of the constriction ring in order to deliver the fetus or the placenta, and the inhalation of 1 ampoule of amyl nitrite, or the administration of 10 ml. of a 20 per cent solution of magnesium sulphate intravenously, is sometimes successful in relieving the spasm. A general anæsthetic may on occasions be necessary.

CERVICAL DYSTOCIA

RIGID CERVIX

In this rare condition the external os dilates very slowly although the uterine action is normal. The condition occurs mainly in primigravidæ; the first stage of labour is prolonged and painful, backache is severe and persistent.

On vaginal examination the cervix feels thin, tight and unyielding, but may become thick and œdematous later.

The fetus suffers the usual dangers of prolonged, difficult labour; a large caput forms on the presenting part.

Treatment

The treatment is as for hypertonic uterine action.

Cæsarean section is performed in most cases.

Dührssen's incisions of the cervix are rarely made (see Glossary).

N.B.—Cervical rigidity may occasionally be due to other causes, e.g. scarring due to previous injury or infection.

ŒDEMATOUS ANTERIOR LIP OF CERVIX

In cases of disproportion when the cervix is nipped between the fetal head and the brim of the pelvis the lip of cervix becomes swollen and œdematous; it does not stretch well and gives rise to delay and much suffering. Œdema of the cervix may also be caused by the woman bearing down during the first stage.

DIAGNOSIS

The œdematous anterior lip is felt on vaginal or rectal examination as a firm ridge, sometimes as thick as a finger. On occasions, when the condition is not recognised and treated, the glistening cervix may be seen at the vulva between the occiput and the lower border of the symphysis pubis. Partial detachment of cervix may occur.

TREATMENT

The woman is told to breathe rhythmically with her mouth open, throat relaxed, without accentuating expiration during contractions, in order to refrain from pushing; a midwife should be in constant attendance to ensure this. Turning the woman on her side and elevating the foot of the bed may help to take the pressure of the fetal head off the cervix.

Pethidine, or inhalational analgesia, may be helpful, but in persistent cases an attempt is made between contractions to push the cervix up over the head. This must be done very gradually to avoid lacerations.

ANNULAR DETACHMENT OF CERVIX

This occurs in rare instances due to prolonged pressure of a large head on a rigid cervix producing an ischæmic area which inhibits dilatation: bearing down during the first stage may be conducive to this. The necrosed ring of cervix becomes detached and is expelled. Medical aid must be obtained.

CONTRACTED PELVIS

A pelvis is contracted when one or more diameters are less than the minimal normal range by over 1 cm., thereby making the delivery of an average-sized baby by the natural route difficult or impossible.

If undiagnosed, contracted pelvis will give rise to prolonged, difficult and possibly obstructed labour, which may result in injury or death of mother and child.

The recognition of signs which indicate possible contraction of the pelvis is one of the fundamental duties of a midwife.

DIAGNOSIS

Contracted pelvis is more commonly seen in women whose height is less than 1·54 metres (5 feet 1 inch). The more gross deformities may be due to diseases such as rickets, and tuberculosis of spine or hip.

Diminutive height, if due to disease such as rickets, is more serious than when occurring in the small woman with fine bones. A limp, waddling gait, bony deformity of the hips or spine, and any sign of rickets, will arouse suspicion of serious pelvic malformation.

A medical history of injury or disease of spine or pelvis is significant.

OBSTETRICAL HISTORY

If the patient gives a history of difficult labour, forceps delivery, Cæsarean section, or stillbirth, the cause must be sifted. A woman who has given birth spontaneously to a 3,629 G. (8 lb.) baby is likely to have an adequate pelvis, but subsequent babies may give rise to difficulty if over that weight.

EXAMINATION OF THE PREGNANT WOMAN

Every woman must be examined for cephalo-pelvic disproportion at the 37th week, even when her pelvis is of normal shape and dimensions; when a high head or malpresentation is found further investigation is essential.

Pelvimetry by the use of X-rays is resorted to after the 32nd week, if clinical signs of contraction are manifest. **Digital exploration of the pelvic canal will reveal pelvic size and shape** (p. 104).

A pendulous abdomen in a primigravid woman near term usually indicates pelvic contraction or spinal deformity which diminishes the accommodation between the ribs and pelvis and so causes the uterus to become anteverted.

Medical assistance must be obtained by the midwife when she suspects pelvic contraction or cephalo-pelvic disproportion.

The obstetrician will decide whether trial labour or Cæsarean section is indicated, depending on the degree of disproportion; admission to hospital at term will be arranged.

THE JUSTO MINOR PELVIS

This pelvis has been likened to a gynæcoid pelvis in miniature. All the pelvic measurements are diminished but are in correct proportion.

These women are petite, usually under 1·57 m. (5 feet 2 inches) in height, with small hands and feet, shoes size 3 or less, but occasionally the justo minor pelvis may be present in a woman of normal stature.

EFFECT ON LABOUR

The difficulty encountered will depend on the degree of cephalo-pelvic disproportion, and will persist throughout the first and second stages. The mechanism proceeds in the usual way, but there will be exaggerated flexion of the head. If vaginal delivery is possible, a trial labour is carried out.

Cæsarean section may be necessary, but fortunately these women often have small babies.

THE FOUR BASIC TYPES OF PELVES

Female pelves have been classified by Caldwell and Moloy into four basic types, each being designated according to the shape of the brim. The four types are:

GYNÆCOID.   ANTHROPOID.
ANDROID.   PLATYPELLOID.

Gross abnormalities, due to developmental errors and accidents, as well as deformities brought about by diseases such as rickets and tuberculosis of the spine or hip, may be superimposed on any of the four basic types.

GYNÆCOID

This, the true female pelvis, is normal in size and shape. (It has been described under the Normal Pelvis (p. 9).)

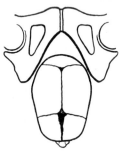

FIG. 285

OUTLET OF ANDROID PELVIS.
The head does not fit into the acute pubic arch and is forced backwards on to the perineum.

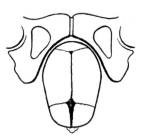

FIG. 286

OUTLET OF GYNÆCOID PELVIS.
The head fits snugly into the pubic arch.

THE ANDROID PELVIS

This pelvis has a heart-shaped brim, and because the cavity is deep and the outlet narrow it has been likened to a funnel. It is no longer believed to be male in type.

Marked contraction of the intertuberischial and the bispinous diameters is the outstanding characteristic.

The subpubic angle and the sacro-sciatic notches are found to be acute on vaginal examination; the ischial spines prominent. Because of the depth of the cavity the diagonal conjugate may be greater than 12·1 cm. (4¾ inches), giving a misleading impression regarding the obstetrical conjugate.

Effect on labour

Posterior positions of the vertex are more common, because the biparietal diameter is more easily accommodated in the posterior segment of the heart-shaped brim.

Deep transverse arrest of the head sometimes occurs.

The head may be forced back into the posterior segment of the outlet, because it cannot be accommodated in the acute pubic arch; much bruising or laceration of the pelvic floor and perineum results.

The fetus does not stand up well to the stress and delay which may occur during the second stage. An episiotomy and forceps delivery are usually necessary.

THE ANTHROPOID PELVIS

In this pelvis the brim is oval, with the transverse diameter less than the anteroposterior.

THE PLATYPELLOID OR SIMPLE FLAT PELVIS

The brim is kidney-shaped, with a diminished antero-posterior diameter and an enlarged transverse. The antero-posterior diameters of the cavity and outlet are also reduced, the whole sacrum being displaced forwards. This **simple flat pelvis** is said to be due to a subclinical form of rickets.

The effect on labour is similar to that in the rachitic flat pelvis, but the difficulty persists throughout labour, as the antero-posterior diameters of the brim, cavity and outlet are all diminished.

THE RACHITIC FLAT PELVIS

This deformed pelvis is due to rickets in early childhood, and is rarely encountered in pronounced form because of the facilities now provided for child health.

Clinical signs of rickets may be evident, such as bow legs and deformities of the spine which, in conjunction with defective growth of bone, tend to diminish stature.

The only diameters diminished in the rachitic flat pelvis are the obstetrical conjugate and the sacro-cotyloid. All the other diameters are increased.

The brim is kidney-shaped because the sacral promontory projects so far forwards. The sacrum lacks the normal curve, and in some cases is straight, with the coccyx bending acutely forwards. The ischial tuberosities are farther apart, so the pubic arch may be greater than a right angle: **the outlet is therefore capacious.**

EFFECT OF FLAT PELVIS ON LABOUR

Cæsarean section will be necessary if the degree of contraction is severe. In minor or moderate degrees a **trial labour** may be carried out (see p. 403). Many hours will elapse before the head passes through the pelvic brim, but when this is accomplished the remainder of the labour will be unusually rapid in the rachitic pelvis.

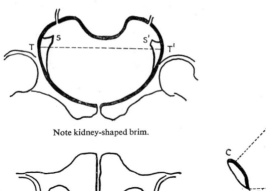

Note kidney-shaped brim.

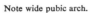

Note wide pubic arch.

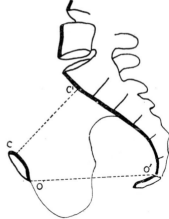

The lateral view shows the diminished antero-posterior diameter of the brim and the increased antero-posterior diameter of the outlet.

FIGS. 287 AND 288

RACHITIC FLAT PELVIS.

Face presentation, prolapse of cord and fetal distress are complications to be anticipated during labour.

MECHANISM OF LABOUR

The fetal head enters in the transverse diameter of the brim and moves to the side of the pelvis on which the occiput lies. This movement permits the bitemporal diameter, instead of the biparietal diameter to pass through the diminished obstetrical conjugate. Increased flexion does not take place, and both fontanelles remain on the same level. The head negotiates the pelvic brim in the following manner.

Anterior asynclitism or Nægele's obliquity.—This is a lateral tilting of the head, so that the super-subparietal diameter, which is less than the biparietal diameter, engages. The anterior parietal bone moves slowly down behind the symphysis pubis until the parietal eminence has passed through the brim. The movement is then reversed, the head tilting in the opposite direction until the posterior parietal bone is pushed past the promontory. Flexion, internal rotation and extension then take place in the usual way.

Posterior asynclitism or Litzmann's obliquity is similar to anterior asynclitism, but the movements are reversed. The posterior parietal bone enters first and is driven past the promontory of the sacrum; then the anterior parietal bone passes down behind the symphysis pubis. This mechanism is less common and occurs in the more severe degrees of flat pelvis.

RARE PELVIC DEFORMITIES

Necessitating Cæsarean Section

1. OSTEOMALACIC OR MALACOSTEON PELVIS

This extreme deformity is due to the disease, osteomalacia, which is found in certain localities but is rarely seen in Britain or America. It occurs in multigravidæ and is due to gross deficiency of minerals and vitamins in the diet. All the bones of the skeleton soften and the sides of the pelvic canal are squashed together until the brim becomes a mere Y-shaped slit.

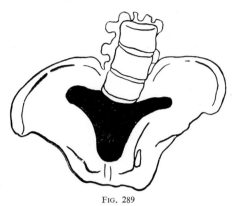

Fig. 289

Osteomalacic or malacosteon pelvis.

2. NÆGELE'S PELVIS

In this instance the sacrum has only one wing, probably due to maldevelopment or disease of the sacro-iliac joint with ankylosis, occurring during infancy. The brim is obliquely contracted.

3. ROBERT'S PELVIS

This is one in which there are no wings to the sacrum and the brim consists of a narrow opening.

SPINAL DEFORMITIES

When kyphosis (forward angulation) or scoliosis (lateral curvature) is evident, or any limp or deformity is present, the midwife must refer the woman to a doctor. Such marked deformities are readily diagnosed, but **greater vigilance is needed in detecting the lesser degrees of pelvic contraction or of cephalo-pelvic disproportion.**

TRIAL LABOUR

A trial or test of labour is carried out in cases where there is a moderate degree of cephalo-pelvic disproportion, in which it is difficult to decide whether delivery *per vaginam* is possible.

The outcome depends on such factors as:

THE STRENGTH OF THE UTERINE CONTRACTIONS.

THE GIVE OF THE PELVIC JOINTS.

THE DEGREE OF MOULDING OF THE HEAD.

THE PHYSICAL AND EMOTIONAL FORTITUDE OF THE MOTHER.

The effect of these factors cannot be predicted, so judgment is withheld as to whether Cæsarean section will be necessary, until labour has been in progress for some hours.

Trial labour is not a test of how much the woman or the fetus can endure, and must not be permitted to continue until signs of fetal or maternal exhaustion are exhibited; nor should it ever reach the stage of obstruction. **The outcome ought to be a live mother and child who have sustained the minimal amount of trauma.**

It is a searching test of the judgment of those in charge during labour, and successful management rests heavily on the labour ward sister. Practical experience and knowledge are needed, but wisdom, which is the faculty of applying knowledge and experience judiciously, is indispensable in such circumstances.

MANAGEMENT

The woman, usually a primigravida, is allowed to go to term, because the spontaneous onset of labour is more likely to result in efficient uterine action; the mature fetus is better equipped to withstand prolonged labour. But disordered uterine action sometimes occurs when disproportion exists.

Labour is conducted in hospital, where constant supervision, expert care and provision for operative procedures are available.

Lower segment Cæsarean section should be anticipated: it is usually performed in preference to a difficult forceps delivery.

THE LENGTH OF TRIAL LABOUR

Opinions differ regarding this. So many factors have to be considered that " *time in hours* " can be a treacherous criterion on which to make the decision. Some authorities consider that, on weighing up the situation after **six or eight hours of good contractions,** they can predict whether a safe vaginal delivery is possible. If the cervix dilates slowly with good contractions or if the contractions are poor the outlook is gloomy.

The decision rests with the obstetrician.

THE MIDWIFE'S DUTIES

1. Careful Abdominal Examination on Admission

(*a*) **The presentation will be the vertex;** the position should be diagnosed, L.O.A. being most favourable.

(*b*) **The head will not be engaged,** but its level in relation to the pelvic brim should be assessed. This can be checked by rectal examination.

(*c*) **The degree of flexion** of the head and the amount of overlap at the brim is noted.

(*d*) **The fetal heart rate** is carefully counted and recorded in graph form.

2. Vigilant Observation

The midwife remains in constant attendance—observing, recording, and maintaining the woman's morale.

(*a*) **Uterine action.**—The time of the onset of contractions, their frequency, length and strength should be recorded. A monitoring device may be employed.

(*b*) **Fetal condition.**—The fetal heart rate should be taken every 15 minutes or electrically monitored and recorded in graph form.

Signs of fetal distress are watched for, and these may arise early in labour because of the excessive moulding necessary to allow the head to engage. Fetal scalp blood sampling may be done.

(*c*) **Progress.**—The midwife should note what is accomplished in a given time, *i.e.* every two hours, taking into consideration the type of uterine contractions.

The maternal condition needs close supervision but does not usually cause anxiety during the first 18 hours, as ketosis is not as a rule manifest until then.

The nursing care is similar to that which is given for prolonged labour : a fluid balance and urine analysis chart is kept (see p. 410).

ON ABDOMINAL EXAMINATION

Increase of flexion and descent of the head should be noted.

ON VAGINAL OR RECTAL EXAMINATION

(*a*) Level of the head and degree of flexion; (*b*) dilatation of the os; (*c*) consistency of cervix; (*d*) membranes intact or ruptured; (*e*) excessive moulding; a large caput.

CONDITIONS TO BE REPORTED TO THE DOCTOR

Rupture of membranes, colour of amniotic fluid.—Time of occurrence and number of hours in labour.

Unsatisfactory advance when contractions are good, *e.g.* head still high after six to eight hours in labour.

Hypotonic inertia, or inco-ordinate uterine action.

Signs of fetal or maternal distress.

Change of vertex presentation to brow or face.

OBSTRUCTED LABOUR

Obstructed labour is present when there is no advance of the presenting part in spite of strong uterine contractions and is due to some fault in the passages or passenger (but not in the powers) producing an impassable barrier. Obstruction should not occur, as the cause should have been detected during pregnancy or early in labour.

Obstruction usually occurs at the pelvic inlet but can take place at the outlet, as in cases of android pelvis and when undiagnosed deep transverse arrest of the head occurs.

CAUSES

1. CONTRACTED PELVIS 2. PELVIC TUMOURS

(*a*) Fibroid tumours rarely give rise to obstruction unless situated in the lower pole of the uterus; (*b*) bony tumours are rarer still.

3. MALPRESENTATION. Shoulder. Brow. Face. (*persistent mento-posterior*).

4. LARGE BABY

When the fetus is over 4·5 kg. (10 lb.) and the pelvis average in size, there will be delay and difficulty, but actual obstruction is more likely with a baby weighing over 5·46 kg. (12 lb.).

5. GROSS FETAL ABNORMALITIES

Hydrocephaly is the most common cause ; tumours and conjoined twins are rare.

EARLY SIGNS

The presenting part does not enter the pelvic brim, in spite of good contractions. It should be remembered that a full bladder and a large bag of membranes may prevent the head from engaging.

The os dilates slowly and the cervix hangs loosely like " an empty sleeve " because the presenting part cannot descend and become applied to it.

The membranes tend to rupture.

25

LATER SIGNS

(a) **The uterus becomes moulded round the fetus** and does not relax properly between contractions.

(b) **The presenting part becomes wedged** and immovable when it descends partly into the pelvis.

(c) **The cranial bones overlap excessively** and a large caput forms.

(d) **Uterine exhaustion ; contractions may cease for a period** to recommence with renewed vigour, usually in primigravid women.

(e) **Bandl's ring may occasionally be seen abdominally,** rising nearer the umbilicus as the lower uterine segment becomes progressively thinner.

Evidence of maternal ketosis and fetal distress are usually manifest

DANGERS

1. MATERNAL

Rupture of the uterus, due to excessive thinning of the lower uterine segment.

Death of the mother.—In neglected cases the woman may die from exhaustion, undelivered, or from shock following urgent operative delivery especially when ketosis and dehydration have not been combated. She may die from rupture of the uterus. (Sepsis and haemorrhage can usually be dealt with by modern methods.)

Vesico-vaginal fistula may occur, due to bruising of the bladder, or to injury during a difficult instrumental delivery.

2. FETAL

Stillbirth. Neonatal death, due to asphyxia or intracranial hæmorrhage.

TREATMENT OF OBSTRUCTED LABOUR

1. During Pregnancy (prophylaxis)

Recognition of, and reporting to the doctor, conditions which would give rise to obstruction.

Examination of every woman at the 37th week by a doctor, to exclude cephalo-pelvic disproportion.

External version for shoulder presentation.

Making arrangements in cases of hydrocephaly for admission to hospital, where craniotomy will be done during labour when the os is 5 cm. dilated.

2. During Labour

Lower segment Cæsarean section is performed if conditions are present which would cause obstruction or if early signs of obstruction are manifest. **It is the duty of the midwife to recognize these and summon medical assistance.**

Intravenous dextrose, 5 or 10 per cent, is given prior to, and during operative delivery. Preparations are made to treat a shocked mother and baby. Blood should be at hand.

Embryotomy may be necessary in neglected cases.

TONIC CONTRACTION AND RETRACTION

This serious condition arises during the uterine effort to overcome an obstruction; the contractions occurring more frequently and more strongly, until one long contraction is maintained. Retraction is extreme and the upper segment becomes hard and excessively thick: the lower uterine segment is abnormally thin, tender to touch, and may rupture, particularly in multigravid patients.

The fetus dies of anoxia, due to the constant contractions diminishing its supply of oxygen.

Treatment of Tonic Contractions

Medical assistance must be summoned urgently.

Papaveretum, 20 mg., will relieve pain but a general anæsthetic is needed to damp down uterine activity and prevent rupture. The uterus is emptied without delay and Cæsarean section is usually performed but if not practicable embryotomy may be necessary.

Such a state of affairs should not arise; the midwife ought to have diagnosed the condition causing obstructed labour and obtained medical assistance prior to the onset of tonic contractions.

QUESTIONS FOR REVISION

DISORDERED UTERINE ACTION

What is the cause of constriction ring occurring during the third stage ? Give the treatment of constriction ring.

C.M.B.(Scot.) paper.—What are the types of disordered uterine action during labour ? Give the nursing care of prolonged labour.

C.M.B.(Scot.) paper.—What are the dangers of uterine inertia ? Outline the nursing care of such a case.

CONTRACTED PELVIS

Rearrange Correctly

DESCRIPTION	TERM		
1. Funnel shaped pelvis	**Justo minor**	(	)
2. Small pelvis	**Gynæcoid**	(	)
3. Narrow transverse diameters	**Platypelloid**	(	)
4. Round brim	**Anthropoid**	(	)
5. All antero-posterior diameters diminished	**Android**	(	)
6. Y shaped brim	**Roberts**	(	)
7. One ala to sacrum	**Malacosteon**	(	)

C.M.B.(Scot.) paper.—(*a*) What is a contracted pelvis ? (*b*) What would lead you to suspect this deformity ? (*c*) What effects might it have on the course of the patient's pregnancy and labour ?

C.M.B.(Scot.) paper.—Describe the main characteristics of the following types of pelvis (*a*) justo minor (*b*) simple flat, (*c*) rachitic flat. Discuss the care of a patient having a trial labour.

TRIAL LABOUR

Define Trial Labour.—On what four unpredictable factors does the outcome depend ? Describe the abdominal examination you would carry out at the beginning of labour, What observations would you make and record during labour ? What would you report to the doctor ?

C.M.B.(N. Ireland) paper.—What steps would you take to maintain a mother's good condition during a trial labour ? What signs and symptoms would lead you to suppose that her condition was deteriorating ?

C.M.B.(N. Ireland) paper.—What are the important points in the nursing of a case of " trial labour " ?

C.M.B.(Scot.) paper.—Describe the nursing care of a patient who is having a trial labour. How would you recognize the development of (*a*) maternal exhaustion and (*b*) fetal distress ?

C.M.B.(Scot.) paper.—Describe the management of a patient during a trial labour.

OBSTRUCTED LABOUR

C.M.B.(Scot.) paper.—What are the causes of obstructed labour ? How can these be prevented by proper antenatal care ?

23

Prolonged Labour

CAUSES; MANAGEMENT; DANGERS

Labour is said to be prolonged when it exceeds the normal limit of 24 hours; false labour should not be included. But delay can be inferred prior to then if, with good contractions, the presenting part remains high or descends slowly, and when dilatation of the os is retarded.

Student midwives sometimes confuse prolonged labour with obstructed labour. Cephalo-pelvic disproportion lengthens labour and the more serious degrees give rise to obstruction; weak uterine contractions prolong, but never obstruct, labour.

The midwife should be aware of the conditions which lengthen labour, in order that special precautions can be taken from the onset to avert the hazards to which mother and fetus are subjected.

The more common causes of prolonged labour are given below; diagnosis and treatment are considered under their respective headings.

CAUSES OF DELAY

First Stage	*Second Stage*
Disordered uterine action	**Hypotonic uterine action.**
Contracted pelvis.	**Rigid perineum. Android pelvis.**
Impacted lip of cervix.	**Unreduced occipito - posterior**
Occipito-posterior position.	**position: deep transverse arrest.**
Big baby, face presentation.	**Big baby, face presentation.**

Admission to Hospital

The modern tendency is to admit patients to hospital if the first stage is still in progress after 18 hours and there is no likelihood of the early completion of labour.

The woman needs constant supervision, and unless good nursing care is provided ketosis develops; her condition begins to deteriorate after about 36 hours, and when 48 hours have elapsed the danger zone is reached. Mother, uterus and fetus are all exhausted. The domiciliary midwife, however willing, becomes tired, her judgment is impaired and she is no longer capable of giving the high standard of obstetrical nursing care necessary in such cases.

Midwives in developing countries should be taught the old maxim: that " *the sun should not set twice on the woman in labour* " Medical aid should be obtained.

INVESTIGATION OF PATIENT ADMITTED WITH PROLONGED LABOUR

1. **A history of labour, including records, is obtained** from doctor or midwife: (*a*) labour—length of, type and frequency of contractions; (*b*) When membranes ruptured;? **this is significant because after 24 hours the risk of puerperal sepsis or neonatal pneumonia is very great.**

Tranquillisers and analgesic drugs given; sleep or rest obtained; food and fluid taken; vomiting; bowel and bladder function; maternal and fetal condition.

2. **Examination of woman:** (*a*) general appearance—distressed, dispirited, exhausted, dehydrated; (*b*) **temperature and pulse—an increase in either would be significant indicating the possible need for antibiotics;** (*c*) **urine analysis—concentrated urine suggests fluid imbalance and dehydration.** Ketostix reagent strips will detect ketones.

3. **Abdominal examination:** (*a*) uterine tonus—strength, length and frequency of contractions; (*b*) presentation, position, engagement, size of baby, disproportion, fetal heart rate.

4. **Vaginal examination:** (*a*) dilatation and consistency of cervix, membranes ruptured, level of presenting part, presentation, position, moulding and caput formation.

MANAGEMENT

Sedation.—Drugs are given for the relief of pain and to induce sleep which is usually very much needed: papaveretum, 20 mg., or pethidine, 100 mg., with 25 mg. promazine (Sparine) are effective. For severe backache paracervical block or epidural anæsthesia may be resorted to.

Electrolyte replacement and fluid balance control is carried out.

Mechanical devices to monitor uterine contractions, fetal heart and blood gases are usually employed (see p. 396).

Operative measures should be anticipated: Cæsarean section; ventouse extraction; episiotomy and forceps delivery. The baby may need respiratory resuscitation and maintenance with the intermittent positive pressure respirator.

NURSING CARE

In addition to the nursing care prescribed for normal labour, the following recommendations are made.

URINE ANALYSIS

The bladder is emptied and the urine is examined every four hours for ketones, to detect ketosis, and when present indicate the need for a full review of fluid balance and electrolytes. It is also advisable to test for protein every four hours. After 12 hours in labour every specimen is tested.

FLUID

A fluid balance chart should be kept and at least 1,800 ml. of fluid given in 24 hours; if ketones are present in the urine, 5 per cent dextrose should be administered intravenously. After 18 hours fluid is usually administered by the intravenous route. The woman should lie on her side to facilitate the excretion of fluid by the kidneys.

FOOD MAY BE DANGEROUS

Dilatation of the stomach with fluid, or the retention of undigested food, must be avoided. Withholding food by mouth and the administration of dextrose 5 per cent intravenously is imperative.

PATIENCE

During the first stage the best treatment is patience so long as the membranes are intact, the condition of mother and fetus good and progress is taking place. Tact is also needed; cases of " premature interference," often subsequently sent into hospital, are in some measure due to faulty handling of the situation by an inexperienced midwife.

COMPANIONSHIP AND SUPERVISION

The woman should not be left alone unless in sound sleep and during this time she must be closely observed.

ENCOURAGEMENT

Much encouragement is needed, for when the woman becomes tired she clamours for her labour to be brought to an end. It is here that management often breaks down, especially in posterior position of the vertex in domiciliary practice. Relatives implore the midwife to send for the doctor, but she should explain that " the neck of the womb " must be completely opened up before the baby can be born or instruments used.

CHANGE OF POSITION

During a tedious first stage, change of position often brings relief and sometimes stimulates uterine action. She should be permitted to get up and walk about, sit or lie down, as she feels inclined, but if liquor is draining freely she ought to be kept in bed.

PERSONAL TOILET

A bath or shower is very soothing and should be repeated in 12 hours. Help in cleaning her teeth and brushing her hair will be appreciated by the tired woman.

UNREMITTING OBSERVATION

1. CONSTANT DESCENT

The midwife must note whether constant, even if slow, descent of the fetus is taking place. This is observed abdominally during the first stage, and from " below " during the second stage.

Progressive dilatation of the os should also be taking place.

2. THE MATERNAL CONDITION

Blood pressure, pulse and temperature are taken and recorded every four hours, more frequently if necessary.

The woman's general condition should be under constant surveillance. It is not good midwifery to wait until maternal distress is apparent before sending for medical assistance. Such a state should be anticipated by taking into consideration:

(a) The woman's general vitality.

(b) The time she has been in labour and whether the membranes are intact.

(c) How much sleep she has had.

(d) The amount of pain experienced.

(e) Whether dehydration and ketosis are present.

SIGNS OF MATERNAL DISTRESS – KETOSIS
EARLY SIGNS

(a) A rising pulse is one of the earliest signs of distress, and when over 90, constitutes a definite warning: it may be 120.

(b) Increase in temperature.—The temperature will probably be over 37·2° C. (99° F.).

(c) The woman feels weak; she is apathetic. (d) Vomiting commonly occurs.

(e) Ketonuria is present.

LATER SIGNS

(*a*) **Anxious expression.**—The woman has a drawn, anxious expression with a degree of circumoral pallor; her nose and mouth look pinched, and with an imploring glance she appeals for help.

(*b*) **The woman looks and feels ill.** She senses that something is wrong.

(*c*) **Beads of perspiration are seen on the upper lip.**

(*d*) **Signs of dehydration are manifest,** *e.g.* dry lips, parched tongue, concentrated urine.

(*e*) **Marked restlessness.**—Between uterine contractions she does not relax; she is distracted and restless.

(*f*) **Vomiting when persistent,** with dark-coloured vomitus welling up into the mouth, is an ominous sign.

Treatment

Medical aid is summoned.

Intravenous fluid and electrolytes will be given. Dextrose 10 per cent 540 ml. ×2 then 5 per cent.

The cause of distress is dealt with and may necessitate operative procedure.

3. THE FETAL CONDITION

In cases of prolonged labour the fetal condition needs assiduous supervision, especially, as previously stated, when the membranes rupture early. Recording the fetal heart in graph form draws attention to an increase or decrease in rate: continuous recording by cardiotocograph enables early warning signs of distress to be detected.

FETAL ANOXIA

This occurs when conditions are present which interfere with the supply of oxygen to the fetus. The supply may be cut off in the cord, placenta, uterine wall, or in the mother's blood vessels, *e.g.*

THE CORD	THE PLACENTA	THE UTERUS	MATERNAL CONDITIONS
Prolapse	Premature separation		Pre-eclampsia Hypertension
Nipping	Multiple infarcts Dysfunction— (*a*) Pre-eclampsia (*b*) Post-maturity (*c*) Diabetes	Hypertonic action	Severe cardiac or pulmonary disease. Hb below 8·4G
Tightening knots	Early rupture of membranes	Tonic contractions	Effect of analgesic drugs and anæsthetics given

FIG. 290

Signs of Fetal Distress

(*a*) THE FETAL HEART-SOUNDS

RAPID FETAL HEART RATE

When the rate increases by 20 beats this is a sign of mild oxygen lack and is the earliest sign of fetal distress. A rate of over 160 should give rise to concern.

SLOW FETAL HEART RATE

When the rate decreases by 20 beats this usually indicates oxygen lack.

The heart-beat becomes progressively slower, and may be as slow as 80 beats per minute, but a fetal heart rate under 110 gives rise to concern; when below 100 the fetus is in the danger zone.

If the fetal heart takes progressively longer to recover its normal rate or a slow beat persists for over 15 seconds, after each uterine contraction has ceased, the possibility of cardiac weakness is likely.

Any alteration in rhythm, such as a long first sound and a short second sound, instead of the reverse, may indicate that distress is imminent. An irregular or intermittent beat is equally serious, but a weak fetal heart-sound is not always significant, as it may be due to a change in the position of the fetus, causing the chest or scapula to be less accessible to the fetal stethoscope.

The fetal heart may remain quite good and then suddenly fail, but, on the other hand, the baby may be born in a satisfactory condition after having shown what were believed to be signs of distress.

(*b*) THE PASSAGE OF MECONIUM

Except during the second stage in cases of breech presentation this should be considered a serious sign. In 30 per cent of cases fetal distress is present. It is due to the relaxed state of the intestine and anal sphincter because of the poor muscle tone induced by anoxia. Slight green staining of the liquor may be due to previous distress from which the fetus has now recovered. Thick fresh meconium denotes distress which needs urgent attention except as already stated.

In cases of early fetal distress some obstetricians puncture the membranes to find out whether meconium is present.

(*c*) EXCESSIVE FETAL MOVEMENTS

These may be of serious import, and are due to convulsions of the anoxic fetus that sometimes precede intra-uterine death. As a general rule, very little fetal movement is felt during normal labour.

(*d*) THE FUNIC SOUFFLE (p. 120).

This is sometimes heard when the cord circulation is impeded, as would occur in prolapse or nipping of the cord or a tightening knot. It can and does occur in the absence of fetal distress, but should be considered a warning sign until proved otherwise.

THE FETAL HEART MONITOR

Continuous monitoring of the fetal heart provides an added safeguard in cases where fetal distress may be anticipated. It is particularly useful during the first stage, and at night, to avoid disturbing the patient.

The transducer is secured to the woman's abdomen over the area of fetal heart maximal intensity. Fetal heart rate and amplitude are shown on the panel-meter and on a strip chart-recorder.

SALING METHOD OF DETECTING FETAL ANOXIA

When the fetus is anoxic the pH of its blood falls and this is a guide to the oxygenation of the fetus. The normal level is around 7·35.

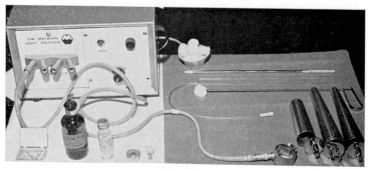

FIG. 291

REQUIREMENTS FOR SALING METHOD OF SAMPLING FETAL SCALP BLOOD.

Non-Sterile	*Sterile*
Light source	**Woolly balls.**
Fibre optic light guide.	**Knife holder** with blade.
Ethyl chloride spray.	**Capillary glass tube** with catheter.
Silicone grease.	**Swab holder.**
Metal rods and magnet for mixing blood.	**3 Sizes of Amnioscope.**
Plasticine to seal tubes.	

Lower Shelf

Gown, gloves; 2 sterile towels; obstetric cream; lotion and swabs.
(*Simpson Memorial Maternity Pavilion, Edinburgh*)

When fetal distress is anticipated or suspected a sample of fetal capillary blood is obtained by passing an amnioscope into the cervical canal, cleansing the scalp and spraying it with ethyl chloride. A small incision is made with a 4 mm. blade and 0·5 ml. blood is sucked through a length of capillary polythene tubing by the obstetrician.

Fetal distress is always accompanied by respiratory and metabolic acidosis with a lowering of the pH of the blood.

The pH of the blood is estimated by the Astrup micro-apparatus; repeated tests being made in suspicious cases, i.e., pH under 7·25. A pH of 7·2 or less is a reliable indication for the consideration of termination of labour in an endeavour to save the baby.

Prophylactic Treatment of Fetal Distress

The fetal heart should be listened to assiduously.

Should conditions exist which would cause anoxia, or intracranial injury, the midwife is required to obtain medical assistance. The experienced midwife does not wait until definite signs of fetal distress are evident, before notifying the doctor; she anticipates them by the amount of stress to which the fetus is being subjected. It is believed that fetal anoxia lasting over 10 minutes may be a **primary cause** of **mental retardation and spastic paralysis.** The midwife must do all in her power to avert such tragic afflictions.

The midwife should be judicious in giving sedatives during premature labour and when conditions exist that give rise to placental dysfunction, or when the fetal condition is causing anxiety. The effect of such drugs in depressing the fetal respiratory centre may inhibit the subsequent establishment of respiration.

The effect of pethidine and trichloroethylene when given together is harmful to the fetus.

ACTIVE TREATMENT OF FETAL DISTRESS

1. ADMINISTRATION OF OXYGEN

When the mother has anoxæmia (*a deficiency of oxygen in the blood*), as occurs in eclampsia, cardiac failure, or in collapse due to severe ante-partum hæmorrhage, oxygen should be administered. (*Some question the value of this.*)

2. CÆSAREAN SECTION

During the first stage of labour Cæsarean section should be anticipated and the necessary preparations made.

3. EPISIOTOMY

Should marked fetal distress occur because the head is held up by a rigid perineum, and there is no possibility of getting the doctor in time, a midwife would make an episiotomy under local anæsthesia.

4. THE PROMPT APPLICATION OF FORCEPS

This will often ensure a live baby, but, when forceps are applied under general anæsthesia in cases of established fetal distress, the baby is liable to be born in a state of severe asphyxia. Pudendal nerve block is preferred.

The pædiatrician should be notified in order that he may be present to resuscitate the baby.

EARLY RUPTURE OF MEMBRANES

The harmful effects of early rupture of membranes have already been discussed under normal labour (p. 288), but in cases of prolonged labour such effects are intensified.

When the liquor has drained away, the uterus may mould round and cling to the fetus, a state of affairs that retards its expulsion. Spasm of uterine muscle may take place, and is extremely painful: if localized, a constriction ring which causes further delay forms.

Intra-uterine anoxia may occur in such circumstances, and there is a risk of fetal pneumonia due to inhalation of infected liquor, as well as the danger of puerperal sepsis.

A high vaginal swab is taken after 24 hours.

Ampicillin 500 mg.+250 mg. 6 hourly may be prescribed when the membranes have been ruptured for 24 hours

Pyrexia of 37·5° C. (99·6° F.) or over during labour is an absolute indication for the administration of antibiotics. A pædiatrician is present at birth when the membranes have ruptured early.

DANGERS OF A PROLONGED SECOND STAGE

1. TO THE FETUS

During the perineal phase the fetal head is being exposed to great pressure; it is being forced downwards by the contracting uterus and resisted by the pelvic floor, and the excessive moulding may give rise to intracranial injury and anoxia. The placenta is compressed between the retracted thickened wall of the upper uterine segment and the buttocks of the fetus, and because much of the amniotic fluid will have drained away, interference with the placental circulation occurs, resulting in fetal anoxia. (*Signs of fetal distress must be watched for.*) (See p. 413.)

2. TO THE UTERUS

If the presenting part does not advance with good contractions, the lower uterine segment may be stretched to such an extent that it ruptures—a serious accident.

3. TO THE PELVIC FLOOR

When the head is pounding on the pelvic floor for longer than three-quarters of an hour, the perineum becomes œdematous and is more likely to tear; in addition, the pelvic floor is unduly stretched and **uterine prolapse, cystocele and stress incontinence are liable to ensue.** When the urethra is persistently compressed by the fetal head it becomes bruised and this may give rise to retention of urine during the puerperium.

When the head does not appear after half an hour of good contractions, a vaginal examination should be made to find the cause of the delay; excessive moulding or a large caput would indicate that the fetal head is being exposed to undue stress.

If, when the head is showing at the vulva, good uterine contractions do not overcome the resistance of the perineum within half an hour, or if no advance is made during that time, it is advisable in the interests of mother and child to obtain medical assistance.

But time is not always the best criterion; much depends on the type of contractions and the condition of mother and fetus.

The Need for Delivery by Forceps

Should delay be due to outlet disproportion, hypotonic inertia, or a rigid perineum the application of forceps may be necessary.

The midwife should not hesitate to send for medical aid, nor should she consider the need for low forceps an admission of failure on her part. There is nothing meritorious in a spontaneous delivery if the mother has endured emotional and physical trauma or the baby suffers intracranial injury or anoxia.

The last hour of labour may do more damage to mother and baby than the whole of the preceding hours, and, if the midwife delays too long in sending for the doctor, the infant's chances of survival are poor.

QUESTIONS FOR REVISION

PROLONGED LABOUR

Differentiate between prolonged and obstructed labour. **What special nursing care is necessary ? Give six signs of maternal ketosis. Mention the dangers** of a prolonged second stage, under the following headings : (*a*) the fetus ; (*b*) the uterus ; (*c*) the pelvic floor.

ORAL QUESTIONS

Why should a woman in labour at home be admitted to hospital after 18 hours ? Which urine tests are made ? How could you give the woman physical and emotional support ?

For what reasons are the following done ? high vaginal swab; pH of fetal blood estimated; fluid balance chart kept; intravenous fluid administered ?

Differentiate between: fetal tachycardia and bradycardia; ketonuria and proteinuria.

How would you try to stimulate poor uterine action ? Why is biochemical control necessary during prolonged labour ?

What precautions are essential when giving an oxytocic drip for hypotonic uterine action ? **Why is hypertonic uterine action more dangerous** than hypotonic action ? **Why is a high vaginal swab taken** when the membranes have been ruptured for 24 hours ?

What are the early signs of obstructed labour ? What would make you suspect contracted pelvis: (a) from the medical and obstetrical histories; (b) from the woman's appearance.

Write not more than 10 lines on: nursing care in prolonged labour; dangers and management of early rupture of membranes; dangers of a prolonged second stage.

Differentiate between: false labour and hypotonic uterine action; constriction ring and retraction ring; simple and rachitic flat pelvis; gynæcoid and android pelvis; hypotonic and hypertonic uterine action; Bandl's ring and a full bladder.

Write not more than 10 lines on: constriction ring dystocia; œdematous anterior lip of cervix; diagnosis of contracted pelvis; deciding factors in length of a trial labour; causes of obstructed labour; tonic contractions.

C.M.B.(Eng.) paper.—Discuss the methods by which the progress of labour can be assessed. What are the common causes of delay in the second stage ?

C.M.B.(Eng.) paper.—What are the causes of delay in the second stage of labour in a woman who has previously had a normal labour ?

C.M.B.(Scot.) paper.—What are possible causes of delay in the first stage of labour ? Under what circumstances would you send for a doctor during the course of such a labour ?

C.M.B. (Scot.) paper.—What are the causes of delay in the first stage of labour ? Describe the management of a patient with delay in the first stage.

C.M.B.(N. Ireland) paper.—What are the causes of delay in the second stage of labour? What are your duties in such a case?

C.M.B.(Eng.) paper, 1969.—Describe the management of a primigravid patient who is not delivered after twenty-four hours in labour.

C.M.B.(Eng.) paper, 1969.—What do you mean by maternal distress? Describe the steps that you would take to prevent and treat this during labour.

FETAL DISTRESS

State what changes may occur in the fetal heart ; rate, rhythm, regularity.

Fill in the causes of intra-uterine anoxia under the following headings :—			
THE CORD	THE PLACENTA	THE UTERUS	MATERNAL CONDITIONS
1.	1.	1.	1.
2.	2.	2.	2.
3.	3.		3.

C.M.B. (N. Ireland) paper.—What are the signs of fetal distress ? What are the duties of a midwife when this condition arises ?

C.M.B.(Eng.) paper.—A primigravida is in early labour, the membranes rupture and the liquor is meconium stained. What may the cause of this be, and what should the midwife do ?

C.M.B.(Eng.) paper.—What are the signs of fetal distress during labour ? Give the causes of this condition and describe how you would deal with it.

C.M.B.(Scot.) paper.—How do you diagnose fetal distress in labour ? How is this condition managed ?

C.M.B.(Scot.) paper.—Describe the methods available for assessing the state of the fetus during pregnancy and labour.

C.M.B.(Eng.) paper, 1969.—What is fetal distress? How is it recognized in labour and how may it be treated.

24

Obstetrical Emergencies

RUPTURE OF THE UTERUS

THIS is one of the most serious accidents in obstetrics, occurring in approximately 1 in 3000 cases.

The four main causes are:

A. WEAK CÆSAREAN SECTION SCAR.
B. OBSTRUCTED LABOUR.
C. TRAUMA DURING OPERATIVE MANIPULATION PER VAGINAM.
D. THE MISUSE OF OXYTOCIC DRUGS.

A. DUE TO WEAK CÆSAREAN SECTION SCAR

Factors causing a weakened scar are:

1. When the wound does not heal by first intention.
2. If another pregnancy occurs within six months.
3. Overdistension as in subsequent twins or hydramnios.

TIME OF RUPTURE

The scar usually ruptures during the last four weeks of pregnancy or at the beginning of labour, and as the signs are not as dramatic as in obstructed labour, the term " silent rupture " is applied.

WARNING SIGNS

The woman may experience intermittent pain in her right side, not necessarily severe, which may persist over a period of four or five days. Pain is due to irritation of the peritoneum by the trickling of blood from the uterine scar which is " giving way."

Low abdominal pain accompanied by vomiting, even when the pulse is below 100, is a significant sign of scar rupture. Shock comes on slowly in some cases, and abruptly in others depending on the degree of rupture and the amount of internal hæmorrhage. (*The baby is rarely found to be alive when the abdomen is opened.*)

MANAGEMENT

All labours subsequent to Cæsarean section should be conducted in hospital because of the danger of scar rupture; the author having seen a case of ruptured scar prior to which the woman had one spontaneous and one forceps delivery subsequent to a classical Cæsarean section for placenta prævia.

These patients should be under the care of an obstetrician, who will admit them to hospital for the last two weeks of pregnancy.

(Oxytocin is rarely given to induce labour in such cases and if so constant monitoring is mandatory.)

DURING LABOUR

The midwife's responsibility is heavy, and she must pay close attention to the following points:

1. Abdominal palpation

This should be reduced to a minimum and performed with great gentleness.

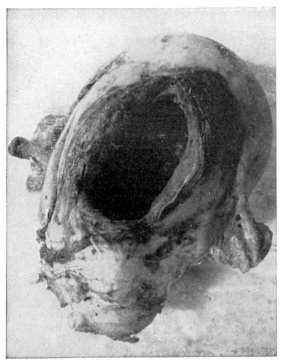

Fig. 292

Rupture of uterus through classical Cæsarean section scar.

2. The following features should be reported to the doctor :

(a) Slight or no advance, with good contractions during first stage.

(b) Increasing tenderness over the scar.

(c) Constant pain in the lower abdomen.

(d) Insufficient advance during second stage.

(e) Vaginal bleeding.

(f) A rising pulse rate.

(g) Signs of shock.

B. DUE TO OBSTRUCTED LABOUR

The uterus ruptures because of excessive thinning of the lower uterine segment, and in view of the possibility of this catastrophe midwives must know the causes of obstructed labour and detect them during pregnancy (p. 402).

Recognition of the signs of obstructed labour is equally important, but such a state of affairs does not arise in the practice of a competent midwife; she detects the conditions causing obstruction and seeks medical assistance.

The patient is usually a grande-multipara whose uterus is liable to have much fibrous tissue that does not stretch well.

Rupture has, to the author's knowledge, occurred when the woman had been one hour in the second stage and less than 12 hours in labour. It occurs more commonly during the second stage.

Warning Signs

1. General and abdominal signs of obstructed labour are manifest, such as a rising pulse rate, tonic contractions and Bandl's ring.

2. The lower segment is exquisitely tender.   3. Vaginal bleeding is an ominous sign.

ACTUAL RUPTURE

The excruciatingly painful uterine contractions cease and the woman may feel that " something has given way ", but not in all cases.

The uterus may be felt as a separate mass.

She feels faint and rapidly becomes profoundly shocked.

Fetal distress and cessation of the fetal heart beat.

The fetus, now in the peritoneal cavity, can be palpated beneath the abdominal wall.

Any abdominal or shoulder pain experienced is due to the presence of blood or of the uterine contents in the peritoneal cavity.

These signs will be less pronounced when uterine rupture is not extensive; shock comes on more slowly.

Treatment of Ruptured Uterus

ON DISTRICT

The " Flying Squad " is summoned and the woman treated for shock (see p. 442).

Blood transfusion will be given if necessary and a sedative administered prior to transferring the patient to hospital as quickly as possible.

IN HOSPITAL

1. The woman is laid flat.   2. Treatment for shock is given.

3. Preparations are made for blood transfusion.

4. Preparations are made for hysterectomy (the rent *may be* sutured in scar rupture and in *other* cases where the tear is not irregular).

The prognosis is less good in cases of obstructed labour, the maternal mortality rate being 50 to 60 per cent. The fetal mortality rate is almost 100 per cent in cases of complete rupture.

C. DUE TO TRAUMA DURING DYSTOCIA

1. INTERNAL VERSION FOR SHOULDER PRESENTATION

When labour has proceeded for some time with a shoulder presentation, the thinned lower uterine segment is unduly stretched, therefore any internal manipulation to rectify the lie carries a grave risk. Cæsarean section is usually preferred.

2. EXTRACTION OF THE AFTER-COMING HEAD OF THE HYDROCEPHALIC BABY

When presenting by the breech a severe cervical tear which extends upwards into the body of the uterus may occur.

3. DURING A DIFFICULT FORCEPS DELIVERY OR DESTRUCTIVE OPERATION

Injury to the uterus may (rarely) occur. In such cases the baby is extracted vaginally; the signs are similar to those of incomplete rupture.

Treatment on District

The treatment is to give ergometrine, 0·5 mg. intramuscularly, and summon the "Flying Squad." A pack will be inserted, a sedative given and the patient transferred to hospital for hysterectomy.

D. THE MISUSE OF OXYTOCIC DRUGS

When given intramuscularly (inadvisedly) to induce labour, **rupture of the uterus may occur:** signs of rupture may not be manifest for a number of hours after its administration. The administration of Buccal Pitocin has been associated with uterine rupture.

Oxytocin is never administered intramuscularly by a midwife during the first stage of labour, except under instructions from a doctor. Oxytocin is equally dangerous during the second stage should obstruction to advance of the fetus be present. (*Intravenous drip is a safer method of administration.*)

INCOMPLETE RUPTURE

In this condition the myometrium and endometrium are ruptured, the perimetrium remains intact and the baby is born vaginally. The diagnosis is made during the third stage of labour, when signs of shock develop.

The treatment is the same as for complete rupture.

(In remote areas the rent and vagina may be packed with gauze to control bleeding and the woman transferred to hospital for hysterectomy.)

N.B.—**Whenever shock during the third stage is more severe than the type of delivery or blood loss warrants,** or if the woman does not recover from shock when given the necessary treatment, the possibility of incomplete rupture of the uterus should be considered.

Presentation and Prolapse of Cord

DEFINITIONS

1. PRESENTATION OF CORD (*funic presentation*).

This term is applied when the umbilical cord lies in front of the presenting part and the membranes are intact.

2. PROLAPSE OF CORD.

The term is applied when the cord lies in front of the presenting part and the membranes are ruptured.

3. OCCULT PROLAPSE OF CORD.

The term is used when the cord lies alongside, but not in front of, the presenting part. (*N.B.*—It does not mean, as the word implies, " unseen.")

CAUSES

Any condition in which the presenting part does not fit accurately into the lower uterine segment will permit the umbilical cord to slip down in front of the presenting part.

Multiparity is a contributory factor because the head may not be engaged when the membranes rupture. Anterior obliquity and malpresentations are both more common in multiparæ.

1. MALPRESENTATIONS

(*b*) **Complete breech presentation is a common cause,** as the umbilicus is so near the buttocks. The prognosis is fairly good, because the presenting part is soft and does not compress the cord as the head would.

(*b*) **Shoulder presentation.**—If in remote areas it is not possible to perform Cæsarean **section internal version is done** and this also succeeds in replacing the prolapsed cord, but the manipulation increases the risk of stillbirth and is not recommended.

(*c*) **Face and brow presentations are less common causes.**

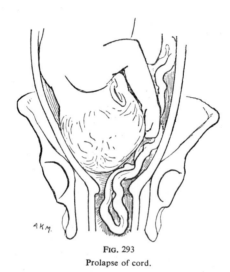

Fig. 293
Prolapse of cord.

2. CONTRACTED PELVIS

In the flat pelvis the cord can slip past the head at the sides of the brim.

3. HYDRAMNIOS

The cord is liable to be swept down in the rush of fluid if the membranes rupture spontaneously: some puncture the membranes at the beginning of labour with due precautions (see p. 157) to prevent this.

4. MULTIPLE PREGNANCY

Malpresentation and hydramnios occur in twins and both cause the cord to prolapse.

5. HIGH HEAD

If the membranes rupture spontaneously with the fetal head high, the cord may prolapse.

Puncture of membranes: because the incidence of prolapse is increased when labour is induced by puncture of membranes this should only be undertaken in a hospital where Cæsarean section can be performed without delay. Close supervision of the fetal heart is recommended.

CORD (Funic) PRESENTATION

Presentation of cord is rarely encountered, because the conditions causing the cord to present tend to produce early rupture of the membranes. It can only be diagnosed by feeling the cord inside the intact fore-waters.

TREATMENT

The midwife should feel if the cord is pulsating, and then withdraw her fingers because of the danger of puncturing the membranes.

If pulsating, the doctor should be sent for urgently, and the woman placed in the exaggerated Sims' left lateral position. Using the Trendelenburg position or having the foot of the bed raised 45·5 cm (18 inches) is less tiring for the woman, but less effective.

Preparations are made to deal with prolapse of cord, which is certain to take place within a short time. The theatre should be set up quickly for Cæsarean section.

PROLAPSE OF CORD

DIAGNOSIS

The cord may be felt in the vagina, or be seen lying outside the vulva. Early diagnosis and prompt treatment may save the baby's life, so the midwife must always be on the alert for the possibility of this complication.

The fetal heart should be auscultated when the membranes rupture, during every labour, but, if conditions liable to cause prolapse of cord exist, a vaginal examination should be made as soon as the membranes rupture, e.g. in hydramnios, breech presentation and contracted pelvis.

Suspicion of prolapsed cord will be aroused when fetal distress occurs for no apparent reason. Any disturbance in the fetal heart rate, particularly slowing, especially during the first stage, is significant; hearing the funic souffle during labour is usually a sign of cord compression.

A vaginal examination will verify the diagnosis; presentation of the fetus and dilatation of the os are noted.

MANAGEMENT

During the first stage.—Cæsarean section is performed if the fetus is alive.
During the second stage.—Episiotomy, application of forceps or breech extraction as indicated.

Active Treatment

Attempts to replace the cord inside the uterus either fail or the cord prolapses again, and valuable time is wasted.

If the cord is outside the vulva it should, after being cleansed with a warm antiseptic solution, be placed in the vagina to keep it clean and warm. Chilling and rough handling of the cord will produce spasm of the umbilical blood vessels and this will further impede the supply of oxygen to the fetus.

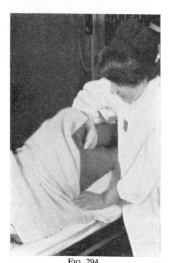

FIG. 294

Manual elevation of the presenting part by domiciliary midwife in ambulance.
(*Bellshill Maternity Hospital.*)

To relieve Pressure on the Cord

(*a*) **The woman is placed in the exaggerated Sims' left lateral position** and two firm pillows are inserted under her buttocks to elevate them still further. This causes the fetus to gravitate towards the diaphragm and takes the pressure off the cord.

(*b*) **The presenting part is elevated manually** by the sterile gloved fingers in the vagina. This procedure is less tiring when maintained for a long period if the woman lies in Sims' position as described above. Elevation of the presenting part should be continued (1) from the time prolapse of cord is diagnosed, (2) during the journey to hospital by ambulance, (3) while being transported in bed or by trolley in hospital from labour ward to operating theatre.

A patient with **prolapse of cord was admitted to the Simpson Maternity Pavilion** after a three-hour journey by ambulance, during which pressure on the cord was reduced by the adoption of Sims' position and manual elevation of the head vaginally. A live baby was born by Cæsarean section. At Bellshill Maternity Hospital, Lanarkshire, five babies during one year were born alive under similar circumstances.

DANGERS

The risks to the baby are anoxia and stillbirth. Head presentations are most serious ; breech most favourable, and 10 minutes is the maximal time the infant can be expected to survive cord compression, but the length of time depends on the degree of compression.

AMNIOTIC FLUID EMBOLISM

This catastrophe usually occurs near the end of the first stage of a labour that is apparently normal but characterized by rapid, strong tumultuous contractions, the membranes having ruptured. The administration of oxytocin may be a predisposing factor. It tends to occur in women over 35 years of age and may result in sudden death.

Amniotic fluid (which is high in thromboplastin) is forced into the maternal circulation via the utero-placental site and this gives rise to blood coagulation disorders, *e.g.* hypofibrinogenæmia.

SIGNS AND SYMPTOMS

Respiratory distress of sudden onset.   Severe dyspnœa.

Cyanosis: Pulmonary œdema.   **Sudden collapse. Rapid heart-beat.**

Oxygen is administered.

A general anæsthetic may be necessary to damp down the tetanic uterine contractions. An anæsthetist will cope with the cardio-respiratory emergency.

Fibrinogen or triple strength plasma is given under the direction of a hæmatologist.

Blood transfusion (fresh, not stored blood) may be given if exsanguinated.

Delivery by forceps.

Torrential uncontrollable postpartum hæmorrhage will occur if the clotting defect is not rectified and the uterus is atonic.

ACUTE INVERSION OF THE UTERUS

Inversion means that the uterus is turned inside out, and is a serious complication of the third stage. In acute cases the inner surface of the fundus appears at the vaginal orifice.

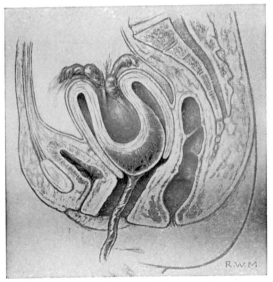

Fig. 295

Acute inversion of the uterus. Note traction on ovaries and Fallopian tubes which gives rise to shock.

The frequency of this condition is said to be about 1 in 100,000 deliveries, and it is only by being aware of and avoiding the causes that it does not occur more often.

CAUSES

1. **Forcibly attempting to expel the placenta by using fundal pressure or Crede's manœuvre when the uterus is atonic.**

2. **Combining fundal expression and cord traction to deliver the placenta** (*Precipitate labour is an unlikely cause as the uterus is contracting strongly.*)

SIGNS AND SYMPTOMS

The uterus may be seen outside the vulva. **The fundus is not palpable abdominally.**

Shock is an outstanding sign and is probably due to traction and compression of the ovaries, Fallopian tubes and broad ligaments (Fig. 295).

Bleeding will be present unless the placenta is completely adherent to the uterine wall.

Pain is usually severe.

In less acute cases the fundus is partially inverted and may or may not pass through the cervical os; it is neither visible at the vulva, nor can it be palpated abdominally.

TREATMENT (*on District*)

The midwife sends urgently for medical assistance " Flying Squad," and if the uterus is outside the vulva it should be wrapped in a towel wrung out of warm Hibitane solution.

Raising the foot of the bed will partly relieve the traction on the ovaries: to alleviate pain the midwife may give an injection of pethidine, 100 mg.

The doctor may attempt to replace the uterus, without removing the placenta, and will undoubtedly order a sedative prior to transferring the patient to hospital.

TREATMENT (*in Hospital*)

1. CONTROLLING HÆMORRHAGE

In doing so it may be necessary to strip off the remainder of the placenta and apply hot towels to the uterus.

2. REPLACING THE UTERUS

Delay increases the difficulty of replacement.

The part which came down last goes back first, *e.g.* the lower segment first, fundus last.

The hydrostatic pressure method of replacement has been used with success in a series of cases. The vagina is douched with Hibitane solution. The solution is then changed to saline, and the vaginal orifice blocked by the forearm or hand. No douche nozzle is used, and to create the necessary pressure the douche-can may have to be raised above the usual level for douching. The pressure exerted by the fluid distends the vagina and reduces the inverted uterus.

3. COMBATING THE SHOCK

The degree of shock does not improve until the uterus is replaced: immediate blood transfusion is essential; Ringer's lactate may be used until blood is available.

4. PREVENTING SUBSEQUENT INVERSION

Ergometrine, 0·5 mg., is given.

The Midwife prepares the equipment for

BLOOD TRANSFUSION.   ANÆSTHESIA.

CATHETERIZATION.   CLEANSING OF THE PARTS.

DOUCHING WITH LARGE VOLUME OF SALINE SOLUTION.

QUESTIONS FOR REVISION

RUPTURE OF THE UTERUS

ORAL QUESTIONS

Give 4 main causes of uterine rupture. Give 4 signs of actual rupture.

Write not more than 10 lines on: (1) how a midwife could try to prevent rupture of the uterus; (2) care of a woman during labour who has had a previous Cæsarean section; (3) obstructed labour as a cause of rupture.

What is meant by: (*a*) silent rupture; (*b*) the misuse of oxytocic drugs; (*c*) grande multipara.

Give three reasons why a Cæsarean scar is likely to rupture :
When does this occur? What are the warning signs ? Which malpresentations, if not diagnosed, might cause rupture ? State the signs of impending rupture due to obstruction. What is meant by incomplete rupture ? How and when is it diagnosed ?

C.M.B.(Scot.) paper.—What factors predispose to and what are the imminent signs of rupture of the uterus ?

Acute inversion of the uterus.—Give two ways in which an incompetent midwife might cause inversion: how would the condition be treated on the district ? What is the reason for raising the foot of the bed ? What preparations would the midwife make for such a case in hospital ? Why is precipitate labour unlikely to cause inversion ?

Give 4 signs of amniotic embolism. During what stage of labour does amniotic embolism occur? Mention 4 procedures you could anticipate being carried out by the doctor. Name 3 substances that may be administered intravenously. If the woman survives the immediate episode what further danger exists?

PROLAPSE OF CORD.

Differentiate between: (*a*) presentation and prolapse of cord; (*b*) treatment during first and second stages of labour.

Explain why: cord prolapse occurs in hydramnios and what a midwife could do to avert or recognize this.

Write not more than 10 lines on: (*a*) causes of prolapse of cord explaining why; (*b*) treatment of prolapse of cord when the cervix is 4 cm. dilated.

C.M.B.(Scot.) paper.—You are attending a patient during labour and you suspect that prolapse of the cord has occurred. How would you confirm your diagnosis and what would you do ?

C.M.B.(Scot.) paper.—Discuss the causation of prolapse of the cord. How would you recognize that this complication had occurred ? What would you do while waiting for medical assistance ?

C.M.B.(N. Ireland) paper.—What conditions predispose to cord prolapse ? What are the midwife's duties pending the arrival of the doctor ?

C.M.B.(Scot.) paper.—Define prolapse of the cord. Describe the predisposing factors and management of such a case.

C.M.B.(Eng.) paper.—Describe the umbilical cord. What should a midwife do if the cord prolapses?

C.M.B.(Eng.) paper. 100 word question.—Prolapse of the umbilical cord.

C.M.B.(Eng.) paper. 50 word question.—Presentation of the umbilical cord.

25

Complications of the Third Stage of Labour

POSTPARTUM HÆMORRHAGE (ATONIC; TRAUMATIC).
ADHERENT PLACENTA. RETAINED PLACENTA. VULVAL HÆMATOMA.
COLLAPSE AND SHOCK. INVERSION OF UTERUS (p. 425).

Other pre-existing conditions may complicate the third stage, such as the sudden collapse of the cardiac patient, or, in the case of pre-eclampsia, an eclamptic convulsion may occur.

POSTPARTUM HÆMORRHAGE

This is one of the most serious complications in obstetrics, and the woman's life depends on the midwife's prompt, intelligent action, for what might become an alarming hæmorrhage can often be checked or kept under control by good management.

DEFINITION.

Postpartum hæmorrhage is severe bleeding during the third stage of labour, or within 24 hours after the expulsion of the placenta. Hæmorrhage occurring after 24 hours and within six weeks of delivery is known as puerperal hæmorrhage. This is considered under complications of the puerperium (p. 486).

Sending for Medical Aid

The amount of blood-loss which constitutes hæmorrhage cannot be gauged entirely in millilitres. Medical aid should be obtained when over 600 ml. is lost, even with no systemic signs, or if the loss of under 600 ml. is accompanied by deterioration in the woman's general condition.

It is the effect of blood-loss rather than the amount of blood lost that matters. In cases of anæmia, whether nutritional or due to antepartum hæmorrhage, the loss of under 300 ml. of blood might be serious.

The average blood-loss during a normal third stage is 120 to 240 ml., and when a woman loses more than 300 ml. the midwife should take action to control the bleeding, but need not send for medical assistance if the woman's general condition is satisfactory and the loss is less than 600 ml. (*In some hospitals the resident doctor is summoned for a blood-loss of 300 ml.*)

All blood should be saved until bleeding is under control.

TYPES

There are two types: ATONIC ; TRAUMATIC.

ATONIC HÆMORRHAGE

This is the more common type and is always from the placental site. As the name implies, it is due to lack of tone in the uterine muscle and any condition that interferes with uterine contraction and retraction will predispose to it.

428

Causes

1. ATONIC UTERUS.   2. FIBROIDS.

3. ANTEPARTUM HÆMORRHAGE.   4. RETAINED PRODUCTS.

5. MISMANAGEMENT OF THE THIRD STAGE.

6. BLOOD COAGULATION DISORDERS. This is an additional hazard.

I. ATONIC UTERUS *due to —*

(a) **Labour being unduly prolonged.**

(b) **The grande multipara** may have a lax uterus : she is anæmic and weak from malnutrition and repeated childbearing.

(c) **Narcosis and anæsthesia.** If large doses of sedative drugs are administered and when deep general anæsthesia is necessary the uterus becomes sluggish.

(d) **Rapid expulsion of a large baby.** It may be that the muscle fibres in the upper segment do not have time to retract properly during rapid expulsion of the baby.

(e) **Twins. The overdistended uterus may not contract well** and the large placental site provides a more extensive bleeding area.

2. FIBROIDS.

Where a number of small fibroids are present, they interfere with good muscular action and prevent the closure of the blood sinuses.

3. ANTEPARTUM HÆMORRHAGE.

In cases of abruptio placentæ, blood percolates amongst the muscle fibres and inhibits their contractility. **In placenta prævia** the circular muscle fibres do not furnish the " livin ligature " action as do those in the upper segment,

4. RETAINED PRODUCTS.

When blood clot, pieces of placenta or membrane are retained they interfere with uterine contractions.

5. MISMANAGEMENT OF THE THIRD STAGE.

This is probably the most common cause of postpartum hæmorrhage and one which is under the control of the person conducting the labour.

(a) A DISTENDED BLADDER.

If the woman is permitted to come into the third stage of labour with a full bladder, this inhibits proper placental separation, and as a result hæmorrhage is liable to follow. It is reprehensible to have to pass a catheter when postpartum hæmorrhage occurs; the need should not exist; the bladder should have been emptied at the end of the first stage.

(b) MEDDLING.

Massaging, kneading, squeezing and pushing over-stimulate the uterus and cause irregular contractions and partial separation of the placenta. Such contractions are inadequate to control the bleeding from the separated areas. Too much massage may prevent clot formation in the blood sinuses of the placental site.

(c) RETAINED PRODUCTS.

The uterus cannot retract completely until it is empty; blood clot in the cavity of the uterus interferes with uterine action, and a partially separated placenta has the same effect. When a piece of placenta is left adhering to the uterine wall, it inhibits the effective closure of the surrounding blood sinuses. Later it may slough off, giving rise to serious puerperal hæmorrhage.

6. BLOOD COAGULATION DISORDERS.

If in the presence of this condition the uterus is atonic, torrential and uncontrollable hæmorrhage will occur.

SIGNS

BLEEDING.	PULSE RAPID.
BIG UTERUS.	PALLOR (*a later sign*).
BOGGY UTERUS.	COLLAPSE (*see p. 438*).

BLEEDING.

In atonic hæmorrhage the bleeding does not as a rule begin until a few minutes after the birth of the baby, and there is no difficulty in making the diagnosis when blood is seen pouring from the vagina. It tends to come in gushes, because the inert uterus fills up with blood and the large clots which collect in the uterus or vagina are expelled when a contraction occurs.

BIG UTERUS

When the fundus rises above the level of the umbilicus or feels large the cause must be investigated (p. 323). On rare occasions the fundus has been known to reach the xiphisternum, because the inert uterus was filled with clot and no blood was escaping from the vagina. This could only happen when there was **ignorance or gross negligence** on the part of the person in charge of the case.

BOGGY UTERUS.

A uterus distended with blood lacks the firm consistency of the well contracted uterus. In severe cases the uterus may be so soft and flabby that it is impossible to detect its outline.

PULSE.

When the pulse rate rises to 90 beats per minute it is abnormally rapid, but the midwife should realize that one or more minutes may elapse before the pulse increases, even when 600 ml. of blood has been lost.

PALLOR.

This is usually noticed in the face, and is a later sign; a striking feature often indicating collapse (p. 438).

PROPHYLAXIS

1. HOSPITALIZATION FOR SUSCEPTIBLE CASES.

The following women should be delivered in hospital :

(a) **Women who have a history of postpartum hæmorrhage** or adherent placentæ as they are liable to have a recurrence.

(b) **The grande multipara** (*more than five confinements*) is particularly likely to bleed.

(c) **Those who have had antepartum hæmorrhage.**

(d) **The woman with fibroid tumours.**

2. GOOD MANAGEMENT OF THE SECOND STAGE OF LABOUR.
The bladder should be emptied at the end of the first stage.
Slow delivery of the baby's body during a contraction.

3. GOOD MANAGEMENT OF THE THIRD STAGE OF LABOUR. (See p. 321, also Mismanagement p. 429.)

4. ANTICIPATION OF BLOOD COAGULATION DISORDERS.
This condition may exist in cases of abruptio placentæ, prolonged retention of a dead fetus, or amniotic embolism, and if the uterus is atonic, may cause torrential hæmorrhage.

5. USE OF OXYTOCIC DRUGS

(a) **Intramuscular injection of Syntometrine, 1 ml.,** is given by most British doctors and midwives as soon as the anterior shoulder is born.

(b) **Oxytocin drip.**—This would be set up as a prophylactic measure in cases when postpartum hæmorrhage is anticipated, and kept running for one hour after completion of the third stage.

Principles of Treatment

1. **Stop the bleeding.** 2. **Replace fluid lost.** 3. **Treat circulatory failure (shock).**

ACTIVE TREATMENT *(prior to expulsion of placenta)*

To stop the bleeding the uterus must be stimulated to contract, and this can best be accomplished when it is empty, so blood clot and placenta must be expelled.

1. MASSAGE AND KNEAD THE UTERUS UNTIL IT CONTRACTS.
Then squeeze out the blood clots. Remove the placenta by controlled cord traction.

2. SEND FOR THE DOCTOR OR THE "FLYING SQUAD."
But never leave the patient while doing so. Send a responsible person, if available, and make it clear that the doctor is urgently needed.

If the blood group and Rh factor are known notify this to the "Flying Squad."

Instruct the person to give the name and address clearly, and, if remote, directions for finding the house or flat. Valuable time will be saved at night by having a lighted window to attract attention; in multistoried blocks of flats some person should be strategically placed to direct the "team".

3. ADMINISTRATION OF OXYTOCIC DRUGS.
If the placenta cannot be expelled because it is not completely separated, the midwife should give Syntometrine, 1 ml. which consists of **ergometrine, 0·5 mg., and oxytocin (Syntocinon), 5 units.** Given intramuscularly Syntocinon acts in $2\frac{1}{2}$ minutes, ergometrine acts in 6 to 7 minutes. **Syntometrine may be given intravenously unless the patient is of doubtful cardiac status.**

The left hand is kept on the fundus, and when the contraction induced by the Syntometrine occurs the midwife should deliver the placenta by controlled cord traction.

If the placenta does not separate completely, she should not meddle any further; the Syntometrine already given ought to control the bleeding; but if not and the loss is profuse a second dose may be administered in ten minutes. If hæmorrhage continues and medical assistance cannot be obtained in time, manual removal of the placenta will have to be performed by the midwife.

4. MANUAL REMOVAL OF PLACENTA.

This formidable procedure should not be undertaken by the midwife except in a grave emergency, for when done without a general anæsthetic the risk of shock is intensified. But when the need arises, the procedure should be carried out before the patient is exsanguinated.

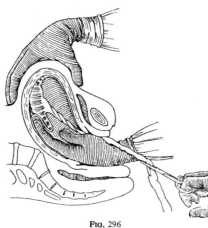

FIG. 296

MANUAL REMOVAL OF PLACENTA

Fingers, inside amnion, separating the placenta.

When serious postpartum hæmorrhage occurs in hospital, manual removal of placenta is carried out under general anæsthesia without delay, usually within one minute following the intravenous injection of ergometrine, 0·5 mg. Syntometrine 1 ml. may be given intravenously unless the patient is of doubtful cardiac status.

Method

The patient is placed in the lithotomy position. An assistant cleanses the vulva quickly with a suitable disinfectant, and smears the labia with obstetric cream.

The midwife makes her hands as aseptic as possible in the very short time at her disposal, e.g. she washes them quickly, draws on a sterile gauntlet glove (if available) and smears her hand with Hibitane cream.

The left hand holds the umbilical cord taut while the right hand, with the thumb in the palm, shaped like a cone, is inserted into the vagina and follows the cord up to the placenta.

The left hand now steadies the uterus abdominally, holding it down within reach of the hand in utero. On finding the separated area the ulnar border of the extended fingers is insinuated between placenta and decidua, the palm facing the placenta. With a sideways slicing movement the placenta is gently detached.

The left hand rubs up a contraction and expels the hand with the placenta within its grasp.

TREATMENT OF ATONIC POSTPARTUM HÆMORRHAGE
(after the placenta is expelled)

1. THE UTERUS SHOULD BE MASSAGED UNTIL IT CONTRACTS.
Blood clots are then expelled.

2. MEDICAL AID OR "FLYING SQUAD" IS SUMMONED.

3. OXYTOCIC DRUGS ARE GIVEN.

Syntometrine, 1 ml., given intramuscularly acts in two and a half minutes.

Ergometrine 0·5 mg. given intramuscularly acts in seven minutes;

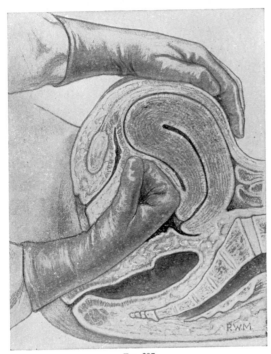

FIG. 297

Internal bimanual compression of the placental site.
The left hand is on the abdomen.

The doctor may give ergometrine intravenously; by this route it acts in 45 seconds, dose 0·25 to 0·5 mg, but may cause the placenta to be trapped.

Midwives may use the intravenous route but if inexperienced in the technique of intravenous injection they will waste valuable time in attempting to inject the vein of a collapsed patient (p. 672).

If bleeding continues, an oxytocin intravenous drip is given; *i.e.* dextrose (5 per cent) 540 ml., with 10 units Pitocin or Syntocinon at 40 drops per minute.

The midwife should not discard any blood until the hæmorrhage is under control, and the amount of blood lost should always be measured and recorded. (For treatment of collapse due to hæmorrhage, see p. 439.)

4. BIMANUAL COMPRESSION OF THE PLACENTAL SITE.

This method is useful in controlling severe hæmorrhage until oxytocic drugs take effect.

(a) THE INTERNAL METHOD

The patient is in the dorsal position. An assistant, if available, cleanses the vulva. The right hand is made as aseptic as possible in the manner described for manual removal of placenta and inserted into the vagina like a cone; the hand is closed and the flat part of the closed fist is placed into the anterior vaginal fornix and against the anterior uterine wall. The right elbow rests on the bed between the woman's thighs.

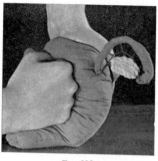

The left hand is placed down behind the uterus abdominally, with the fingers directed towards the cervix. The uterus is brought forwards and with the palm of the left hand it is pressed on to the fist in the vagina. In this way the placental site is compressed between the two hands.

Bimanual compression must be maintained until the uterus contracts and retracts, even although the bleeding has stopped.

FIG. 298

DEMONSTRATION OF INTERNAL BIMANUAL COMPRESSION OF THE UTERUS.

Model of uterus used at Aberdeen Maternity Hospital for student midwives. *Note.*—Ovaries are not being compressed.

(b) THE EXTERNAL METHOD

Although the internal method is the more efficacious, an inexperienced midwife may hesitate to attempt it. The external method can be done quickly and entails no risks of sepsis, and as it can be demonstrated clinically for teaching purposes, the midwife feels more confident in performing it. Although the external method may not stop the hæmorrhage completely, it will control it, and is most successful in the multiparous patient with a hin abdominal wall.

The patient is in the dorsal position. The uterus is massaged to induce a contraction and then grasped with the left hand and drawn up towards the umbilicus.

The right hand is made into a fist and placed on the lower abdomen against the lower uterine segment, as far down as possible, behind the symphysis pubis. The left hand is placed behind the uterus, with finger tips pointing towards the cervix, and the uterus is brought forwards and compressed between the two hands. Pressure is maintained until uterine contractions and retractions are established. If the bladder is distended, it will not be possible to carry out this manœuvre successfully.

TRAUMATIC POSTPARTUM HÆMORRHAGE

Traumatic hæmorrhage is usually due to lacerations of the cervix or upper vagina. (Bleeding from a lacerated perineum is readily controlled, but when from the region of the clitoris the flow may be profuse and necessitate the insertion of sutures. The midwife should apply pressure with a sterile pad in an endeavour to control bleeding.)

CAUSES

Traumatic hæmorrhage can take place during the spontaneous delivery of a large baby, or when a large diameter presents as in face to pubes, or during extraction of the after-coming head in a breech presentation, but is more commonly associated with a difficult instrumental delivery.

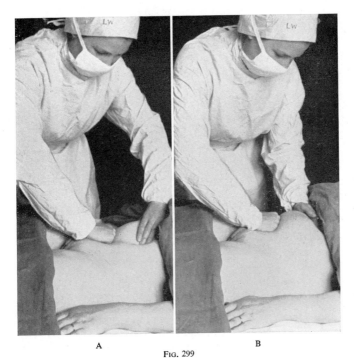

A   B

Fig. 299

DEMONSTRATION OF EXTERNAL BIMANUAL COMPRESSION OF THE PLACENTAL SITE

(A) shows the uterus being drawn upwards with the left hand so that the right hand can be laid against the anterior wall. (B) shows the left hand behind the uterus which is compressed between the two hands.

(*Simpson Memorial Maternity Pavilion, Edinburgh.*)

SIGNS

1. **Bleeding starts immediately after the baby is born.**

2. **The flow of blood is continuous,** often a heavy trickle, although it may collect and form clots in the vagina, especially when the woman is lying on a sagging bed.

3. **The uterus is in good tone** and may be firmly contracted.

TREATMENT

The only satisfactory treatment is suturing of the lacerations, so medical aid should be obtained. The requirements for suturing are outlined on page 623. The woman is anæsthetized and the vagina swabbed as dry as possible. For visual inspection a Sims-Ferguson's speculum and a good light are essential.

The anterior and posterior lips of the cervix are grasped with sponge-holding forceps, as teneculæ are liable to tear the soft cervix. The bleeding points are tied, and the lacerated edges sutured with catgut.

Treatment by the Midwife

There is usually sufficient time to wait for medical assistance as the bleeding in traumatic hæmorrhage is a heavy continuous trickle rather than the profuse gushing of atonic hæmorrhage.

Oxytocic drugs are not effective for traumatic hæmorrhage.

PACKING THE VAGINA

Only in very remote areas will the midwife have to cope with traumatic hæmorrhage alone, and in such circumstances she may have to resort to packing the vagina in order to compress the bleeding vessels. Such packing will not control bleeding from an atonic uterus.

Method

If a sterile gauze pack is not available sterile perineal pads smeared with obstetric cream may be used.

Clots should be swabbed out of the vagina and the bladder emptied.

If no speculum is available, the woman is placed in Sims' left lateral position and, while using the first and second fingers of her left hand as a perineal retractor, the midwife should pack the vagina snugly and then apply a perineal pad which is held firmly in position by being attached to a T-binder. The recorded number of pads are removed in six hours.

VULVAL HÆMATOMA

Vulval hæmatoma is a condition which may give rise to a form of traumatic hæmorrhage. It is caused by rupture of the subcutaneous veins of the vagina which produces an effusion of blood into the connective tissue of the vulva and vaginal wall. A small hæmatoma may be associated with the repair of a medio-lateral episiotomy or perineal laceration. It may be a few hours after labour before signs are manifest.

The woman complains of discomfort and pain in the perineum and/or labia; the labia majora may be distended to such a degree that the skin is glistening; the hæmatoma may bulge into the vagina.

Treatment

Under a general anæsthetic an incision is made into the hæmatoma by the doctor, the blood clot removed and the bleeding vessels tied or the tissues sutured. Otherwise the wound is firmly packed with gauze wrung out of hot saline. In a case seen by the author 450 ml. (15 oz.) of blood clot were removed.

Blood transfusion may be required; antibiotics are sometimes prescribed to avoid abscess formation.

ADHERENT PLACENTA

The placenta is said to be adherent if, 30 minutes after the birth of the baby, there are no signs that it has left the upper uterine segment.

CAUSES

1. The most likely cause is that the uterus is not contracting and retracting strongly enough to diminish the area of the placental site sufficiently to separate it from the placenta. A full bladder may predispose to weak uterine action.

2. **Very rarely the placenta is morbidly adherent,** because there is no spongy layer of decidua and the chorionic villi are embedded into the uterine muscle. This is known as **placenta accreta** and the treatment is hysterectomy, but it occurs so seldom that the midwife need not anticipate such an unlikely event.

Treatment
See manual removal, p. 432.

The midwife should seek medical assistance, the " Flying Squad."

If there is no separation of the placenta there will be no bleeding and on no account should the midwife attempt to detach the adherent placenta or she will cause partial separation and hæmorrhage, as well as shock.

When the doctor is not immediately available, the midwife should give the woman a sedative and remain with her until medical assistance can be obtained.

Many authorities consider that the woman must not be transferred to hospital with the placenta *in situ* lest partial separation and profuse hæmorrhage occur *en route.* The " Flying Squad " will remove the placenta and give a blood transfusion if necessary.

In hospital practice manual removal of the placenta will be performed even in the absence of bleeding, in 30 minutes, under a general anæsthetic.

Ergometrine, 0·5 mg., is usually administered intravenously as soon as the placenta is removed, and if bleeding is free 0·5 mg. is given intramuscularly at the same time; otherwise it may be administered half an hour later.

Hæmorrhage is usually present, and the treatment is therefore that of atonic postpartum hæmorrhage: the placenta, in the majority of cases, being partially adherent.

RETAINED PLACENTA

In this condition the placenta has left the upper uterine segment but is not expelled from the vagina.

1. FAULTY TECHNIQUE.
An inexperienced midwife may be trying to expel the placenta, abdominally, *e.g.* downwards but not backwards. It is conceivable that she may be trying to expel the placenta before it has separated completely.

This may induce spasm of the lower uterine segment.

2. A FULL BLADDER.
This will prevent descent of the placenta or interfere with the midwife's efforts to expel it.

3. CONSTRICTION RING (HOUR-GLASS CONTRACTION).
This condition usually arises during treatment of third stage hæmorrhage.

Too vigorous massaging and squeezing of the uterus may cause spasm of the circular muscle fibres at the level of the physiological retraction ring or at the internal os, and prevent the expulsion of the placenta.

A constriction ring is diagnosed vaginally, usually when an attempt is being made to remove the placenta manually.

26

If it is imperative to remove the placenta because of hæmorrhage, a drug to relax the spasm will be administered, *e.g.*

(*a*) **The inhalation of one ampoule of amyl-nitrite.**

(*b*) **A general anæsthetic may be administered** to relax the spasm.

Treatment of Retained Placenta

If after 30 minutes, with no bleeding, the placenta is still retained in spite of using controlled cord traction, medical aid should be obtained.

The placenta will be removed manually under aseptic precautions. *Pushing on the fundus is not recommended.*

By the Midwife

The midwife on district should, before summoning the " Flying Squad " determine by vaginal examination whether the placenta is partly trapped in the cervix or lower uterine segment. In such circumstances she could apply controlled cord traction or grasp the placenta and remove it.

COLLAPSE DUE TO HÆMORRHAGE

Hypovolaemic Shock

This condition is also known as low cardiac output state.

Shock in obstetrics occurs most frequently during the third stage of labour and is usually associated with hæmorrhage.

When blood loss is rapid and severe the situation becomes extremely grave, and if not remedied promptly an irreversible stage is reached from which the woman may not recover even after the transfusion of several litres of blood.

SIGNS

1. THE PULSE IS RAPID (over 120), thready and soft; it may be imperceptible.

2. THE BLOOD PRESSURE FALLS

    (*a*) **In a moderate degree of shock the systolic pressure will be below 100 mm. Hg.**

    (*b*) **In a severe degree of shock the systolic pressure will be below 90 mm. Hg.**

    (*c*) **In a very severe degree of shock the systolic pressure will be below 80 mm. Hg**

    (*d*) **When the systolic pressure is below 60 the condition is critical.**

    (*e*) **In desperate cases it cannot be estimated.**

3. MARKED PALLOR OR AN ASHEN GREY HUE OF THE FACE IS NOTICED; the mucous membranes become blanched; the skin feels cold and clammy.

4. RESPIRATIONS ARE AT FIRST SHALLOW AND LATER DEEP AND IRREGULAR (air hunger).

5. THE WOMAN IS APATHETIC WITH OCCASIONAL BOUTS OF RESTLESSNESS.

PROPHYLAXIS

1. GOOD PHYSICAL CONDITION.

During pregnancy the woman should be brought into good physical condition to enable her to withstand the unavoidable blood loss that will occur postpartum ; the prognosis in cases of hæmorrhage always being more grave when the woman's health is poor.

2. RECTIFICATION OF ANÆMIA.

Whether nutritional or due to blood loss, anæmia should always be rectified. It is prudent to repeat the hæmoglobin test at the 36th week to ensure that it is at a safe level for delivery, *i.e.* 12·6 G. (85 per cent).

TREATMENT

1. **Hæmorrhage must first be brought under control** (p. 431). (*The doctor will have been summoned on account of postpartum bleeding.*)

FIRST-AID TREATMENT BY THE DISTRICT MIDWIFE

2. **Reassure the patient by keeping calm,** handling her gently, working quietly and expeditiously, so that the woman is not aware that an urgent situation has arisen.

3. **Remove the blood-stained linen.** Excessive heat should not be applied in these circumstances: sufficient warmth for comfort is all that is required.

4. **Elevate the foot of the bed 30·5 cm (12 inches)** as treatment for shock; **it does not control hæmorrhage.** Raising the legs is more effective than lowering the head. **This measure will raise the blood pressure 10 mm** and, by gravity, blood will flow to the vital centres in the brain. (The hand should always be kept on the fundus while the patient is in this position because, if bleeding recommences, the uterus may fill up with blood clot and the inexperienced midwife may not be aware of this.)

5. **Administer fluid.**—If facilities for giving an intravenous drip are not available tap water (600 ml.) may be given rectally. If run in slowly with a catheter, the dehydrated patient will readily absorb that amount, and as the foot of the bed is elevated, she ought to be able to retain it. To give fluid by mouth is not advisable, even if the patient is thirsty; sips of water are useless and, if sufficient is given to be of any avail, vomiting will be induced.

ACTIVE TREATMENT

1. **SPEED.** *This is vital in :—*

(*a*) The first-aid measures instituted by the midwife.

(*b*) Obtaining medical assistance. (*c*) Arranging for blood replacement.

2. RESTORATION OF BLOOD VOLUME.

The "Flying Squad" will give the patient blood of the correct group and Rh classification, otherwise Rh negative group O. Synthetic blood substitutes such as Macrodex, Intradex or Dextraven are used to restore blood volume until whole blood is available. Dextrose, 10 per cent. or Ringer's lactate solution may be used.

The first 1,200 ml. of blood are given rapidly, *i.e.* in 30 minutes, using the Baxter disposable blood administration set with pressure pump, or the Martin transfusion pump. The central venous pressure is monitored. The doctor remains with the patient during this time.

(*In remote areas, in desperate cases as a first aid measure, the lower limbs may be bandaged from the feet to the thighs, and the legs elevated to direct more blood to the brain, heart and lungs.*)

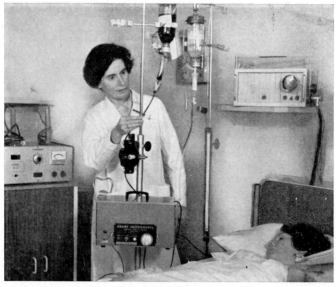

Fig. 300

Resuscitation of Patient with Severe Post-partum Haemorrhage.

Left to Right

(1) **Oscilloscope** to monitor cardiac rhythm.
(2) **Grant Heat Exchanger** warms blood to temperature selected by control thermostat dial. Useful when large volume of blood is given rapidly.
(3) **Capon Heaton pump** to increase speed at which blood transfusion is given.
(4) **Central venous pressure manometer.** When in use, zero on manometer scale should be at the level of the right atrium.
(5) **D. C. Defibrillator:** used if cardiac arrest due to ventricular fibrillation occurs.

(*Royal Maternity Hospital, Rottenrow, Glasgow.*)

3. TRANSFER TO HOSPITAL.

Blood is always given prior to, and in some cases during, her removal by ambulance. The woman will not be transferred to hospital while in a state of collapse.

4. DRUGS.

Hydrocortisone, 100 mg., is given in a slow intravenous drip, of dextrose, 5 per cent, if suprarenal failure is present or suspected. This occurs most commonly in cases of prolonged labour when dehydration, ketosis and electrolyte imbalance have not been corrected.

A sedative may be necessary to calm a restless or apprehensive patient. Morphine has no beneficial action in the treatment of shock; some think it is harmful.

5. For duties re transfusion, see page 444. 6. Oxygen is administered in severe cases.

OBSERVATION

The pulse should be recorded in graph form every five minutes.

The blood pressure is recorded every 15 to 20 minutes.

INTRAVENOUS BLOOD TRANSFUSION REQUIREMENTS

Only on rare occasions are instruments for cutting down required, but they should always be in readiness because for the collapsed patient they may be urgently needed.

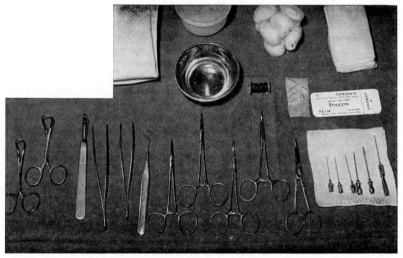

FIG. 307

INTRAVENOUS PACK SET (CUTTING DOWN)
(Simpson Memorial Maternity Pavilion, Edinburgh.)

INSTRUMENTS

2 towel clips.
1 Bard Parker handle No. 3, blade No. 10.
2 fine dissecting forceps, toothed, plain.
1 small aneurysm needle.
2 mosquito forceps.
2 Spencer Wells' forceps.
1 fine scissors curved on the flat.

LINEN: DRESSINGS

1 gown, cap, mask, gloves.
2 dressing towels.
5 gauze swabs, 10 wool swabs.

NEEDLES: SUTURES

3 hypodermic needles.
1 intravenous needle, B.G.W. 16.
1 intravenous cannula, B.G.W. 16.
1 curved fine triangular needle, No. 1.
1 curved fine triangular needle, No. 8.
1 cutting fistula needle, No. 2.
(Needles in rust-proof paper)
Chromic catgut, size 2/0. Mersilk, size 2/0.
1 gallipot for local anæsthetic.
1 polypropylene gallipot for Hibitane in spirit.
1 syringe, 2 ml.

NON-STERILE TABLE

Two Baxter giving-sets with pressure pump for blood. Flasks of dextrose, blood or blood substitute as required. Tourniquet, sphygmomanometer and stethoscope, C.V.P. manometer. Stand for flasks of blood, equipment for examining blood. Hibitane 0.5 per cent in spirit. lignocaine (Duncaine), 1 per cent. Bag for soiled swabs. 5 cm bandage. Adhesive tape, 2.5 cm.

CAUSES OF SHOCK IN OBSTETRICS

1. **Hypovolæmia** (*low blood volume*): due to hæmorrhage is the commonest cause.

2. **Tissue trauma**: due to rupture or inversion of the uterus and difficult instrumental delivery.

3. **Oxygen deprivation**: this may occur due to serious obstruction of the pulmonary artery by an embolus, *i.e.* blood clot, amniotic fluid.

4. **Endotoxic** (bacteræmic): this type of shock occurs more commonly in association with septic abortion (see p. 148).

THE "FLYING SQUAD"
Obstetrical Emergency Service

Doctors and midwives are now encouraged to call the " flying squad " for potential as well as actual emergencies.

When hæmorrhage has occurred a blood transfusion is given prior to her removal. Emergencies such as obstructed labour, failed forceps (now rare) would be transferred to and dealt with in hospital.

The team consists of an obstetrician, resident obstetric officer, an experienced midwife and student midwife. If local anæsthesia is not employed, an anæsthetist should be one of the team.

Speed in answering calls and dealing with the situation is imperative, and an ambulance equipped for the purpose is ideal (Fig. 302).

THE MIDWIFE'S DUTIES

CARE OF EQUIPMENT

Three midwives delegated as members of the team are responsible for packing the equipment according to a pre-arranged plan so that any drug or appliance can be produced without delay. They are also responsible for maintaining the equipment in first-class order.

CARE OF BLOOD

The midwife should have some knowledge of the care of blood to avoid wastage of this very precious fluid. To avoid delay the Blood Transfusion Service maintains a supply of blood in most large maternity hospitals. Double checking is imperative to ensure that compatible blood is given.

Blood can only be used for three weeks after withdrawal from the donor and should not be removed from the refrigerator or insulated box for longer than 30 minutes.

It is sometimes necessary to warm the blood prior to transfusion in circumstances in which shivering would be induced in a shocked patient; room temperature is usually adequate; overheated blood may cause death.

DUTIES OF MIDWIFE ON DISTRICT

The district midwife should, while awaiting arrival of the team, **prepare adequate supplies of hot and, more especially, cold sterile water. The bedroom should be cleared** as far as possible and arranged so that one good-sized table is available for sterile packs, a smaller one or dressing chest for non-sterile equipment, and two kitchen chairs or boxes for packs, hand-lotion, etc.

The midwife should keep a five-minute pulse chart and record the blood pressure every 15 minutes. **A concise history of the case** should be written. Placenta, blood and blood-stained linen are kept for inspection.

Resident doctor takes blood to the ambulance in insulated carrier:

2 bottles blood, patient's group

or

2 bottles group O Rh negative.

2 bottles group O Rh positive.

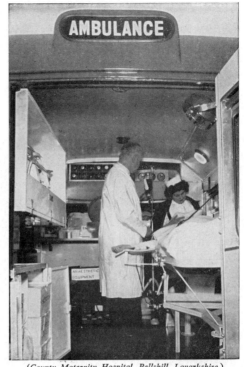

Fig. 302

AMBULANCE EQUIPPED EXCLUSIVELY FOR OBSTETRIC EMERGENCIES.

Note blood transfusion being given. Midwife holding baby.

By two-way radio control, contact with labour ward is maintained.

TOP LEFT

PORTABLE INCUBATOR; ANÆSTHETIC CASE.

(County Maternity Hospital, Bellshill, Lanarkshire.)

BOTTOM LEFT

Box No. 1. **Scrub up and prep. pack; 2 polythene sheets; 6 paper towels; 6 paper masks; 6 paper caps; 2 plastic aprons; sphygmomanometer; stethoscope; thermometer; gastric suction equipment; Pinard's stethoscope.**

Box No. 2. **Transfusion equipment; I.V. puncture set; cut down set; box of syringes, needles; dressing pack. C.V.P. manometer.**

Box No. 3. **Drugs; lotions; locked drug box; bowl pack; linen pack; delivery pack.**

Box No. 4. **Instruments; sutures; 6 pairs gloves; pudendal needles; perineal repair set; catheter pack.**

Box No. 5. **Spare gowns, drapes, dressings; catheter pack.**

Box No. 6. **Eclampsia requirements.**

Box No. 7. **Baby resuscitation equipment; neonatal laryngoscope; disposable mucus extractors; endotracheal tubes; fine suction catheters; syringes; drugs; swabs.**

TOP RIGHT

Powerful light.

BOTTOM RIGHT

Anæsthetic machine and equipment.

UNDER COUCH

Bed clothes (in polythene wrap) Oxygen cylinders.

OVER DRIVER'S CABIN

Infusion fluids; spare cylinders;

UNDER SHELF

Centrifuge; suction apparatus; dripstand.

Bottle basket with 2 plasma, 1 sterile water; 1 × 5 per cent Dextrose.

A complete detailed list of equipment is not given.

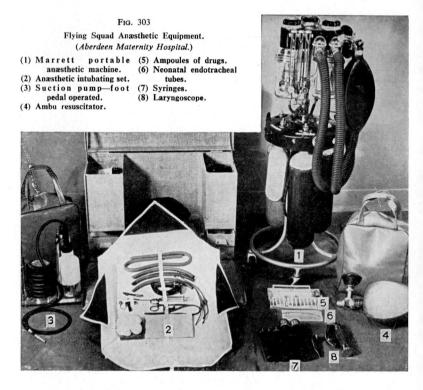

Fig. 303

Flying Squad Anæsthetic Equipment.
(*Aberdeen Maternity Hospital.*)

(1) **Marrett portable** anæsthetic machine.
(2) Anæsthetic intubating set.
(3) **Suction pump—foot** pedal operated.
(4) Ambu resuscitator.

(5) Ampoules of drugs.
(6) Neonatal endotracheal tubes.
(7) Syringes.
(8) Laryngoscope.

Management by Midwife during Drip Transfusion

1. **Strict asepsis** to be maintained.

2. **Flow of blood** as directed, usually 1·2 to 2·4 ml. (20 to 40 drops) per minute.

3. **To facilitate the flow of blood** the limb should be kept warm by a well-wrapped hot-water bottle.

4. **Displacement of needle** to be avoided.

5. **Pulse to be recorded** every 5, 15 or 30 minutes ⎫ depending on condition
   Temperature every 1 or 2 hours ⎬ of patient.
   Blood pressure every 15 or 30 minutes ⎭

6. **Colour of woman to be noted.**

7. **Fluid balance** to be recorded during and for 24 hours after transfusion.

8. **Urine Analysis.** Observe for hæmaturia and test each specimen for protein and specific gravity during, and for 24 hours after, transfusion.

9. **Watch for signs of reaction.**

TRANSFUSION REACTION

This may be due to giving incompatible blood or using outdated blood or blood hæmolysed by overheating, freezing or infection. The reaction usually occurs during the transfusion, but may be delayed for some hours.

In a severe case of incompatibility the following may occur.

Shock; acute lumbar pain; rigor; a feeling of constriction of the chest; dyspnœa; pyrexia. Hæmaturia follows soon after the preceding signs. Anuria may occur.

Jaundice occurs a few hours or days later.

Rapid improvement may take place, but acute renal failure may ensue, sometimes resulting in death. Recovery from this phase is heralded by diuresis.

Treatment

The midwife must stop the transfusion immediately, send for the doctor, and prepare for treatment of shock if present. Alternative fluid will be given using a fresh giving set.

A fluid balance chart is kept; each specimen of urine is saved for analysis.

Piriton 10 to 20 mg. may be administered for a mild reaction.

For treatment of acute renal failure see p. 203.

QUESTIONS FOR REVISION

COMPLICATIONS OF THE THIRD STAGE

ORAL QUESTIONS

Which women are more likely to have post-partum hæmorrhage ?

How by good management of the second stage could you try to prevent post-partum hæmorrhage ?

How may blood coagulation disorders complicate the third stage ?

Why is undue kneading and squeezing of the uterus harmful ?

What is the average blood loss during the third stage ?

What constitutes post-partum hæmorrhage ?

How would you know that a succenturiate lobe had been retained ? what are the dangers ?; what would you do ?

Differentiate between: atonic and traumatic post-partum hæmorrhage; adherent and retained placenta; hypovolæmic and endotoxic shock.

Write not more than 10 lines on:
1. Mismanagement of the third stage as a cause of hæmorrhage.
2. The midwives' duties as a member of the " flying squad " team.
3. Vulval hæmatoma.
4. The use of oxytocic drugs in the prevention and treatment of post-partum hæmorrhage.

Explain in not more than 10 lines how you would:
1. Do manual removal of placenta.
2. Do internal bi-manual compression.
3. Cope with traumatic post-partum hæmorrhage in a remote area.
4. Recognize a transfusion reaction.

C.M.B.(N. Ireland) paper.—How would you distinguish between atonic and traumatic postpartum hæmorrhage ? Give the treatment of the atonic variety.

C.M.B.(N. Ireland) paper.—What are the possible causes of severe hæmorrhage from the uterus half an hour after the placenta has been delivered ? What is the management of such a case ?

C.M.B.(Scot.) paper.—Discuss the treatment of a patient in whom hæmorrhage occurs shortly after the delivery of the baby.

C.M.B.(Scot.) paper.—What natural processes prevent hæmorrhage after delivery ? Give the management of 3rd stage hæmorrhage.

C.M.B.(N. Ireland) paper.—Immediately following the delivery of the baby the mother has a severe blood loss of 600 ml., per vaginam. What are the causes and what is the management ?

C.M.B.(Scot.) paper.—Describe the causes, prevention and management of third stage hæmorrhage.

C.M.B.(Eng.) paper. 50 word question.—Discuss the importance of the obstetric emergency service (Flying Squad).

C.M.B.(Scot.) paper.—What signs during the third stage would lead you to believe the placenta had separated ? What is meant by (a) retained placenta ; (b) adherent placenta ? What are the dangers associated with these two conditions ?

C.M.B.(Eng.) paper.—There are no signs of separation of the placenta after an hour in the third stage. Describe your management of the case.

C.M.B.(N. Ireland) paper.—How does the placenta separate during the third stage of labour ? What complications may occur and how would you deal with them ?

C.M.B.(N. Ireland) paper.—Give the predisposing causes of shock during labour and state what you would do to avoid them. How would you treat shock due to postpartum hæmorrhage on district ?

C.M.B.(Scot.) paper.—A patient collapses suddenly after delivery. What emergency treatment would you carry out pending the arrival of the doctor ?

C.M.B.(Scot.) paper.—Discuss the causes of severe collapse in a patient within twenty-four hours of delivery.

26

The Normal Puerperium

The puerperium is the period following labour, characterized by the following three features:

1. THE GENERATIVE ORGANS RETURN TO THEIR PREGRAVID STATE.
2. LACTATION IS INITIATED (p. 506).
3. RECUPERATION from the physical and emotional experience of parturition takes place.

The puerperium begins as soon as the placenta is expelled, and lasts for six to eight weeks. The period, during which the woman takes adequate rest should be 7 to 10 days. The Central Midwives Boards require midwives to attend for 10 days post-partum.

1. RETURN OF THE GENERATIVE ORGANS TO NORMAL

The process by which the generative organs return to their pregravid state is known as " involution." The main changes occur in the uterine muscle and decidua, but the ligaments also return to the condition they were in prior to pregnancy. The stretched vagina, pelvic floor and perineum regain their tone, but in some instances a degree of laxity persists.

INVOLUTION OF THE UTERUS

On the completion of labour, the uterus measures $15 \cdot 2 \times 11 \cdot 4 \times 8 \cdot 9$ cm. and weighs 907 G.

At the end of the puerperium it has almost returned to its pregravid size of $7 \cdot 6 \times 5 \cdot 1 \times 2 \cdot 5$ cm. and weight of 57 G.

The marked reduction in size is most rapid during the first week, the uterus losing half of its bulk during that time; this being brought about by two factors: autolysis of the muscle fibres, ischæmia of the uterus.

Autolysis (*self digestion*).

The muscle fibres, which during pregnancy increase 10 times in length and 5 times in thickness, are reduced to normal dimensions. Whether the factor producing autolysis is a uterine hormone or enzyme is not known, but some of the protoplasm in the fibres is broken down, absorbed into the blood-stream and excreted by the kidneys.

ISCHÆMIA (*localized anæmia*)

The contraction and retraction of the uterine muscle fibres compress the blood-vessels and reduce the uterine blood supply. During pregnancy the increased blood supply causes uterine hypertrophy; the diminished blood supply in the puerperium produces atrophy.

REDUCTION IN SIZE OF THE UTERUS

At the completion of labour the fundus is 5·1 cm. below the umbilicus or 12·7 cm. above the symphysis pubis.

Twenty-four hours later it has risen to the level of the umbilicus. This occurs because the collapsed lower pole of the uterus is regaining its tone and because there is some relaxation of the upper segment.

One week after labour the fundus is 7·6 cm. above the symphysis pubis.

Twelve days after labour the fundus is not usually palpable.

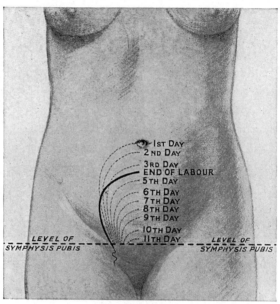

FIG. 304

Showing fundal height during the postnatal period.

The following list gives comparative findings:

	Weight of uterus	Diameter of placental site	Cervix
End of labour	907 G.	12·7 cm.	Soft, flabby
End of 1 week	454 G.	7·6 cm.	Admits 2 fingers
End of 2 weeks	312 G.	5·1 cm.	Admits 1 finger
End of 6 weeks	71 G.	2·5 cm.	A slit

THE DECIDUA

The remains of the spongy layer of the decidua, to which the placenta and membranes were attached, are shed; the basal or unaltered layer regenerates a new endometrium and at the end of eight weeks the placental site is healed. A further four weeks or longer may elapse before menstruation recommences.

THE LOCHIA

Lochia is the term given to the discharge from the uterus during the puerperium. They have an alkaline reaction in which organisms flourish more readily than in the acid vaginal secretion. The amount of lochia varies in different women and is rather more in quantity than what is lost during the menstrual flow; the odour is heavy and unpleasant, but not offensive.

LOCHIA RUBRA (red), 1 to 4 days.

For the first three days the lochia consist mainly of blood. They also contain shreds of decidua and fragments of chorion, liquor amnii, lanugo; vernix caseosa and meconium may also be present.

LOCHIA SEROSA (pink), 5 to 9 days.

The discharge is paler and brownish in colour, containing less blood and more serum as well as leucocytes and organisms.

LOCHIA ALBA (white), 10 to 15 days.

The discharge is creamy-greenish in colour and contains leucocytes, organisms, cervical mucus and debris from the healing process in the uterus and vagina. Slight blood discoloration may be seen for as long as three weeks.

Persistent red lochia (fresh blood) is a warning sign that products of conception have been retained *in utero,* and of the likelihood of severe puerperal hæmorrhage occurring. **It is important that midwives realize the danger of retained products** and that persistent red lochia be reported to the doctor.

THE PSYCHOLOGY OF THE PUERPERAL WOMAN

The midwife should have some appreciation of the sensitivity of the woman's nervous system and the emotional turmoil to which she is subjected during the puerperium. Her nervous, as well as her physical energy may have been depleted by the stress of labour, and while in this weakened condition she is faced with the care of what appears to her to be a very fragile human being.

THE MATERNAL INSTINCT

The young mother is overwhelmed with joy in having her precious infant safely in her arms: rather awed at being entrusted with such responsibility and acutely aware of the inadequacy of her knowledge and experience of babies.

It is to the midwife she looks for guidance and advice, and, if neither is forthcoming, she becomes apprehensive and dismayed.

The maternal instinct at this time may be very strong, and the mother should be given ample opportunities to express this by handling and cuddling her baby. But this natural urge, which should be loving and protective, may very readily develop into a state of acute anxiety, particularly if the infant does not appear to her to be thriving.

Any bad news should be withheld, if possible, and especially regarding the baby: the father being told when serious illness occurs.

THE ATTITUDE OF THE MIDWIFE

The psychological and educational aspects of puerperal care must be woven into the very fabric of the student midwife's education and become an integral part of her practical training.

It is essential that, by attitude, word and action, the midwife shows her deep understanding and her willingness to be helpful. A kindly approach is appreciated by all women on occasions such as these, and any advice or counsel regarding the baby's or her own welfare will be received with gratitude and appreciation.

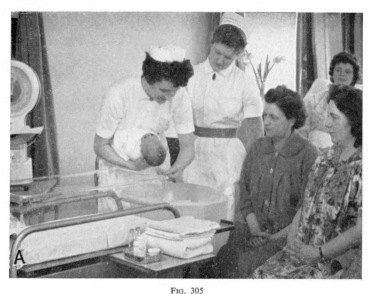

FIG. 305
BABY-CARE TEACHING.
Sister demonstrates to mothers in four-bed ward; student midwife observes.
(*County Maternity Hospital, Bellshill, Lanarkshire.*)

Assurance and assistance should be given when necessary, with all procedures concerning the baby, and a certain flexibility of mind should be exhibited. The midwife must refrain from dictating or dominating.

The midwife should encourage mothers to change napkins, bath and dress their babies; this builds up their morale and gives them confidence in their ability to cope with their infants at home.

A TRANQUIL ATMOSPHERE

Student midwives who are trained nurses, when assigned to care for puerperal women require to alter their conception of what they may consider to be good ward administration.

The ward should have a home-like quality in which mothers with a feeling of contentment can relax and enjoy their babies. Although it is a school for inexperienced mothers, discipline is not evident, the routine is flexible and learning a happy experience.

The ward should be a pleasant, even casual place where mothers move at their own pace while tending their infants. Rigid routine, rush and bustle are detrimental to the calm atmosphere which should prevail. Where rooming-in is practised, it is not possible to have an immaculately tidy ward, but the contentment of the mothers and the quietness of the babies more than compensate for this.

THE MOTHER'S EMOTIONAL REACTIONS

Women react during the postpartum period in different ways. The majority are happy and contented unless for some niggling fear or anxiety regarding their babies.

The temperament of the woman has an important bearing on her reactions. The happy-go-lucky woman of average intelligence is usually a successful mother. The ultra-intelligent, the imaginative or the highly-strung types are more likely to encounter or create difficulties.

Certain mothers may desire to carry out ideas that they have used on previous occasions, or which have been recommended to them. A minority feel very deeply regarding having to conform to hospital ideas and methods which concern the baby, *e.g.* whether he should be beside her all the time ; on self-regulated, three-hourly or four- hourly feeding.

If " reasons why " are given and advantages explained, such mothers would be less resentful than when they are dominated without being consulted. The midwife should try to see the mother's point of view, guiding rather than directing her.

Some women are slower and more awkward in handling their babies than others. Allowance must be made for this. If made to feel incompetent they become perturbed, even depressed.

A Process of Adjustment

The woman with her first baby goes through a process of adjustment that for the well-balanced woman presents no problem. The pampered type may resent the transfer of attention from herself to the baby, and such feelings may be manifest as tantrums or in the making of unjustifiable complaints to redirect attention towards herself. The immature may tend to reject the responsibilities involved in parenthood and object to the curtailment of their social activities. **Patience is needed in handling such women.**

POSTPARTUM TEARS

The susceptibility to tears is undoubtedly present during the puerperium, and it is the duty of the midwife to do all in her power to prevent the occurrence of this.

During the first week of the puerperium the woman should lead a quiet sheltered existence, free from worry or excitement. The baby may be the main cause of worry: the visitors the cause of excitement.

Causes

Having been on the staff of maternity hospitals in the United States and in Great Britain, the following causes are, in the writer's opinion, the most outstanding.

1. TOO MANY VISITORS

Relatives, friends and sometimes acquaintances are eager to offer personal congratulations to the mother and to see the new baby. When, as happens in some countries, there are practically no restrictions on visiting hours, the patient is deprived of the recuperative power of rest and quietness and subjected to a protracted social experience that her nervous system is not in a state to cope with.

Visiting during the first week should be judiciously rationed to not more than two hours daily and visitors limited to near relatives and intimate friends for whom no special social effort need be made. Husbands usually visit in the evening, but should not remain too late.

2. TOO LITTLE SOUND SLEEP

In hospital this is a common complaint. The baby requires food early in the morning and late in the evening. The depletion of the nursing staff on duty at those periods delays settling down for the night and necessitates an early start which shortens the period available for sleep. The remedy is obvious.

3. NOISE

Inevitable and unavoidable maternity hospital noises bombard the nervous system. Most midwives remove crying babies from puerperal wards at night to allow the short period of sleep available to be sound.

4. ANXIETY ABOUT THE BABY

If there is difficulty with breast feeding the mother is certain to be upset : the good midwife will spend extra time with mother and baby at feeding times, and by encouragement and competent handling overcome the problem and eradicate the anxiety.

TEARS AFTER DISCHARGE

Husbands are often warned to expect this : they should be instructed in how to prevent them.

1. Building up confidence in her ability to care for her baby : by knowledge, *e.g.* teaching given at the prenatal clinic and in the puerperal ward.

2. The provision of extra help in the home : by the husband if none other is available : sufficient rest, sleep, and good food.

3. Encouragement, patience and understanding from the husband.

MODERN IDEAS REGARDING PUERPERAL CARE

Ideas are changing regarding the type of care required by, and to be provided for, the woman during the postpartum period. She is no longer regarded as an invalid but a normal woman recuperating from a natural physiological process.

Supervision of the recuperative processes that follow childbirth is necessary in order to detect and correct the abnormal, but actual nursing care is not required after the first 48 hours unless complications arise.

Planned 48 hour discharge from hospital is discussed on page 463.

THE NEEDS OF THE PUERPERAL WOMAN

The mother's needs are physical, psychological, social and educational, and in many respects they dovetail into each other. Her physical requirements are well catered for, but her psychological needs are neither fully recognized nor met on all occasions. Her educational needs, as the inexperienced mother of a young baby, are sometimes ignored.

NEW OUTLOOK FOR MIDWIVES

The need for the education of puerperal mothers is a challenge and student midwives should be orientated during their midwifery training to the role of teacher-supervisor and counsellor.

Good human relationships are most important and must be maintained.

Early ambulation has transferred many of the midwife's nursing duties to the patients themselves. This will entail lucid instruction and unremitting supervision.

Intelligent and assiduous observation must still proceed, daily routine examination of breasts, bladder, lochia and the perineal suture line is most necessary.

INSTRUCTION OF INEXPERIENCED MOTHERS

It would seem reasonable to instruct new mothers regarding the care of their babies. During pregnancy, labour and the puerperium doctors foster and supervise the health and wellbeing of the baby, yet he is permitted to go home under the complete jurisdiction and care of a mother with neither knowledge of baby behaviour nor experience of baby care.

With the discharge of women from hospital during the first week of the puerperium, it is even more urgent that prenatal and intranatal teaching programmes be inaugurated to enable them to cope successfully with their babies at home. A follow-up system whereby mothers are visited daily by midwives until the 10th day is being established.

EDUCATION WITH A PSYCHOLOGICAL BIAS

The psychological aspect is dealt with on page 446.

Young mothers need advice in regard to refraining from devoting all their time and affection to their babies. Father must get his share of love and attention.

Most young mothers are perturbed because of their lack of knowledge and experience of baby care, and have a feeling of inferiority regarding their ability to take charge of their infants at home. Physical weakness and emotional instability add to the problem.

EDUCATION GEARED TO MEET SOCIAL NEEDS

The social aspect of puerperal care should deeply concern the midwife; the adjustment from wife to mother and the establishment of the family unit should be kept in mind and the mother advised as to coping with her new responsibilities.

The fact that babies are going home with inexperienced parents is an urgent social problem, and more should be done to prepare for and deal with this.

1. **By trying to establish a satisfactory feeding-sleeping routine.** The baby who is fed satisfactorily during the day usually sleeps at night. It is most distressing for the parents to have to cope with a crying baby at night when they do not understand the cause or know the remedy.

2. **By making an endeavour to have the baby established on either breast or bottle feeding prior to discharge.** The hospital staff should prescribe the strength and amount of milk and demonstrate the correct procedure in the preparation of feeds. It is asking too much to expect the mother to cope with unsuccessful breast feeding at home.

3. **By using equipment similar to what will be found in the homes** when demonstrating baby-care procedures in hospital.

4. **By advocating techniques applicable in the home,** *e.g.* bathing baby on the knee rather than on a table.

Much of the teaching on baby care given during pregnancy can be revised and consolidated during the puerperium, and when applied to the mother's own baby it becomes real, worthwhile, and infinitely more effective.

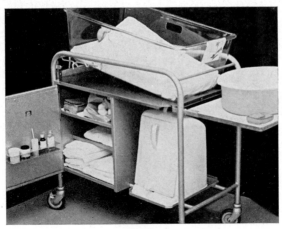

Fig. 306

Locker with individual bath, baby linen and equipment for " rooming-in."

(*Simpson Memorial Maternity Pavilion, Edinburgh.*)

THE ROOMING-IN PLAN

Under this system the baby in his cot remains at the mother's bedside for the greater part of the 24 hours ; mother and baby being treated as a unit.

At its best rooming-in is an excellent educational project with psychological and physical advantages to both mother and baby.

ADVANTAGES

1. EDUCATIONAL

(*a*) **The inexperienced mother can study her baby,** and so gain knowledge, experience and assurance that will be invaluable when she goes home. Confidence is engendered by handling her infant and in carrying out procedures such as changing napkins, bathing and dressing.

(*b*) **By observing his behaviour** she notes and can enquire about incidents, *e.g.* the pallor of the sleeping baby, irregular or shallow breathing, hiccough, green stools, that would worry her at home.

(*c*) **She sees her baby handled, napkins changed, bathed,** and does all those things herself prior to going home.

(*d*) **Her questions can be answered** as the need arises; problems would otherwise remain unsolved at home with no adviser available.

(*e*) **Rooming-in is a real-life situation** which provides the best possible environment for the learning process.

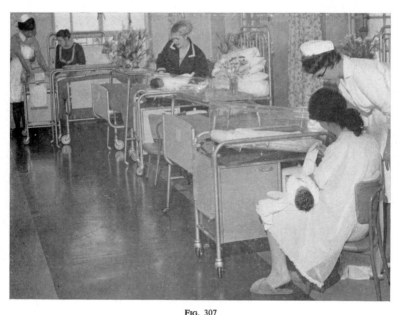

FIG. 307

ROOMING-IN WARD.

(*Simpson Memorial Maternity Pavilion, Edinburgh.*)

2. PSYCHOLOGICAL

(*a*) **The infant gets more mothering** than he would get in a nursery: cuddling, warmth and physical contact are necessary as an expression of love and to give emotional security to the baby.

(*b*) **A more satisfactory and satisfying mother-child relationship can be established.**

(*c*) **The mother is happy and contented** to have her babe near her, to see him when she wishes and to be given the opportunity to express her maternal instinct.

(*d*) **Reduction in the length of hunger-crying** and frustration, by the proximity of the mother and the prompt provision of food, may have a beneficial influence on the temperament of the child.

(*e*) **During visits of the father both parents are more conscious of the family unit.**

3. PHYSICAL

(*a*) **Breast feeding is more successfully initiated.**

(*b*) **The dangers of neonatal cross-infection are lessened** if adequate individual equipment is provided. The contact of baby and nursing staff is reduced to a minimum and this also reduces cross-infection.

THE MIDWIFE, A TEACHER

The midwife is well endowed with obstetric knowledge, skill and experience, and the tuition in parentcraft teaching now required, during training, by the Central Midwives Boards will enable her to instruct mothers in a practical manner.

Teaching requires patience (1) to allow for lack of comprehension, and (2) because of the inevitability of much repetition.

Fortunately more teaching time is now available since midwives are relieved of many of the nursing duties incumbent on those who care for patients confined to bed.

Zeal and an abiding interest in mothers and babies make the effort worth while; the satisfaction in preparing mothers to care for and enjoy their babies is immense.

A curriculum should be drawn up giving daily talk-demonstrations of at least thirty minutes' duration to groups of mothers. **Incidental teaching should proceed throughout the day,** mainly in a supervisory capacity. Rounds should also be made to discuss non-urgent individual difficulties and to give advice where indicated.

The following subjects would no doubt prove beneficial and acceptable:

1. **Advice when mother goes home.**—Food, sleep, rest, tranquillity, recreation.
2. **Baby care.**—Feeding, fresh air, sleep, exercise, stools, sore buttocks, crying.
3. **Bathing baby as in the home.**—(*Talk demonstration.*)
4. **Attending the child health clinic.**—(*By Health Visitor*).
5. **Attending for postnatal examination.**—(*By doctor*).
6. **The new father.**   7. **Enjoy your baby.**
8. **Planning baby's day.**—(*Now we are three—or four.*)

SUBJECTS FOR DISCUSSION

Subjects other than those given below can be brought up for consideration and discussion and multiparæ could contribute from their practical experience, *e.g.*—

1. **Morning or evening bath times.**   2. **Self-demand feeding;** three or four hourly feeding.
3. **How long vaginal discharge persists. When menstruation recommences.**
4. **Family planning.**   5. **How to deal with the toddler.**

MANAGEMENT OF THE PUERPERIUM

The management of the puerperium consists in providing the means whereby the woman can recuperate physically and emotionally, and gain supervised experience in the feeding and care of her infant; this **embraces the following principles:**

1. **The advancement of physical well-being—**
   Good nutrition: correction of anæmia: comfort: cleanliness: sufficient physical activity to ensure good muscle tone.

2. **The establishment of emotional well-being—**
   Quietness: freedom from excitement and worry: the proper psychological approach.

3. **The prevention of infection and other avoidable complications.**

4. **The promotion of breast-feeding** (p. 506).

5. **The provision of baby-care teaching.**

IMMEDIATE CARE

Although the puerperium begins immediately the placenta is born, the first hour is usually included under the management of labour. The woman is made comfortable, a light meal served and a sedative given to ensure rest and sleep.

The uterus should be of cricket-ball consistency, the blood loss normal in amount, the pulse below 90.

Should bleeding occur, or if the uterus is believed to contain blood clots, it should be massaged until it contracts, the clots expressed and an oxytocic preparation, such as ergometrine, 0·5 mg. or Syntometrine 1 ml. given intramuscularly. If the bleeding is not brought under control, medical aid must be summoned.

ASEPSIS AND ANTISEPSIS

Asepsis must be maintained, especially during the first week of the puerperium. The woman is particularly vulnerable to infection at this time, for the following reasons:

1. **The uterus provides an ideal environment for the multiplication of organisms.**

2. **The lacerated or bruised tissues of the vulva and vagina, being devitalized, are unable to resist the invasion of organisms.**

3. **The vaginal orifice is gaping and organisms can readily enter.**

4. **The woman's resistance is lowered because of depletion of energy,** lack of sleep and food.

5. **Blood loss may have been excessive.**

DOMESTIC CLEANLINESS

The adequate use of soap and water is the first requirement. In hospital modern appliances are used to minimize the spread of infected dust.

The room and bed-linen, the woman's skin and clothing should be clean.

The midwife must wear a mask when the vulva is exposed during the first week of the puerperium.

TEMPERATURE AND PULSE

Temperature and pulse are two excellent guides as to the woman's condition, and both should be normal throughout the puerperium.

A slight rise of temperature within 24 hours of delivery is commonly said to be reactionary, but, unless following a difficult delivery, should be viewed with suspicion. Any rise in temperature during the first week should be attributed to puerperal sepsis until proved otherwise.

The temperature is unstable during the puerperium and tends to rise because of minor disorders, such as engorgement of the breasts, the discomfort of a full bladder or due to excitement, but such an elevation is transient and should not be above 37·7° C. (100° F.).

The pulse rate should be slow, ranging between 60 and 80, but, if over 90, it is advisable to record it on the chart in red to draw attention to the fact. Excitement and fatigue may accelerate the pulse temporarily, but when pulse and temperature are both increased, puerperal sepsis or other infection is the most likely cause.

Temperature and pulse are taken every morning and evening, and if the temperature is 38° C. (100·4° F.) once, or 37·4° C. (99·4° F.) on two occasions, or if the pulse is over 90 on more than two instances, temperature and pulse should be taken four-hourly. (*In some hospitals the temperature is taken twice daily for three days and then once daily, in the evening.*)

CENTRAL MIDWIVES BOARDS' RULES

C.M.B.(Scot.) rule.—If a rise of temperature after the first 24 hours or any other condition requiring close supervision be found at the morning or evening visit a registered medical practitioner must be summoned and the Local Supervising Authority notified.

C.M.B.(Eng.) code of practice.—If the patient has a continuously rapid or rising pulse rate, or if she has a rise of temperature above 37·4° C. (99·4° F.) on three successive days, or a rise of temperature to 38° C. (100·4° F.) a registered medical practitioner must be summoned.

ESTIMATING THE FUNDAL HEIGHT

The uterus is palpated daily and any tenderness noted. The regular decrease in fundal height, approximately 1·3 cm. (½ in.) every day, is a means of determining that involution is proceeding normally; although the measurement may not be accurate unless always taken by the same person, it gives the novice some idea of what is taking place. (*Some authorities consider the procedure has little value.*) Not until the 11th or 12th day is the fundus no longer palpable, and only on such occasions as following premature labour does it reach the symphysis pubis on the seventh day.

Measuring the height of the fundus also draws attention to a full bladder.

The author is aware of a puerperal patient in 1965 being admitted to hospital on the fourth day with acute abdominal pain: 3 litres 360 ml. of urine were withdrawn by catheter. Another hospital patient in 1965 had 1 litre 860 ml. of urine withdrawn on the fifth day post-partum.

The bladder should be emptied first, because a full bladder may displace the uterus upwards, as will a loaded rectum. If the fundal height remains stationary, or is higher than on the previous day, the bladder should be percussed to ascertain whether it contains residual urine. A plastic 15 cm. ruler should be used, being more accurate than a tape measure which may curve down behind the fundus.

THE LOCHIA

Lochia should be handled like pus and never touched with the bare fingers. Pads should be removed by using forceps, then wrapped in paper or grasped with the hand inserted into a 15 cm. plastic bag, and burned as soon as possible. They should always be kept for the doctor's inspection when there is some abnormal finding to report.

ABNORMALITIES OF THE LOCHIA

Note and record	Report to Doctor	Significance
The amount .	Excessive	Retained products.
	Scanty	Due to poor drainage.
	Scanty (*with pyrexia*) . . .	Puerperal sepsis (*septicæmia*).
The colour .	Persistently red	Danger of hæmorrhage
	Brown and profuse (*with bulky uterus*)	Sub-involution.
The consistence .	Pieces of membrane or placenta .	Retained products.
The odour .	Offensive	Retained products.
	Offensive (*with pyrexia*) . .	Puerperal sepsis (*local uterine infection*).

The skin is very active during the puerperium, and a daily bath or shower is necessary. Night sweats may be so profuse as to necessitate changing the nightgown, but the woman can be assured that this is a normal state of affairs.

THE BLADDER

Large amounts of urine are secreted during the first few days, due to the discarding of the increased amount of blood plasma and tissue fluid present during pregnancy.

Retention of urine (p. 466).

RESIDUAL URINE

The inexperienced midwife may overlook the possibility of residual urine, because the woman is apparently passing adequate amounts. The bladder should be percussed every day.

The woman should be encouraged to void within 12 hours of confinement, but must never be forced to wait for that period before catheterization is carried out. The experienced midwife is never eager to pass a catheter unnecessarily, and will do all in her power to avoid this. Nevertheless, the woman must not suffer, and if the simple remedies do not succeed and she is obviously in pain the catheter should be passed. It is the overdistended bladder as much as the procedure of catheterization which gives rise to lower urinary tract infection.

The instillation of chlorhexidine, 1 in 5,000, 30 ml., before withdrawing the catheter will help to combat infection. The doctor's wishes should be ascertained.

THE BOWELS

The bowels tend to be sluggish during the puerperium, for the following reasons:

1. **The woman is losing fluid** from her body in the large quantities of urine she is passing, in perspiration and in milk if breast-feeding.

2. **The anus may be insensitive** to stimulation, having been forcibly dilated by the pressure of the baby's head.

It is customary to give some mild laxative 36 hours after delivery such as Senokot.

When the diet contains sufficient roughage and fluid, the bowels need less artificial stimulation, but a small prepacked enema, a glycerine, or Dulcolax suppository, is usually given if the bowels do not move 48 hours after delivery and on every subsequent third day. The modern tendency is to pay less attention to the bowels if the woman is well and comfortable.

Whether any particular laxative affects the baby is a moot point. Dulcolax, Senokot, or vegetable laxative pills are as a rule efficacious and do not cause the baby to have loose stools.

The traditional idea that fruit and vegetables upset the baby is no longer recognized.

DIET

The nursing mother needs a liberal nourishing diet to build up her strength and to enable her to produce sufficient breast milk. Good wholesome food is essential, containing sufficient proteins (100 G.) daily, minerals and vitamins, as the production of an adequate supply of breast milk is believed to be influenced by the intake of protein and vitamin B.

As so many women are anæmic at this time the midwife must ensure that **foods rich in iron** are included in the diet. The hæmoglobin is estimated on the 1st day and if low this is repeated on the 8th or 9th day. Iron supplements are usually prescribed for one month.

Additional fluid is required, but excessive quantities of fluid will not increase the milk supply. Milk is high in proteins and calcium, and as the woman is losing calcium from her body when she produces milk, 1,200 ml. should be taken in her diet every day. Fruit or vegetables should be served at every meal.

POSITION

Immediately after labour the woman lies in the recumbent position, usually under the influence of a sedative, until she is rested.

She is advised to move in bed as she feels inclined: sitting up encourages drainage from the uterus. Free movement of the legs is essential to avoid venous thrombosis.

REST AND SLEEP

A sedative, such as amylobarbitone sodium 200 mg. (Sodium Amytal) or butobarbitone 100 mg. (Soneryl), is usually necessary to ensure sleep the first night; rarely should it be necessary after then, except in cases of high blood pressure. If kept awake by some discomfort, such as after-pains, hæmorrhoids, or engorged breasts, the midwife should treat the cause before giving analgesics.

Persistent insomnia in the absence of pain should be viewed with concern as a warning sign of oncoming mental illness.

The woman needs adequate rest, quietness and sleep, because of the hypersensitive state of her nervous system, but without organization this is not easily achieved in a puerperal ward. The day begins early and ends late, with an almost incessant round of routine visits and treatment. The ward should be closed morning and afternoon for one hour; the patients requested to relax and keep silent if they cannot sleep.

What to Report to the Doctor

The midwife should be prepared to report on the following points. (Reporting on the baby is considered under Care of the Newborn, p. 499.)

Temperature and pulse.	Condition of sutured perineum.
Appetite: sleep.	Pain, *e.g.* in the breast; abdomen; leg; head.
Bowels: bladder.	
Character of lochia.	Any peculiarity in behaviour.

VULVAL TOILET

For non-ambulant patients swabbing should be carried out prior to bed-making, sweeping and dusting, or not less than one hour afterwards, because of the danger of dust as a medium of cross-infection. The groins, thighs and buttocks should be thoroughly washed with soap and water prior to swabbing.

Details in swabbing technique will vary from hospital to hospital. Opinions differ as to how frequently swabbing should be carried out, the modern tendency being to limit the procedure to twice in 24 hours during the first few days if the woman is not fit to go to the bathroom or shower.

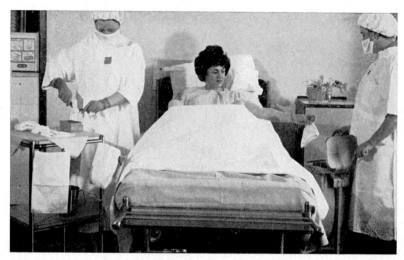

Fig. 308

PERINEAL TOILET FOR NON-AMBULANT PATIENT.

Disposable individual packs used.

Patient puts pad in paper bag and drops it into portable sack holder. Cardboard container for swabbing lotion. Two disposable dissecting forceps used by midwife. Buttocks dried with Kleenex paper towel. Gloved hands washed between patients. Nursing auxiliary gives and removes bed-pan

(*County Maternity Hospital, Bellshill, Lanarkshire.*)

Mask-wearing is imperative, because the hæmolytic streptococcus and *Staphylococcus pyogenes* are harboured in the nose and throat. All utensils and dressings must be sterilized, including bed-pans.

Newly delivered women and those who have had Cæsarean sections are swabbed first; those with offensive lochia are swabbed last.

EARLY AMBULATION

Normal patients are allowed to be out of bed on the first day of the puerperium; they may have a shower (with mobile hand spray) six hours after delivery.

The practice appears to have no immediate deleterious effect. Primitive women get up early with no harmful results.

SELF-VULVAL SWABBING

In most maternity hospitals the woman carries out her own perineal toilet on the first postpartum day by taking a shower with a mobile hand spray. In others swabbing is discontinued then and tub-baths in the kneeling position given. (See also bidet with mobile hand spray.) See fig. 310.

The project should be planned and well organized for vulval swabbing must be executed by the mothers in such a way that puerperal sepsis does not result. This will entail lucid instruction and unremitting supervision.

OBSERVATION BY MIDWIVES

It is important that observation of the suture line be carried out daily during the first few days : pads must be inspected daily.

Scrupulous cleanliness of toilets, baths and hand basins must be rigorously attended to.

FACILITIES TO BE PROVIDED

These will vary, and structural alterations may have to be made to ensure a safe technique and some degree of privacy. The provision of cubicles each with wash basin and toilet ; a bidet with a mobile hand spray is excellent.

The following accessories would be convenient:

1. CONTAINERS ON THE WALLS FOR :
   (a) **Wrapped sterile pads** (one pad, six wool balls).   (b) **Paper towels : tissue wipes.**
   (c) **Bags, for soiled dressings.**
2. A shelf on which to open sterile dressings.
3. A shelf for wrapping soiled dressings.   4. Sani-bin for dressings.

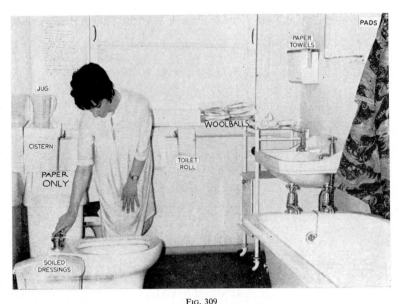

FIG. 309

" SET-UP " FOR SELF-PERINEAL CARE.

(Maternity Unit. Central Hospital, Irvine, Ayrshire.)

INSTRUCTIONS ON SWABBING

Talks to groups of mothers should be given, explaining in simple language the following :
1. **How germs are spread.**
2. **The need for hand washing** even although hands look clean.
3. **Why pads must be removed and applied in a certain way.**
4. **Why swabbing is done from front to back.**
The opening of a sterile packet should be demonstrated.

TECHNIQUE EMPLOYED

The swabbing procedure should be simple, instructions given ought to be clear and a typed copy exhibited in each cubicle. Supervision must be adequate with a midwife or senior student in attendance to assist each woman until she is confident in doing it alone.

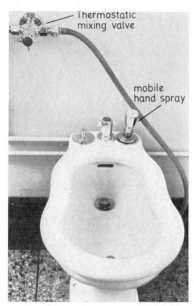

FIG. 310
BIDET WITH MOBILE HAND SPRAY.
Queen Mother's Maternity Hospital, Glasgow.)

Paper towels to be used after hand washing.

Pads are unpinned, front first, removed from behind.

SWABBING.

One stroke one swab, front to back; tissue wipes to be used for inner sides of thighs. **Tissue wipes are used for the " back passage "** (*always from behind*), wiping from front to back. **Clean pad applied from the front.** Surface of pad which will be in contact with the vulva must not be touched.

TREATMENT OF THIRD DEGREE TEAR

The sutured perineum must be kept clean, antiseptic and dry. The vulva is swabbed in the usual way and dried carefully. A piece of gauze is placed between the labia.

Exposure to light.—The vulva may be exposed to the air or to the light of an ordinary electric lamp, the anglepoise type being very convenient. With the woman's legs in the position for swabbing, the light is placed 30·4 cm. from the vulva ; the gentle heat is soothing to inflamed tissues, dries the area and the light aids healing. The exposure is given for 15 minutes and repeated every eight hours.

Avoidance of strain on the sutures.—The woman should not sit bolt upright; she may roll over on to her side to feed her baby. Non-absorbable sutures are removed on the 6th or 7th day.

Pain in the wound.—Marked inflammation or œdema should be reported; (*the application of magnesium sulphate or saline soaks will lessen such inflammation and swelling*). Bromelain (Ananase) 20 mg. every 6 hours for 48 hours is useful to relieve inflammation, bruising and œdema. Rikospray Benzocaine or Nestosyl ointment is useful to relieve pain. Codis or Panasorb or pentazocine (Fortral) tablets (2) may be necessary. If there are signs of sloughing, if the wound is infected, or when the tissues are being cut by the sutures they should be removed. Fæces passed vaginally indicate lack of healing by first intention and the formation of a **recto-vaginal fistula.**

The bowels need not be confined: giving small doses of Senokot granules or milk of magnesia, 8 ml. twice daily, beginning on the second day and increasing the dose to 15 ml. on the third day. A small, water enema given with a catheter, a prepacked enema or a Dulcolax suppository will result in an easy evacuation of the bowels.

No dietary restrictions are necessary.

REMOVAL OF SUTURES

Non-absorbable sutures are removed on the sixth or seventh day, depending on the wishes of the obstetrician.

A mask is worn, gloves are not absolutely necessary. The perineum is first swabbed with Hibitane 1-2,000, the knot held with dissecting forceps, and the stitch snipped and gently removed.

The number of sutures should be checked with the record of the number inserted.

THE BREAK-DOWN OF A SUTURED PERINEUM

If clean

Hibitane sitz baths are given twice daily for not longer than five minutes.

Exposure to an ordinary electric light four-hourly (see p. 462).

If septic

In addition to Hibitane sitz baths a small piece of gauze soaked in Eusol is inserted into the broken-down area.

While resuturing the perineum most obstetricians prefer a general anæsthetic. **The wound is** subsequently treated as a third degree tear.

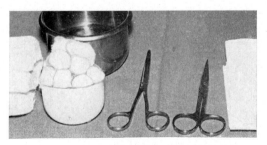

FIG. 311
REMOVAL OF PERINEAL SUTURES

1 pair stitch scissors.	Wool swabs.
1 pair dressing forceps.	Sterile towel.
	Perineal pad.
Disposable bag.	Lotion bowl.

(*Simpson Memorial Maternity Pavilion, Edinburgh.*)

EARLY DISCHARGE FROM HOSPITAL

Planned 48 Hour Discharge

To provide more beds for abnormal prenatal patients suitable normal puerperal women are being discharged from hospital 48 hours after confinement.

When the woman attends the prenatal clinic the question is discussed with her and, if home conditions are satisfactory and provision can be made for domestic help, " early discharge " is planned. Arrangements are made for her own doctor and the domiciliary midwife to take over supervision and care of mother and baby at home. If non-absorbable perineal sutures are present arrangements must be made for their removal. (Some hospitals insert subcuticular catgut.)

To avoid unsettling other puerperal patients these women are nursed together in a separate ward for 48 hours. Careful screening of babies is carried out prior to discharge.

Good liaison between hospital, family doctor and local authority is necessary for the success of " early discharge "; **close co-operation** between hospital and domiciliary midwives being an important factor.

GOOD POSTURE FOR AMBULANT MOTHERS

Notes to Midwives

Since most mothers are ambulant from the first postpartum day, bed exercises are unnecessary: group teaching is now more readily accomplished so a programme of health education combined with good posture and rehabilitating exercises should be inaugurated.

For patients confined to bed deep breathing exercises are beneficial. To prevent venous thrombosis, raising and lowering the knees, flexing and rotating the ankles, flexing and stretching the toes can be done repeatedly during the day.

The approach with greatest appeal to young mothers is via health and beauty, special emphasis being laid on restoration of the figure and the creation of a feeling of well-being. To arouse and maintain interest the exercises should be linked with some domestic or baby-care activity rather than being presented as bald physical exercises.

HEALTH EDUCATION

Good nutrition plays a very important part in the maintenance of good health so a diet high in proteins, minerals (including iron) and vitamins should be advocated and, when possible, displayed. **Mental and emotional health contribute to physical well-being** as well as the enjoyment of life and good human relationships. This aspect of health education should not be neglected.

At home, working surfaces, *i.e.* kitchen table and sink, are not at the correct height for all women, and they should be made aware that after the birth of a baby they are vulnerable to low backache and unnecessary strain and fatigue due to prolonged stooping while working at a table or sink which is too low.

Specific instructions regarding the lifting of heavy weights should be given (see p. 753) and the method of avoiding back strain while so doing demonstrated.

The nursing chair should be without arms and low enough to make a comfortable lap for baby without the need for a foot-stool. **Baby's bath could be placed on a stool to bring the edge to knee level.**

ADVICE ON PERSONAL MATTERS

Many women are reluctant to mention certain subjects although they are eager for advice concerning them :

1. *When may sexual intercourse be resumed?* Six weeks should elapse after childbirth in order that the womb is healed and in its normal position.

2. *Family Planning?* Clinics exist or this purpose and the midwife should know the address and their functions (p. 469). Attendance not later than 3 weeks after delivery is necessary for advice *re* contraception.

3. *How long will vaginal discharge continue?* Slight blood stained discharge may continue for three or more weeks after childbirth.

4. *When does menstruation restart?* Usually menstruation returns in two or three months after childbirth : pregnancy may occur prior to this.

5. *Is it necessary to wear firm corsets?* Heavy corsets are not necessary unless ordered by the doctor for some particular reason. Elastic " roll ons " give slight support and allow the abdominal muscles to function normally.

POSTNATAL EXERCISES

All movements should be made gently, smoothly and rhythmically.

The midwife should grade the exercises carefully, beginning with " deep breathing " the day after delivery; then " strengthening of the abdominal muscles " : then " exercises for the pelvic floor muscles."

On the third postpartum day ambulant exercises may be started. They need not be complicated by exhortations to breathe in or breathe out. Deep breathing facilitates the circulation of blood and may diminish the risk of venous thrombosis: this should be practised prior to each lesson.

When demonstrating correct posture this should be followed by an exaggerated display of wrong posture to stress the fault to be remedied.

The wearing of " tights " with night-gown tucked inside them provides suitable attractive attire that appears to have a tonic effect on the women. Outdoor shoes with low heels are more desirable than the soft fuzzy bedroom slippers that tend to encourage a shuffling gait. (*The exercises are described on p. 751.*)

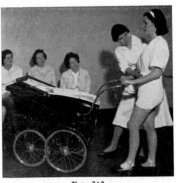

FIG. 312

Physiotherapist demonstrating correct posture when pushing the pram—Shoulders relaxed ; elbows in contact with body ; back straight ; pram handle close to mother's body ; hands relaxed.

(*Royal Maternity Hospital Rottenrow Glasgow.*)

MINOR DISORDERS

FTER-PAINS

These are due to spasmodic uterine contractions, and have been likened to dysmenorrhœa. They occur during the first 48 hours of the puerperium and are more commonly experienced by multiparæ. In some cases they are due to the presence of blood clots in the uterus ; if the uterus is bulky, clots are usually present and should be expressed. When a piece of membrane is known to have been left *in utero* one of the ergot preparations should be given.

To relieve the pain an analgesic drug will be necessary. Panasorb or pentazocine (Fortral) tablets (2) are good. Pethidine, 50 mg. by mouth, repeated in two hours, if necessary, is also effective.

HÆMORRHOIDS

With the pressure of the baby's head on the anus during the perineal phase of labour, hæmorrhoids sometimes prolapse and give rise to pain and intense discomfort.

To relieve the engorgement, magnesium sulphate or hypertonic saline soaks may be applied for 48 hours. The application of some soothing ointment such as Nupercainal is very comforting ; Anusol or other suppositories may be inserted later, when the hæmorrhoids have been reduced.

RETENTION OF URINE

Retention of urine is less common since the puerperal woman has been permitted to get out of bed early, but occasionally occurs following a difficult delivery.

Causes :

1. **Reduced tone in the bladder.**—This may be due to the dominance of progesterone when œstrogens are reduced after the placenta is expelled. Lack of tone allows the bladder to become overdistended; such overdistension may occur during or after labour.

(2) **Trauma.**

(*a*) **An overdistended bladder** may have been bruised by the fetal head, and the tissue at the *base of the bladder is sometimes œdematous.*

(*b*) **Bruising of the urethra and bladder neck.** This may take place if the second stage has been prolonged, and the subsequent œdema of the vulva, as well as the suturing of the perineum, interfere with the act of micturition. The pain and discomfort in the vulva prevent relaxation of the urethral sphincter, which may go into spasm.

To avoid urinary tract infection, retention of urine should be treated actively.

If not successful the doctor must be consulted before passing a catheter.

SUBINVOLUTION

In this condition there is delay in the return of the uterus to normal; The fundal height remains stationary for a few days (check for full bladder); the uterus is soft and boggy, the lochia are reddish brown and profuse.

CAUSES

1. **Any condition which interferes with good uterine contractions,** such as retained products, fibroids, **or which interferes with the ischæmic state of the uterus,** e.g. local uterine infection.

TREATMENT

The midwife should ensure that the uterus is empty at the end of labour and facilitate good uterine drainage by early ambulation and avoiding a distended bladder or loaded bowel.

RETROVERSION

Retroversion, which is usually associated with subinvolution, does not occur until after the seventh day of the puerperium as the uterus is too big to enter the pelvic brim until then. It is more commonly found at the post-natal clinic.

The woman complains of a bearing-down or dragging sensation in the pelvis. Pelvic floor exercises are recommended.

POSTNATAL EXAMINATION

The object of postnatal examination is to detect and rectify any abnormal condition resulting from the recent pregnancy, labour or puerperium. By treating minor lesions or ailments, much suffering and chronic ill health will be prevented.

The examination is not confined to purely obstetrical aspects. The woman's general condition is also considered, and the higher the standards of prenatal and intranatal care, the better will be the state of the woman's health at the postnatal examination.

POSTNATAL EXAMINATION (*on discharge*)

The first postnatal examination is carried out by the doctor on the day prior to discharge. A laxative is given on the previous day, so that the rectum is empty; the woman passes urine immediately before the examination.

REQUIREMENTS.

Sterile gloves; lubricant.	**Mask; wool swabs; perineal pad.**
Basin of swabbing lotion.	**Paper bag for soiled swabs.**

The doctor notes whether the perineum and vaginal walls are healed; the size, mobility and position of the uterus; the presence of red lochia: any tenderness in the appendages.

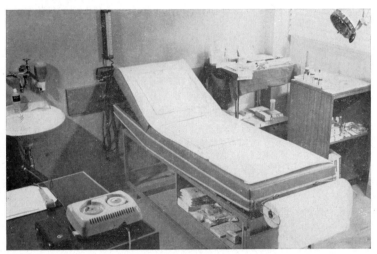

Fig. 313
WELL-EQUIPPED EXAMINATION CUBICLE: POST-NATAL CLINIC.
(*Aberdeen Maternity Hospital.*)

The woman should be advised to take a liberal nourishing diet, and the need for " body building " foods, iron and vitamins stressed. When necessary, iron is prescribed in tablet form.

The need for adequate rest should be impressed on her as well as the avoidance of lifting heavy weights. Many hospitals provide a leaflet or give advice on attending the family planning clinic.

An appointment for a second examination, six weeks postpartum, is made.

At the Simpson Maternity Pavilion each patient is interviewed by a Health Visitor on the day preceding her discharge.

POSTNATAL EXAMINATION (*sixth week or later*)

This examination may be delegated to the patient's family doctor under the general practitioner co-operation scheme.

Prior to examination the bladder is emptied and the urine tested for protein: if a urinary infection occurred during pregnancy a mid-stream specimen is obtained for bacteriological examination; the woman is weighed, blood pressure taken. A hæmoglobin estimation is made and iron therapy prescribed if necessary. The patient's records should be at hand. It is a psychological error not to ask how the baby is progressing (having first made sure it survived). **The woman's abdominal muscles are inspected.**

A vaginal examination is made on the same lines as on the day prior to discharge. The tone of the pelvic floor muscles is noted, a speculum examination made to detect cervical lacerations or erosion. (**A Papanicolaou smear for cervical cytology is made** at some clinics to detect early cancer.)

REQUIREMENTS.

Sterile gloves.	Pessaries: Hodge, Ring.
Swabbing lotion: obstetric cream.	Bivalve and Sims' specula.
Wool swabs.	Uterine dressing forceps.

Paper bag, for used instruments and dressings.

Special follow-up clinics are conducted in some centres for women who have had pre-eclampsia or who have such conditions as tuberculosis, cardiac disease, anæmia or urinary tract infection.

Common Postnatal Complaints and Clinical Findings

Erosion of cervix is considered by some to be hormonal in origin. It may regress spontaneously within two months of confinement. If persistent, with an offensive discharge, thorough cauterization under general anæsthesia is carried out.

Vaginal discharge may be due to infection or erosion of the cervix.

Slight red lochia may still be present for three or four weeks. Bleeding may be due to the resumption of menstruation, but this is not usual until two or three months after childbirth or even later.

Prolapse and retroversion of the uterus are often associated with cystocele and rectocele. The woman complains of pelvic discomfort with a dragging or bearing-down feeling. The knee elbow position for 10 minutes twice daily and the adoption of the prone position for sleep may prove beneficial. If not a pessary is inserted at the 12th week and worn for two months. Additional rest is essential, and constipation should be corrected if present.

Conditions such as frequency, urgency, dysuria, if due to infection, respond well to sulphonamides or antibiotics; in some centres the woman is referred to the Urological Department. Stress incontinence is usually associated with a lax pelvic floor and cystocele.

BACKACHE

This is a common complaint among poorly nourished, overworked multiparous women whose muscles are lax and easily fatigued. The remedy (*not easily provided*) is good food, rest and fresh air; a well-fitting corset gives much relief.

Sacro-iliac strain, due to laxity of the sacro-iliac ligaments, causes severe backache, which is often relieved by physiotherapy, *e.g.* radiant heat, massage, remedial exercises and the rectification of faulty posture. A suitable supporting belt is sometimes advocated but orthopædic advice may be necessary.

Pelvic conditions are no longer considered to be the cause of lumbo-sacral backache.

An introduction to family planning

It would seem to be a fundamental human right that parents should control the size and spacing of their family, for involuntary parenthood creates many problems, social and financial as well as physical and emotional.

In the past mothers of large families endeavoured to welcome each baby in spite of poverty and the tremendous strain of repeated childbearing and rearing. The infant mortality rate was high; mothers suffered much ill-health; many died prematurely.

ESTABLISHING A FAMILY

This is still the earnest desire of most married couples although the modern idea is to limit the number of children. Four is suggested as a satisfactory number and they are usually spaced at intervals of about two years. This concentrated period of childbearing enables the mother to resume her career at an earlier date than was previously possible.

FAMILY PLANNING CLINICS

Under the National Health Service (Family Planning) Act 1967 local authorities have power to provide advice, medical examination and contraceptive substances and appliances. These will be available on social grounds (not only on medical grounds) and to the unmarried as well as the married. The service should be free for medical cases but a charge made for non-medical cases where a person can afford it. The services of the Family Planning Association and other voluntary bodies will continue to be used.

Hospital Boards have been requested by the Dept. of Health and Social Security to provide family planning advice in their hospitals to all women patients.

Leaflets on the subject of family planning could be made available in maternity hospitals, and advice given regarding attending family planning clinics.

METHODS OF CONTRACEPTION

No contraceptive appliance is absolutely reliable so it is essential that the woman fully understands the instructions she is given and carries them out faithfully.

1. THE OCCLUSIVE RUBBER CAP
(Failure rate is said to be 12 per cent)

There are various types of cap that are inserted into the vagina prior to coitus and removed not less than eight hours afterwards; the diaphragm or Dutch cap being most frequently

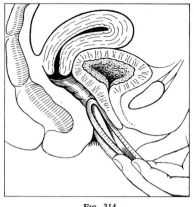 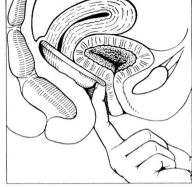

Fig. 314   Fig. 315

Inserting the rubber cap.   Removing the rubber cap.
(Ortho Pharmaceutical Ltd.)

27

prescribed. It consists of a thin rubber dome encircled by a coiled wire-spring 50 to 100 mm. (2 to 4 inches) in diameter and by covering the cervix and fitting snugly against the walls of the vagina it prevents the spermatozoa from entering the cervical os. At the clinic the correct size of cap is selected, and the woman is shown how to insert and remove it. She is told to avoid constipation.

HOW TO INSERT THE CAP.

The woman usually stands with the left foot on a chair, thigh at right angles to the body. Spermicidal jelly is smeared on the diaphragm as an additional safeguard. The rim is squeezed and the cap directed along the posterior vaginal wall, into the posterior fornix; then the anterior rim is pushed up behind the symphysis pubis.

HOW TO REMOVE THE CAP.

The finger is hooked into the rim behind the symphysis pubis and the cap is pulled downwards.

In some cases the vaginal walls and pelvic floor muscles are lax, not having recovered from the effects of parturition, and the cap will not remain in position. Another type of cap **must then be used.**

2 THE CONDOM OR RUBBER SHEATH

This thin rubber appliance (like a finger stall) is worn by the husband. **For maximal safety spermicidal jelly is introduced into the vagina** as well as being smeared on the outside of the condom. The failure rate when used with spermicidal jelly is 5 per cent.

Condoms are often recommended.

1. Until the woman can insert the diaphragm satisfactorily.

2. Until the vaginal walls are involuted after childbirth.

Neither cap nor condom is absolutely reliable, but detailed advice on their use is given at the F.P.A. clinic.

3. THE RHYTHM METHOD
(erroneously known as the safe period)

This method limits coitus to the periods when no ovum is available for fertilization, ten days prior to and five days after menstruation. The nine days surrounding the day of ovulation are unsafe, so coitus must not take place on the five days before, on

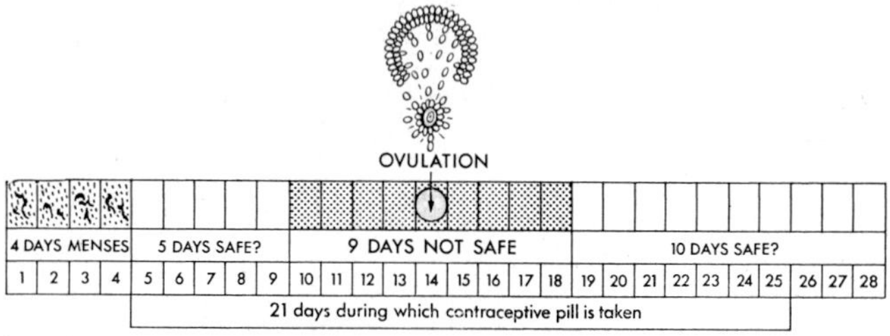

OVULATION

4 DAYS MENSES				5 DAYS SAFE?					9 DAYS NOT SAFE									10 DAYS SAFE?									
1	2	3	4	5	6	7	8	9	10	11	12	13	14	15	16	17	18	19	20	21	22	23	24	25	26	27	28

21 days during which contraceptive pill is taken

FIG. 316

Diagrammatic representation of the 15 safe days and of the 21 days during which the contraceptive pill is taken. The pills are started on the 5th day: the first day of the menstrual period being day no. 1.

the day of, and on the three days after ovulation, a total of nine days. Ovulation usually occurs 14 days prior to the first day of the menstrual period but may occur earlier or later.

Determining the day of ovulation

A slight rise in temperature 0·34° C. (0·6° F.,) occurs on the day following ovulation and is sustained for a few days, so by taking the temperature in the mouth every morning on awakening for a few months the day of ovulation can be established; the temperature is recorded in graph form.

A detailed menstrual record is kept for at least six months ; the days of abstinence from coitus are then adjusted to allow for irregularities in the time of ovulation.

Limiting coitus to the safe period is acceptable where other methods are condemned on religious grounds.

4. ORAL CONTRACEPTIVE PILLS

Oral contraceptive pills provide maximal safety against conception; if the tablets are taken exactly as prescribed the woman will very rarely become pregnant.

The pills act by inhibiting ovulation in the menstrual cycle during which they are administered. For the purpose of taking the pill the first day is calculated from the first day of the menstrual period. One pill is prescribed daily for 21 days from the 5th to the 25th day. They are dispensed in packs of 21 and 22. The menstrual periods continue. The pills should not be used for intermittent periods of time and may be taken for one menstrual cycle prior to marriage.

In order to detect cancerous cells in the cervix a Papanicolaou smear is taken prior to starting the course.

Following childbirth the pills should be taken at one month from the day of delivery. Some prefer to wait until the 5th day of the first menstrual period.

Eighty per cent of women of proven fertility who wish to conceive did so within two months of stopping the " pill ".

LOWER RISK PILLS AVAILABLE

Because of the incidence of venous thrombosis oral contraceptives containing not more than 50 micrograms of oestrogen are now prescribed.

Orthonovin 1/50; Gynovlar 21; Minilyn Minovlar; Norinyl-1; Anovlar 21; Volidan 20; Volidan 21; Norlestrin 21; Ovulen 50.

They are prescribed only under strict medical supervision and are on the Schedule 4 Poisons List. Unless the woman agrees that her general practitioner be informed by the F.P.A. clinic they do not prescribe oral contraceptive pills.

The lower-risk pills have an oestrogen content so small that lactation is rarely inhibited.

Side effects are nausea, headaches, breast discomfort; break through bleeding always occurs when the tablets are withdrawn.

ABSOLUTE CONTRAINDICATIONS

Oral contraceptive pills are not prescribed in the following circumstances:

1. History of deep venous thrombosis.

2. History of severe liver disease especially when jaundice is manifest during pregnancy.

3. Malignant disease of the breast.

Episodes of motor or sensory loss should be reported at once.

27 A

5. INTRA-UTERINE DEVICE (I.U.D.)

This method has its greatest advantage in developing countries to control population explosions, minimal co-operation being required from those using it.

A pliable plastic loop is introduced into the uterine cavity by straightening and passing it through a 3 mm. plastic cannula. The device remains *in utero*: Lippes loop and the Saf. T. Coil are both effective. That the loop is still *in utero* is indicated by the strand of thread hanging from the cervix.

One month after insertion the woman is examined, and again after 6 and 12 months. Expulsion of the device occurs in some cases during the first year. Pregnancy has occurred while the loop was *in situ*: in rare cases it has perforated the uterine wall and entered the pelvic cavity. Some women experience abdominal pain, backache and profuse menstrual periods, with staining up to 10 days, during the first three or four cycles.

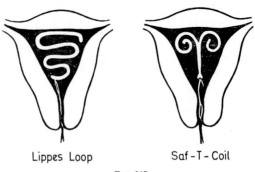

Lippes Loop   Saf - T - Coil

Fig. 317

Intra-uterine contraceptive devices.

Insertion of the device is recommended at the end of a menstrual period when some cervical dilatation exists; after confinement, not sooner than the sixth postpartum week.

The mode of action is not completely understood; fertilization occurs but embedding is inhibited. **The doctor is responsible for the insertion of these devices.**

TUBAL LIGATION

Surgical sterilization of the woman may be carried out by ligation of the Fallopian tubes within 48 hours of delivery or by laparoscopy 6 weeks after confinement (see p. 631).

VASECTOMY

Husbands can now be sterilized, free of charge, on the National Health Service, for medical reasons. The consent of their wives must be given in writing.

The vas, the tube that carries the spermatozoa from the testes, unites with the duct of the seminal vesicle from which the seminal fluid is derived. If the vas on both sides is ligated and cut the sperms produced cannot mingle with the semen and enter the ejaculatory duct; they eventually become absorbed.

The operation can be done under local anæsthesia; a small incision being made on each side of the scrotum. It is not effective for 2 or 3 months until any sperms already in the tube have been passed.

The Role of the Midwife

The midwife must always respect any religious objection to contraception.

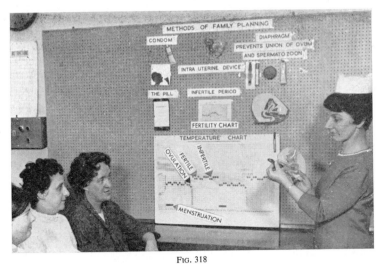

Fig. 318

Lesson to Mothers on Family Planning.
(County Maternity Hospital, Bellshill, Lanarkshire.)

Oral contraceptive pills are prescribed by the doctor who will make the necessary investigations and see the woman at regular intervals. Any advice given by the midwife must be under the direction of a doctor.

Midwives appointed to participate in family planning programmes may attend courses to widen their knowledge of all aspects of the situation and to acquire technical skill in the insertion of intra-uterine devices. They will work under medical direction.

QUESTIONS FOR REVISION

ORAL QUESTIONS

How does nursing in a puerperal ward differ from that in a gynæcological ward ?

What do you understand by rooming in ?: state the advantages?

What would you report to the doctor regarding the puerperel woman ?

For how many days must a domiciliary midwife visit her patients ?

Why are temperature and pulse important during the puerperium ?

What abnormalities of lochia may occur and what is their significance ?

What can you learn from palpating the lower abdomen of the puerperal woman?

How soon can a woman, delivered normally, have a shower bath ?

On which occasions during the puerperium must you wear a mask ? Why is this important ?

What advice or help could you give for the following: (*a*) after pains; (*b*) œdema and bruising of the perineum; (*c*) backache; (*d*) restoration of the figure.

What would you do in the following circumstances:

If the pulse was 90 one hour after delivery ?

If the uterus was larger than you thought it ought to be on the 3rd post-partum day ?

If the lochia were bright red on the 8th day ?

If the woman is upset and crying? If the perineal sutures are cutting out ?

Terminology

DESCRIPTION	TERM
Cervical cytology to detect early cancer..	
Raw area of cervix..	
Bladder prolapsed into vagina..	
Localised anæmia of the uterus..	
Fæces being passed vaginally..	
Delay in return of the uterus to normal size..	
Breaking down of uterine fibres by hormone or enzyme..................................	

Write not more than 10 lines on: (*a*) the psychology of the puerperal woman; (*b*) the social aspects of puerperal care; (*c*) the education of the young mother; (*d*) treatment of a third degree tear.

Family planning: (1) Who is responsible for providing family planning clinics ? (2) Which women are entitled to free contraceptive advice ? (3) What are the risks associated with: (*a*) using the rhythm method ? (*b*) intra-uterine devices ? (*c*) the oral pill ? (4) How is the day of ovulation determined ? (5) When should the woman attend the F.P. clinic after confinement ?

48 hour discharge: (1) In which cases would this not be advisable ? (2) What previous arrangements must be made ? (3) Between whom is liaison necessary ? (4) For which reasons might the baby not be permitted to go home on the morning of intended discharge ? (5) What advice is given regarding a sutured perineum ?

Post-natal examination: What reasons would you give to persuade a woman to have a post-natal examination ? If you were attached to a general practitioner clinic what would you set out in readiness for: (*a*) a post-natal examination; (*b*) Papanicolaou smear; (*c*) insertion of a Hodge pessary ?

C.M.B.(N. Ireland) paper.—A primigravida has been delivered spontaneously 24 hours previously. What points would you report to the doctor on his first visit ?

C.M.B.(Eng.) paper.—Describe the nursing care of the patient in the lying-in period who has incurred: (*a*) a severe perineal tear; (*b*) engorgement of the breasts.

C.M.B.(Scot.) paper.—What is the puerperium ? Describe the nursing care of a patient in the first week after delivery.

C.M.B.(Eng.) paper.—Discuss the emotional stresses of the puerperium.

C.M.B.(Eng.) paper.—What disorders of micturition may occur in the puerperium ? Describe the management of each.

C.M.B.(Eng.) paper.—What is meant by the Lochia ? What lochial changes occur during the puerperium ?

C.M.B.(Eng.) paper.—Describe the physiological changes which occur during the puerperium.

C.M.B.(N. Ireland) paper.—What is a complete tear of the perineum ? Give in detail the nursing " after-care " in such a case.

C.M.B.(N. Ireland) paper.—What are the advantages of: (a) mothers and babies " rooming in " together ? (b) breast feeding ?

C.M.B.(Eng.) paper.—Outline the basic needs and nursing care of the mother during the first ten days after delivery. What fears does the mother commonly experience during this time ?

C.M.B.(Scot.) paper.—Describe the nursing care of a patient during the first 48 hours after a forceps delivery.

C.M.B.(Scot.) paper.—Describe the management of a patient during the first 10 days following delivery.

C.M.B.(Eng.) paper.—Discuss the advantages and disadvantages to mother and baby of planned early discharge from hospital. What preparations would you make to ensure continuity of care ?

C.M.B.(N. Ireland) paper.—What are the observations made on a patient during the early post-natal period ? Explain why each one is important.

C.M.B.(Eng.) paper.—What investigations and examinations of a mother should be carried out about six weeks after delivery ? What is their purpose ?

C.M.B.(Eng.) paper. 50 word question.—What facilities for family planning are available in your area ?

C.M.B.(Eng.) paper.—What methods of family planning may be suggested to a grande multipara ?

C.M.B.(Eng.) paper. 50 word question.—How does the local authority fulfil its obligations under the Family Planning Act ?

27

Complications of the Puerperium

PUERPERAL SEPSIS

Puerperal sepsis is an infection of the genital tract by organisms, occurring within 14 days (Eng. and Wales) and 21 days (Scot.) after abortion or childbirth. The infection may be confined to the uterus—local uterine infection—or the organisms may invade and multiply in the blood stream and give rise to septicæmia.

The maternal mortality rate from puerperal sepsis has been lowered since the introduction of sulphonamides and antibiotics, but this should not give rise to an attitude of complacency, nor should there by any lowering of the high standards of aseptic technique necessary for the protection of the woman.

CONTROL OF THE SPREAD OF INFECTION

Efficient mask wearing. The use of paper handkerchiefs followed by hand-washing.

Scrupulous domestic cleanliness. Fresh air. Modern methods of dust control.

Impeccable obstetric aseptic and antiseptic technique.

Staphylococcal infection tends to be localized, and abscess formation is common, but fatal septicæmia may occur.

The hæmolytic streptococcus group A is still potentially the most dangerous organism for the postpartum woman because of its ability to invade the blood stream. Fortunately it is sensitive to certain antibiotics, and if treated promptly the infection can usually be brought under control. The habitat of the hæmolytic streptococcus group A is in the nose and throat.

OTHER PATHOGENS

The *Clostridium welchii* is occasionally found in the vagina and in the presence of bruised or necrosed tissue may become aggressive and cause septicæmia. Hæmolysis of red cells occurs, resulting in profound anæmia. Liver destruction occurs and jaundice is frequently manifest, anuria is sometimes present, and the infection may become rapidly fatal.

The *Escherichia coli*. Genital tract infection by this organism is usually confined to the uterus and gives rise to foul-smelling lochia. Septicæmia sometimes occurs.

SIGNS AND SYMPTOMS

The outstanding signs are a rise in temperature to over 38° C. (100·4° F.) and an increase in pulse rate to over 90, commonly occurring on or before the third day of the puerperium. Following prolonged labour and especially in virulent cases of septicæmia the onset may be on the first day.

The clinical features and the outcome will depend on (1) whether the infection is local or general; (2) the virulence of the organism; (3) the resistance of the patient.

LOCAL UTERINE INFECTION

The temperature steps up gradually and rarely goes beyond 38·8° C. (102° F.).

The pulse is over 90 and rarely over 120.

The lochia are profuse, brownish, offensive and frequently contain pieces of chorion.

The uterus is large (subinvoluted), soft in consistence and tender to touch.

The woman may complain of headache and general malaise; she is constipated and has a furred tongue.

In this condition the leucocytes in the wall of the inflamed uterus destroy many of the invading organisms and limit the spread of infection. With prompt antibiotic treatment the condition usually resolves within three or four days.

PERITONITIS

When pelvic peritonitis occurs there is pain and tenderness in the lower abdomen, the temperature ranging from 38·3° to 39·4° C. (101° to 103° F.) and when generalized peritonitis occurs, the situation becomes grave.

The abdomen is distended, rigid, painful and tender.

Vomiting is persistent; dark-coloured vomitus welling up without effort. The patient is restless and apprehensive. **Paralytic ileus** may further complicate the situation.

GENERAL OR BLOOD-STREAM INFECTION
SEPTICÆMIA

The temperature rises sharply to 39·4° C. (103° F.) or over and may be continuous or remittent. Rigors are common, especially with anaerobic organisms.

The pulse in sever ases may be 140 to 160 and is the best guide to the patient's condition. (A fall i ʰemperature with a rapid pulse is not a sign of improvement.)

The lochia are sometimes pale and scanty; they may have a fetid odour.

The uterus involutes normally and may not be tender to touch.

The patient looks ill, but does not complain unduly.

Pallor, due to anæmia, becomes marked, and the skin sometimes has an icteric tinge; skin rashes may be evident.

Vomiting may be persistent, and, on occasions, diarrhœa is troublesome.

Loss of appetite and sleeplessness are usual, delirium is not uncommon.

Endotoxic (bacteræmic) shock may occur (see p. 148).

MANAGEMENT OF PUERPERAL SEPSIS

Barrier nursing should be employed by the midwife in cases of puerperal pyrexia, prior to the patient being seen by the doctor, who will then order isolation of the patient.

ISOLATION

A midwife must never nurse a clean and an infected puerperal patient at the same time, even if the septic patient is isolated. The infection of a puerperal woman has a legal as well as an ethical aspect and in a court of law the infection of one patient from another is considered to be criminal negligence unless all due precautions have been taken to prevent such a spread of infection. Some years ago in England a woman was admitted to a puerperal ward where another patient was suffering from a mild degree of puerperal sepsis. The newly delivered woman became infected and died. Her husband successfully sued the maternity home for £2,000.

INVESTIGATION OF PUERPERAL SEPSIS

(a) CLINICAL

The type of labour and delivery, including any vaginal interference, is noted. The temperature and pulse chart is studied. The breasts, chest, throat and legs are examined for signs of infection. The abdomen, lochia, and vulva are inspected.

(b) BACTERIOLOGICAL

A high vaginal swab for culture, mid-stream specimen of urine, nose and throat swabs and, in some cases, blood culture are taken. The sensitivity of the infecting organism to the sulphonamides and antibiotics is also tested. When taking a high vaginal swab the woman is placed in the lithotomy or cross-bed position and the vulva swabbed with sterile water to which no antiseptic has been added. The use of a speculum is essential, to avoid contamination from the lower vagina.

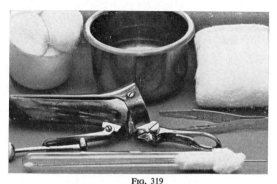

FIG. 319

EQUIPMENT FOR HIGH VAGINAL SWAB.

Swabbing lotion without antiseptic. Vaginal speculum, tissue forceps. Test-tube for swab.

(*Simpson Memorial Maternity Pavilion, Edinburgh.*)

(c) HÆMATOLOGICAL

Blood investigation is made because anæmia is common in puerperal sepsis, due to blood loss and to the hæmolysis of red cells by certain organisms and toxins.

NOTIFICATION

The clinical condition of Puerperal Sepsis (*known legally as Puerperal Fever*) is no longer a notifiable infectious disease in England. In Scotland the doctor notifies the Medical Officer of Health.

England and Wales.—*Puerperal Sepsis is included under the term Puerperal Pyrexia, which is defined as " any febrile condition occurring in a woman in whom a temperature of 38° C. (100·4° F.) or more has occurred within 14 days after childbirth or miscarriage."*

Scotland.—*Puerperal Sepsis and Puerperal Pyrexia are regarded separately under existing Regulations, and each must be notified. Puerperal Pyrexia is defined as " any febrile condition (other than a condition requiring to be notified as Puerperal Fever) occurring in a woman within 21 days after childbirth or miscarriage in which a temperature of 38° C. (100·4° F.) or more has been sustained during a period of 24 hours or has recurred during that period."*

DISINFECTION

The wearing of a gown and concurrent disinfection help to limit the spread of infection. Before attending another patient, the midwife must disinfect:

1. **Her equipment.** 2. **Her person by taking a bath, washing her hair and putting on clean clothing and uniform: bed linen changed.**

C.M.B. rule "If a midwife in domiciliary practice has been in contact with a person, whether or not a patient, suffering from any condition which is or may reasonably be suspected to be infectious, or if she herself is liable to be a source of infection, she must, without delay, notify the Local Supervising Authority or Authorities of the fact, using for the purpose the prescribed form.

MEDICAL TREATMENT

The administration of ampicillin (Penbritin) is started as soon as high-vaginal swab, throat swab and mid-stream specimen of urine have been obtained. The initial bacteriological report, usually received in 24 hours, states to which of the antibiotics the infecting organism is most sensitive; the appropriate antibiotic is then prescribed.

Ampicillin (Penbritin) 500 mg. + 250 mg. six-hourly is given until the infection is controlled.

Cloxacillin (Orbenin) 250 mg. six-hourly intramuscularly, is useful for resistant staphylococcal infections.

Some give streptomycin also 1 G. daily for 5 days.

Benzylpenicillin (Solupen) is useful for penicillin sensitive infections.

The need for iron is great. A transfusion of packed cells is given if the hæmoglobin is under 7·4 G. (50 per cent).

The high vaginal swab is repeated 24 hours after antibiotic therapy is stopped, and if positive, therapy is continued.

NURSING CARE

Good nursing is absolutely essential and may be a life-saving measure. The room should be bright and airy. With plenty of fresh air the patient sleeps better, her appetite is improved and her mental outlook more cheerful.

Sleep is imperative and sedatives are usually necessary, even after all means to promote comfort and induce sleep have been tried.

The bowels:—Drastic purgatives must be avoided. They dehydrate and exhaust the woman and the frequent use of the bed-pan interferes with rest : they may also initiate diarrhœa which is difficult to control. It is advisable to give a mild laxative such as Senokot tablets (2) at night followed by a Dulcolax suppository or small prepacked enema, next morning.

The bladder:—A fluid balance chart should be kept, and the bladder gently palpated and percussed daily to detect residual urine.

Electrolyte control is carried out.

The patient is propped upright with pillows to encourage uterine drainage; the adoption of the prone position for half an hour twice daily will also facilitate drainage from the uterus.

The diet should have a high caloric, high vitamin content, and must be easily digested. Adequate protein is essential. **The appetite is usually poor, so the food should be nicely cooked, daintily served,** and the woman coaxed to eat. Vitamins are very necessary. Vitamin C aids healing and blood formation.

OBSERVATION

Temperature and pulse are recorded every four hours, also following a rigor.

Appetite, sleep, mental outlook should be charted.

The midwife should be on the alert for signs that would indicate spreading of the infection or a worsening of the patient's condition.

EXTRA-GENITAL INFECTIONS

(Notified as Puerperal Pyrexia)

URINARY TRACT INFECTION

Pyelonephritis occurs in a number of cases during the puerperium, but the efficient treatment of pyelonephritis during pregnancy helps to prevent recrudescence of the condition. It may sometimes follow prolonged difficult labour. **Rigors may occur;** pain and tenderness in the kidney region are present.

Treatment is similar to that given during pregnancy: prophylactic measures are:— (1) the avoidance of (*a*) anæmia, (*b*) prolonged labour, (*c*) catheterization, (2) the active treatment of retention of urine.

RESPIRATORY INFECTIONS

Respiratory infections and tonsillitis may cause puerperal pyrexia, but the possibility of puerperal sepsis must not be disregarded even when signs of other infections are apparent, for both might be present.

BREAST INFECTIONS

Mastitis is inflammation of the breast, which if not treated may proceed to abscess formation. In mild cases which are superficial and localized the term " flushed breast " is commonly applied. The condition rarely occurs prior to the eighth day of the puerperium and most frequently arises during the second or third week.

CAUSE

The most common infecting organism is the *Staphylococcus aureus*: the infant's eyes and nose may be the source of infection.

1. The multiplication of organisms which are always present in the breast. This is commonly due to **stasis of milk** brought about by (*a*) **engorgement;** (*b*) **imperfect emptying** of the breast; (*c*) **bruising of breast tissue** by rough or prolonged expression of milk.

2. Cracked nipple which permits the introduction of organisms, sometimes from the baby's nose.

SIGNS AND SYMPTOMS

A sharp rise in temperature, 38·3° to 40° C. (101° to 104° F.).

Rapid pulse. Throbbing pain and tenderness in the breast.

A diffuse or wedge-shaped, indurated, reddened area.

General malaise with headache and shivering.

TREATMENT

Prompt recognition of the early signs and immediate administration of antibiotics offer the greatest hope in the prevention of abscess formation.

Antibiotics such as cloxacillin are most effective when given early. In hospital the *Staphylococcus aureus*, the common infecting organism, is penicillin resistant, so methicillin (Celbenin) is usually prescribed.

To relieve pain and induce sleep analgesics are given, *e.g.* Codis tablets (2); Pana-sorb tablets (2); Pentazocine (Fortral) tablets (2).

Lactation is suppressed. **A supporting binder should be applied** (*while the woman is lying flat on her back*, the breasts being supported by large pads of cotton wool. It is definitely harmful to apply a firm binder over unsupported inflamed breasts; stasis in the dependent area results, and this favours abscess formation which is treated in the Surgical Department.

VENOUS THROMBOSIS

In this condition clot formation occurs in the veins usually of the lower limbs.

Susceptibility of puerperal women to thrombosis

1. INCREASED VISCOSITY OF THE BLOOD AFTER THE 28th WEEK.

    This is often intensified because of dehydration and hæmorrhage during labour.

2. STASIS OF BLOOD IN THE VEINS.

    Varicose veins predispose to stasis. The recumbent position and disinclination to move, *e.g.* following Cæsarean section, hæmorrhage, shock.

3. CHANGES IN THE WALLS OF THE VEINS.

    These may be due to varicosities, inflammation or trauma.

4. AGE OVER 35 AND HIGH PARITY.

PROPHYLAXIS

(A) DURING PREGNANCY.

The treatment of varicose veins.

(B) DURING LABOUR.

1. **The avoidance of exhaustion, dehydration and hæmorrhage.**

2. **The avoidance of trauma to limbs, due to:**

    (*a*) Pressure by stirrup rods, when in the lithotomy position.

    (*b*) Pressure under the knees while in the Trendelenburg position.

    (*c*) Bruising of limbs in moving unconscious patient on to trolley.

(C) DURING THE PUERPERIUM

1. THE AVOIDANCE OF STASIS

Movement of the whole leg, every two hours should be inaugurated on the second postpartum day to stimulate blood flow in the calf muscles. Deep breathing facilitates venous flow. Some raise the foot of the bed 22·9 cm. (9 in.)

A leg elevator (Fig. 322) gives excellent facility for free movement and should be used in susceptible cases.

2. EARLY AMBULATION

This has reduced but has not eliminated thrombosis. Patients who need assistance must be helped and encouraged to walk along the ward. **Merely sitting immobile in a low arm-chair has less therapeutic value than ankle exercises, leg elevation and freedom of leg movement in bed.**

OBSERVATION

Successful treatment depends on early diagnosis. The midwife must be " leg conscious " in susceptible cases. The legs should be examined, while bathing or bed-making, without producing a phobia.

Localized pain or tenderness in the calf or groin should be reported to the doctor.

SUPERFICIAL VEIN THROMBOSIS

Mild cases in which the superficial leg veins are affected may be associated with varicose veins which can be palpated and are tender to touch. Redness of the overlying skin may be evident. Temperature and pulse are both slightly increased. The condition may be manifest as early as the fourth day postpartum, but usually around the 10th day. The risk of pulmonary embolism is slight.

TREATMENT

Usually no anticoagulants are necessary.

The leg is elevated and its muscle activity encouraged.

Oxyphenbutazone (Tanderil) is sometimes prescribed for marked inflammation.

When the temperature subsides and the area is non-tender, usually in four or five days, a strip of orthopædic felt is applied over the affected vein and the patient is allowed to walk about wearing a crepe bandage, elastic stocking or elastic tights.

DEEP VEIN THROMBOSIS

SIGNS AND SYMPTOMS

Deep vein thrombosis is usually manifest during the second week of the puerperium, but may arise during the first week. The danger of a portion of the blood clot becoming detached and giving rise to pulmonary embolism exists.

ULTRASONIC SCREENING

Ultrasonic investigation is employed in screening patients with suspected deep vein thrombosis. The transducer of the pulse detector is placed over the femoral vein. If the leg veins are not thrombosed, when the calf is squeezed a pulse wave of blood passes up to the femoral vein and is detected by the ultrasonic beam and represented by an audible signal. If no signal is elicited a thrombosis is probably present.

The patient may complain of a slight tingling or cramp-like pain in the leg; an early symptom. **Tenderness in the groin is a significant sign.**

The calf or thigh feels tender and tense in comparison with the other leg.

Homans' sign, *i.e. pain felt in the calf-muscles when the foot is dorsiflexed with the leg extended at the knee is only present in a minority of cases.*

Swelling of the limb may be apparent, with an increase of 2·5 to 5·1 cm. (1 or 2 in.) in the girth of the calf and mid-thigh of the affected leg. In some cases pitting œdema extends from the groin to the toes: a bluish flush may be noted.

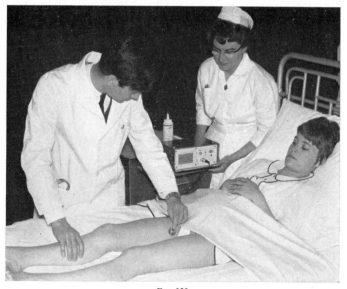

FIG. 320
Ultrasonic screening for deep vein thrombosis.
(*Simpson Memorial Maternity Pavilion, Edinburgh.*)

Temperature and pulse.—A slight rise in temperature 37·2° C. (99° F.) and pulse around 90, occurring on two or three evenings, is very suspicious.

Pain in the chest should be reported immediately: chest radiography and electro-cardiography will be carried out.

TREATMENT
Anticoagulant Drugs

Heparin is used therapeutically as a powerful anticoagulant which will prevent massive clotting in the early stage and inhibit further clot formation in cases of established thrombosis. Heparin is administered intravenously; the initial dose is 15,000 units followed every six hours by doses of 10,000 to 12,000 units, and continued until anticoagulant drugs given orally have had time to take effect (24 to 48 hours).

The blood clotting time is taken immediately prior to giving, and one hour after, each injection, and should be prolonged to 20 minutes (two or three times the normal, which is five to eight minutes).

Side Effects

Heparin may, if given for longer than four days during the first week of the puerperium, **cause hæmorrhage from the placental site** or the formation of a hæmatoma in an abdominal incision. The doctor is notified and he will, if other means of controlling hæmorrhage fail, give the antidote, 1 per cent **protamine sulphate solution,** 5 to 10 ml. intravenously, to counteract the effect of heparin. A blood transfusion is given.

Reactions such as rigor or sudden rise in temperature indicate the need for immediate cessation of the heparin drip or injection.

Antibiotics may be employed to combat infection.

Phenindione (Dindevan), a synthetic anticoagulant, or warfarin sodium (Marevan) can be given orally in conjunction with heparin for 24 to 48 hours, and continued alone

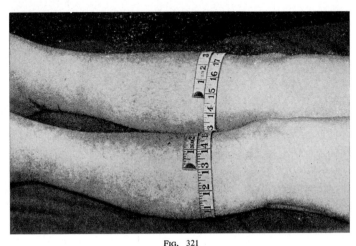

FIG. 321
VENOUS THROMBOSIS.
Girth of affected leg almost 5·1 cm. (2 in.) greater than normal leg.

usually for about 3 weeks after that time, the patient being fully ambulant. The dose is regulated according to the prothrombin activity, which should be maintained at 25 to 30 per cent; 100 per cent being normal, and this is determined by prothrombin time estimations on alternate days until controlled and then two or three times weekly.

Side Effects

Severe bleeding should be treated by giving vitamin K$_1$ *e.g.* slow intravenous injection of mephyton, 100 mg.; blood transfusion is effective and rapid in action.

Phenindione (Dindevan) is not given during pregnancy because of risk to the fetus.

Leg Elevation and Movement

The limb must be elevated to above heart level to facilitate the venous flow of blood. This must be done in such a manner that the leg is not immobilized and free movement is possible. A cradle to support the bedclothes is necessary.

Flexion and extension ankle exercises are started.

Deep breathing aids the venous return of blood to the heart.

Leg muscle movement is allowed when the acute pain subsides, usually in 48 hours. This is supervised by the physiotherapist. **Passive leg movement is commenced** within a few days and active leg exercises gradually instituted.

The patient is usually allowed up in about two weeks when œdema has dispersed, having had an effective supporting bandage applied. Prior to discharge she is wearing an elastic stocking or elastic tights.

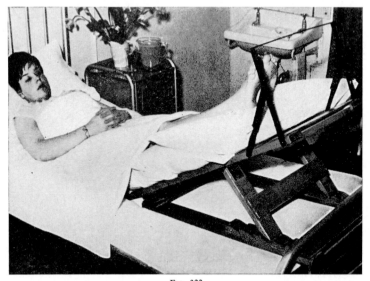

FIG. 322

LEG ELEVATOR.

Used in cases predisposed to or having developed venous thrombosis.

Note.—(1) Elevation of feet to above heart level. (2) Provision by metal cradle for freedom of movement (3) Affords maximal comfort.

(Photographed at Aberdeen Maternity Hospital.)

PULMONARY THROMBO-EMBOLISM

A piece of blood clot becomes detached from a thrombus in the veins of the pelvis or lower limbs and travels by the inferior vena cava to the right side of the heart and via the pulmonary artery to the lung. The outcome will depend on the size of the embolus; in rare cases death occurs in a few moments.

SIGNS AND SYMPTOMS

Acute pain in chest, intense dyspnœa, blood-stained sputum.

Collapse with grey cyanosed colour, rapid pulse.

When suspected, chest radiological and electrocardiographic evidence help to confirm the diagnosis.

Treatment

Send urgently for medical aid. Give oxygen, extra pillows. Screen the bed.

Prepare tray for intravenous administration of morphine, 15 mg. and heparin, 15,000 or 20,000 units. Phenindione (Dindevan) is also given, and heparin continued six-hourly for 24 hours. An antibiotic is given to diminish the risk of pulmonary infection. Notify the relatives of dangerous illness.

PUERPERAL HÆMORRHAGE
(Secondary Postpartum Hæmorrhage)

Bleeding may take place from the 24th hour up to the sixth week of the puerperium, but commonly occurs between the 10th and 14th days.

CAUSE

Retention of a piece of placenta, which when it sloughs off opens up the large uterine sinuses. In some cases no products of conception have been retained. The hæmorrhage may or may not be associated with sepsis.

WARNING SIGN
Persistent Red Lochia

Severe hæmorrhage is usually due to the presence of a succenturiate lobe or large cotyledon of placenta. The author has known of three fatal cases from this cause, two of which occurred after the women had been discharged. In another case, 12 litres (20 pints) of blood were given over a period of days to replace the blood lost. One patient lost 1,200 ml. of blood while in the " toilet " on the ninth day of the puerperium. Hysterectomy was performed in a case in which the bleeding could not be controlled.

TREATMENT OF SEVERE HÆMORRHAGE BY THE MIDWIFE

She should massage the uterus, squeeze out clots, send urgently for medical assistance (" Flying Squad "), give ergometrine, 0·5 mg. or Syntometrine, 1 ml. intramuscularly, and repeat if necessary. If the situation is critical bimanual compression of the uterus must be carried out to control the bleeding and ergometrine given I.V.

The " Flying Squad " will, if necessary, give blood (to which oxytocin may be added); **when the woman has rallied she will be transferred to hospital for digital exploration of the uterus.**

INCONTINENCE OF URINE

(1) **Paradoxical incontinence** due to retention of urine with overflow may not be diagnosed by the inexperienced midwife.

(2) **Stress incontinence** occurs in multiparous women with laxity of the pelvic floor and urethral orifice which has occurred during parturition; cystocele may also be present. Incontinence in such cases is not complete, and consists in the dribbling of urine during coughing, sneezing or sudden exertion. The condition sometimes clears up as the woman's health improves. Nourishing food, iron, and pelvic floor exercises will help to increase muscle tone. If incontinence persists, operation may be necessary.

(3) VESICO-VAGINAL FISTULA

This is an artificial opening between the bladder or urethra and vagina. The condition is rare in countries where good obstetric care is available.

When incontinence occurs immediately after the birth of the baby, it is usually due to laceration of the bladder during a difficult instrumental delivery.

When incontinence begins five or six days after labour, it is due to sloughing of a bruised area of bladder, caused by prolonged pressure by the fetal head during labour.

To avoid such an occurrence the bladder should be emptied every two hours throughout labour and prolonged labour should be avoided; more especially the second stage.

Treatment

A self-retaining catheter is inserted and left *in situ* for eight or ten days with sealed drainage. Fluids are given up to 3 litres daily; antibiotics are prescribed. The fistula usually heals without operation, but if it persists the woman is referred to the gynæcological department for operation, usually about three months later when her health has been built up.

PSYCHIATRIC DISORDERS

These occur in about 1 per 1,000 births, more commonly in primigravidæ, and may be manifest during pregnancy, labour, the puerperium, and later during the ensuing year.

There is no special type of mental disorder peculiar to the childbearing woman.

Normal pregnancy and labour may impose a degree of emotional strain on the woman of nervous temperament, and severe stress may precipitate psychiatric disorders, especially if she has a family history of mental instability. But many such women go through the experience of childbearing without a mental breakdown if other contributory factors are not superimposed. If the woman is happy in her home life and is not subjected to severe conflict or anxiety she is less likely to develop psychiatric symptoms.

The maladjusted personality when subjected to gross disharmony is liable to break down.

THE ROLE OF THE MIDWIFE

The midwife should try to inculcate in all her patients a serene outlook regarding childbearing. When necessary, she must assist the pregnant woman to understand her misapprehensions and help her to dispel her fears. She should also recognize the early signs of mental and nervous illness and refer the woman to her doctor, who will consult a psychiatrist.

DURING PREGNANCY

Fifteen per cent of cases occur during pregnancy : usually the woman is depressed, sometimes suicidal, and the prognosis is more serious when the onset occurs after the 24th week. Should the condition recur in a subsequent pregnancy, the obstetrician and the psychiatrist may consider it advisable to terminate the pregnancy.

Psychiatric disorders arising during labour are rare but not unknown.

DURING THE PUERPERIUM

Mental illness in the puerperium usually occurs during the first two weeks, and depression is probably the most common manifestation. Depression that persists or is associated with abnormal thought processes or behaviour requires specialist attention.

The very mild depression (postpartum " blues "), experienced by some women around the third or fourth day is probably endocrine in origin and clears up rapidly with adequate rest and sleep, assurance and " TENDER LOVING CARE."

Confusional states which in the past were often manifest in cases of severe eclampsia or puerperal sepsis are no longer considered to be psychotic episodes. They respond to modern drug therapy.

SIGNS AND SYMPTOMS

Persistent insomnia for no apparent reason is a warning sign. At first the woman may seem slightly peculiar, imagining that the other patients don't like her or are talking about her. At this early stage the doctor should be informed, so that treatment may be commenced without delay.

She may take a dislike to her husband, baby or midwife and become restless, talkative and elated with rapid incoherent speech. Sudden outbursts of mania occur, and she may be uncontrollably violent; suicidal and homicidal tendencies may be manifest and such threats should be taken seriously.

Food and fluid are refused, wasting and exhaustion ensue; the pulse is rapid.

Temporary Nursing Care by the Midwife

Until arrangements are made for the woman to be transferred to a psychiatric hospital, attention should be paid to the following nursing points:—

Sedatives are administered if the patient is acutely disturbed, sodium amylobarbitone (Sodium Amytal), 200 mg., four-hourly, orally, being useful at the onset; more powerful sedatives are given intramuscularly or intravenously.

The patient should be nursed on the ground floor, in a quiet, single room, and never left alone for one instant. Scissors, knives and forks are not taken into the room, the woman being fed with a spoon. The danger of matches, gas and antiseptics must be constantly kept in mind, but such precautions should not be obvious to the patient.

Attractive digestible food should be served and the woman coaxed to eat and drink, 3 litres of fluid being given daily; the bladder must be emptied regularly.

Persuasion and patient reassurance are required: it is useless trying to convince the woman by argument.

SPECIALIZED TREATMENT

The medical and nursing techniques are highly specialized, and early treatment in suitable surroundings, by experts, gives the greatest opportunity for rapid and complete recovery.

Mother and baby units are advocated by some authorities and the mother sees her baby and can look after him under supervision if this is considered advisable by the psychiatrist.

For depression, thymoleptic drugs, such as amitriptyline (Tryptizol), or phenelzine (Nardil), are given, but not during early pregnancy because of possible effects on the developing embryo. If after three weeks' administration no improvement is evident **electro-convulsive therapy is used.**

Midwives should be aware that certain anti-depressant drugs such as phenelzine (Nardil) are believed to potentiate the action of pethidine and may produce coma. Enquiry should be made during labour in such cases, prior to administering pethidine.

Eighty per cent of women recover, and in favourable cases this takes place within **four to six months.** If no improvement is apparent after nine months the prognosis **is gloomy.** Ten per cent become chronic and 10 per cent die.

QUESTIONS FOR REVISION

COMPLICATIONS OF THE PUERPERIUM

For what reasons are the following drugs prescribed ? Nardil; heparin; Orbenin; Dindevan; Tryptizol.

What are the causes of vesico-vaginal fistula ? What is the treatment ? What are the signs of pulmonary embolism ? What could the midwife do pending the arrival of the doctor ? What precautions would you take when nursing a puerperal patient with depression ? How would you apply a supporting breast binder ? How would you take a high vaginal swab ?

Define the words: stasis; flushed breast; anaerobic organism; concurrent disinfection; puerperal hæmorrhage.

C.M.B.(Scot.) paper.—Name the complications which may arise during the first two weeks of the puerperium. What could the midwife do to prevent them ?

C.M.B.(Scot.) paper.—On the ninth day of the puerperium the patient has a sudden vaginal hæmorrhage. What is the cause of this ? Give the emergency and subsequent treatment.

C.M.B.(N. Ireland) paper.—What are the predisposing factors leading to thrombophlebitis in obstetric practice ? What can be done to reduce the incidence of this condition ?

C.M.B.(Eng.) paper.—What urinary tract complications may occur in the puerperium? Indicate briefly how these might be avoided and treated.

C.M.B.(Eng.) paper, 1969.—What factors predispose to deep venous thrombosis in the puerperium? What are the clinical signs and symptoms of this condition?

C.M.B.(N. Ireland) paper, 1969.—What are the dangers of venous thrombosis in the puerperium? How would this condition be recognized? Outline the management.

C.M.B.(Eng.) paper, 1969.—Write short answers to each part of the question: (a) define the puerperium; (b) what is meant by involution of the uterus? (c) what factors may predispose to deep vein thrombosis in the puerperium?

C.M.B.(Eng.) paper, 1969.—How would you recognize that a mother is mentally disturbed during the early post-natal period? What urinary problems may occur after delivery? Describe how you would recognize each condition.

PUERPERAL PYREXIA AND SEPSIS

Differentiate between: puerperal sepsis and puerperal pyrexia; local uterine infection and septicæmia; venous thrombosis and thrombophlebitis; thrombus and embolus; paradoxical incontinence and stress incontinence.

Write not more than 10 lines on: hæmolytic streptococcus group A; investigation of puerperal sepsis; nursing care in puerperal sepsis; incontinence of urine; the rôle of the midwife in psychiatric disorders; efficient mask wearing.

C.M.B.(Scot.) paper.—What conditions may cause a rise of temperature to 38·3° C. (101° F.) on the fifth day of the puerperium ? Give the nursing care of any one.

C.M.B.(Eng.) paper.—What is the cause of a raised temperature in the lying-in period ? What observations and investigations would help to determine the cause ?

C.M.B.(Eng.) paper.—What abnormal conditions may occur in the breast during the lying-in period ? How would you recognize them ?

C.M.B.(N. Ireland) paper.—What is the cause of mastitis ? Give the signs and symptoms and outline the prevention and treatment of this condition.

C.M.B.(Eng.) paper.—Enumerate the main causes of pyrexia during the puerperium. Describe the diagnosis and treatment of one condition you mention.

C.M.B.(N. Ireland) paper.—Infection in a maternity hospital is extremely serious. What are the usual precautions taken to prevent this?

C.M.B.(Eng.) paper, 1969.—Briefly describe the main causes of pyrexia in the puerperium. What investigations should be carried out?

C.M.B.(N. Ireland) paper, 1969.—Enumerate the possible causes of pyrexia during the puerperium. Describe the investigations which should be made.

28

Physiology and Management of the Newborn

In order to appreciate the need for gentleness and patience in handling the newborn baby student midwives should consider:

1. THE SHELTERED LIFE HE HAS LED *IN UTERO*.

2. THE ORDEAL TO WHICH HE HAS BEEN SUBJECTED.

3. THE PHYSICAL ADJUSTMENTS HE MUST MAKE TO EXTRA-UTERINE LIFE.

1. **For nine months the fetus has lived in a warm environment,** protected by fluid, obtaining nourishment without using the intestinal tract and receiving oxygen without pulmonary respiration. The fetus has not been called on to produce heat, and has encountered only a very few organisms.

2. **The process of labour causes injury and death to many babies,** so because of the strenuous ordeal to which the infant has been subjected, involving pressure on the brain and some degree of anoxia, he should be handled with infinite gentleness, wrapped up warmly and left quietly in his heated cot to recover from the trauma of birth.

3. **The main physiological adjustments to be made are the initiation of pulmonary respiration,** the establishment of changes in the circulation, the inauguration of digestion, the regulation of heat and the reaction to organisms.

THE INITIATION OF RESPIRATION

Breathing is the first function to be established.—The lungs *in utero* are solid, because they have not been inflated and aerated; the alveolar cells secrete a substance, surfactant, that prevents the walls of the alveoli from adhering. Breathing is initiated in response to lack of oxygen and the high level of carbon dioxide in the blood stream, which stimulates the respiratory centre in the medulla. But if the CO_2 level is too high it depresses instead of stimulates.

Respiration is aided by compression of the chest wall during actual birth, the impact of cool air on the face and the handling of the limbs and body. The healthy baby cries almost as soon as he is born, but he must breathe in order to cry: with the first breath the blood vessels in the lungs expand.

The initial respiratory movements are shallow and almost imperceptible, then comes a gasp, followed by crying. The respirations are rapid (around 40 per minute) and may be irregular for some hours. To facilitate lung expansion *healthy babies are encouraged to cry* lustily at birth; otherwise complete aeration of the lungs may be delayed for hours or days, as occurs in premature and asphyxiated babies. Breathing in the newborn is almost entirely abdominal.

DIGESTION

The baby has to suck, swallow, digest and absorb food as well as defæcate.

491

Colostrum.—Nature has wisely provided this food which is easily digested, the protein consisting of lactalbumin but not caseinogen as in milk. It is nutritive, quenches thirst, is laxative in effect, and contains immune bodies and vitamins.

Meconium.—The baby's first stool is meconium which is present in the intestine from about the 16th week of intra-uterine life. It is dark green in colour, being composed of bile-pigment, fatty acids, mucus and epithelial cells.

HEART BEAT

The pulse rate is 120-140 beats per minute usually ascertained by ausculating the apex beat. The heart is higher in the newborn than in the adult so the bell of the stethoscope is placed at the left sternal edge in the midclavicular line but the point of maximal intensity is variable, sometimes over and above the left nipple. There is little difference between the sounds at apex or base in the newborn.

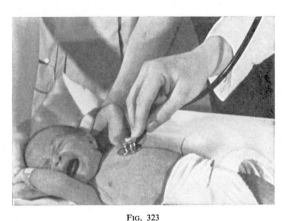

FIG. 323
Auscultating the Apex Beat

TEMPERATURE REGULATION

Heat regulation in the newborn is unstable and because of the low metabolic rate heat production is poor.

The baby leaves an environment of 37·7° C. (100° F.) and enters one of about 21·1° C. (70° F.); being wet, he will lose heat by evaporation. The baby should therefore be received into a warm turkish towel, dried, wrapped in a cotton cellular blanket which covers the head and laid into a warmed cot.

Even with such treatment his temperature may fall to around 35° C. (95° F.) within an hour and it may be eight hours before it rises to the normal level, 36·6° to 37·2° C. (98° to 99° F.).

The first bath should be carried out in a room at a temperature of 21·1° to 26·6° C. (70° to 80° F.), with water at 37·7° C. (100° F.). Towels and clothing should also be warmed. If the baby's hands, feet and lips are blue after the first bath, it has been carried out too soon or the baby has been chilled.

NEONATAL HYPOTHERMIA
Cold Injury

This condition, in which the baby's temperature may fall as low as 29·4° to 32·2° C. (85° to 90° F.), is the result of exposure to cold (see p. 560). Low-reading rectal thermometers, ranging from 21·1° to 37·7° C. (70° to 100° F.) should always be used for newborn babies in order to detect temperatures below 35° C. (95° F.).

REACTION TO ORGANISMS

Passive immunity to many specific infectious diseases is inherited from the mother, but some weeks elapse before the baby produces an active immunity to various organisms.

During passage through the birth canal skin abrasions may occur and the baby's face is exposed to organisms.

The eyes, umbilicus and skin are all vulnerable to infection.

The staphylococcus aureus is the organism to which babies have least resistance.

Thorough domestic cleanliness when handling babies is the finest safeguard against infection.

BLOOD

The number of red cells necessary during intra-uterine life is in excess of what is required after birth, so the extra cells are broken down and the hæmoglobin stored by the liver. The number of red cells at birth is approximately 6,000,000 per ml. and hæmoglobin 18 G. (120 per cent).

The clotting power is low because newborn infants are nearly always deficient in vitamin K, a substance needed by the liver in the production of prothrombin, one of the elements necessary for the clotting of blood.

Urinary Function

The bladder of the baby at term contains urine which is usually expelled during birth. No concern need be felt if the baby does not pass urine for 24 hours, but student midwives are often agitated when babies do not do so. The author has only once seen a case of urethral obstruction, and in that instance the dribbling from the over-distended bladder was misinterpreted, the diagnosis being made on a marked gain in weight and abdominal swelling. Catheterization was necessary for some weeks.

The kidneys of the newborn do not excrete fluids nor chlorides efficiently, and if insufficient fluid is given, the urine may be dark yellow in colour and may leave a brick-dust-like deposit on the napkins which at first glance appears to be blood.

WEIGHT

The average weight at birth is 3·1 kg. (7 lb.), but babies at term may weigh from 2·2 to 5·4 kg. (5 to 12 lb.). Boys are slightly heavier than girls, and in the third and subsequent babies the weight tends to increase.

During the first three days a physiological loss of 113 to 227 G. occurs. The bigger the baby the more it will lose, and when feeding is not satisfactory the loss may be as much as 454 G.

The decrease in weight is due to the loss of tissue fluid, a deficient food and fluid intake as well as the loss of meconium. When the milk supply becomes adequate, a slow steady increase in weight occurs, but infants do not all regain their birth weights by the 10th day. **170 G. weekly is the usual amount gained during the first months.**

LENGTH

The average length of the baby at term is 49·5 to 52·1 cm. (19½ to 20½ inches), and may be as much as 58·4 cm. (23 inches) in babies over 4·5 kg. (10 lb.). A plastic ruler should be used and the baby measured from the vertex to the heels. To undo flexion it may be necessary to hold the infant upside down.

Two midwives are necessary to ensure accuracy. Using a measuring-tape, which follows the body curves, gives misleading information.

THE SPECIAL SENSES

Parents often ask when the baby will see, hear, etc., and for that reason the following facts are given :—

Taste :—The lips and tongue are very sensitive ; the sense of taste is not very well developed, but babies seem to prefer sweeter foods.

Hearing :—Loud noises cause the baby to cry, but the ability to discriminate between sounds is not developed for two or three months.

Sight :—True vision is not present at birth, but at one month the baby looks towards a bright light. The eyes do not focus properly for some weeks, and squint may persist for as long as six months.

The eyes are of a bluish-grey colour and may change to brown during the first year. Tears are not present unless the eyes are inflamed ; smiles and tears appear at from four to six weeks.

THE UMBILICAL CORD

The stump of umbilical cord shrivels by a process of necrosis or dry gangrene, and separates from the skin at a line of demarcation. The umbilical vein inside the abdomen becomes thrombosed. **To aid separation of the cord,** it is kept clean and dry.

THE SKIN

The skin is very delicate, easily irritated, abraded and infected. It is covered at birth with a substance—**vernix caseosa,** secreted by the sebaceous glands—which acts as a lubricant during birth, protects the skin and retains heat.

To remove the vernix the finger tips smeared with mild soap should gently massage the area and the substance will rapidly dissolve.

Some authorities do not remove the vernix, they believe it should be left alone to act as a protection against infection, but the babies develop an unpleasant odour after a few days. Any excess vernix should be removed from areas such as the axillæ and groins, as it tends to produce irritation where skin surfaces meet.

Lanugo, a downy fluff, is seen mostly on the skin of the premature baby.

PSYCHOLOGY OF THE NEWBORN BABY

Midwives and mothers are apt to consider the baby's welfare entirely from the physical angle ; but the health and happiness of each individual is dependent on psychological and mental as well as physical factors. Psychological defects account for more of life's failures than do physical defects.

The newborn baby is an individual, having certain inherited tendencies which will to some extent influence his behaviour, but he is also influenced by the environment into which he is born. He has no knowledge of the world, and he will build up his impression of it and form habits of reacting to it, according to whether he finds it pleasant or otherwise.

Certain primal needs must be met in order to survive. The baby's reaction to hunger and thirst is vociferous crying, and when these needs are not met the response is one of uncontrolled frustration ; crying is his only language. The persistent thwarting of a natural urge which the infant is unable to satisfy may sow the seed of a disgruntled personality.

NEWBORN BABIES NEED LOVE

Nature has provided the mother with a maternal instinct which she expresses by cuddling and caressing her infant. Much of a baby's experience is centred round feeding, and when nestled in the mother's arms he feels warm, comfortable and infinitely secure.

The average baby is more likely to develop into a well-balanced personality under the care of a mother who gives expression to her maternal instinct rather than one who subordinates her instinct to scientific principles (see Self-regulated Feeding, p. 511).

Babies will not thrive without mothering (*mother love*); though there are mothers who give too much love, they can be guided and it is safer to give too much than too little.

Midwives should try to foster a happy relationship between mother and baby by helping with the difficulties of feeding and creating a serene atmosphere, for it seems reasonable to expect the baby who finds the world a pleasant place to respond to it positively.

Midwives should give mothers scope for the expression of their love. Some condemn any attempt to comfort a crying baby as " spoiling," but much harm can accrue from leaving a baby alone crying for long periods.

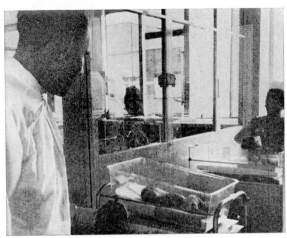

Fig. 334

Father viewing his baby daughter (4 hours old) through glass in corridor of neonatal pædiatric department.

(*Royal Maternity Hospital, Rottenrow, Glasgow.*)

THE BABY'S NEEDS

1. WARMTH

This is very necessary until the infant has recovered from the ordeal of birth and food is being taken. Loss of heat by evaporation from the baby's head at birth should be avoided. The room should be between 21·1° and 23·8° C. (70° and 75° F.) and the cot clothing light but warm. There is a tendency to over-heat babies in summer; on the other hand, they are not always kept warm enough during the winter nights, especially at home. Chilling must be avoided to prevent neonatal hypothermia.

2. NOURISHMENT

See Breast and Bottle Feeding, page 506.

3. FLUID

The need for fluid is imperative during the first two days. About 10 per cent of babies will develop dehydration fever unless given sufficient fluid during the first two days; 150 ml. fluid per kg. body weight are required daily after the third day.

4. SLEEP

Babies sleep for 20 out of the 24 hours during the first two months. Mothers should be advised to avoid noises such as a blaring radio, to which the infant will become accustomed, but which by bombarding the nervous system may produce irritability.

5. FRESH AIR

This is necessary but draughts must be excluded. Nurseries should be aired at feeding times. In warm weather healthy babies can be taken out of doors after the first few days.

6. EXERCISE

The need for newborn babies to exercise is not always appreciated: arms and legs should have freedom to move, and babies should not be tightly bound up. They must be allowed to squirm, wriggle and kick, to stimulate the circulation of blood and strengthen their muscles for sitting, standing and walking later on.

7. MOTHERING

The newborn baby needs love and affection (p. 494.)

8. PROTECTION

Babies need protection from infection, suffocation, bright lights and strong wind.

To avoid suffocation by inhalation of vomitus, babies should be laid on their sides after feeds, as vomitus may be inhaled if lying on their backs. At home the young baby should sleep in the same room as the mother.

Choking may occur when milk flows too quickly through a rubber teat, therefore propping of bottles during feeding is strongly condemned.

Smothering on a soft pillow. Babies who are tightly wrapped up are very likely to roll over on their faces, which they burrow into the pillow. A young baby does not require a pillow and, because of the risk of suffocation, it should not be used. **Plastic bibs** are also potentially dangerous.

Overlaying:—This will only occur in the home, and the mother should have been instructed to provide a separate cot. She must be warned of the danger should she inadvertently lay her arm or the blankets over the baby's face. The midwife must always improvise a cot when one is not provided. The danger of cats must be kept in mind; they have been known to lie on the baby's face, with fatal results due to suffocation.

Bright lights:—Babies' eyes should be shaded from brilliant sunshine; glaring ceiling lights should be dimmed when possible.

Strong wind blowing on a baby's face will " take its breath away." Mothers should be advised to arrange the shawl loosely round the head when taking the baby home from hospital on a windy day.

EXAMINATION OF THE NEWBORN BABY

On admission from the delivery ward. (Babies who need special care are admitted to the neonatal intensive care unit.) The need for warmth at this time must be observed; *i.e.* room, cot, clothing, towels.

Note: Appearance, activity, regular breathing. Any abnormality in colour such as cyanosis, pallor or jaundice should be reported to the doctor.

Check: Name and identification bracelet, sex, Apgar score, weight, length and other relevant facts *re* baby from the delivery chart (see p. 333). Check cord for bleeding and religature if necessary.

A detailed examination is carried out, usually prior to the first bath, beginning at the head and working downwards. Unless deliberately and systematically done some abnormality may be overlooked.

THE HEAD

Excessive moulding and a large caput arise during difficult labour and suggest the possibility of intracranial injury. Depressed skull fractures are very rare. The mongoloid appearance of a baby with Down's syndrome is characteristic.

The eyes:—Nystagmus is not uncommon in normal babies. Small subconjunctival hæmorrhages, bright red in colour, are frequently seen; they disappear spontaneously within a week.

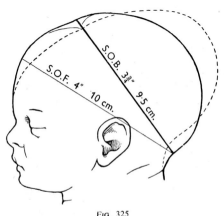

FIG. 325

The type of moulding in a vertex presentation, head well flexed, is shown by the dotted line.

The mouth should be inspected in a good light for cleft palate, which may only involve the soft palate. Cleft lip is readily seen. The mouth may be drawn to one side, due to facial paralysis. Excessive frothy mucus suggests an œsophageal atresia.

Tongue-tie.—In this condition the frenulum of the tongue is attached almost to the tip. Pædiatricians do not advocate snipping it unless sucking is interfered with, which is rare. The mother should be told that it will be all right, as older relatives are apt to advise having it cut.

Teeth.—Very occasionally babies are born with the two lower incisors erupted. They are sometimes soft and loose, and are always easily extracted.

THE ARMS AND HANDS

The infant should be moving both arms freely, and, if not, the question of fracture, dislocation or paralysis must be considered.

Fingers should be counted, the hand being opened out, as an extra little finger attached by skin may be lying in the palm: the application of a tight ligature (by the doctor) will remove it by necrosis. Webbed fingers are rare, and are operated on some months later.

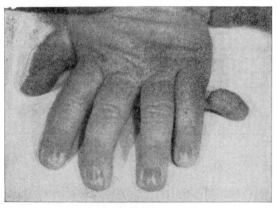

FIG. 326
Extra digit.

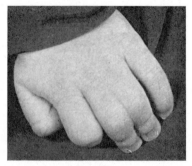

FIG. 327
WEBBED FINGERS.
Hand of newborn baby.

THE BODY

The cord should be examined for oozing, and a clamp or ligature applied if necessary.

The external genitalia:—More than a cursory glance is needed to establish the sex; pseudohermaphroditism may be present and conditions such as hypospadias.

The penis:—A degree of narrowing of the foreskin (phimosis) **is natural** and the prepuce is non-retractable during the first year. Forcibly pulling back the foreskin is apt to cause minor lacerations, and is not advocated: the orifice grows satisfactorily during the first year. **Pædiatricians do not recommend circumcision as frequently as they did in former years.**

The anus may be imperforate, and to prevent this being overlooked the first temperature should be taken rectally—gentleness is essential to avoid injury.

The back is inspected for spina bifida (*meningocele*).

THE LEGS

Fractures are rare: paralysis, if present, usually accompanies spina bifida. Talipes and congenital dislocation of the hips should be recognized early so that corrective treatment is given as soon as possible. The legs may appear to be bent, but this is normal. The toes should be counted: webbed toes are not uncommon and are usually ignored. The pad of fat on the instep gives an erroneous impression of flat foot.

DAILY OBSERVATION OF THE NEWBORN BABY

To the inexperienced student midwife newborn babies look very much alike until she is shown the variations in appearance and behaviour of the normal baby and how to recognize evidence of health or otherwise.

SIGNS OF A THRIVING BABY

The baby has a clear, pink and often mottled skin, firm muscles, a vigorous kick and a lusty cry. He takes his food eagerly, has a clean tongue, normal stools, bright eyes, gains in weight and sleeps well. (*Signs of illness are described under their respective headings.*)

CHARTING OF OBSERVATIONS

The doctor depends on the vigilant observation of the midwife to detect abnormalities and early signs of illness, and on the careful recording of her findings.

1. Respirations:—The rate and type of respirations are most important during the first 48 hours of life; the normal rate being around 40 per minute.

Periods of apnœa, grunting respirations, flaring of the nasal alæ or indrawing of the chest wall should be reported to the doctor at once.

2. Temperature taken once or twice daily.   **3. Weight daily.**

4. Feeding.

    (*a*) **Time, whether three-hourly or four-hourly or self-regulated.**

    (*b*) **Breast-fed,** whether wholly or partly; amount of milk in any test feeds.

    (*c*) **Bottle-fed,** type of milk and the amount taken.

Cyanosis or exhaustion during or after feeding should be reported; regurgitation noted.

5. Medicines, oxygen and treatment.

6. Other facts such as the passage of urine; the number and character of the stools; day on which the cord comes off; excessive crying, anorexia, any signs of illness.

THE STOOLS

Meconium (see p. 492). **When the baby is given milk the meconium stool becomes greenish-brown,** then yellowish-brown.

After the fourth day the typical soft, yellow semi-fluid stool of the breast-fed baby is usual, the bowels moving three or four times daily. **Cow's milk produces a firmer, paler stool of putty-like consistency, with a slightly offensive odour.**

Occasional green stools occur in healthy babies, and if the infant is hungry and not feverish they may be ignored. Persistent green stools with mucus should be reported.

Greenish-yellow, frothy, loose stools, with a sour odour, are due to too much sugar. Greenish-yellow, loose, frequent stools, with fine curds, are due to overfeeding. Both cause sore buttocks.

Bluish-green stools are due to the addition of alkalis to cow's milk, or to the action of certain organisms, but in the latter case the colour appears some time after the stool is passed and does not permeate it.

Yellow or green frequent watery stools may be due to epidemic gastro-enteritis (p. 568).

Small dark brownish-yellow stools, often accompanied by mucus, are due to gross underfeeding.

Pale, greasy, offensive, bulky stools, often accompanied by vomiting, may be due to cow's milk too rich in fat.

Pasty stools with tough curds are due to too much protein from giving whole cow's milk too soon. Colic may be present.

Mucus.—A trace of mucus is normal; mucus may be due to underfeeding and, if excessive, usually denotes enteritis.

Melæna (see p. 580).

DAILY CARE

The eyes:—Because of the risk of ophthalmia neonatorum the eyes must be inspected several times daily and inflammation and any discharge noted.

C.M.B.(Eng.) Code of Practice; C.M.B.(Scot.) Rule.—*A midwife must call in medical aid without delay if there is any discharge from the eyes of an infant, however slight this discharge may be.*

To avoid infecting the eyes it is advisable to wash and dry the face with cotton wool, using a small bowl of sterile water.

The mouth does not require cleansing, but should be examined daily for thrush after the fourth day: the small glistening spots sometimes seen on the posterior area of the palate are not due to thrush.

The nose needs no attention, unless to wipe away any visible smudges with a piece of cotton wool.

THE UMBILICAL CORD

Daily inspection is advisable, as a thick cord may be very moist and this predisposes to infection. The umbilical area is cleansed with Hibitane, 0·5 per cent, in spirit 70 per cent, and dusted with Ster Zac cord powder.

Thorough cleansing with an efficient antiseptic, and spraying with a plastic solution such as Octaflex or Nobecutane at birth is also recommended.

Some authorities consider that the baby should not be placed in water until the cord is off; others recommend immersing the baby, drying and powdering the cord.

The cord should come off about the sixth day, delay usually being due to a low-grade infection.

Inflammation, discharge, or an offensive odour should be reported.

THE TEMPERATURE

This is taken every day and each infant in hospital should have his own low reading thermometer (C.M.B. Rule). The axilla or groin may be used instead of the rectum.

To detect neonatal hypothermia the temperature should be taken daily during the winter months, even by those who think this is otherwise unnecessary.

Bathing, handling and dressing the baby are described under Baby Care (pp. 736 to 748).

The buttocks (see Prophylactic Care, p. 501).

CRYING

Crying is the baby's only language, and the newborn baby cries vigorously, looking as though he is suffering extreme pain. But babies cry because of the slightest discomfort, and the midwife can merely surmise the cause, for different cries are not easily recognized in the first two weeks of life, except the high-pitched cry of the baby who has sustained intra-cranial injury.

The following are common reasons :—

The baby is hungry, thirsty, in pain, wet, too hot, too cold, uncomfortable.

If the baby is neither hungry nor wet, changing his position is usually sufficient to quieten him. Wind is seldom troublesome during the first 14 days. After crying for some time he will be thirsty, and 30 ml of water should be given.

Minor Disorders of the Newborn

1. SORE BUTTOCKS

Reddening of the napkin area is caused by the napkins not being changed frequently enough; material too rough (*e.g.* Turkish towelling, dried too quickly); using strong soaps in washing napkins and not properly rinsing them.

Localized excoriation and ulceration of the area between the buttocks is usually caused by frequent loose irritating stools; (*a*) acid, frothy stools due to too much sugar; (*b*) frequent green stools due to overfeeding; (*c*) epidemic gastro-enteritis.

Monilial rash (*thrush*). A scraping should be taken from any resistant napkin rash and sent for culture. If positive the application of nystatin cream is curative.

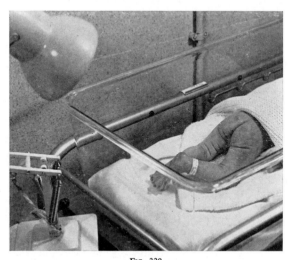

FIG. 328

TREATMENT OF SORE BUTTOCKS
(*ordinary electric light bulb*).

(*Aberdeen Maternity Hospital.*)

Prophylactic Care of the Buttocks

Meconium should not be permitted to dry on the buttocks as it becomes firmly adherent to the skin. Even if the napkin feels dry, it should be inspected for meconium. The application of a square of gauze spread with an emollient substance will prevent meconium from adhering to the buttocks.

The practice at the Simpson Memorial Pavilion during the first 10 days is to change the napkins, if soiled or wet, before and after feeds, to wash the buttocks with soap or hexachlorophane (Phisohex) and water, gently mop them dry, and massage a very little ointment into the buttocks.

CURATIVE TREATMENT

The cause, if known, should be remedied. To avoid urine and stool irritating the lesions, napkins should be changed as soon as possible if the baby is awake. The buttocks are gently washed with soap and water, the excoriated area may be wiped with olive oil if preferred.

If the skin is red, Thovaline ung., Massé or benzalkonium (Drapolene) cream, Eucerin anhydrous or titanium (Metanium) ung. are soothing. White of egg promotes rapid healing; *albumin powder is available*, 15 G. *to water* 150 *ml.*

Exposure of the buttocks to the air.—The infant is laid on his side upon a napkin, for an hour or two, three times daily and an Anglepoise type of lamp, at least 35·6 cm. (14 in.) distant, is directed on to the buttocks; the light aids healing and provides warmth. (*The lamp should be alongside and not above the buttocks in case it slips downwards.*) Exposure to sunshine for 10 minutes daily is also helpful.

Marking ink poisoning

Deaths have occurred by absorption through the skin of marking ink on napkins that have been issued without having been boiled to fix the aniline dye. **Cyanosis is manifest.**

2. SKIN RASHES

Because of the risk of staphylococcal infections, babies should be examined daily and segregated, if necessary, to avoid epidemics.

A wool rash consists of blotchy red patches which make the infant cross. The affected area should be dabbed with calamine lotion.

A heat or sweat rash is evident as pin-point spots, sometimes having a hard transparent centre also reddened areas between skin folds. It is more common in summer when babies are sometimes swaddled in layers of wool. After bathing, a bland antiseptic dusting powder is applied.

Nail-fold injuries, scratches.—Babies' fingers should be dried gently, as the nail-folds are easily torn. To prevent babies from scratching their faces the use of cotton mittens is favoured by some experienced nursery midwives, but precautions are necessary to avoid loose threads becoming wound round the fingers and causing gangrene (see p. 741).

3. DEHYDRATION FEVER

When given insufficient fluid and kept too warm the temperature rises to 38·3° C. (101° F.) and over; the mouth and skin are dry, the baby is flushed, thirsty and cross. The urine, being concentrated, leaves a stain on the napkin, which feels gritty. Blood electrolytes should always be determined. In such cases equal parts of Hartmann's solution and dextrose 10 per cent every four hours will rapidly alleviate the condition.

4. JAUNDICE OF IMMATURITY

About 20 per cent of newborn babies develop jaundice during the third or fourth day, due to inefficient hepatic function; bilirubin in the blood rises and this is evident as jaundice.

Extra fluid should be given because the bile in the blood stream makes the infant drowsy and disinclined to suck. The condition clears within the first week. Occasionally a replacement blood transfusion may be neccessary if the serum bilirubin reaches 18 to 20 mg. per 100 ml.

5. ENGORGED BREASTS

The breasts of male, as well as female, babies may become swollen, hard and hot, most commonly on the third day. The condition is due to breast stimulation by the withdrawal of maternal œstrogen and this releases luteotrophin from the fetal pituitary. This condition is rarely seen in premature babies.

The breasts should not be squeezed or compressed. The condition will subside spontaneously.

6. PSEUDO-MENSTRUATION

A blood-stained vaginal discharge is occasionally seen in girl babies, and is thought to be due to the withdrawal of œstrogen which has passed into the fetal blood stream from the placenta.

7. CONSTIPATION

Constipation is rare in breast-fed babies.—The term should only be applied when the stools are infrequent and hard, causing the infant to strain in passing them. No concern need be felt if the bowels only move once in two or three days, so long as the motion is soft and easily passed. **It is better to avoid using laxatives;** extra water and orange juice are usually effective; milk of magnesia, 4 ml. (one teaspoonful), is suitable if these fail. Midwives should not resort to the drastic stimulus of inserting catheters or soap suppositories into the rectum.

8. VOMITING

Vomiting is common in young babies, and during the first 24 hours the vomitus may consist of mucus, sometimes streaked with blood, which the infant has swallowed during labour: giving 30 ml. of glucose water, 5 per cent, may act as a stomach lavage. Vomiting, occurring at intervals of a few days, in a thriving infant may be ignored.

Possetting, which is the return of a few ml. of milk after feeds should not be described as vomiting.

Faulty technique in feeding is probably the commonest cause. The infant gulps the milk too quickly, is not given an opportunity to bring up wind, or is handled roughly after feeding. If bottle fed, the amount or the strength of the food may be excessive.

Vomiting may be mechanical, in that the cardiac sphincter of the stomach is too relaxed, a condition which usually improves in a week or two. If persistent, thickening the feed with Nestargel is, as a rule, effective.

Vomiting may be a serious sign and sometimes accompanies grave conditions, such as infections of the alimentary or urinary tract and organic obstructions. Bile staining almost always indicates intestinal obstruction.

If persistent, electrolyte imbalance must be corrected.

The following should be noted:

The day of onset ? Are other signs of illness present ? The colour of the vomitus (*particularly bile*). **Is the vomiting forcible ? Is the whole feed returned ? Is the baby constipated ? Is the appetite poor ? Is diarrhœa present ?**

QUESTIONS FOR REVISION

MINOR DISORDERS OF THE NEWBORN

How would you (*a*) prevent ? (*b*) treat sore buttocks ? Describe the various skin rashes which may occur and state how they may be prevented. **How would you** recognize and treat the following: engorged breasts; constipation in an artificially fed baby ? **What are the common** (*not serious*) causes of vomiting ? What observations would you make and report to the doctor regarding this sign ?

C.M.B.(N. Ireland) paper.—Discuss the care of the skin in the neonatal period, mentioning the commoner abnormalities which may be met.

C.M.B.(N. Ireland) paper.—How would you recognize and treat the following conditions ? (*a*) Thrush stomatitis, (*b*) A napkin rash.

C.M.B.(Scot.) paper.—What are the causes of vomiting in the baby during the first week of life ? Describe the investigation and management of such a case.

C.M.B.(Scot.) paper.—State the causes of vomiting in the newborn. What observations should be made and how may these conditions be treated ?

PHYSIOLOGY AND MANAGEMENT OF THE NEWBORN BABY

State a normal baby's temperature, respirations, heart rate, length, weight.

Write not more than 10 lines on each of the following:

The psychology of the newborn baby; the establishment of respiration; the thriving baby; the baby's needs; examination of the newborn baby; daily observation of the new born.

What would make you surmise that a baby crying in the night during the second week of life is: too hot; thirsty; too cold; in pain; hungry ? Give other reasons for discomfort.

Define the following terms: surfactant; hypothermia; passive immunity; phimosis; nystagmus; vernix caseosa; overlaying; frenulum; lanugo; webbed fingers; meconium; tongue-tie.

CARE OF THE UMBILICAL CORD

The cord comes off about the .... day; keeping the stump dry aids ....; the cord separates by a process of ....; plastic clamp is removed on the .... day; inflammation of the umbilicus is known as ....; delay in separation may be due to ....

State why the following substances are applied: SterZac; Nobecutane; Hibitane 0·5 per cent in spirit; Octaflex.

BABIES' STOOLS

PLACE NUMBER OF CAUSE AGAINST SIGN		
Cause	Signs	Number
1 gross underfeeding	tough curds, mucus	
2 meconium	black stool	
3 too much sugar	offensive, bulky pale	
4 breast fed	slightly offensive odour, pale yellow	
5 overfeeding	yellowish-green, watery	
6 too much fat	greenish-yellow, loose small curds	
7 gastro-enteritis	greenish, frothy, loose	
8 melæna	dark green	
9 fed on cows milk	yellow, semi-fluid	
10 too much protein	small, dark green with mucus	

C.M.B.(Eng.) paper.—What abnormal conditions may develop in an apparently normal baby in the first forty-eight hours following its birth ? Briefly discuss their management.

C.M.B.(Eng.) paper.—Describe the normal stools in the first 10 days of life. What abnormalities may occur in the stools during this time ?

C.M.B.(Scot.) paper.—Describe the umbilical cord. Give details of the treatment of the cord at birth and during the lying-in period.

C.M.B.(Eng.) paper.—A baby loses weight during the second week of the puerperium. Discuss the causes of this and outline the management of the baby.

C.M.B.(N. Ireland) paper.—A week old infant fails to gain weight. What steps would you take to determine the cause and to correct this ?

C.M.B.(Scot.) paper.—Describe the routine examination of a newborn child to exclude developmental abnormalities.

C.M.B.(N. Ireland) paper.—Describe the midwife's routine examination of a newborn baby. What abnormalities might she find ?

C.M.B.(Eng.) paper.—Describe how you would examine a newborn baby. What congenital abnormalities might you find ?

C.M.B.(Scot.) paper.—Describe in detail the examination of a newborn baby.

C.M.B.(Eng.) paper.—A baby fails to gain weight during the first week of life. What may be the causes and what treatment may be required ?

29

29

Breast Feeding—Bottle Feeding

It is universally agreed that breast milk cannot be excelled as a food for babies.

Breast milk is suited to the baby's needs and digestion. It is almost germ-free when produced; goes directly to the consumer without being handled and is always fresh.

Breast milk contains protective antibodies and vitamins.

Breast-fed babies get more mothering and when cuddled at the breast they feel loved and secure. **They have fewer illnesses during the first year of life.**

Breast feeding is beneficial from the psychological aspect.

Breast feeding causes less work: no modification of milk, no cleaning of pans and bottles, no heating of feeds. **Breast milk is cheap to produce, but expensive to buy.**

ANATOMY AND PHYSIOLOGY OF THE BREAST

The breasts are compound secreting glands, composed mainly of glandular tissue which is arranged in lobes, approximately 20 in number. Each lobe is divided into lobules: these form alveoli or cavities lined with secreting cells which produce milk. The breasts are richly supplied with blood.

Small lactiferous ducts, carrying milk from the alveoli of each lobe, unite to form about 20 larger ducts. These, before opening on the surface of the nipple, widen to form ampullæ which act as temporary reservoirs for milk.

The nipple, composed of erectile tissue, is covered with epithelium and contains plain muscle fibres which have a sphincter-like action in controlling the flow of milk. Surrounding the nipple is an area of loose skin known as the areola.

The pituitary growth hormone has lactogenic properties and in conjunction with œstrogen and progesterone induces alveolar and duct growth as well as stimulating localized milk secretion.

The production of milk is held in abeyance during pregnancy by the high level of œstrogen, which keeps the anterior pituitary lactogenic hormone in check. Œstrogen is produced by the placenta as well as the ovary, and when the placenta is expelled, the œstrogen level falls and luteotrophin (*prolactin*) from the anterior pituitary initiates the production of milk and maintains lactation.

The act of sucking also stimulates the production and the flow of milk, probably by some neuro-hormonal reflex mechanism which activates the anterior pituitary to produce luteotrophin (*prolactin*) and the posterior lobe to produce oxytocin.

The emptying of the breast by sucking stimulates the glands to produce more milk: the expulsion of the milk is influenced by oxytocin.

PREPARATION FOR LACTATION

The maternal instinct is not always dominant until after the birth of the baby, and the woman during pregnancy may have no inclination towards breast feeding. If the mother-to-be states that she has no intention of attempting breast feeding, she may be persuaded to try, but she should not be forced to do so against her will.

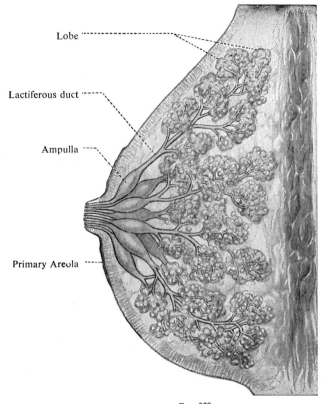

Fig. 329
Diagram of the lactating breast.

To give the woman confidence the midwife should advise her regarding preparation for and the general management of breast feeding. The minor details of management are best taught when actually feeding the baby.

The breasts should be supported with a firm brassiere which does not depress the nipples.

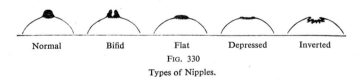

| Normal | Bifid | Flat | Depressed | Inverted |

Fig. 330
Types of Nipples.

Breast treatment should be as simple as possible: if too elaborate or time-consuming the woman may decide that breast feeding is not worth the trouble.

Inverted nipples.—The nipples may be below the level of the skin surface and great difficulty experienced in everting them. Sometimes they are " flat " (on a level with the skin surface) and in both cases they may be improved by the use of plastic Woolwich shells.

PREVENTION OF CRACKS

During pregnancy an effort should be made to toughen the nipples and get them accustomed to friction, in readiness for the vigorous sucking to which they will be subjected.

1. The nipples should be massaged by rolling them between the finger and thumb and drawing them out every day during the last two months, using a good face-soap and water.

2. Lanoline or other suitable ointment such as Massé cream may be applied twice weekly. Spirit dries the natural oil (from Montgomery's tubercles) and is apt to produce cracks.

MANAGEMENT OF BREAST FEEDING

Cleanliness is the first essential, the midwife explaining to each mother that her nails should be short and clean and that she must not touch her nipples with unwashed hands nor wipe them with her handkerchief. The woman's hands are washed before each feed, and the midwife must always wash her hands before touching the breasts.

The modern tendency is to reduce nipple cleansing to a minimum and to wash the breasts once daily only. Spirit and antiseptics should not be used: they dry and irritate the epithelium of the nipple and predispose to excoriation.

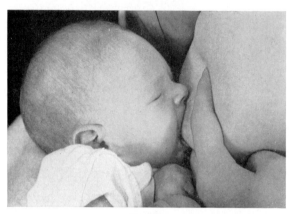

FIG. 331

Note that the areola is in the baby's mouth and that his lips are wide apart.

Clean supporting brassières should be worn. Keybak dressings 7·6 cm. × 7·6 cm. (3 by 3 inches) are absorbent and non-irritating to the nipples.

Before the infant is taken to the breast, any discharge from its eyes or nose ought to be removed; the napkin must be changed, and the gown should not be stained with stool.

Attention to such details will reduce the number of breast infections. Midwives should remember that the mother who develops mastitis is unlikely to feed this or any subsequent baby or to recommend breast feeding to others.

LENGTH OF TIME AT THE BREAST

The baby is offered 60 ml. dextrose 5 or 10 per cent. four hours after birth.

First and second days.—Beginning 6 to 8 hours after birth, the infant goes to the breast every six hours during the day; 3 minutes at each side on the first day and 5 minutes on the second day.

Third day.—The infant goes to the breast every three (or four) hours, and should feed from both breasts not more than 10 minutes at each; longer than that will blister the nipples. He must not be cajoled to suck for 20 minutes in case over-feeding occurs.

It is important that the first breast is emptied before the infant is transferred to the second. This usually means 10 minutes at the first breast and five minutes at the second, the baby commencing with the second breast next time in order to empty it completely.

THE TECHNIQUE OF BREAST FEEDING

The first feed.—The woman should be given a few moments to admire her baby before putting him to the breast, unless he is crying. The breast feeding experience ought to be one of pleasure as well as business for mother and baby, the midwife giving help and advice, if necessary, but not dominating the situation.

Serenity and quietness.—The mother ought to be serene and calm, and there should be no bustle, hurry or tension; she should give her undivided attention to her infant and should not read or talk to anyone.

Mother and baby should be in a comfortable position.—If the baby is held almost upright the swallowing of air is minimal and eructation facilitated; his cheek in contact with the breast stimulates the " search " reflex. The mother, sitting up and leaning slightly forwards, supports the breast in the palm of her hand, allowing the nipple to pass between her first two fingers. In this way she directs the nipple into the baby's mouth and keeps the breast away from the baby's nose.

FIXING AND SUCKING

The baby draws the nipple back to the posterior region of the tongue; the loose tissue around the nipple (the areola) is in the baby's mouth, therefore the ampullæ are also in the mouth. The lips are wide apart, not pursed. The gums compress the ampullæ and the milk flows along the tongue.

The baby's neck should not be hampered by blankets, in order that free movement of the lower jaw is possible. The head should be at such a level that too much pull is not exerted on the nipple. There is no necessity to bind the baby's arms firmly except when he is struggling and refusing to fix, but once having got hold of the nipple the infant should be given freedom to squirm and kick.

DIFFICULTIES DUE TO THE MOTHER

She may, because of perineal sutures, be unable to sit up to handle her baby properly. The baby can feed equally well when the mother is lying on her side (see Fig. 332).

She might be highly strung and nervous, especially if the baby is proving difficult. Calmness and reassurance are necessary.

The nipples may be flat.—If so, the areola should be gently stroked and stretched away from the nipple which is then pulled out with the fingers or a breast pump used to draw it out. To encourage the baby to persevere, some colostrum should be expressed into his mouth.

If the areola and the baby's face become wet and slippery, the baby won't be able to get hold of the nipple; so the face and breast should be dried. Nipple shields, whether made of rubber, or glass and rubber, are of little value; the baby can rarely suck sufficient milk through them. (Flattened nipples, due to acute engorgement, are discussed on page 513.)

DIFFICULTIES DUE TO THE BABY

Conditions such as cleft lip, a receding chin, or marked tongue tie. The baby may be excessively sleepy for no apparent reason or because he has been crying for some time and is exhausted.

The baby should be soothed and quietened.—After a reasonable attempt, the effort should be abandoned until three hours later and the baby given a mixture of milk, water and dextrose. The mixture should be less sweet, therefore less attractive than breast milk, and

29A

sufficient in amount to satisfy the immediate needs without satiating the natural urges of hunger and thirst.

The cause should be investigated, and for the tense highly strung infant the doctor may order chloral hydrate, 30 mg. three times daily, between feeds.

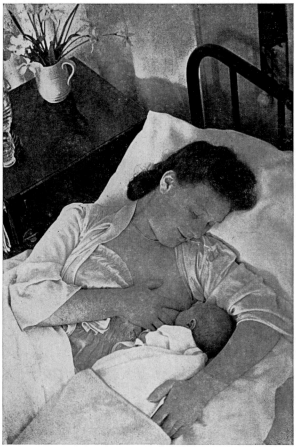

FIG. 332

A mother comfortably feeding her baby while lying on her side.
(Note how the breast is being held away from the baby's nose.)
(*Simpson Memorial Maternity Pavilion, Edinburgh.*)

Prevention of Cracked Nipples during the Puerperium

Do not allow the baby to suck for longer than three minutes every six hours during the first day, five minutes at each breast during the second day. Tell the mother there is only about 4 ml. of "milk" in the breast and that the baby will only blister the nipple if he sucks too long.

Ensure that the baby has "fixed" properly, to avoid bruising the nipple with his gums. The nostrils must be clear, or the baby will let go of the nipple in order to breathe, and repeated catching hold of the nipple will bruise it.

Do not pull the baby off the breast when he has finished sucking; press the cheeks and depress the lower jaw to avoid trauma to the nipple or lift the outer border of the upper lip to break the suction; holding the nostrils is unkind.

The nipples should be dried thoroughly after each feed and a soothing ointment such as Massé cream applied during the first weeks, especially in the case of the blonde or red-haired primipara.

The baby should not sleep at the breast in any case, but, if the nipple is in his mouth, breathing on it will cause it to become excoriated in the same way that improperly dried hands become chapped.

THE FREQUENCY OF FEEDING TIMES

Many pædiatricians recommend, and it is a good working rule, that **6 to 8 hours should elapse** before the baby is put to the breast, in order that both mother and child have an opportunity to rest after the stress of labour: a crying restless baby should not be forced to wait 8 hours.

When lactation is initiated, generally on the third day, it is usual to feed the normal full term infant according to a plan, either **three hourly or four hourly,** but a number of pædiatricians favour self-regulated feeding in which the clock is ignored (see below). The baby's welfare should be the deciding factor in selecting a time schedule.

THREE-HOURLY FEEDING *(6 feeds)*

If the baby weighs less than 2·9 kg. (6½ lb.), it would be prudent to use three-hourly feeding until it has been proved that the breast can produce sufficient milk and that the infant can get it.

FOUR-HOURLY FEEDING *(5 feeds)*

This gives the mother more time between feeds for housework and shopping, and it is easier to run a hospital nursery on that régime, but the initial weight loss is usually greater, sometimes as much as 454 G. (1 lb.).

SELF REGULATED FEEDING
(on demand)

By this method feeding times are regulated according to the baby's appetite and his nutritional needs are met in a satisfying manner. It is a revival of the " natural way " in which the woman responds to her instinctive urge to comfort and feed her crying infant.

Making a young, hungry or thirsty infant cry for an hour before getting a feed teaches him nothing and creates frustration which destroys the happy relationship that should exist between mother and baby. Admittedly many babies are quite satisfied on three-hourly or four-hourly feeding, but some refuse to be limited by the clock. They appear to need more frequent feeds and extra soothing and cuddling. If such babies are forced to abide by the clock they use up so much energy crying and kicking that they fall asleep at the breast; almost invariably they are underfed.

The infant should not be fed every time he cries, and causes other than hunger should of course be considered, feeds being limited to eight during 24 hours.

A certain amount of give and take is necessary during the early days, allowing him to sleep for half an hour beyond the usual feeding time, or feeding him half an hour sooner if awake and crying. The mother studies his habits and tries to build up an acceptable routine. Babies vary in their feeding characteristics.

The infant will gradually put himself on to a four-hourly schedule as soon as he takes sufficient milk to satisfy him for that period of time.

NIGHT FEEDS

Babies have no cognizance of day and night, and it may be some weeks before they settle into a rhythm of convenient feeding times, but if adequately fed during the day, babies are more likely to sleep throughout the night.

A young, inexperienced mother, with little knowledge of babies is faced during the night with her screaming infant. She has never fed him between 22.00 hours and 05.00 hours in hospital, and she has no idea why he is crying or what to do. She probably

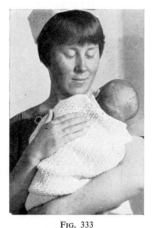

imagines her milk is upsetting the baby or that the trouble is wind or colic, when it is in reality sheer hunger, due to underfeeding. After a few nights of broken sleep, the mother is worn out and worried beyond measure, so her supply of breast milk diminishes still further.

Night feeds should neither be condemned nor forbidden.

If an infant will not settle after being made comfortable and given water, he is probably hungry and should be fed, for water does not pacify a hungry baby and he will not learn to sleep at night by screaming for hours. There is no danger of the baby forming a habit of waking to be fed in the night. When an infant gets enough food during the day he will tend to sleep for longer periods at night until eventually he sleeps from 22.00 hours to 05.00 hours.

Fig. 333

Breaking the wind.

(*Aberdeen Maternity Hospital*)

BREAKING THE WIND

All babies swallow air while sucking, and the baby who is not fixed properly or who sucks an empty breast swallows more than usual.

To bring up wind the baby is held upright against the left chest, and when the back is gently patted the slight jogging movement releases the air in the stomach; as the air escapes the baby belches. The advantage of the upright position is that no milk is expelled.

Some sit the baby on the mother's lap making him bend forwards and to the left to bring the air bubble under the cardiac orifice of the stomach. If the infant is laid in his

cot without first bringing up wind, he will bring it up later and milk as well, or it will pass down and give rise to " colicky pain."

Wind should be broken half-way through the feed, because if the stomach is distended with air the infant will not take a sufficient amount of milk. The procedure is repeated at the end of the feed.

Possetting is the regurgitating of a mouthful of milk by the baby and should not be described as vomiting. It may occur when wind is broken, with hiccoughs, or because of clumsy or rough handling after a feed. Possetting is also a safety valve when the infant has taken too much.

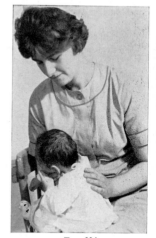

Fig. 334

Breaking the wind.

(*Aberdeen Maternity Hospital*)

DIFFICULTIES IN BREAST FEEDING
(Maternal)

Many of the difficulties are preventable and surmountable.

1. **Attitude.**

(*a*) **Unwillingness.**—A mother who is unwilling to breast feed her baby rarely succeeds, but if handled with tact and understanding she may be persuaded to do so.

(*b*) **Over-anxiety.**—In cases where breast feeding has previously failed, or in the older primipara, the woman's anxiety to succeed may inhibit successful lactation. The midwife can impart knowledge and try to instil a placid and hopeful outlook.

2. **General health.**—The woman may be in poor health. (See Contra-indications to Breast Feeding, p. 514.)

3. **The breasts.**—The difficulty may be functional when the breasts are incapable of secreting an adequate amount of milk. The supply is sometimes scanty from the beginning, or it fails after two or three weeks. This may be due to mismanagement.

ENGORGED BREASTS

This is a condition varying in degree from slight to severe, commonly occurring between the third and fifth day of the puerperium.

The breasts are full, heavy and hard, due to venous and lymphatic engorgement and œdema and not to an abundant supply of milk. The muscular mechanism by which milk is expelled is inhibited and when breast tension rises excessively the cells cease to produce milk.

Treatment

SLIGHT ENGORGEMENT

Bathe the breasts in hot water before feeds and gently stroke them with soapy hands towards the nipple.

Put baby to the breasts for a few minutes and then express the remaining milk.

Apply ointment (Massé cream) to the nipples and use a firm supporting brassière.

SEVERE ENGORGEMENT

Do not put the baby to the breast or use manual expression if the breasts are so tense, hard and swollen that the nipple is flattened and the baby cannot grasp the areola.

Stilboestrol is not prescribed by as many obstetricians as formerly. The dose, 10 mg. followed by 5 mg. four-hourly to a total of 40 mg.

It may be necessary to give an analgesic such as Panasorb or pentazocine (Fortral) tablets (2) at night to relieve pain. The baby is put to the breast as soon as the nipple can be grasped, and an effort made to keep the milk flowing and the breasts soft.

CRACKED NIPPLES

The mother should be told to report if her nipples are tender, and, if so, they should be examined under a magnifying glass for fissures. Early recognition and prompt treatment will result in more rapid healing.

The baby should be taken off that breast for 24 hours if the nipple is tender, and for 48 to 72 hours if cracked. In the interval the milk is expressed manually.

Exposure to an electric lamp 30·5 cm. (12 inches) distant for 20 minutes every six hours will promote healing.

VARIOUS REMEDIES ARE ADVOCATED AND MANY ARE SUCCESSFUL

Ointments are soothing, but must be applied sparingly or the nipple will become soggy, *e.g.* Massé cream. Cicatrin cream contains two antibiotics and is believed to be effective in preventing infection.

The midwife should be aware that cracked nipples often bleed during sucking and cause melæna; the infant may vomit the blood.

DIFFICULTIES DUE TO THE BABY

Serious defects, such as cleft lip or cleft palate, prevent the infant from sucking, but breast milk should be expressed and fed by bottle or spoon. A sore tongue, due to thrush, makes the child disinclined to feed. Snuffles, usually due to a nasal infection, interferes with breathing during sucking. Mentally subnormal babies do not use their tongues effectively.

Premature babies below 2,041 G. (4½ lb.) in weight may be too weak to nurse at the breast and should not be taken out of the warm nursery in any case. They are given expressed breast milk if available.

Asphyxia and intracranial injury may necessitate the administration of oxygen and the infant may be too ill to be moved from the cot.

Jaundice causes lethargy and disinclination to suck.

CONTRA-INDICATIONS TO BREAST FEEDING

PSYCHIATRIC DISORDERS. **Because of the danger of the mother doing harm to her child** and because her own nutritional well-being is particularly important the infant may be weaned. **Severe epilepsy** may also result in injury to the child.

TUBERCULOSIS. **In cases of active tuberculosis the baby should be isolated from the mother** because of the risk of infection by handling.

Should a woman who is nursing her baby become pregnant the baby should be weaned.

Mistaken Reasons for Weaning

The breast milk looks blue and weak, or it doesn't agree with the baby.

The baby is vomiting; crying a lot; having green motions; losing weight.

Menstruation has started again.

THE SUPPRESSION OF LACTATION

This is more easily accomplished when treatment is started on the first day of the puerperium, as when stillbirth occurs.

It is much more difficult to suppress lactation when the baby has been sucking the breast for five or six days.

Some authorities do not approve of giving œstrogens to inhibit lactation. Women of high risk, parity over 35 years of age and particularly when having had a major operative delivery are predisposed to thrombo-embolism: œstrogens may intensify this risk.

1. **The baby is taken completely off the breast and under no circumstances must he be allowed to suck the breast again.**

2. **Neither manual expression nor extraction of milk by breast pump should be performed** even although the breasts are hard, heavy and painful. (*The temptation to do so is great but it must be resisted.*) The removal of milk by either sucking, expression or extraction will stimulate the production of milk.

3. **To prevent stasis in the dependent areas of the breasts** they are elevated by pads of cotton wool and supported by a firm brassière or binder. This must be applied while the woman lies flat on her back holding her breasts inwards and upwards.

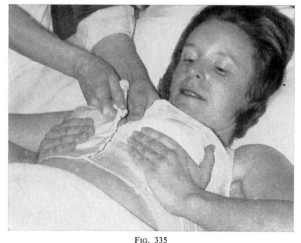

FIG. 335
APPLYING BRASSIÈRE WHEN SUPPRESSING LACTATION.
Breasts elevated; brassière fastened from bottom upwards.
(*Maternity Section, Central Hospital, Irvine, Ayrshire.*)

Applying a firm binder to breasts, without first elevating them, produces stasis in the lower area and this may predispose to mastitis due to multiplication of the organisms that are inevitably present in the breasts.

4. **Analgesics are given for pain,** *e.g.* pentazocine (Fortral) or Panasorb tablets (2).

OVER-FEEDING

Over-feeding is very rare, but is occasionally seen towards the end of the first week. Vomiting may occur and the stools are usually loose and greenish, with undigested curds, the buttocks become excoriated. **The baby behaves as though hungry,** crying and sucking his fist: he may lose weight because of indigestion and frequent loose stools.

Test-weighing (see p. 516) will reveal whether the baby is taking too much food; the infant being weighed after sucking for 5, 10 and 15 minutes. If he gets sufficient milk in five minutes, subsequent feeds will be limited to that time. The interval between feeds should be lengthened.

UNDER-FEEDING

Under-feeding is much more common than over-feeding.

A BREAST-FED BABY MAY BE UNDER-FED IF:
1. **The supply of milk is inadequate. 2. He vomits the milk.**
3. **He does not take the required amount.**

Signs of under-feeding
The baby usually, but not always, cries a great deal and fails to gain weight.
The stools may be dark yellow and small, occasionally they contain mucus: the urine may be insufficient in quantity.

Investigation

Is the tongue clean and the baby eager for food? Does he vomit? Are the stools normal?

The midwife should supervise a feed, watching if the baby is sucking and swallowing properly. Manual expression of both breasts is carried out to see if the baby has emptied the breasts.

TEST-FEEDS

These should be carried out over a period of at least 24 hours. Accurate scales are necessary. The infant is weighed with his clothes on before being fed at the breast and again in the same clothes at the conclusion of the feed, without changing the napkin if it is soiled. The difference between the two weights indicates the amount of milk obtained from the breast.

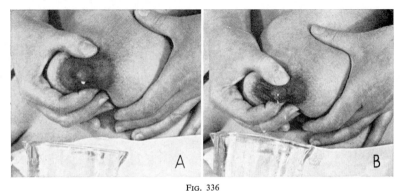

FIG. 336

MANUAL EXPRESSION OF MILK

A, Fingers directed inwards and backwards.
B, Fingers brought slightly forwards without moving them on the skin.

The midwife washes her hands and stands behind the woman, who is sitting up; lifts up the breast by placing the fingers of the right hand under it and the thumb above, grasping the outer border of the primary areola.

With a deep, inward compressing movement she squeezes the reservoirs about thirty times per minute, moving the areola but not the fingers and avoiding touching the nipple. The milk flows from a lactating breast in a steady stream.

TREATMENT OF UNDER-FEEDING

Reassurance should be given and a confident attitude maintained.

Complementary feeds are given temporarily (see p. 517).

If the milk supply is inadequate, an endeavour is made to stimulate the breasts to produce more milk.

1. **See that the woman is having three substantial meals** daily with sufficient proteins and vitamin B with **an adequate but not excessive fluid intake.**

2. **Change to three-hourly** if the baby is on four-hourly feeding.

COMPLEMENTARY FEEDING

This method consists in giving the baby additional milk immediately after a deficient breast feed to complete it. The milk should not be too sweet, or the baby may prefer it to breast milk.

He should be offered 60 ml. (2 oz.) (*or more*) **of reconstituted dried or evaporated milk,** and permitted to take as much as he wants.

SUPPLEMENTARY FEEDING

This method consists in giving milk in place of a breast feed, and should not be used in cases of under-feeding as it tends to inhibit the production of breast milk. Occasionally it may be used if breast feeding is well established and the mother wishes to be absent at feeding time.

BOTTLE FEEDING

There is no perfect substitute for breast milk. Cow's milk can be modified so that the percentage of its constituents approximates to those of human milk, and although it does not completely meet the nutritional requirements of the infant it provides a satisfactory food.

BASIC PRINCIPLES

1. **The milk must be clean and free from organisms.**

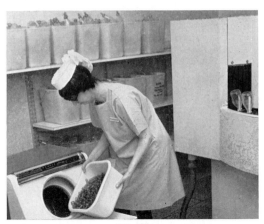

FIG. 337
TEAT AND BOTTLE WASHING MACHINES.
(*Simpson Memorial Maternity Pavilion, Edinburgh.*)

2. **The milk should be modified to meet the infant's requirements** for growth, energy and heat. It ought to be capable of digestion by the infant.

3. **The amount** given should be in a concentration to satisfy the infant's needs without giving an excessive amount of water.

EXPERT ADVICE IS NEEDED

Inexperienced midwives should not take full responsibility for the bottle feeding of babies; no two babies require exactly the same amount and strength of food, and it may be weeks before the infant shows evidence of wrong feeding. It is an expert's job, and much experience of babies and baby-feeding is necessary.

Comparison of Colostrum, Human and Cow's Milk

	% SUGAR	% FAT	% PROTEIN	% MINERALS	% WATER	CALORIES
Colostrum	3·5	2·5	8·5	0·4	85·1	21 per 30 ml.
Human milk	7	3·5	1·5	0·2	87·8	20 per 30 ml.
Cow's milk	4·5	3·5	3·5	0·75	87·75	20 per 30 ml.

The amount of sugar in cow's milk is less than in human milk, therefore sugar must be added.

The percentage of fat in human and cow's milk is the same, but the fat globule in cow's milk is coarse, more difficult to digest and liable to cause vomiting and diarrhœa. On that account " half cream " dried cow's milk is usually given during the first week or two.

There is more than twice as much protein in cow's as in human milk, and the ratio of caseinogen to lactalbumin is six times greater. The tough caseinogen curd of cow's milk must be made more digestible for babies.

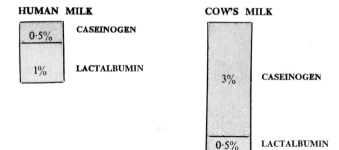

HUMAN MILK — 0·5% CASEINOGEN, 1% LACTALBUMIN. COW'S MILK — 3% CASEINOGEN, 0·5% LACTALBUMIN.

CALCULATION OF AMOUNT OF MILK REQUIRED

The amount given should be regulated by the infant's appetite, as in breast feeding: the active, fretful baby uses up more energy and therefore requires more food than the placid infant.

Babies should not be urged to finish the amount prescribed, or, conversely, if not satisfied, they should be given more food.

Any method of calculating the dietary requirements of an infant is but a guide suitable for the baby who is of average weight for his age: viz. 3·1 kg. (7 lb.) at birth: 3·6 kg. (8 lb.) at one month: 5·4 kg. (12 lb.) at three months.

If a baby weighs 4·5 kg. (10 lb.) at birth, which is the usual weight at six weeks, the food requirements are calculated by splitting the difference between normal birth-weight and actual weight, $7 + 10 = 17 \div 2 = 3·8$ kg. (8½ lb.) Thus the newborn 4·5-kg. (10-lb.) baby is given the amount required by a baby weighing 3·8 kg. (8½ lb.).

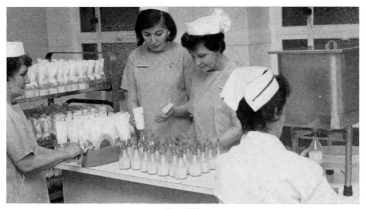

FIG. 338

MILK KITCHEN FOR PREPARATION OF BABIES' FEEDS.
(*Simpson Memorial Maternity Pavilion, Edinburgh.*)

The fluid requirements after the first few days are at least 150 ml. per kg. of body-weight per day. In hot weather or when the stools are loose the infant will require more fluid.

One hundred and ten calories per kg. of body weight per day are said to be required by the newborn infant, but calories alone are not a physiological method of calculating the amount of infant food needed. Thirty millilitres of human or cow's milk = 20 calories; 4 G of sugar = 15 calories.

FORMS OF COWS MILK

Cow's milk is available in 3 forms, dried, evaporated and fresh

Fresh cow's milk is not now recommended as a food for infants under one year old. Modification and sterilization have to be carried out in the home and these may be neither adequate nor accurate. The casein curd is tough, the fat globule large and coarse, so digestive upsets are more common. The essential vitamins and iron are deficient.

DRIED MILK

Dried or powdered milk is produced from fresh cow's milk which is subjected to heat; the fluid being removed by evaporation. The process renders the casein curd and the fat more digestible. The milk powder is free from bacteria; it should be protected from flies by placing the opened carton in a glass jar or tin with a lid.

Sugar has been added to all the proprietary brands of dried milk to bring the carbo-hydrate content up to that of human milk. National dried milk contains no additional sugar so this must be added when the feeds are being made up. 4 G. (one level teaspoon) to 90 ml. water. Vitamin D 100 i.u. per 30 oz. is used to fortify all dried milk baby foods. Some proprietary brands contain added Vitamins A and C, iron and calcium. The only addition to National Dried milk is Vitamin D.

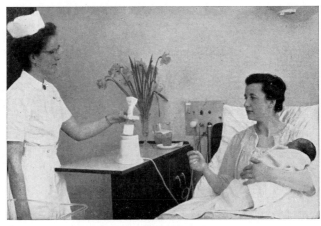

FIG. 339

Individual Dee Gee electric bottle warmer for baby's feed.
(*Obtainable from David Griffin, Wimborne Road, Poole, Dorset.*)
(*Photographed at County Maternity Hospital, Bellshill, Lanarkshire*)

TO RECONSTITUTE DRIED MILK

The scoop provided in the carton must be used to measure the powder. It is essential that the less intelligent mothers are shown how, and understand the importance of accurately measuring the dried milk and the water. (For demonstration see p. 754.) One level measure of powder is added to each 30 ml. water.

(Two mothers used the powder scoop to measure the water with fatal results due to grossly concentrated feeds.)

Sugar must be added to National Dried milk 4 G. (one level teaspoonful) to 90 ml. water.

Each feed should be poured into a separate bottle because if made up in a jug for the day the fat separates out and will not remix. The infant might get all the fat in one feed and be upset.

STRENGTH OF FEEDS

Weight of baby approx. 3,000 G.

The baby is given 20 ml. 10 per cent dextrose = one feed, six to eight hours after birth.

Half strength half cream dried milk may be given 12 hours after birth. 25 ml. = three feeds.

Half cream dried milk 40 ml. is given on the second day = **six feeds.** The amount is increased by 15 ml. daily depending on appetite. If not satisfied when 120 ml are given, full cream dried milk should be introduced by using equal parts of half cream and full cream powder, or by replacing one scoop of half cream by one scoop of full cream powder. The change-over takes 2 days: the baby then being given full cream dried milk. This is usually possible prior to discharge from hospital.

Three-hourly feeds are given to start with = six feeds. When on full cream milk 4 hourly feeds **five feeds** are given. An extra feed at night may be necessary but an effort is made to satisfy the infant during the day time.

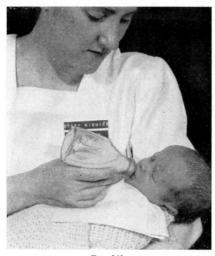

Fig. 340

STUDENT MIDWIFE FEEDING BABY AS INSTRUCTED.

Giving her undivided attention to baby.
Holding bottle " as a pencil ".
Bottle neck full of milk.
Baby's head well supported.
Bib in position.

(*Aberdeen Maternity Hospital.*)

EVAPORATED MILK

This is full cream cows milk that has been condensed by evaporation and fortified by the addition of vitamin D. Sugar has not been added. The fat is in a fine emulsion, the protein curd flocculent, therefore babies digest it readily. Because of its smooth consistency it is preferred by some for naso-gastric feeding.

TO RECONSTITUTE EVAPORATED MILK

To reconstitute milk from the tin to approximately the consistence of full cream cows milk, 1 part of milk is added to 2 parts of water with 4 G. of sugar to every 120 ml. of reconstituted milk.

Further dilution is necessary in feeding the new born: *e.g.* 1 part of evaporated milk and 3 parts of water sugar 4 G. (one level teaspoonful) to 120 ml. of the milk and water mixture or as directed by the pædiatrician.

DISADVANTAGES OF EVAPORATED MILK

The tins are heavy to carry when shopping, bulky for storage and more expensive than dried milk. Contamination by flies can occur if the opened tin is left exposed. (The top of the tin and the tin opener should be washed prior to use.)

30

VITAMIN SUPPLEMENTS

It is advisable to give all babies additional vitamins, beginning on the 14th day, but they need not be introduced into the diet until the infant is coping successfully with the digestion of milk.

COD-LIVER OIL

Four ml. cod-liver oil contains 400 i.u. vitamin D which is the daily amount required to provide adequate protection from rickets.

Mothers should be warned that too much may be harmful. A high intake of vitamin D will cause excess absorption of calcium (hypercalcæmia) with deposition of calcium in the kidneys and walls of blood vessels.

Babies having breast milk should be given 2 ml. cod-liver oil twice daily.

Babies having National Dried Milk (which contains added vitamin D) require 0·5 ml. daily (50 i.u.). Do not give oil in bottle feeds, it adheres to the glass and the baby does not get it all.

ORANGE JUICE

This should be started one week later, giving 4 ml. of fresh orange juice diluted with 15 ml. of water and a few grains of sugar. The daily amount is increased by 4 ml. per month, until the juice of a whole orange is taken. Synthetic vitamin C tablets can be given (one 25 mg. tablet daily).

QUESTIONS FOR REVISION

BREAST FEEDING

How would you persuade a woman to breast feed her baby ? What are the benefits to the baby ? **How would you " fix "** a baby at the breast ? **How often** does the baby go to the breast during the first 3 days ? **How long** should the baby suck at each breast ?

Write not more than 10 lines on: (*a*) prevention and treatment of cracked nipples; (*b*) treatment of engorged breasts; (*c*) the modern attitude to breast feeding; (*d*) advantages of breast feeding.

Define the following terms: colostrum; luteotrophin; lactiferous ducts; search reflex.

How would you differentiate between: (*a*) overfeeding and underfeeding; (*b*) vomiting and possetting; (*c*) weighing and test weighing.

C.M.B.(Eng.) paper.—Describe your routine management of breast feeding in the first ten days of life. What do you understand by the term " engorgement of the breasts." ?

C.M.B.(N. Ireland) paper.—What would make you think that a breast fed baby was being underfed ? How would you deal with this problem ?

C.M.B.(Eng.) paper.—What are the advantages and disadvantages of breast feeding ? How would you assist the mother to achieve success in breast feeding ?

C.M.B.(N. Ireland) paper, 1969.—A primipara has breast-fed her baby while in hospital. What advice would you give her about the feeding and general care of the baby when she returns home on the 9th day.

C.M.B.(Eng.) paper, 1969.—What are the advantages of breast feeding ? Discuss the attitudes of modern mothers to breast feeding.

C.M.B.(N. Ireland) paper, 1969.—Describe the anatomy of the female breast. What physiological changes occur during pregnancy and the puerperium ?

C.M.B.(N. Ireland) paper, 1969.—What do you consider to be the advantages of breast feeding ? Why do you think so few mothers breast feed their infants today ?

C.M.B.(N. Ireland) paper, 1969.—What guidance would you give to a young primipara on infant feeding ?

BOTTLE FEEDING

Discuss the advantages and disadvantages of:

1. Three-hourly, four-hourly and self demand feeding.
2. Fresh cow's milk; dried milk; evaporated milk.

Differentiate between: (*a*) half cream dried milk, full cream dried milk, half strength half cream dried milk; (*b*) complementary and supplementary feeding; (*c*) caseinogen in cows and human milk; (*d*) vitamins A, C and D.

What advice would you give to a mother: (*a*) whose baby cried for long periods during the night ? (*b*) whose baby was bottle fed, appeared to be healthy but was not gaining weight ? How would you apply a supporting breast brassiere while inhibiting lactation ?

C.M.B.(N. Ireland) paper.—What types of artificial foods may be used for a healthy full-term baby ? Describe in detail the preparation of *one* of them.

C.M.B.(N. Ireland) paper.—What detailed feeding instructions would you give to a mother who wishes to feed her ten-day old baby weighing 8 lbs., on Full Cream National Dried Milk ?

C.M.B.(Eng.) paper. 50 word question.—Engorgement of the breasts.

C.M.B.(Eng.) paper. 50 word question.—Cow's milk must be altered for use in infant feeding. How is this done ?

C.M.B.(N. Ireland) paper.—A baby weighs 8 lbs. at birth. How would you organise artificial feeding during the first week of his life. Describe in detail the preparation of one feed.

Low Birth Weight	**Light for Dates**
Premature Baby	*Dysmature Baby*

The management of premature babies, being highly specialized is usually directed by a **pædiatrician.** Nevertheless a grave responsibility rests on the midwife, for the survival of these infants, whose hold on life is slender, depends greatly on expert nursing: because of their immaturity they need special care in regard to environment and feeding. This can be given with greater efficiency in a neonatal intensive care unit where incubators and mechanical monitoring devices are available and skilled midwives and pædiatricians are on constant duty. The first 48 hours are the most dangerous.

In a recent national survey 8 per cent of babies were found to weigh 2500 G. or less.

DEFINITION

The accepted international definition of a premature baby is based on weight— 2,495 G. (5½ lb.) or less—regardless of the estimated period of gestation.

Preterm. This applies to the gestational age of 36 completed weeks or less from the onset of the last menstrual period.

But not all babies of low birth weight are preterm: some are light for dates (dysmature) (see p. 546). Differentiating between the two is important because the treatment and the complications are not similar.

Light for dates babies total approx. one third of all low birth weight babies.

Certain neurological tests which elicit reflex behaviour are utilized; e.g. **the traction reflex:** when the baby is raised, by traction on the arms, the premature does not attempt to raise his head, the light for dates does. **The Moro reflex** may be incomplete or absent in the premature baby:—when the body and head are supported in the supine position and the head is allowed to drop back a cm. or two (with the baby relaxed) he throws out his arms with extension of elbows and fingers.

The plantar skin creases are less well defined in the premature baby when the skin is stretched from toes to heel.

CONDITIONS ASSOCIATED WITH LOW BIRTH WEIGHT

SERIOUS	COMMON	LESS COMMON	
Eclampsia.	**Severe Pre-**	Fetal Malformations :	Hydramnios ;
Antepartum Hæmor-	**eclampsia.**	Maternal Cyanosis ;	Acute Infection.
rhage.	Twins.		

In 50 per cent of cases no cause is apparent. (*Socio-economic factors may be important, e.g. insufficient rest during the last 8 weeks of pregnancy*).

SIGNS OF PREMATURITY

Length, 45·6 cm. (18 inches) or less.	**Skull bones** soft.	Eyes closed.
Weight, 2,495 G. (5½ lb.) or less.	**Skin red** and loose.	*Nails are soft but not always short.*
Sutures and fontanelles wide.	**Lanugo** plentiful.	*Under 36 weeks no plantar creases are visible.*
Pinnæ of ears soft and flat.	**Vernix** scanty.	

Within a few hours the skin is shiny with œdema.

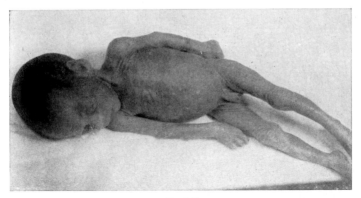

Fig. 341

Premature baby weighing 709 G. (1 lb. 9 oz.) at birth. Weight on discharge at 16 weeks 2,410 G. (5 lb. 5 oz.).

Extension of limbs is common in babies of low birth weight.

(*Simpson Memorial Maternity Pavilion, Edinburgh.*)

Average Weights and Lengths

Weeks	Grammes	Pounds	Centimetres	Inches
28	1,134	2½	35·6	14
32	1,588	3½	40·6	16
36	2,268	5	45·7	18

Eighty per cent of premature babies are over 1,184 G. (4 lb.) in weight.

THE PRINCIPLES OF TREATMENT ARE

1. PREVENTION. 2. GOOD MANAGEMENT DURING LABOUR.
3. EFFICIENT CARE OF THE BABY AT BIRTH.
4. MAINTENANCE OF BODY TEMPERATURE. 5. SUITABLE FEEDING.
6. EXPERT NURSING. 7. AVOIDANCE OF INFECTION.

1. PREVENTION

Because of the serious loss of life in premature babies, an effort should be made to recognize and treat early the medical and obstetrical conditions which induce premature labour. Expectant mothers should be advised regarding good nutrition and to cease outside employment at 28 weeks.

2. GOOD MANAGEMENT DURING LABOUR

When a woman goes into labour prior to the 37th week she should be admitted to hospital.

To avoid depression of the fetal respiratory centre, sedatives of the opium and barbiturate groups should not be used. Cyanosis must be avoided.

An episiotomy is made under local anæsthesia, when the fetus is expected to weigh under 2,268 G. (5 lb.), to shorten the perineal phase and so prevent the intracranial congestion or injury which may occur because of the soft skull bones and wide sutures.

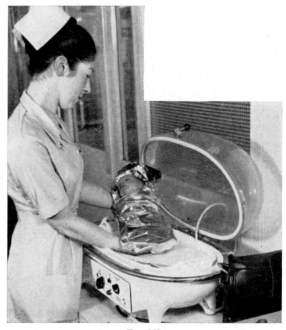

FIG. 342
SILVER SWADDLER PREVENTS LOSS OF HEAT.
(*Neonatal Intensive Care Unit, Royal Maternity Hospital, Rottenrow, Glasgow.*)

Preparations for the Baby

If the woman in premature labour cannot be transferred to hospital, the baby should be admitted to a special baby-care unit if he weighs less than 1,814 G. (4 lb.). It is recommended that a resuscitation team (neonatal Flying Squad), consisting of a pædiatrician and nursery midwife. be available to treat and transport to hospital for further supervision premature babies and other neonatal emergencies.

Wrapping the infant in a Silver Swaddler (aluminium coated plastic) prevents loss of heat if the incubator must be opened en route to suck out mucus from the pharynx.

The portable incubator should have the temperature constantly maintained at 26·6° C. (80° F.) in readiness to transport a baby from labour ward to nursery or from the home to the hospital neonatal resuscitation unit.

3. EFFICIENT CARE OF THE BABY AT BIRTH

WARMTH

The delivery room should be at a temperature of 26·6° C. (80° F.). Two warm towels should be in readiness, one into which the baby is received and the other with

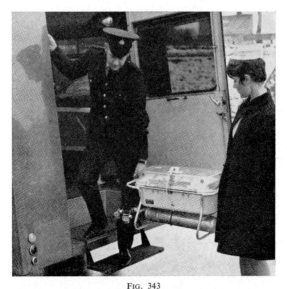

FIG. 343

TRANSPORTING PREMATURE BABY BY AMBULANCE.
(*County Maternity Hospital, Bellshill, Lanarkshire.*)

which to dry him: the head being large must not be exposed while wet. The infant should be wrapped and warm while any necessary treatment is being carried out.

A pædiatrician is present when the baby is expected to weigh less than 1,814 G. (4 lb.) or if not immediately available, a midwife from the neonatal intensive care unit.

ESTABLISHMENT OF RESPIRATION

Preparations should be made to assist in the establishment of respiration, for the respiratory centre in the medulla is immature. The lungs tend to be atelectatic and are not well developed; the diaphragm and chest muscles are weak, therefore the baby is often asphyxiated. Fine mucus catheters are used to clear the air passages, and mucus must be repeatedly removed. The gastric contents may also be aspirated by using a 5-ml. syringe and No. 5 Jaques catheter.

The cord is clamped and cut.

The infant is transferred to the nursery in the portable incubator, placed in an incubator, given oxygen, 30 per cent. if necessary, and allowed to recover from the stress of birth.

Bathing is contra-indicated. There is no need to smear the skin with oil, a procedure that predisposes to the eruption of pustules.

An aqueous solution of vitamin K_1, 1 mg. (Konakion), may be injected intramuscularly to minimize the risk of hæmorrhage. (Some do not approve of giving vitamin K_1.)

4. THE MAINTENANCE OF BODY TEMPERATURE

Premature babies are unable to maintain body temperature because of an immature heat regulating centre in the medulla. Heat production is poor because of the limited food intake and low metabolic rate; heat loss is excessive because of the large surface area, lack of subcutaneous fat and sluggish muscular activity.

The midwife must do all in her power to prevent heat loss at birth or a dangerously low temperature level will be reached. Babies under 1,361 G. (3 lb.) may have a temperature of 33·8° to 34·4° C. (93° to 94° F.) or less within one hour of birth, those weighing 1,814 G. (4 lb.) 35° to 35·5° C. (95° to 96° F.). A fall of two to three degrees occurs even when the baby is wrapped immediately he is born and all precautions taken to avoid heat loss.

No attempt should be made to raise the temperature rapidly (*overheating is harmful*), nor to endeavour to achieve the temperature level of the mature infant. Concern need not be felt when the 1,361 G. (3 lb.) baby maintains a temperature of 35° to 35·5° C. (95° to 96° F.) and the 1,814 G. (4 lb.) 35·5° to 36·1° C. (96° to 97° F.), if the condition is otherwise satisfactory.

INCUBATOR TEMPERATURE

The smaller babies are usually naked so the temperature should be 32·2° C. (90° F.) with relative humidity maintained at 65 per cent. The temperature may be 5 to 10 degrees lower when clothing is worn.

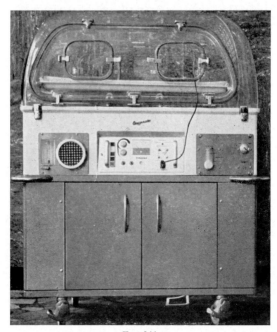

Fig. 344

SERVO-CONTROLLED INCUBATOR (VICKERS).

The air temperature within the incubator is controlled by a thermistor probe which is attached to the baby's abdominal skin. The incubator responds via the thermistor probe to the baby's body temperature.

(*Vickers Ltd., Basingstoke, Hampshire.*)

When incubators are not available the room temperature should be 26·6° C. (80° F.) for the smaller babies and 21·1° C. (70° F.) for the larger ones. A kettle boiling constantly in a small room will provide the required humidity.

The cot temperature should not be higher than 29·4° C. (85° F.) for the clothed infant. In developing countries heat may be provided by the use of three well-wrapped new hot-water bottles in pockets at the sides and foot of the cot; one bottle being refilled every hour.

Electric blankets should be used with great caution if at all, because of the risk of burns and electric shock.

Cooling rooms 15·5° to 18·3° C. (60° to 65° F.) are necessary to acclimatize the baby to ordinary temperature.

CLOTHING

Clothing is necessary for warmth if no incubator is available. Garments must be light in weight and loose in style to permit free movement and facilitate changing. The premature baby's head is large and should be covered. The napkin is laid under the buttocks (not pinned on).

5. FEEDING

The sucking and swallowing reflexes are sometimes poorly developed, and fluid placed in the mouth may run down the trachea. The vomiting and coughing reflexes are also inadequate and regurgitated food is inhaled into the lungs; vomiting must therefore be avoided.

A guide to the daily nutritional and fluid requirements of premature babies: 1·5 kg. in weight excepting those who have respiratory distress syndrome and those who require intravenous therapy.

Simpson Maternity Pavilion

ALL FORMULÆ CONTAIN 5% ADDED GLUCOSE

DAY OF LIFE	DAILY FLUID INTAKE	CALORIES PER KG. PER DAY		G. PROTEIN PER KG. PER DAY	
	ml./kg.	evaporated milk 1-6	dried whole milk 1 scoop -60 ml.	evaporated milk 1-6	dried whole milk 1 scoop -60 ml.
1	75	36	40	1·1	1·3
2	100	48	53	1·4	1·7
3	125	60	66	1·8	2·1
4	150	72	80	2·1	2·6
5	175	84	93	2·5	3·0
6, 7	200	96	106	2·8	3·4
Second week		evaporated milk 1-3	dried whole milk 3 scoops to 120 ml.	evaporated milk 1-3	dried whole milk 3 scoops to 120 ml.
	200	150	140	5·6	5·2
Schedule for feeding a baby 1588 G.					

Feeds are given 3 hourly = 8 feeds.

First week. Evaporated milk 1-6: day 1 = 14 ml.; day 2 = 18 ml.; day 3 = 23 ml.; day 4 = 28 ml.; day 5 = 33 ml.; days 6 and 7 = 37 ml.

Second week: 37 ml. evaporated milk 1-3.

This schedule is only a guide; the volume being increased or decreased depending on how the baby tolerates the feeds.

A simple working rule, that can be used as a guide, is to give **9 ml. of diluted milk per kg. of body-weight** at each feed to start with and gradually increase it.

The amount of food necessary is governed by the baby's appetite, ability to digest the food and general condition.

It is not advisable to increase the amount and the strength of feeds on the same day.

The practice of withholding oral fluid or food for 24 or more hours is no longer approved of: the dehydration and hypoglycæmia that ensues is believed to produce impairment of the cerebral circulation which may adversely affect intellectual function.

Dextrose 10 per cent is given I.V. 72 ml. per kg. bodyweight per 24 hrs. by some pædiatricians to ill babies or those of 1,361 G. (3 lb.) or under.

The feeding of very small premature infants should be undertaken only by skilled experienced nursery midwives.

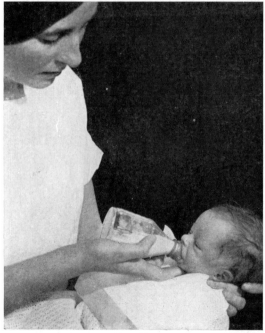

FIG. 345

Note forefinger under chin to assist the up and down movement of
the lower jaw when a baby is reluctant to feed.
(*Aberdeen Maternity Hospital*)

Choice of Milk

Breast milk is ideal, because of its digestibility, but in some cases of premature labour the mother is unable to produce a satisfactory supply of milk, and if pooled breast milk is not available other milk must be used.

Evaporated milk is frequently used because of its smooth consistency for tube feeding: one part of milk to six of water during the first week, then 1-3 dilution.

National Dried Milk Half-cream is also used, starting at half strength: others give diluted full cream dried milk, 1 scoop to 60 ml. during the first week, then 3 scoops to 120 ml.

METHOD OF FEEDING

The method used depends on the size and vitality of the infant and his ability to suck and swallow.

BABIES OVER 2,041 G. (4½ lb.)

After 6 hours these babies may be given breast milk or ½ strength half-cream dried milk (next day full-strength half-cream).

A FEEDING-BOTTLE

This may be used if the baby does not become exhausted by sucking it. An admirable method of holding the bottle, with the forefinger under the tip of the chin to assist the " up and down " movement of the lower jaw is shown in Fig. 345.

BABIES UNDER 2,041 G. (4½ lb.)

Judgment is needed in deciding on the most suitable method of feeding these babies. Many of them suffer from some degree of respiratory distress syndrome, or intracranial injury, and **the effort of feeding may increase cyanosis and induce exhaustion.** The method used should (*a*) reduce exertion, (*b*) avoid any interference with breathing and (*c*) prevent vomiting and inhalation of food.

TUBE FEEDING (*every three or four hours*).

This method meets the preceding requirements, and its use is recommended in the following circumstances:

(*a*) **When the baby weighs 1,588 G. (3½ lb.) or under.**

(*b*) **If sucking or swallowing produces cyanosis or exhaustion.**

(*c*) **If the baby will neither suck nor swallow.**

(*d*) **When the time taken for a feed exceeds 30 minutes.**

(*e*) **In cases of illness,** e.g. respiratory distress, i.e. respiratory rate above 60/min. or intracranial hæmorrhage, in full-term babies.

A midwife without experience in tube feeding should not attempt it before having had a practical demonstration and having carried out the procedure under supervision. The dangers are inhalation pneumonia and over-feeding, both of which are preventable.

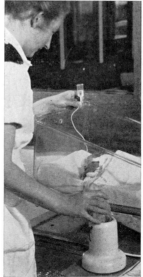

FIG. 346
TUBE FEEDING.
Using Alexa disposable infant feeding set and Dee Gee heater.
(*Aberdeen Maternity Hospital.*)

Midwives are often apprehensive in case they pass the catheter into the trachea. If due care is taken this is unlikely, as the opening of the larynx is very small. The baby would cough and become cyanosed.

Method

The catheter, funnel, milk and measure are sterile. Disposable infant feeding sets, funnel and feeding tube size 10 FG are available. The head of the cot is raised; the baby's arms wrapped in. The neck should be extended not hyperextended.

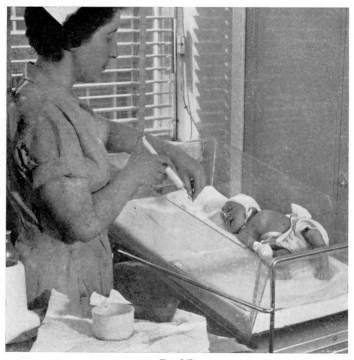

FIG. 347
SISTER GIVING NASO-GASTRIC FEED.
(*Neonatal Intensive Care Unit, Royal Maternity Hospital, Rottenrow, Glasgow.*)

The midwife washes her hands. By depressing the lower jaw the mouth is opened and the empty catheter passed by sight; otherwise it may coil in the pharynx.

When the catheter enters the stomach a slight plop (escaping air) **is heard.** The feed is poured into the funnel, which is lowered or raised to control the rate of flow and not allowed to become empty until the whole feed is given. **When withdrawing the catheter it should be pinched** (near the baby's lips) to avoid fluid dripping into the pharynx, and removed with deliberation, not whisked out.

Sucking lip movements do not necessarily mean that the baby should be permitted to suck a bottle, for unless he is vigorous enough he is liable to collapse. The first attempt at sucking should be short, and if signs of distress develop it should be abandoned at once and resumed again in a few days. *The change from tube to bottle should take about one week.*

NASO-GASTRIC FEEDING

This method is preferred for babies 1,134 G. to 1,588 G. (2½-3lb.) as it carries the least risk of bronchial aspiration.

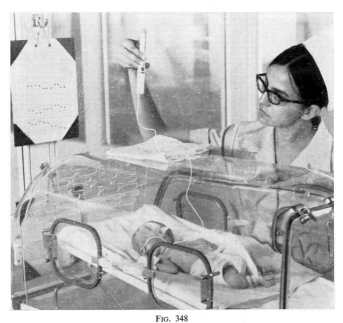

Fig. 348
MIDWIFE GIVING NASO-GASTRIC FEED.

The Argyle naso-gastric tube is brought through an aperture in the top of the incubator. Feeds are given every 15, 30 or 60 minutes and may be continued for 72 hours or longer.
(*Neonatal Intensive Care Unit, Royal Maternity Hospital, Rottenrow, Glasgow.*)

Requirements
1 **Plastic indwelling infant feeding tube.** Luer fitting 53 cm. 3½ to 5 F.G.
1 **Syringe,** 5 or 10 ml: **1 gallipot with sterile water:** receiver and 2 gauze swabs: bottle of milk.

With the head slightly extended, the tube is introduced via the nostril into the stomach (see method of tube feeding above). The tube is attached to the nose and forehead with strips of J. & J. clear tape 1 cm. wide.

Milk is injected by syringe every 1, 2, 3 hours or as directed, and followed by 1 cm. sterile water to rinse the tube. Every 4 days the tube is changed and another inserted into the other nostril.

Some wrap the tube in a gauze swab and place it under a cap worn by the baby. Mitts and cap help to prevent the tube being inadvertently pulled out by the infant.

Cambric mitts are applied with the precaution that no loose threads will wind around the fingers causing gangrene.

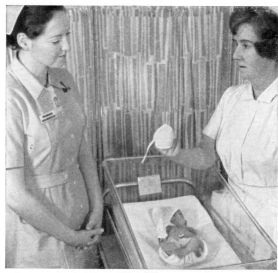

FIG. 349

CAMBRIC MITT THAT AVOIDS INJURY TO BABY'S FINGERS.

Sister stressing the importance of mitts with no loose threads that could wind round baby's fingers as with wool, gauze, lint. A number of babies have lost the terminal phalanx of one finger in this way.

These mitts have a French seam, *i.e.* the two halves are stitched together, turned inside out and stitched again.

(*Neonatal Intensive Care Unit, Royal Maternity Hospital, Rottenrow, Glasgow.*)

INTRAVENOUS FLUIDS

Babies weighing 1,588 G. or less and those suffering from respiratory distress syndrome may be given, at birth, dextrose or fructose 10 per cent intravenously for a few days. The amount administered is approximately 72 ml. per kg. body-weight per day and the flow may be regulated by a micro-infusion roller pump which allows slow rates of flow to be accurately controlled.

An Argyle feeding tube 5 F gauge or a Tizzard catheter is inserted into the umbilical vein. Strict aseptic precautions must be observed. The scalp vein is preferred by some to avoid the risk of infection and thrombosis.

Intravenous fluids are as a rule continued for 24 to 72 hours and the infant is having oral feeds.

PIPETTE FEEDING

This method is not recommended but is sometimes used by midwives not experienced in tube feeding. Only about 0·6 ml. should be given at a time ; this must be swallowed before the next 0·6 ml. is given. It is a slow process, so the milk should be kept warm. The pipette should have a bulbous tip.

GENERAL POINTS ON FEEDING

(*a*) **Scrupulous cleanliness should be observed.**

(*b*) **The baby should be held in the arms** with head and shoulders raised except for tube feeding.

(*c*) **Wind is brought up** by raising baby to the sitting position or by gently rolling him over on to the left hand and rubbing his back with the right hand.

Tube-fed babies do not require to have wind brought up.

(*d*) **After feeds the baby should be laid on his right side,** with the head of the cot raised, for half an hour, to facilitate emptying of the stomach and to allow any vomited milk to run out of his mouth.

(*e*) **An aspirator ought to be readily available** to remove regurgitated milk from the nasopharynx.

(*f*) **The amount of food actually taken should be recorded** not the amount offered.

VITAMIN REQUIREMENTS

The premature baby requires vitamin A 300 μg. daily **(1,000 i.u.) vitamin D 800 i.u. daily after the second week** (*this amount must not be exceeded because of the risk of hypercalcæmia*).

To avoid the risk of aspirating oily vitamin preparations, water miscible or concentrated forms should be used.

Vitamin C is given as early as the fourth day, and Celin or Redoxin, 25 mg. b.i.d., is tolerated better than orange juice which can be given when 2,275 G. (5 lb.) weight is reached. A useful preparation containing vitamins A, B, C and D is Abidec, 0·125 ml. is given on the 10th day if baby is feeding well, and increased until 0·25 ml. is being given twice daily.

Protovite (vitamins A, B_1, B_2, C, D) 7 drops daily is used in some centres.

Folic acid 1 mg. daily is given to infants 1,588 G. or less starting at 12 days and finishing at 12 weeks.

6. EXPERT NURSING

Infinite patience and devoted care are essential; meticulous attention to detail imperative. The midwife must understand the basic principles of treatment, if she is to carry them out intelligently and be able in the doctor's absence to change or withhold treatment when necessary.

All changes should be made tentatively and gradually whether in feeding or the environmental temperature.

The infant should be handled as little as possible and with great gentleness; dexterity comes with practice.

The baby should lie on alternate sides following feeds: a folded towel behind the back helps to maintain position which should be changed at hourly intervals.

It is advisable to allow a period of rest between undressing and feeding, as the necessary handling, followed by the effort of sucking and swallowing, may produce cyanosis and exhaustion.

The cord is swabbed four-hourly with Hibitane in spirit: Ster Zac powder is applied.
Daily the face and buttocks are washed.

MOTHERING

Even tiny babies thrive better when cuddled. The mother should be permitted to do this, but if she is not available this should be done by the midwife as soon as the baby is well established. While giving devoted care nursery midwives must avoid being too possessive as some mothers resent this.

OBSERVATION

During the critical first 48 hours the small baby needs constant supervision.

Prompt recognition, accurate observation and timely reporting of abnormal signs will enable the doctor to interpret their significance and prescribe the appropriate and often life-saving treatment.

(*a*) COLOUR.

Cyanosis, greyness, pallor, jaundice should be reported.

(*b*) RESPIRATIONS.

The respirations may be 50 to 60 per minute recorded when quiet, sometimes shallow, frequently irregular and occasionally Cheyne Stokes.

Any sudden difficulty in breathing should arouse suspicion of food or vomitus having been inhaled; aspiration of the naso-pharynx should be carried out and the baby held upside down if necessary.

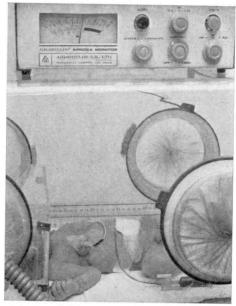

FIG. 350

APNOEA MONITOR ON TOP OF INCUBATOR, WITH ELECTRODES
ATTACHED TO BABY'S CHEST.

Perspex box over baby's head to achieve accurate regulation
of O_2 and high humidity (from nebuliser).

(*Simpson Memorial Maternity Pavilion, Edinburgh.*)

ATTACKS OF APNŒA SHOULD BE REPORTED AT ONCE

Such episodes lasting over 30 seconds or recurring at frequent intervals are of serious importance. They may be associated with low levels of calcium or glucose in the blood.

Flicking the sole of the foot or directing a stream of oxygen on the face will usually stimulate respiration.

The airway is cleared and if breathing does not start an endotracheal tube is passed and a mechanical ventilator used if necessary. The infant is nursed in an incubator with 30 to 40 per cent oxygen.

Apnoea alarm mattresses give a bleep signal when non-breathing episodes arise.

Apnœa monitors with 2 leads attached to the baby's chest sound an alarm when breathing stops.

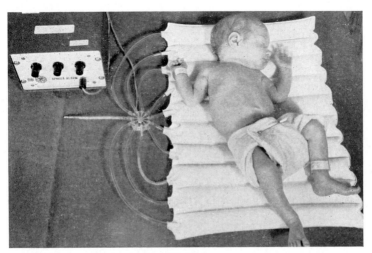

Fig. 351

APNOEA ALARM MATTRESS.
(Neonatal Intensive Care Unit, Aberdeen Maternity Hospital.)

(c) TEMPERATURE.

The temperature is taken morning and evening, with a low-reading thermometer, per rectum, axilla, or groin ; the usual range is 35·5° to 36·1° C. (96° to 97° F.). If below 34·4° C. (94° F.) or above 37·2° C. (99° F.) the temperature is taken four-hourly.

(d) STOOLS.

The stools are inspected, their frequency and consistency noted : meconium tends to persist for three or four days.

(e) ŒDEMA.

Œdema of the face, abdomen and legs is common; if severe, this should be reported

(f) WEIGHT-GAIN

Premature babies gain weight slowly and very little useful information is obtained from repeated weighing during the first week. Retention of tissue-fluid causes weight-gain, and this may give a misleading impression of well-being; when such fluid is excreted weight-loss occurs.

It would be reasonable to weigh the baby after birth, as soon as his condition warrants the handling involved, then twice weekly.

The midwife with limited experience of premature babies may become perturbed at loss of weight, or failure to gain, and may be tempted to overfeed him. Signs of well-being, other than weight-gain, are recognizable (see favourable signs).

Babies of 1,361 G. (3 lb.) regain their birth-weights in two to three weeks.

Babies of 1,814 G. (4 lb.) regain their birth-weights in one to two weeks.

(g) FAVOURABLE SIGNS

Pink colour with absence of cyanosis.

Good muscle tone, increasing vigour in movements.

Hearing the cry in very small babies, lusty crying in larger ones.

Eagerness for food; gain in weight.   Lessening of œdema.

(h) LESS FAVOURABLE SIGNS

1. CYANOSIS

This may be due to some serious condition such as respiratory distress syndrome, intracranial injury, or both.   **Increasing cyanosis should be reported at once.**

Greyness is due to a combination of cyanosis and pallor, and when the baby is limp, indicates collapse, extreme exhaustion or severe infection.

Fleeting cyanotic attacks may follow activities such as sucking and swallowing, or by being chilled, handled inexpertly, or too much.

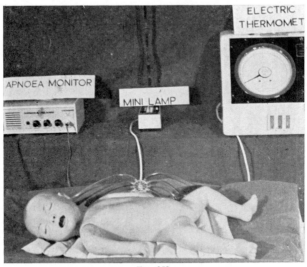

Fig. 352

Equipment for intensive care of premature babies.
(*Aberdeen Maternity Hospital.*)

2. RESPIRATORY DISTRESS

Tachypnœa (above 60 per min.).

Cyanosis of face and body, or grey colour with cyanosis of lips, hands and feet.

Indrawing of lateral chest wall.   Inspiratory recession of sternum.

Dyspnœa and irregular respiratory rhythm: periods of apnœa.

Moist grunting respirations (expiratory): head may be extended.

OXYGEN THERAPY

Midwives should be aware of the potential dangers in administering oxygen in concentrations of over 30 per cent.   Blindness in premature babies due to retrolental fibroplasia appears to be related to the administration of oxygen; nevertheless the baby must get sufficient oxygen to relieve cyanosis.   The concentration should be reduced to the lowest that will maintain a pink colour.

REGULATION OF OXYGEN CONCENTRATION.

This should be carried out at four-hourly intervals as a routine measure to ensure that the concentration does not exceed 30 per cent.   The Beckman analyser is preferred by some pædiatricians.

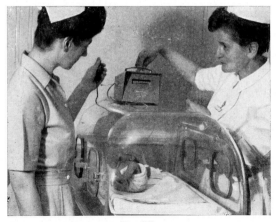

Fig. 353

BECKMAN PORTABLE OXYGEN ANALYSER.

Sister demonstrating use of the analyser.   A connecting piece of rubber tubing is inserted into the incubator.   Student midwife will squeeze rubber bulb 5 times to withdraw air from the incubator at level of baby's face.   Sister will press button and read the oxygen percentage on the gauge.

(*Neonatal Pædiatric Unit, Royal Maternity Hospital, Rottenrow, Glasgow.*)

The most accurate method of controlling oxygen therapy is to measure the partial pressure of oxygen in arterial blood and to adjust the inspired oxygen concentration accordingly.   An Argyle feeding tube $3\frac{1}{2}$ F.G. is introduced through an umbilical artery into the aorta with strict aseptic precautions; then sutured in position.

Samples of blood 0·3 ml. are withdrawn into a heparinized syringe and analysed. For convenience a 3-way tap is attached to the catheter which is flushed after the sample has been obtained and kept filled with a heparinised saline solution.

Routine antibiotic therapy with Ampicillin and Cloxacillin is given on account of the risk of infection.

Oxygen withdrawal should be done gradually by reducing the amount of oxygen by 0·25 ($\frac{1}{4}$) litre every few hours.

7. AVOIDANCE OF INFECTION

Infection is one of the greatest dangers to premature babies, and is preventable. In addition to the precautions taken to avoid infection of all newborn babies (p. 562), the following are recommended for prematures.

Hand washing is vitally important. Phisohex may be used to wash hands between handling each baby and always after changing napkins and before feeding. Paper or other individual towels should be used.

Feeds should be prepared and given under conditions similar to surgical asepsis; midwives who change napkins should not feed babies.

Disposable napkins are placed in destructible containers and removed from the nursery as soon as possible.

The value of wearing masks is questioned by many pædiatricians except when surgical procedures are being undertaken.

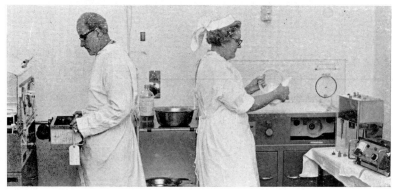

Fig. 354

CLEANING INCUBATORS.

Electrician replacing motor after soaking in tank of disinfectant.   Nursing auxiliary spends 65 minutes washing each incubator.

(*Simpson Memorial Maternity Pavilion, Edinburgh.*)

PSEUDOMONAS ÆRUGINOSA *(Pyocyanea)*

The pyocyanea group of organisms is causing serious infections in premature babies: urinary, gastro-intestinal and other lesions. Pseudomonas aeruginosa have been found in incubators, aspirators and resuscitating machines; humidity and moisture favour growth. They are resistant to the hexochlorophane antiseptics. Sudol (phenol 50 per cent) is bactericidal to pyocyanea.

DISINFECTION OF INCUBATORS

The inside of the incubator should be cleaned and the water changed daily; they should be replaced every week and on discharge of the baby, in order to cleanse and disinfect them thoroughly after which they are aired for 48 hours. Cleansing should always precede disinfection because gases will not penetrate " dirt." An incubator provides an ideal environment for organisms as well as for premature babies.

INSTRUCTION OF MOTHERS

Before the infant is discharged the mother should be given repeated and adequate instruction in feeding, bathing and the general care of her infant. She should be shown how to give iron and vitamin supplements, and advised on how to avoid respiratory and gastro-intestinal infections.

Some hospitals have furnished a room in which the mother can reside with her baby for a few days while gaining supervised experience under home-like conditions: an admirable educational project.

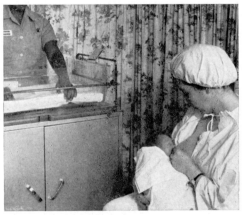

FIG. 355

Discharged mother of premature baby visits daily to feed and maintain contact with her baby.
(Royal Maternity Hospital, Rottenrow, Glasgow.)

DISORDERS OF PREMATURE BABIES

RESPIRATORY DISTRESS SYNDROME

This condition occurs mainly in premature babies weighing less than 1,588 G. (3½ lb.) at birth, also some babies of diabetic mothers and those delivered by Cæsarean section. In fatal cases hyaline membrane is found plastered on the smaller bronchioles and on the alveolar ducts.

Atelectasis occurs due to failure of the alveolar cells to produce surfactant: hyaline membrane develops and this impairs alveolar gas exchange.

Biochemical abnormalities ensue—respiratory and metabolic acidosis, a rise in serum potassium and low-blood-oxygen concentration.

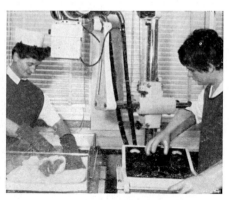

Fig. 356

Portable X-ray used for baby with respiratory distress. Note leaded protective apron and mitts worn by sister.

(*Neonatal Pædiatric Unit, Royal Maternity Hospital, Rottenrow, Glasgow.*)

SIGNS

The baby may be apparently well at birth, but difficulty in establishing respiration is more common.

Within the first hour the respirations tend to become laboured, moist and rapid, with expiratory grunting and marked intercostal and sternal recession: a respiratory rate of over 60, one hour after birth, is suspicious.

A chest X-ray is taken as an aid to diagnosis and characteristic ground glass mottling of the lungs and the unduly clear outline of the bronchial tree is manifest.

Cyanosis becomes pronounced, and if untreated respiratory distress increases, attacks of apnœa ensue, with exhaustion, and within about 48 hours the infant may die.

Acidotic breathing is deep and rapid, with a grey colour and perspiration.

SILVERMAN RETRACTION SCORING

This method is concerned with the degree of retraction; in cases of respiratory distress, a score of 10 at a single observation indicates maximal retraction: a serious state of affairs. **The criteria A, B, C, D, E, are scored 0—1—2** depending on the severity.

A.	**See-saw sinking of upper chest** with rising abdomen .	2
B.	**Marked sinking of intercostal spaces** on inspiration .	2
C.	**Marked xiphoid retraction**	2
D.	**Chin descends,** lips apart	2
E.	**Expiratory grunt audible**	2

$\overline{10}$ = serious

Absence of all of these signs would give a score of 0 = favourable.

Sternal recession may persist for days after respiratory distress syndrome.

Treatment of Respiratory Distress Syndrome

1. **The infant is nursed in a warm incubator with 30 to 40 per cent oxygen and high humidity.**

Suction to clear the airway is essential.

2. **Umbilical arterial and venous catheterization is carried out** as soon as the clinical diagnosis of respiratory distress syndrome is made, *i.e.* one or two hours after birth.

Into one of the umbilical arteries an Argyle feeding tube $3\frac{1}{2}$ F.G., with 3-way tap, is inserted. By syringe blood samples are obtained for the estimation of pH, PCO_2, $PaCO_2$, base excess (see p. 792) and electrolytes as required. From the findings

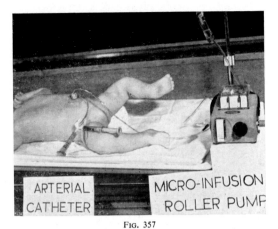

Fig. 357

Monitoring Blood Gases.

(*Neonatal Intensive Care Unit, Aberdeen Maternity Hospital.*

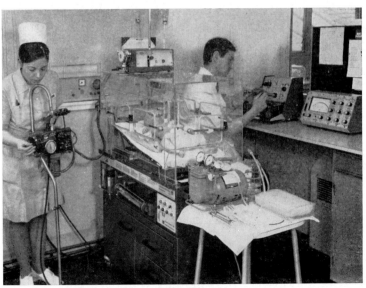

Fig. 358

Treatment of Baby with Respiratory Distress Syndrome.

Baby in Draeger incubator: Pædiatrician carrying out blood-gas determination.

Resuscitating equipment: Dia-Pump for suction, in foreground; electrocardiograph monitor behind nurse who is adjusting Bird mark 8 respirator. Peristaltic pump for accurate control of slow drip intravenous infusion, on top of incubator.

(*Neonatal Intensive Care Unit, Royal Maternity Hospital, Rottenrow, Glasgow.*)

respiratory and metabolic acidosis are diagnosed and rectified; oxygen therapy accurately controlled.

Into the umbilical vein an Argyle feeding tube 5 F.G. is introduced for the administration of fluid, fructose, sod. bicarb and other electrolytes.

The Astrup micro-apparatus permits calculation of the pH of the blood and other biochemical factors in 30 minutes.   Acidosis and other disturbances can be combated promptly by the administration of fructose 10 per cent and sodium bicarbonate 5 to 8·4 per cent.   The I.V. drip is regulated by means of a peristaltic pump the amount usually being 72 ml./kg body-weight/24 hours.   Some give sod. bicarb and fructose via the scalp vein.

3. **No oral food for 6 or more hours.**   4. **Avoidance of over-feeding.**

5. **Removal of excess mucus.**

6. **Turning the infant from side to side** at hourly intervals and supporting him in the position that affords greatest respiratory ease.   Clothing must not impede respiration.

7. **Administration of antibiotics.** Ampiclox, which is a combination of ampicillin 25 mg. and cloxacillin, 50 mg. in each ampoule, is given intramuscularly 6-hourly for 5 to 7 days.

8. **The midwife records the baby's pulse rate, temperature and respirations 4-hourly;** the incubator temperature, hourly.   Warmth is essential.

INFECTIONS

Infections of the respiratory tract and pneumonia due to inhalation of food are serious.   Thrush can be fatal to premature infants.   Gastro-enteritis is particularly lethal.

ŒDEMA

Œdema in which the tissues are hard is sometimes present in small premature babies. This is probably due to electrolyte imbalance, and immaturity of kidney function.

JAUNDICE

Jaundice is more severe and prolonged in premature babies and when persistent over 36 hours the serum bilirubin test is made.   Earlier feeding of premature babies has reduced the need for replacement transfusion.

PHOTOTHERAPY

To reduce hyper-bilirubinaemia the baby with " jaundice of prematurity " is exposed (naked) to high density fluorescent light.   The light chamber attached to the roof of the incubator emits " blue light " (from the violet end of the spectrum) and a fall of about 3-4 mg./100 ml. serum bilirubin can be expected after 12 hours' exposure.

This treatment is not adequate for the overwhelming jaundice of Rh hæmolytic disease but is occasionally used when there is delay in giving a replacement transfusion.

Phototherapy should be commenced as soon as possible and the hours of exposure recorded.   The baby should be turned at intervals and the eyes must be protected by a black shield or a bandage.   To avoid hypothermia adequate warmth and monitoring of body and cot temperatures are necessary.

HYPOCALCÆMIA

In premature babies fed on cow's milk the blood calcium may fall below the safe level of 9 mg./100 ml. **Signs:** Fine muscular twitching of fingers, waving arm movements; a high pitched cry. After a period of agitation the infant is pale, exhausted, limbs straightened. Between attacks the baby's appearance is normal. The response to calcium is rapid. If below 6 mg./100 ml. calcium gluconate is given by slow injection I.V. If between 6 and 8 mg./ 100 ml. a calcium syrup is prescribed.

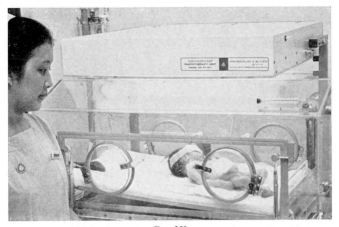

Fig. 359
PHOTOTHERAPY UNIT.
(*Simpson Memorial Maternity Pavilion, Edinburgh.*

ANÆMIA

The small premature baby is deprived of the store of iron that the mature infant obtains during the last 12 weeks of intra-uterine life. This state of affairs is rectified before the fourth or fifth month unless illness supervenes.

Some authorities estimate the hæmoglobin at birth, then every two weeks and, if it is less than 7·4 G. (50 per cent), a blood transfusion is given.

Because of the possibility of megaloblastic anæmia folic acid is given to babies weighing under 1,588 G. in some centres.

The administration of iron is of no value until the second month of life as it is not utilized for hæmoglobin formation before that time, but it is imperative that iron supplements are given after the fourth week and continued throughout the first year of life.

Ferric ammonium citrate, 60 mg., or Ferrous Sulphate, 30 to 60 mg. are given daily, starting with smaller doses to avoid digestive upsets. Fersamal syrup, 2 to 4 ml., is well tolerated. Sytron, 2 ml. daily, is suitable for small babies. **Iron should always be given after feeds to avoid gastric irritation.**

RICKETS

This condition is liable to occur in premature babies so vitamin D must be given after the second week to aid the absorption of calcium and maintain the concentration of phosphorus.

RETROLENTAL FIBROPLASIA

This serious eye condition, in which an opaque membrane forms behind the lens **resulting in blindness,** occurs in premature babies under 2,041 G. (4½ lbs.) in weight. **The iris changes in colour** from fetal blue to a grey or a dull brown.

The cause is related to the **administration of concentrations of oxygen above 40 per cent over an extended period.** The skilful administration of oxygen has decreased the incidence of this catastrophe in recent years.

LIGHT FOR DATES *(Dysmaturity)*

The term " small for dates " or " light for dates " sometimes known as " dysmaturity " refers to mature babies born after the 37th week of pregnancy weighing less than 2,500 G.: the birth weight is below the tenth percentile for its estimated maturity, this being obtained from a graph (see Fig. 362). This concept has been extended to include premature babies who may also be small for their dates.

The condition reflects intra-uterine malnutrition and growth retardation of the fetus, which may be due to placental dysfunction, as might occur in pre-eclampsia, essential hypertension and diabetes.

CLINICAL FEATURES DURING PREGNANCY

Small Baby Syndrome. After the 30th week, on abdominal palpation, the fetus appears to be small for dates and does not increase in size at the normal rate. The amount of liquor amnii is below average and maternal weight and abdominal girth are stationary.

Urinary œstriol assays are made after the 34th week to assess feto-placental vitality.

Ultrasonic cephalometry is employed to measure fetal growth rate. If the bi-parietal diameter does not show a normal increase, intra-uterine growth retardation is suspected.

Fetal blood sampling and **electrocardiograph monitoring** of the fetal heart are usually advisable during labour. Caesarean section may be necessary.

DIAGNOSIS OF LIGHT FOR DATES BABY AT BIRTH

It is imperative that the midwife recognizes the light for dates baby early at birth so that treatment can be given without delay.

(*a*) **A history of pre-eclampsia** during pregnancy would arouse suspicion.

(*b*) **If the small baby syndrome syndrome had been suggested.**

(*c*) **The clinical appearance of the baby.**

The skin is dry and wrinkled giving a wizened " old man " look in severe cases. The baby is long and thin.

The breasts are more developed than in the premature baby: a nodule of breast tissue being palpable.

The plantar creases are well defined on stroking the sole of the foot from toes to heel and the Moro and the traction reflexes are present. In the premature baby they are not.

Gross discrepancy between the weights of twin babies, one 10 per cent less than the other is strongly suggestive that the smaller baby is light for dates.

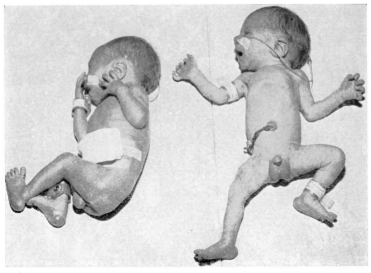

FIG. 360

| Low Birth Weight Baby. | Light for Dates Baby. |
| 30 weeks' gestation 1,474 G. | 39 weeks' gestation 1,474 G. |

(*Simpson Memorial Maternity Pavilion, Edinburgh.*)

COMPLICATIONS

Asphyxia. There is a high incidence of asphyxia but respiratory distress syndrome does not occur as in the premature baby.

Hypoglycæmia. This is a very hazardous state that must be diagnosed and dealt with at once because if low blood glucose persists for more than 36 hours it may cause permanent brain damage. Delayed or low glucose feeds favour hypoglycæmia.

Hypothermia. Light for dates babies are more liable to hypothermia especially if environmental warmth is inadequate and feeding delayed.

TREATMENT OF POTENTIAL HYPOGLYCÆMIA

1. Dextrostix Glucose Screening Test

The midwife carries out this test in suspected babies within 2 hours of birth and if negative, every six hours for 48 hours. The risk of hypoglycæmia is even greater on the second day.

Blood is obtained by heel prick. The foot should be warm; the heel cleansed with Hibitane 0·5 per cent in spirit 70 per cent and dried. With a sterile disposable pricker a puncture 3 mm. deep is made parallel to the sole, avoiding bone. One large drop of blood is allowed to drip on to the reagent area and after exactly 60 seconds it is washed off. The strip area is compared with the colour chart according to instructions on the bottle. If the result is under 45 mg., the lowest reading on the chart, the doctor does a blood glucose estimation.

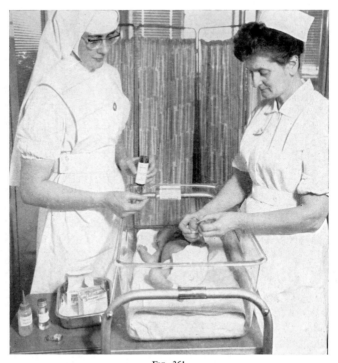

Fig. 361

Dextrostix Blood Glucose Screening Test.

Sister pricks heel to obtain blood. Student midwife holds reagent strip. Note watch on
table for accurate timing.

(*Neonatal Intensive Care Unit, Royal Maternity Hospital, Rottenrow, Glasgow.*)

2. Early Feeding

The baby should be given a feed of 10 per cent dextrose within 3 hours after birth;
repeat in 3 hours then give two feeds ½ strength half cream milk with 10 per cent
dextrose.

Signs of Established Hypoglycæmia

The baby is jittery; twitching or convulsions may occur; apnoeic episodes are
common; muscle tone is poor, the baby is lethargic and reluctant to feed.

TREATMENT OF HYPOGLYCÆMIA

When the blood level glucose is below 20 mg./100 ml. intravenous dextrose 10 per
cent solution is given by I.V. constant infusion pump or micro-drip set to achieve an
accurate fluid and glucose intake.

The response is usually rapid, and oral feeds with 10 per cent dextrose are recommended
before the I.V. infusion is discontinued.

Light for dates babies are on the " at risk " register and their mental development
followed closely.

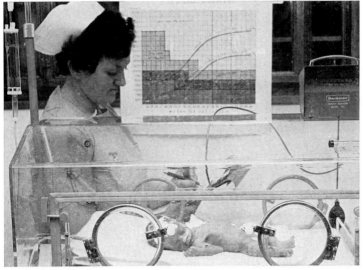

FIG. 362

" Light for Dates " Infant Receiving 10 per cent Dextrose by intravenous scalp-vein infusion in addition to milk feeds to correct hypoglycæmia. The wall chart indicates the appropriate birth weight for gestational age of normally grown infants.

(*Neonatal Intensive Care Unit, Simpson Memorial Maternity Pavilion, Edinburgh.*)

THE BABY OF THE DIABETIC MOTHER

Expert care is needed in looking after these babies, as the mortality rate is high during the first few days of life. The infant is sometimes excessively large, and may weigh 4,536 G. (10 lb.) although only of 37 weeks' gestation. Besides being fat and flabby, he is overgrown, but in spite of size and weight the midwife must remember that **this baby is premature** and requires special care.

The first 48 hours are the most hazardous; inhalation of regurgitated stomach contents may be an avoidable cause of respiratory complications. Respiratory distress syndrome may occur. The baby's condition, which at birth appears to be good, deteriorates in a matter of hours; the lungs fill with fluid, and foamy mucus exudes from the nose and mouth.

Lung expansion is poor, the breathing rapid and laboured with marked indrawing of the lower ribs and sternum on inspiration, and an audible grunt or moan on expiration; the infant may become cyanosed or limp and pale.

MANAGEMENT
PREVENTION OF RESPIRATORY COMPLICATIONS

As soon as the child is born, and before the cord is severed, mucus is aspirated from the throat and nose. At the Simpson Maternity Hospital gastric suction is no longer considered to be necessary. The infant is dried, received into a warm towel by an

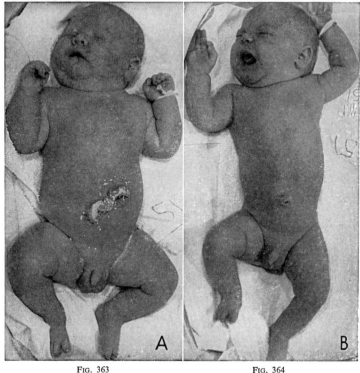

Fig. 363   Fig. 364

Baby of diabetic mother.

Weight 4,875 G. (10 lb. 12 oz.) at birth.   Weight 4,200 G. (9 lb. 4 oz.) on eighth day,
                                              a loss of 690 G. (1½ lb.).

experienced nursery midwife and placed in an incubator with a humidified environmental temperature of 30 to 32·2° C. (86 to 90° F.). Oxygen of adequate concentration
to relieve any existing cyanosis is administered as required.

Vitamin K₁ (Konakion), 1 mg., is given by intramuscular injection.

A marked and rapid fall in blood glucose, from over 100 mg. per cent to as low as
15 mg. per cent occurs within two hours of birth. When signs suggestive of hypoglycæmia (twitching and limpness) are associated with a " true glucose " reading
below 30 mg. per cent, or by Dextrostix, after 12 hours, measures are taken to raise
the blood glucose, but if the condition of the infant does not improve, blood serum
is examined for abnormally high potassium and low calcium concentrations. *Intravenous dextrose solution* 10 *per cent is given into a scalp vein which will remain patent
for three or four days if carefully managed. Blood glucose and potassium levels are
estimated every six hours while the drip is being given. Over-hydration should be
avoided.*

The infant is turned from side to side at hourly intervals, otherwise left undisturbed
as far as possible. A midwife sits constantly at the cot-side removing mucus when
necessary, observing the colour, and condition in general and recording respirations

and the apex beat as directed by the pædiatrician. Equipment for intubation should be readily available.

Jaundice may develop after the first day. Phototherapy can be used and may lessen the need for blood transfusion.

Every precaution must be taken to prevent infection. These babies perspire a great deal, which may predispose to the staphylococcal infections so prevalent in the folds of skin and on their boggy scalps. Ster Zac powder has proved to be effective.

They pass large quantities of urine and lose weight rapidly (*i.e.* 690 G. in one week).

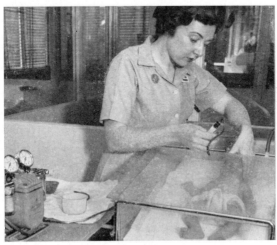

FIG. 365

GASTRIC ASPIRATION

| 10 ml. syringe. | 14 F.G. Warne catheter. |
| Gauze swab. | Gallipot for aspirate. |

Dia-Pump in readiness for tracheal aspiration of mucus or vomitus.
(*Neonatal Paediatric Unit, Royal Maternity Hospital, Glasgow.*)

Most babies can be transferred to a cot on the fifth day.

These babies are not diabetic, but there is a slightly higher incidence of diabetic children from diabetic parents.

FEEDING

Feeding is directed by the pædiatrician. After a period of 2 hours a 10 per cent solution of dextrose is given (10 ml. per kg. body weight per feed). Milk feeds are advocated earlier than formerly: as soon as the baby is hungry, and every 3 or 4 hours: half cream dried milk with 10 per cent dextrose.

A midwife experienced in the handling of premature infants gives all feeds during the first week, because over-feeding and vomiting must be avoided to prevent aspiration of food.

If not inclined to suck or distressed by so doing, naso-gastric feeding is resorted to.

Breast feeding is not as a rule successful; the babies are inclined to be lethargic and are not usually fit to go to the breast for five or six days. Furthermore, premature birth militates against the production of a good supply of milk.

QUESTIONS FOR REVISION

PREMATURE BABY

What percentage of babies are of low birth weight ? How could a midwife try to prevent premature labour ? Why is delayed feeding no longer practised ? How would you transfer a premature baby 20 miles to hospital ? What incubator temperature is advisable for a baby 1,361 G. ?

Write 10 lines on: (1) advice to a mother on taking her baby home weighing 2,500 G.; (2) incubator nursing; (3) prevention of infection; (4) feeding a baby weighing 1,361 G.

For what reason may the following drugs be given to premature babies: Konakion; Redoxin; Sytron; Abidec ?

For what reason might the following appliances be used and what are the midwives' responsibilities: (1) Beckman oxygen analyser; (2) apnœa monitor; (3) silver swaddler; (4) constant I.V. infusion pump; (5) phototherapy unit; (6) arterial catheter ?

Why are the following carried out: (1) Silverman retraction scoring; (2) positive pressure respiration ?

What do you suspect from the following observations and what would you do: (1) baby twitching; (2) cyanosed: (*a*) with frothy mucus (*b*) after a feed; (3) apnœic episode lasting 15 seconds; (4) respirations 80 per minute; (5) inspiratory recession.

Discuss as a means of preventing infection: (*a*) mask wearing; (*b*) use of disposable napkins; (*c*) use of pHisoHex on baby's skin; (*d*) the method you prefer in cleaning incubators.

Why may premature babies develop the following ? What can be done to prevent them ? (*a*) Anæmia; (*b*) rickets; (*c*) retrolental fibroplasia; (*d*) kernicterus; (*e*) hypothermia.

What precautions would you take during premature labour to preserve the life of the fetus ?

Why should an inexperienced midwife not take charge of the feeding of a premature baby ? How would you (*a*) pass the naso-gastric tube ? (*b*) use a pipette ?

What would you note and record regarding a premature baby ? What are you responsibilities when administering oxygen ?

C.M.B.(Scot.) paper.—What are the risks associated with prematurity ? Describe the management of a premature baby weighing 1,680 grams (3½ lb.) at birth.

C.M.B.(Scot.) paper.—Describe the respiratory distress syndrome and its management.

C.M.B.(N. Ireland) paper.—What are the chief risks to a baby in having been born prematurely ? In what way (apart from prevention of prematurity) can these risks be reduced ?

C.M.B.(Eng.) paper. 100 word question.—" Small for dates " babies.

C.M.B.(Eng.) paper. 100 word question.—Respiratory distress syndrome.

C.M.B.(Eng.) paper.—Describe the care of a baby weighing 1,580 grams (approximately 3½ lb.) at birth, for the first 10 days of its life.

C.M.B.(N. Ireland) paper.—What are the special risks to which a premature baby is exposed ? Describe the nursing care of such an infant.

C.M.B.(Eng.) paper.—Discuss the main reasons for an increased mortality in premature infants.

C.M.B.(Scot.) paper.—Describe the nursing care of a premature infant weighing 1,600 G. during the first week of life.

C.M.B.(Scot.) paper, 1970.—Describe the care of a premature baby.

LIGHT FOR DATES BABY

What do you mean by a light for dates baby ? In what conditions would you: (*a* anticipate; (*b*) recognize a light for dates baby ? What complications may arise ? Describe the feeding of such a baby. What is the normal newborn blood glucose level ?

Write not more than 10 lines on: (1) the Dextrostix test; (2) signs and treatment of hypoglycæmia; (3) nursing care of a light for dates baby.

For what reasons are the following carried out during pregnancy: œstriol assay; ultrasonic cephalometry ?

Define: (*a*) intra-uterine-growth retardation; (*b*) " at risk " register; (*c*) small baby syndrome; (*d*) hypoglycæmia; (*e*) hypothermia.

BABY OF DIABETIC MOTHER

Describe the appearance of the baby of a diabetic mother. Are these babies always over-weight ? Why are they often nursed in an incubator ? What are the dangers of the first 48 hours ?

Write not more than 10 lines on each of the following: (*a*) observation; (*b*) feeding; (*c*) nursing care of the baby of the diabetic mother.

C.M.B.(N. Ireland) paper.—What are the special risks to which the infant of a diabetic mother is exposed ? Outline the management of the respiratory distress which often affects these infants.

31

Serious Neonatal Disorders

ASPHYXIA; INFECTIONS; HÆMOLYTIC DISEASE

During intra-uterine life the mechanism of pulmonary respiration is held in abeyance by the fore-brain (slight respiratory movements do take place). If, during labour, the oxygen supply to the fetus is diminished, the respiratory centre is stimulated and the fetus breathes and inhales liquor amnii which may be meconium stained: should oxygen-lack continue the baby will die of anoxia.

The main signs of intra-uterine anoxia are slowing of the fetal heart rate and the passage of meconium (*causes and signs are discussed under Fetal Distress, page* 413).

INITIATION OF PULMONARY RESPIRATION

Pulmonary respiration is initiated when the respiratory centre in the medulla is stimulated by oxygen-lack This occurs when the uterine contraction that expels the baby's body causes the placenta to become partly detached from the uterine

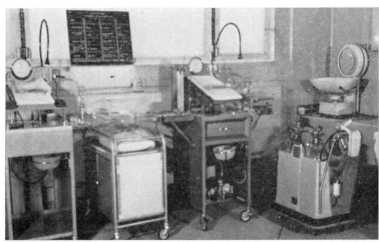

FIG. 366

RESUSCITATION AREA FOR NEWBORN IN LABOUR WARD.

Equipment

Endotracheal tubes, Warne, disposable, bore 3 mm.	2 syringes, 2 ml.; needles, size 12.
Baby laryngoscope, Magill.	Neonatal nalorphine (Lethidrone), levallorphan (Lorfan).
3 baby Portex Guedel airways, size 0, 00, 000.	10 gauze swabs (green).
1 nasal catheter (F.G. No. 8).	1 roll adhesive tape; scissors.

(*Aberdeen Maternity Hospital.*)

wall. The mechanism of respiration is also aided by compression of the thorax during the expulsion of the body, and the impact of the relatively cool air on the baby's skin (see p. 491).

ASPHYXIA NEONATORUM

In this condition the baby at birth does not breathe. Asphyxia is usually classified under two main types which are in actual fact clinical stages of the same condition.

MILD ASPHYXIA (*livida*)

The **descriptive term** "livida" **is applied to the less severe stage** in which response to treatment is usually prompt.

SEVERE ASPHYXIA (*pallida*)

The **descriptive term** "pallida" **is applied to the serious stage** in which the infant is profoundly shocked.

CAUSES

1. DYSFUNCTION OF THE RESPIRATORY CENTRE.

(*a*) **Immaturity**—as occurs in the very premature baby.

(*b*) **Depression**—due to general anæsthetics and narcotic drugs.

(*c*) **Damage**—increased pressure due to intracranial hæmorrhage or œdema.

2. OXYGEN LACK.

(*a*) **Blockage of the airway** by thick mucus, meconium-stained liquor, blood.

(*b*) **Maternal cyanosis**—as in eclampsia.

(*c*) **Placental**—insufficiency as in pre-eclampsia and postmaturity.

        „   —separation as in antepartum hæmorrhage.

(*d*) **Cord**—Prolapse of or true knots in.

Anoxia produces venous engorgement and capillary hæmorrhage in the brain, lungs, heart, liver and other tissues: biochemical changes in the blood occur.

MILD ASPHYXIA (ASPHYXIA LIVIDA)

This condition may be due to any of the causes mentioned, which have been of short duration or mild. It is frequently due to blockage of the airway with mucus.

Signs

1. **The period of apnœa is usually short** (less than 30 seconds); the infant may make an attempt to breathe.

2. **The colour is a dusky, bluish red.**   3. **The muscle tone is good.**

4. **The cord is pulsating strongly and feels firm.**   5. Apgar score 5 to 7.

TREATMENT

1. **Clear the airway immediately** with mucus extractors using short sharp sucks to prevent the inhalation of mucus during the first gasp and to allow the infant to obtain air. Mechanical suction is ideal, and should be readily available; holding the baby upside down will drain fluid but not thick mucus.

2. **Stimulate crying by flicking the sole of the foot.**

3. **Clamp and cut the cord.**   4. **Place the infant in a warmed cot.**

31A

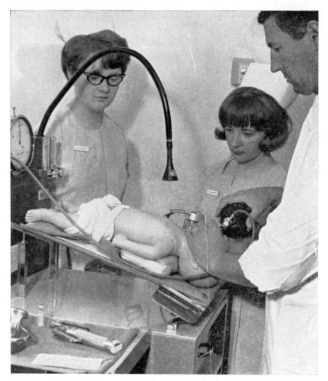

Fig. 367

INTERMITTENT POSITIVE PRESSURE VENTILATION.

Using the Resuscitaire machine. I.P.P.V. is being administered by bag and mask as to a moderately asphyxiated infant. Pharynx and nostrils cleared first, an airway introduced; shoulders raised to hyperextend the head; angle of jaw supported.

Note stop clock and also apparatus available for immediate intubation.

(*Neonatal Pædiatric Unit, Royal Maternity Hospital, Rottenrow, Glasgow.*)

5. *Administer oxygen.*

By baby funnel or mask, not closely applied to the face, at 2 litres per minute.

A stream of oxygen directed on the baby's face will stimulate respiration and provide high O_2 for the baby's first breaths.

6. *Respiratory stimulants* are not now recommended. **Vandid and nikethamide** are given by some, but should only be administered in mild cases when the baby has gasped. Other authorities condemn the use of analeptic drugs because there are other less dangerous methods of resuscitation.

7. **If pethidine or morphine has been administered to the mother within three hours of birth** give levallorphan (Lorfan) 0·25 mg., or neonatal nalorphine (Lethidrone) 0·25 mg.

8. **Summon medical aid** if the baby does not respond in one minute to the treatment given; prolonged oxygen lack will give rise to asphyxia pallida.

SEVERE ASPHYXIA
(ASPHYXIA PALLIDA)

When profound shock is present at birth it is possible that intra-uterine anoxia has existed or intracranial injury occurred.

Prolonged anoxia (over 10 minutes) will damage the brain cells and may give rise to mental retardation and physical disabilities.

SIGNS

The baby is not breathing. (Later, shallow breaths with occasional gasps.)

The colour is bluish-white or grey.

Muscle tone is poor; the infant is limp and cold.

Cord pulsation is feeble and slow; the cord feels flabby. **Apex beat weak. Apgar score 0 to 2.**

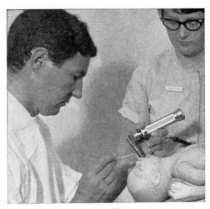

FIG. 368

Pædiatrician demonstrating position for holding the laryngoscope prior to insertion of endotracheal tube. Note pillow under shoulders to hyperextend the head. (*Neonatal Pædiatric Unit, Royal Maternity Hospital Rottenrow, Glasgow.*)

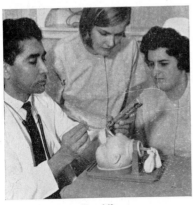

FIG. 369

USING RESUSCI INTUBATION MODEL (INFANT)

Doctor demonstrating the technique of intubation to student midwives.
(*Neonatal Pædiatric Unit, Royal Maternity Hospital, Rottenrow, Glasgow.*)

TREATMENT

Medical aid is summoned. **Clear the airway at once.**

Clamp and cut the cord. Remove baby to resuscitation table.

Prepare for intubation without delay to avoid acidosis which will inhibit respiratory activity.

Provide warmth.

METHOD OF INTUBATION

Baby placed on Resuscitaire or high table, head slightly extended.

Magill infant laryngoscope passed, any mucus in glottis removed with a fine suction catheter.

Endotracheal tube is inserted into glottis; fine mechanical suction catheter used to clear trachea and bronchii.

Inflate the lungs and administer oxygen.

Oxygen at 30 cm. water pressure is administered by intermittent positive pressure (short half-second puffs) to aid expansion of lungs. Pressure is then reduced to 10 cm.

The Central Midwives Boards permit the midwife to carry out intubation in appropriate cases if she has been properly trained in the procedure and has obtained prior approval of the medical authority under whom she is working.

RISKS OF INTUBATION

Midwives should be aware that endotracheal intubation should not be undertaken without due need as well as adequate instruction and practice under supervision. During 1966-1967, five babies were admitted to one children's hospital with a Portsmouth endotracheal tube inadvertently introduced into the stomach (*a Cardiff connector fitted to the tube would prevent this*). **Inexpert intubation** may cause soft tissue damage or induce laryngeal spasm.

Place baby in warm cot.

It is not now advocated to lower the head of the cot to allow fluid to drain from the trachea and lungs as the pressure of the liver may embarrass respiration, and the cerebral veins may become engorged.

Suck out and keep the airway clear of mucus. The insertion of a baby airway, Guedel, size 0, 00 or 000, will deal successfully with a sagging tongue.

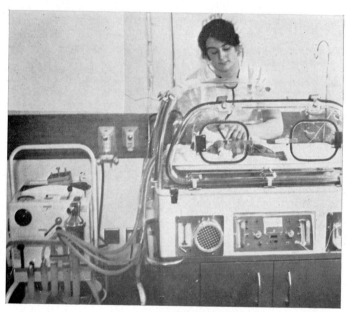

FIG. 370

BABY IN INCUBATOR HAVING ASSISTED RESPIRATION by Radcliffe intermittent positive pressure Ventilator. Midwife taking apex beat.
(*Neonatal Intensive Care Unit, Aberdeen Maternity Hospital.*)

METABOLIC ACIDOSIS

If signs of metabolic acidosis are manifest, *i.e.* low Apgar score at 5 minutes and bradycardia, biochemical monitoring of the blood is carried out. Dextrose 10 per cent and sodium bicarbonate 5 to 8·4 per cent are given intravenously depending on the pH of the blood.

Oxygen is administered in sufficient concentration to relieve cyanosis.

A broad spectrum antibiotic is usually given as a prophylactic measure when inhalation of meconium-stained liquor has occurred, e.g. Ampiclox for 5 days.

Mouth to Mouth breathing may be used when no better method is available. **The airway must first be cleared.** Gauze is placed over the baby's mouth and nose. The midwife expels air into the mouth and nose about 20 times per minute. Undue force could rupture the alveoli of the lungs. The oxygen catheter placed in the midwife's mouth will increase the oxygen content of the air delivered to the baby.

NURSING CARE

1. **Admission to the neonatal intensive care unit.**

2. **Quietness and warmth** are needed for at least 48 hours.

3. **The minimum of handling** is given and with great gentleness; the baby should not be moved from his cot.

4. **The head and shoulders are raised** unless drainage of mucus is necessary. The baby is turned from side to side at two-hourly intervals.

5. **Oxygen, 40 per cent. or more** is administered for cyanosis; frothy mucus is removed from lips and nostrils.

6. **No fluid is given by mouth for at least 4 to 6 hours.**

7. **Observation.** (*a*) **Rate and type of respirations;** (*b*) indrawing of chest wall; (*c*) temperature; (*d*) colour changes; (*e*) apex beat (note bradycardia).

After discharge the baby is "followed up" for neurological damage.

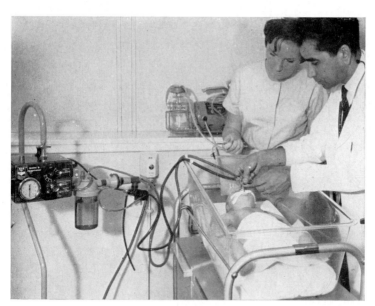

Fig. 371

Bronchial suction being carried out as a routine measure; being part of the essential maintenance of infants on positive-pressure respirators. (*Bird Mark 8 infant Respirator.*) Suction done from Dia-pump (on shelf) using a bronchial catheter passed via the disposable endotracheal tube, 12 FG.

(*Neonatal Pædiatric Unit, Royal Maternity Hospital, Rottenrow, Glasgow.*)

ATELECTASIS NEONATORUM

In this condition there is imperfect expansion of the lungs of the newborn which may be due to a plug of mucus in a bronchus preventing the entrance of air, or the absence of surfactant, which prevents the walls of the alveoli from adhering. Atelectasis occurs in cases of asphyxia and intracranial injury, especially in the premature baby and is often associated with hyaline membrane.

Since diagnostic radiography of chest became routine in all cases of respiratory distress, and respirator therapy has been employed the prognosis is improved.

Signs.   1. Shallow, rapid breathing, with indrawing of the upper abdomen.

2. Cyanosis, often most noticeable during crying or feeding.

Treatment.   This is the same as for respiratory distress syndrome (p. 542).

NEONATAL HYPOTHERMIA

The normal baby's temperature falls to 35° C. (95° F.) or less within one hour of birth, and it may be eight hours before it rises to 36·6° C. (98° F.). If the infant is exposed and chilled a dangerously low temperature level will be reached because heat loss has exceeded heat production. This condition occurs most frequently during the cold winter months.

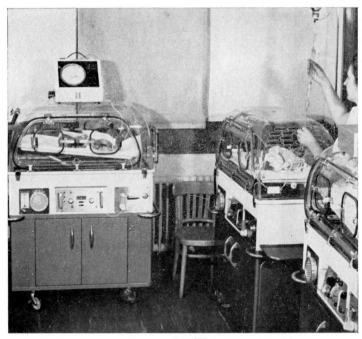

Fig. 372

Electric Thermometer (*on top of incubator*).
(*Aberdeen Maternity Hospital.*)

SIGNS

Baby feels cold to the touch.
Lethargy, reluctance to feed, and a feeble cry are manifest.
Respirations may be very slow.

Rectal temperature is below 32·2 C. (90° F.).

Redness of the face and extremities is marked.

Solid œdema (sclerema) may occur and is an ominous sign.

Prevention

Avoidance of exposure and chilling of babies at birth, particularly during resuscitation.

Temperature of labour ward, 21·1° C. (70° F.).

Babies should be dried, and warmly wrapped, head covered, yet allowing freedom to produce heat by muscular activity.

Bathing should be postponed until the baby has recovered from the trauma of birth; the room, towels and clothing should be warm.

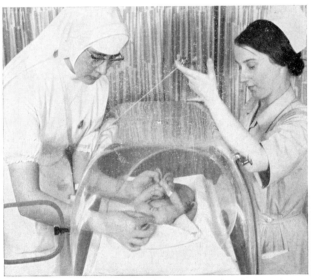

FIG. 373

USE OF RADIATION HEAT SHIELD to improve conservation of heat round infant. Central temperature being recorded per rectum.

(*Neonatal Intensive Care Unit, Royal Maternity Hospital, Rottenrow, Glasgow.*

During transport to hospital a heated portable incubator and a silver swaddler to wrap baby in (see p. 526) are recommended.

Low-reading thermometers, 21·1° to 37·7° C. (70° to 100° F.), ought to be used for the newborn in order to detect the condition early; the baby's temperature should be taken once daily at least. C.M.B. Rule.

Maintaining the nursery temperature at 18·3° to 21·1° C. (65° to 70° F.), and advising mothers to do likewise during cold weather, and particularly at night; wall thermometers should be used.

TREATMENT

Slowly raising the baby's temperature to 36·6° C. (98° F.) over a period of days. To subject the hypothermic baby to sufficient heat to raise the temperature quickly may cause convulsions.

Infections of the Newborn Baby

PREVENTION AND CONTROL

The prevention and control of neonatal infection is a major problem in maternity hospitals in which the common infecting organism, the staphylococcus aureus, is penicillin resistant.

Infection is spread from baby to baby via the hands and clothing of the staff and also by air and dust. Within a few hours of birth staphylococci have colonized on the baby's skin and nasal passages, the umbilicus most readily becoming infected, then nostrils and skin-flexures such as groin and perineum.

The pseudomonas æruginosa (*pyocyanea*) group of organisms, a contaminant of humidifying systems, is causing neonatal infection with increasing frequency: urinary, respiratory and umbilical. The hexachlorophane group of antiseptics is not effective against *ps. æruginosa*; Sudol or Resiguard is recommended for cleansing incubators, sinks and other surfaces.

The provision of a cubicle for mother and baby with individual equipment including toilet and hand basin is ideal. Nurseries should be small with not more than four cots and at least 61 cm. (2 ft.) of space between them.

Admission of patients beyond the optimal number should be avoided: invariably this results in the nursing staff being overworked and unable to carry out good barrier-nursing technique.

No person who is suffering from a respiratory infection, diarrhœa, or who has any septic focus, should be in contact with babies. Visitors should not be permitted to enter nurseries.

THE NEED FOR CLEANLINESS

Domestic and personal cleanliness with the liberal use of soap and water is the first essential. Vacuum cleaners are employed to avoid the dissemination of dust; wet mopping of floors and damp dusting of furniture are essential. Incubators and individual equipment must be cleansed daily and replaced by clean ones at least weekly and on discharge of each infant.

Adequate supplies of clean baby and cot clothing as well as bed linen for the mother should be provided. Cotton blankets have now replaced those of wool.

VIGILANT OBSERVATION

Babies should be inspected thoroughly every day while naked, and isolated for the slightest septic lesion.

Prompt reporting to the doctor is necessary in order that the appropriate investigations and treatment can be carried out.

NURSING TECHNIQUE

HAND WASHING IS MOST IMPORTANT

The hands should be washed for one and a half minutes when coming on duty in the nursery, and hexachlorophane (Phisohex), an antibacterial skin cleanser, has proved effective in inhibiting the growth of staphylococci.

Between the handling of babies the hands are washed for 30 seconds with Phisohex and dried with disposable towels; wrist watches prevent thorough hand washing and should not be worn.

Hand washing should follow immediately after the use of paper handkerchiefs, which are used once only and discarded.

MAKING UP FEEDS

Cleanliness and Surgical Aseptic Technique are essential

Terminal sterilization of feeds is recommended.

Teats on bottles should have individual covers.

The staff who make up or issue feeds should not change napkins or attend to puerperal women.

The use of Hexachlorophane

It has been found that bathing babies within 12 hours of birth and on every second day with hexachlorophane (Phisohex) gives greater protection from infection by staphylococci than the non-bathing regime (the eyes must be avoided) : the film of bacteriostatic material left on the skin giving protection for 48 hours.

Research carried out shows that the repeated application of hexachlorophane dusting powder (Ster Zac) to the umbilicus, groins, perineum and axillæ has greatly reduced the incidence of neonatal staphylococcal infections.

MODIFIED BARRIER NURSING

The rooming-in plan provides a means whereby handling of the baby by the nursing staff and consequent risk of infection is reduced (p. 453). Perspex cots on metal trolleys are available with adequate storage space for equipment and ample linen for the individual baby.

The wearing by nurses of a separate gown for each baby ought to, but has not proved to, be an effective means of limiting the spread of infection, probably because of staff shortage and insufficient time to observe the proper technique of gown-wearing.

If separate gowns are not worn when on duty in the nursery, the wearing of simple short-sleeved dresses, issued once or twice daily, is commendable.

Napkins can be changed and babies sponge-bathed in their cots, and the student midwife should be shown how to do this with the least possible contact between the baby and her clothing.

When a midwife must change the napkins of a series of infants in their cots, she ought to wear a gown which is subsequently discarded : hands must be washed between babies.

The common lap or table used for changing napkins, and the common bathing aprons used in some centres, should be abolished as dangerous means of spreading infection.

MASK WEARING

Mask wearing has not proved an efficient means of reducing neonatal infections. Unless worn intelligently and changed at least every hour they are liable to be an additional source of infection (p. 265). *When worn for long periods the mouth becomes an incubator for organisms.*

Talking should be reduced to the absolute minimum when attending to babies in order to avoid droplet infection ; the unmasked midwife should turn her head away from the baby if talking is necessary.

Handling Napkins

Because the stools of an infant do not have an objectionable odour soiled napkins are sometimes handled carelessly and clean ones used for purposes for which they were never intended. Feeding-bibs used in incubators must not come in contact with the napkin area.

Soiled napkins should be placed immediately in a covered disposable receptacle, removed after a " changing round " and sent directly to the laundry where they are boiled as well as washed, or destroyed if disposable.

Baby clothes should be boilable and laundry methods subjected to critical appraisal. Cotton cellular blankets can be autoclaved.

Isolation

A self-contained unit should be available for babies suffering from an infectious condition, with adequate individual equipment, disposable napkins and other means for limiting the spread of infection. Units for mother and baby are essential for some cases : some recommend removing the baby from the midwifery department.

OPHTHALMIA NEONATORUM

Ophthalmia neonatorum is a notifiable disease, and the doctor notifies the Local Health Authority.

DEFINITION

(England).—" A purulent discharge from the eyes of an infant commencing within 21 days of its birth."

(Scotland).—" Any inflammation that occurs in the eyes of an infant within 21 days of birth and is accompanied by a discharge."

C.M.B.(Eng.) code of practice; C.M.B.(Scot.) rule.

It is the duty of every midwife to inquire from the Local Supervising Authority or from the senior midwife of the institution or organization by whom she is employed, as to the routine she must follow in the care of the eyes of the newborn infant in order to prevent ophthalmia neonatorum.

A midwife must call in medical aid without delay if there is any discharge from the eyes of an infant however slight *this discharge may be.*

Such regulations are necessary because of the danger of impaired vision and blindness, due to gonococcal ophthalmia neonatorum.

CAUSE

The majority of cases of neonatal conjunctivitis are due to the B. proteus and staphylococcus aureus, which produces a profuse yellow discharge. Pneumococci and streptococci are sometimes found, but the **gonococcus is most dreaded because of its destructive action.**

The *ps. æruginosa* causes severe ophthalmia; blindness having been reported: polymyxin (Neosporin) eye drops are recommended.

The baby's eyes may be infected during his passage through the birth canal, or later by the mother's hands.

The midwife may infect the eyes by neglecting to wash her hands prior to touching the baby's face, or by failing to observe the prophylactic measures prescribed on p. 565.

SIGNS

The condition may first be manifest as a sticky, watery discharge, with slight reddening of the conjunctiva. The inflammation quickly spreads, the conjunctiva covering the eyeball and lining the lids being congested and often œdematous ; the discharge becomes copious in amount and purulent. The eyelids also may be inflamed and swollen and are kept tightly shut, due to spasm of the orbicularis oculi muscle.

MANAGEMENT

Prophylaxis

1. The treatment of vaginal discharge during pregnancy.

2. The midwife, with clean hands, should wipe the eyes at birth with large pledgets of dry sterile cotton wool. (Some bacteriologists consider that this procedure is ineffective.)

3. The baby's hands should be washed, and the arms wrapped up in such a way that the hands do not come in contact with the eyes prior to his first bath.

4. When giving the first bath, the face should be washed before the body, preferably with sterile water and using sterile wool. The towel should then be discarded.

5. The midwife should always wash her hands before touching the baby's face, and cleanse the buttocks last. The mother must be told not to use her handkerchief to wipe the baby's eyes.

6. The instillation of sulphacetamide (Albucid), 10 per cent, is used by some, owing to the recent increased incidence of gonorrhœa.

The midwife must carry out the methods of prevention and treatment as laid down by her employer.

ACTIVE TREATMENT

1. Medical aid is sought, the infant isolated.

2. The midwife notifies the Local Supervising Authority.

3. A smear and culture of the discharge is sent to the bacteriological laboratory, where the causal organism is identified and tested for sensitivity to the antibiotics. *Some use Stuarts transport medium. (When the baby of an unbooked mother develops a " sticky eye " a smear and culture is taken immediately and examined for gonococci.)*

In mild cases injections of procaine penicillin, 150,000 units once daily for three to five days, may be adequate.

Polymixin (Neosporin) eye drops are specific for pseudomonas æruginosa.

GONOCOCCAL OPHTHALMIA

The immediate transfer of cases, infected by the gonococcus, from the neonatal department to an isolation unit is imperative.

Soluble penicillin for penicillin-sensitive infections (Crystapen) 50,000 to 150,000 units is injected intramuscularly every four to six hours until 24 hours after inflammation has subsided.

Penicillin 0·125 ml. (2 minims) 2,500 units per ml. may be instilled into the conjunctival sac every five minutes until the purulent discharge ceases.

Neomycin gramicidin or Terramycin or Neobacrin ophthalmic ointment by preventing the eyelids from becoming adherent ensures good drainage from the conjunctival sac.

Bathing the eyes is not necessary unless the discharge is profuse, and should consist in gentle wiping of the lids with large pledgets of wool. Undines should not be used except by an expert, as a stream of water forcibly striking the cornea may damage the eye.

The baby should be laid on the side of the infected eye, so that the pus will drain on to a dressing laid on the pillow.

BLINDNESS

In serious neglected cases of gonococcal ophthalmia milkiness of the cornea ensues, followed by ulceration and subsequent impairment of vision: occasionally perforation of the cornea takes place, giving rise to blindness.

PEMPHIGUS NEONATORUM
(Bullous Impetigo)

Pemphigus, a highly contagious skin disease of the newborn, characterized by watery blisters, is rarely seen in the severe form today. The lesions may be small or as large as 2·5 cm. (1 in.) in diameter.

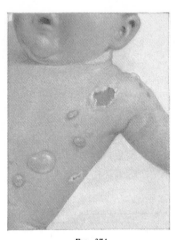

FIG. 374

Pemphigus neonatorum, showing macules, vesicles, one of which is ruptured, and pustules.

The organism is usually the *staphylococcus aureus* and the disease tends to occur in epidemics.

C.M.B.(Eng.) Code of Practice, C.M.B.(Scot.) Rule.—*A midwife must call in medical aid without delay if a watery blister, pustule, or a rash appears on the body of the infant.*

The initial lesions are pink macules, which rapidly form vesicles and then pustules surrounded with a red ring. Later, raw moist areas, partly covered with tags of epidermis, are evident.

TREATMENT

1. **Notify the doctor promptly.**—Taking a smear from one of the blebs; testing the organisms for sensitivity to the antibiotics.

2. **Isolation of infected baby, segregation of contacts.** Newborn babies are not admitted to the unit.

3. **Administration of an antibiotic, both local and systemic,** as indicated by the sensitivity tests. Cloxacillin or erythromycin may be used in severe cases pending the result of sensitivity tests.

4. **Wipe the blebs with Hibitane 0·5 per cent in spirit.** Bathing with Phisohex is effective. **Remove all epidermis from the blebs;** catching the fluid to prevent it from infecting surrounding areas. **Change cot and baby clothing twice daily.**

UMBILICAL INFECTIONS
Omphalitis

The common infecting organism is the *staphylococcus aureus,* but when aseptic precautions are observed serious umbilical infections are rare. **Cases of tetanus have occurred following the use of unsterile cord powder.**

Inflammation, discharge or an offensive odour should be reported to the doctor.

Midwives should always make arrangements for the dressing of the umbilicus if not healed when the infant is discharged from hospital. **The author is aware of a case** in which the baby was discharged with a " sticky " umbilicus and died one week later of septicæmia.

Spread of and Treatment of the Infection

1. **The infection spreads into the cellular tissue,** and an area, the size of a coffee cup, may be red and indurated (in some cases there is no visible inflammation). Neomycin bacitracin (Cicatrin) powder or Hibitane 0·5 per cent in spirit is useful for a newly separated cord with a sticky umbilicus. Warm saline compresses are applied for 24 hours if the cellulitis is acute. The antibiotic to which the organism is sensitive is administered systemically.

Cloxacillin (Orbenin) 62·5 mg. or ampicillin (Penbritin) 62·5 mg. (if sensitive to it) may be given in syrup six-hourly in mild cases if not vomiting.

2. **Infection of the clot in the umbilical vein** may give rise to hæmorrhage before or after the cord is off. A firm pad is applied and medical aid summoned.

3. **Hepatitis. The infection may spread via the umbilical vein to the liver.** Jaundice arising in the second week, even when no local signs of infection are manifest, is suggestive of this condition. Septicæmia usually follows.

4. The association with abdominal distension is particularly ominous; blood culture should be carried out without delay.

UMBILICAL POLYPUS

A reddish brown tag, about 1·25 cm. long and 0·3 cm. in diameter, occasionally develops when there has been a low grade umbilical infection, and is seen three or four weeks after birth. The doctor will apply copper sulphate or ligate it.

URINARY TRACT INFECTION

This gives rise to attacks that look like fainting in which the infant becomes limp and grey. The temperature is raised and vomiting may be present. (*To obtain a specimen of urine the Chironseal urine collector is useful for boy or girl babies.*)

If the infant is vomiting and sensitive to ampicillin it may be given I.M. six-hourly; if not vomiting ampicillin 62·5 mg. (Penbritin syrup) is administered orally six-hourly. The condition may take six weeks or longer to clear up. It may be associated with congenital renal tract abnormality: intravenous pyelography will usually be carried out.

Ps. æruginosa (pyocyanea) is resistant to many antibiotics. Colomycin (Colistin) I.M. 50,000 u. per kg. in 24 hours is effective or carbenicillin (Pyopen).

THRUSH

Oral thrush is characterised by white patches in the mouth, that are composed of epithelial cells; the causal organism is the **candida albicans** which is present in the vagina of 28 per cent of pregnant women.

The baby's mouth and hands, and the midwife's hands are sources of infection. Great care must be exercised in the immediate disposal of napkins and subsequent hand-washing. **Thrush can readily be spread** from baby to baby.

The greyish-white raised patches, often surrounded by a zone of inflammation, are seen inside the cheeks, on the gums, palate and tongue. A milky tongue looks like grey paint and has an even distribution, but spots on the edges of the tongue are diagnostic, as sucking would remove milk curd from that region. **A raw area is left on removing one of these lesions** which are more adherent than milk curds.

Thrush does not occur prior to the fourth day.

In mild cases the infant is not upset, but in severe cases he goes off his feeds, vomits, becomes irritable, looks greyish and may have loose stools. The condition may be fatal to prematures, the lungs and intestinal tract being involved.

TREATMENT

1. **PROPHYLAXIS. Treat vaginal moniliasis in the pregnant woman.**
Good nursery technique, daily inspection of mouths.

2. **Notify the doctor.** 3. **Isolate the baby.**

4. **If the mouth is very dirty it must first be swabbed with sodium bicarbonate solution.** Apply dequalinium (Dequadin) paint, three-hourly, or nystatin 200,000 units per ml. (which must be shaken vigorously prior to each application), four times daily for 4 to 7 days is effective. In resistant cases gentian violet, 0·5 per cent aqueous solution, is applied twice daily for three days and once daily until the lesions disappear; wool on Spencer Wells' forceps is used. Gentian violet 0·06 ml. (one minim) is dropped

with a pipette on the back of the tongue. Staining of tissues and linen is a disadvantage.

N.B.—**Gentian violet is very drying,** and if applied too frequently will cause sloughing of the mucous membrane.

EPIDEMIC GASTRO-ENTERITIS (*Neonatal*)

This is a treacherous scourge because of its insidious onset and rapid course. Unless the midwife recognizes the early signs, other babies will be infected before the disease is diagnosed; successful treatment depends greatly on its being started early. Epidemics still occur.

CLINICAL SIGNS

The condition rarely develops before the end of the first week. The stools are not always green, neither are they invariably offensive. The temperature is seldom elevated.

First day.—The earliest sign is **sudden loss of appetite**; the infant is listless and pale; the stools may or may not be loose at this stage: an abrupt loss of weight occurs.

Second day.—The **stools are watery and yellow, like urine,** as many as 10 daily, or they may be uncountable.

Signs of dehydration occur, such as dry mouth, sunken fontanelle and overlapping of the skull bones; the face is pinched, eyes dull and sunken with dark rings.

Metabolic acidosis is common. Clinically this is manifest by rapid, deep, respirations. **Vomiting may be present;** abdominal distension develops in severe cases. **The infant becomes collapsed, greyish-blue in colour,** and if untreated death may ensue.

TREATMENT

1. **Prophylaxis :**—Breast-feeding ; impeccable nursery technique ; scrupulous cleanliness in preparing bottle feeds.

2. **Strict isolation** and the use of destructible napkins. Preferably the baby is transferred to the isolation unit of a children's hospital.

3. **Rectal swabs** are taken for stool culture and sensitivity tests. (Swabs also taken from contacts.)

4. **Milk is withheld for 24 hours** at least.

5. **Correction of dehydration** is accomplished in mild cases by the oral administration of fluid: *e.g.* Hartmann's solution every two hours; giving 120 ml. per 454 G. body-weight for the first 24 hours.

6. **Replacement of electrolytes** is essential in severe cases and is effected by the administration of equal parts of Hartmann's or Darrow's solution and 5 per cent. dextrose by slow intravenous drip or as indicated by biochemical investigation. Intravenous fluid is given until vomiting ceases.

7. **Kaomycin** (which contains neomycin and kaolin) is excellent in most cases of intestinal infection, dose 4 ml. every six hours. Colomycin (Colistin) syrup is recommended for resistant *E. coli.*

When improvement is noted in about three days, by the diarrhœa lessening and the appetite returning, skimmed breast milk, or National Dried Milk, 1 in 10, is given.

RESPIRATORY INFECTIONS

Babies are readily infected from the mother or a member of the nursery staff who has a " cold," if precautions are not taken. Nasopharyngitis is recognized by snuffles, and if the infection spreads downwards the cry becomes hoarse. The baby should be isolated, given extra fluid and kept comfortably warm. Broncho-pneumonia may develop and is sometimes fatal.

Nose and throat swabs are taken, the usual infecting organism being the staphylococcus aureus.

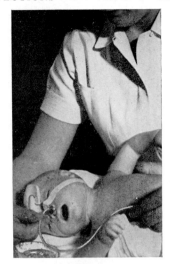

FIG. 375

MIDWIFE PASSING SUCTION CATHETER: **strapping on baby's face** maintains connection for naso-tracheal tube in position.

(*Neonatal Intensive Care Unit, Aberdeen Maternity Hospital.*)

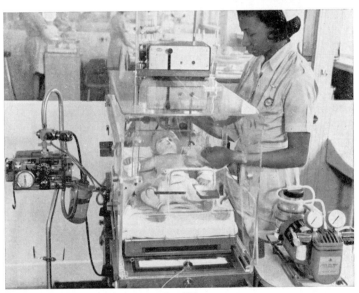

FIG. 376

GIVING BRONCHIAL LAVAGE TO NEONATE WITH RESPIRATORY DISTRESS.

Neonatal staff nurse giving bronchial lavage by inserting fine suction catheter beyond the terminal end of the endo-tracheal tube and injecting 0·5 ml. sodium bicarbonate solution 1·4 per cent (isotonic). This is immediately sucked out using the Dia pump.

The infant is receiving intermittent positive pressure ventilation from a Bird mark 8 respirator. The Draeger intensive care incubator includes an accurate balance for weighing the baby and an access shelf for X-ray plates. The peristaltic pump above the incubator controls the rate of intravenous infusion.

(*Neonatal Intensive Care Unit, Royal Maternity Hospital, Rottenrow, Glasgow.*)

If there is any question of the baby having inhaled meconium-stained liquor, antibiotics are given prophylactically, *e.g.* Ampiclox, four neonatal vials per day for five days; the baby may require oxygen and high humidity.

PNEUMONIA

This condition is more common in premature babies (probably due to inhalation of vomitus), in anoxic babies who have inhaled much liquor amnii, and where the membranes have been ruptured for 36 hours prior to birth.

Respirations are rapid, over 60 per minute, and may be grunting or laboured. **Cyanosis is manifest.**

Cough is not always present. **The temperature** may not be high.

Diarrhœa is sometimes present. **Vomiting** may occur at the onset.

Refusal to feed is common. **Listlessness.**

Treatment

The baby should be isolated in a warm room, 21·1° C. (70° F.), with a humid atmosphere or, if cyanosed, nursed in an incubator (oxygen, 40 per cent).

Antibiotics are administered. Ampicillin 50 mg. cloxacillin 25 mg. (Ampiclox), four neonatal vials per day for five days and longer in severe cases.

The head of the cot is raised and the baby turned from side to side (propped with a small pillow) every hour or two.

Mucus should be removed by suction from mouth and nostrils to keep a clear airway. Bronchial suction and lavage may be needed to remove secretions that might obstruct the bronchii.

Feeding must be carried out by an experienced nursery midwife to avoid choking or exhaustion: feeds should be small; naso-gastric feeding may be advisable if sucking causes respiratory distress or exhaustion.

Clothing must be warm but light to prevent excessive perspiration. The infant should not be tightly wrapped to avoid hampering the movement of the thoracic and abdominal muscles used in respiration.

For apnoeic episodes mechanical ventilation may be employed.

SUPERFICIAL INFECTIONS

These must be controlled as they may be the source of more severe infections.

RHINITIS

To relieve engorgement of the nasal mucosa Ephedrine, 0·5 per cent, or methoxamine (Vasylox), 0·125 ml., may be applied by dropper. Oily drops should never be used.

SEPTIC SPOTS

The baby must be isolated to prevent cross infection. The spots should be wiped with Hibitane 0·5 per cent in spirit, and framycetin (Soframycin) cream applied.

NAILFOLD INFECTIONS (paronychia)

Injury to nailfolds by rough drying and sucking the fingers predispose to infection.

The fingers should be wiped with Hibitane 0·5 per cent in spirit, and the hand enclosed in a cotton mitten. (For the danger of these see p. 534.)

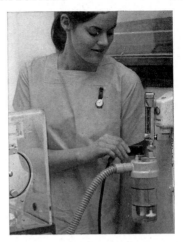

Fig. 377

Student Midwife Regulating Nebuliser.

The oxygen being administered to baby in incubator is passed through the nebuliser. By adequate oxygen humidification the bronchial secretions do not become viscid and block the bronchii and trachea.

The water in the nebuliser must be sterile and should not be allowed to run dry.

(*Neonatal Intensive Care Unit, Simpson Memorial Maternity Pavilion, Edinburgh.*)

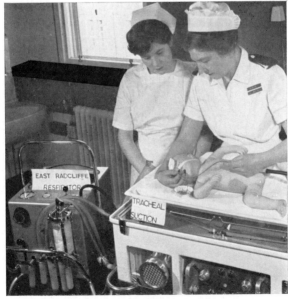

Fig. 378

Clinical Instruction on Tracheal Suction. (*Doll used for demonstration.*) **To remove mucus from trachea of baby** in respirator, the gloved hand inserts a fine suction catheter into the endotracheal tube. Mucus is removed by mechanical suction.

To clear the suction catheter of mucus it is dipped into the gallipot of sterile water placed adjacent to the baby's head, and suction applied.

Neonatal Intensive Care Unit, Aberdeen Maternity Hospital.)

INFECTIVE MASTITIS

Abscess formation may result from squeezing engorged breasts. The area is red, hard, shiny. *Treatment:* Incision and drainage. (The author saw 4 ml. pus evacuated from the breast of a baby two weeks old.)

Hæmolytic Disease of the Newborn Baby
due to Rhesus incompatibility

The Rhesus factor is an antigen present in the red blood cells of 83 per cent of the population: those who have this antigen are known as Rh positive, the 17 per cent who do not have the antigen are known as Rh negative. **If Rh positive blood enters the circulation of an Rh negative individual Rh antibodies may be produced.** These will hæmolyse Rh pos. blood as when antibodies in the blood of an Rh negative pregnant woman pass to the RH pos. fetus and cause hæmolytic disease. Why it only occurs in 10 per cent of such cases is not fully understood. The Rhesus factor is transmitted in the genes of the chromosomes of the spermatozoon and ovum. In 95 per cent of cases it is the D antigen that gives rise to trouble. **96 per cent of affected babies survive.**

ISO-IMMUNIZATION OF MOTHER

About 0·5 to 2 per cent of women at risk are immunized during pregnancy.

An abortion after 12 weeks may cause feto-maternal bleeding and immunize the susceptible woman.

Iso-immunization occurs mainly during the third stage of labour, two ml. (or more) of fetal blood may pass via the placenta into the maternal circulation. If the fetus is Rh pos. and the mother Rh neg. she will produce antibodies to destroy the offending Rh pos. red cells, thereby immunizing herself. These antibodies remain in her blood stream throughout life. **During a subsequent pregnancy** the antibodies in her Rh neg. blood may pass into the Rh pos. fetal blood, hæmolyse the red cells and the fetus develops one or other of the three forms of hæmolytic disease.

The fetus is never affected in a first pregnancy unless the Rh negative woman had at some time previously received a transfusion of Rh positive blood to which she would have produced antibodies. If the fetus *in utero* is Rh negative no Rh incompatibility exists.

THE THREE MANIFESTATIONS OF HÆMOLYTIC DISEASE
1. HYDROPS FETALIS

This is the most serious form of the disease.

The baby at birth is grossly œdematous, with an enlarged abdomen due to ascites.

The placenta is large and pale in colour with fluid oozing out of it, the author having seen one weighing 2,495 G., the baby weighing 3,232 G. (p. 38). Such babies, if at term and therefore large, may give rise to difficulty in labour; if born alive, they only live for a few moments.

During pregnancy the mother will have hydramnios which in an Rh negative woman with antibodies should give rise to suspicion. An X-ray film may (rarely) reveal the large fetus in a frog-like attitude with an œdematous scalp. **(A Buddha-like fetus with a halo round its head.)**

2. HÆMOLYTIC ANÆMIA

This is the rarest and mildest form of hæmolytic disease. Between the 3rd and 10th day tallow wax pallor or pale lemon colour which increases in intensity is noted, but it may not be apparent for three or four weeks. The hæmoglobin may be as low as 5·9 G. (40 per cent); the liver and spleen are enlarged. Blood transfusion of packed cells is given.

3. ICTERUS GRAVIS NEONATORUM

This severe form of jaundice is rarely manifest at birth, because *in utero* the bilirubin from broken down red cells is excreted via the placenta into the mother's circulation. After birth the baby's liver must cope with the elimination of this bilirubin and if unable to detoxicate the bilirubin it accumulates in the blood and jaundice develops.

Golden liquor or a faint green tint in the cord may be present, but this can also be due to meconium staining.

Jaundice usually appears within 24 hours and may be seen as early as one hour. Mild cases may be missed unless the child is examined in strong daylight. Occasionally jaundice does not develop until later.

ADVICE TO THE RH NEGATIVE WOMAN

It is inexcusable to tell a woman she is Rh negative without giving some explanation of what it means, either verbally or by pamphlet. She may have read in popular magazines disturbing and sometimes misleading accounts of the effects of the Rh factor, so the midwife should be prepared to make some simple reassuring statements and to answer questions. The husband also should understand the significance of antibodies.

The following facts should be stated:

1. **The Rh or Rhesus factor is present in the blood of 83 per cent of the population;** 17 per cent are negative.

2. **If the woman is Rh negative and the husband Rh positive, the baby in the womb may be Rh positive.** Because the baby's blood is different from the mother's, her blood may produce antibodies, which will destroy some of the baby's blood and produce anæmia and jaundice.

3. **Only 1 in 20 Rh negative pregnant women will produce antibodies,** and these are detected by examining the woman's blood at intervals throughout every pregnancy.

4. **First babies are rarely affected.**

5. **A blood transfusion** given to the baby at birth is usually successful in treating the anæmia and jaundice.

WHEN ANTIBODIES ARE PRESENT

Arrangements are made for the woman, and her husband if so desired, to see a member of the medical staff having expert knowledge of hæmolytic disease, who will explain the situation, give advice, and answer questions, a procedure designed to allay parental anxiety. **The necessity for delivery in hospital is stressed.**

A specimen of the husband's blood may be required to study the genotype, in order to predict whether all subsequent babies are likely to be affected.

INVESTIGATION DURING PREGNANCY

1. THE RHESUS HISTORY

The Rh negative woman may have had—

(*a*) **a transfusion of Rh positive blood;**

(*b*) **a stillborn baby,** not due to the accidents of birth;

(*c*) **an infant treated for, or who died of, neonatal jaundice.**

2. BLOOD EXAMINATION

The blood of every pregnant woman is examined for the Rh factor and blood group at her first visit to the prenatal clinic or doctor.

If **primigravid** and Rh negative, screen for antibodies and do Coombs' indirect antiglobulin test (I.A.G.T.) at 32 and 38 weeks.

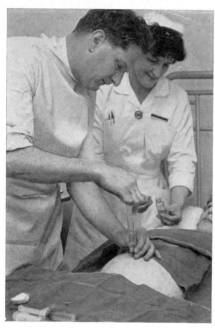

FIG. 379

ABDOMINAL AMNIOCENTESIS.

(*Simpson Memorial Maternity Pavilion, Edinburgh.*)

If **multigravid** and Rh negative, screen for antibodies at 20, 28, 32, 36, 38 and 40 weeks.

If **Rh positive** and history of blood transfusion, unexplained stillbirth, neonatal death or severe jaundice, screen for antibodies and do Coombs' test (I.A.G.T.) at 32 and 38 weeks.

A **rising antibody titre** is not conclusive in diagnosing the severity of the hæmolytic disease but when it reaches a critical level investigation of the amniotic fluid is indicated.

3. AMNIOTIC FLUID SPECTRO-PHOTOMETRIC SCANNING

This is done to assess the severity of the condition by estimating the amount of bilirubin excreted by the fetus into the amniotic fluid. At from 28 weeks an abdominal amniocentesis is performed, using a 5 to 9 cm. 22 G. spinal needle; 5 ml. of amniotic fluid is withdrawn and examined, the placenta being localised by sonar prior to the " tap ". At weekly intervals, or as indicated, the test may be repeated. Light must be excluded from the fluid *en route* to the lab. (*The report states the units of optical density difference, the significance varying with the maturity of the pregnancy.*)

The result obtained enables a decision to be made in selecting patients for (*a*) intrauterine transfusion, or (*b*) premature induction of labour followed by replacement transfusion.

MANAGEMENT

INTRA-UTERINE BLOOD TRANSFUSION
(Feto Intra-Peritoneal)

This highly specialized treatment is given when the Rh history and the result of amniocentesis indicate a severely affected fetus prior to the 32nd week. The procedure is carried out in the radiological department by an Obstetrician and Radiologist. (Sterile pre-set, trolley-top trays are efficient.)

Six to twelve hours previous to the transfusion a radio-opaque substance is injected into the amniotic sac. If the fetus is not hydropic it will swallow the dye which will identify fetal intestine and provide a " target area " for the intra-peritoneal transfusion.

Sedation and local anæsthesia are administered one hour prior to the transfusion. Aided by a television image intensifier a Tuohy 15 cm. needle is introduced through the abdominal wall and the uterus; then inserted into the fetal abdomen (peritoneal cavity). Through the Tuohy needle a polythene I.V. catheter 60 cm. is threaded and the needle removed: 60–120 ml. packed red cells are slowly injected via the catheter. **Most of the blood will be**

absorbed into the fetal circulation within 3 days. Antibiotic cover may be provided. Approx. 40 per cent of babies survive.

PREMATURE INDUCTION OF LABOUR

The Rh negative woman with antibodies, or the history of a previously affected child, is an absolute indication for delivery in a hospital equipped for replacement transfusion.

Labour may be induced at the 35th to 36th week in cases with a bad Rh history, and depending on the findings on amniocentesis. The majority have labour induced at about the expected date of delivery. Pædiatrician, blood transfusion service and laboratory staff are alerted.

At birth, the cord is clamped at once to avoid giving the infant more blood containing the offending antibodies.

Five ml. of cord blood should be allowed to drip from the placental end of the cord via a small funnel into a dry sterile test tube, and into one with anticoagulant. The cord must not be squeezed because Wharton's jelly upsets some of the laboratory tests. Metal or cord clips should not be used.

(Blood may be withdrawn with a dry sterile syringe and needle from the umbilical cord vein. To avoid hæmolysis the needle should be removed before injecting blood into the test tubes.)

No cord powder should be applied to the umbilicus: wet dressings favour sepsis.

THE FOLLOWING BLOOD TESTS ARE CARRIED OUT

1. **Coombs' direct antiglobulin test** (D.A.G.T.) demonstrates the presence of maternal antibodies on the fetal red cells; a positive result signifies hæmolytic disease in the baby and the need for serial estimations of serum bilirubin levels.

2. **Hæmoglobin estimation.** If below 14·8 G. (100 per cent) this suggests red cell destruction. If the level of cord hæmoglobin is below 11 G. immediate replacement transfusion is likely to be necessary.

3. **Rhesus typing.**

4. **Serum bilirubin.** If the cord blood level is over 3·5 mg. per 100 ml., serial estimations are made at 4 to 6 hourly intervals. Should the level reach 10 mg./100 ml. within 24 hours and particularly if the infant is premature, transfusion would be considered. Subsequently, should the level of 20 mg./100 ml. be approached the danger of kernicterus exists, and replacement blood transfusion is indicated.

5. **ABO grouping.**

A post-delivery sample of maternal blood is kept in case antibodies are found later.

CLINICAL EXAMINATION OF THE BABY

Respiration may be slow in being established and frothy mucus troublesome.

Jaundice usually develops within 24 hours and becomes rapidly deeper until the fifth or sixth day. (*Pressure on the skin by the bell of a stethoscope produces a blanched ring which makes the yellow staining obvious.*)

The baby is lethargic and pallor of the mucous membranes is sometimes noted.

Enlargement of the liver and spleen will be detected by the doctor.

REPLACEMENT BLOOD TRANSFUSION

To replace the baby's blood, which contains a reduced number of normal red cells, many hæmolysed red cells, low hæmoglobin, high serum bilirubin and maternal antibodies, a replacement transfusion is carried out.

This should be done within six hours of birth or as soon as possible. The blood is given by plastic catheter via the umbilical vein. Each syringeful of blood taken off is immediately replaced by a similar volume of fresh donor blood. If venous pressure is high 15 ml. are taken off first and replaced by 10 ml., then another 15 ml. off and replaced by 10 ml. The remainder is taken off and replaced in 10 ml. amounts.

Packed cells are given because donor blood may only contain 85 per cent hæmoglobin. Rh negative blood is given because the maternal antibodies in the baby's circulation will destroy Rh positive blood. (It does no harm to give an Rh positive individual Rh negative blood.)

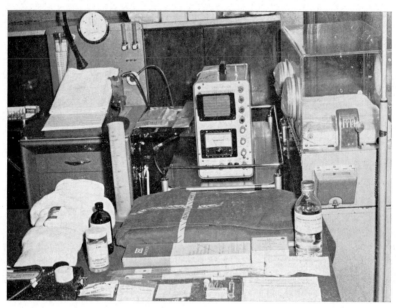

Fig. 380

Requirements for Replacement Transfusion.

Baby Resuscitaire: Cardiac rate meter (Cardiorater): Heated Isolette: Drip stand.

Cruciform padded splint (*sloped*): Kling bandage 10 cm. Blood warmer.

Preset tray (contents in fig. 381): waste blood container 500 ml.

Disposable equipment: adult blood administration set with pump: blood transfusion tubing: ext. tubing Luer fitting, umbilical cannulæ F.G. 6 and 9: stopcock 3-way: syringes 20 ml.: œsophageal tubes F.G. 6: mucus extractors: baby laryngoscope: St. Thomas's endotracheal tubes: eyeless needled sutures with 3/0 silk.

Drugs: Ampoules Lanoxin, frusemide (Lasix), Konakion, neonatal nalorphine (Lethidrone), Calcium, Gluconate 10 per cent, Heparin, dextrose 20 per cent, Hibitane 0·5 per cent in spirit, Vaco-litre isotonic saline, sodium bicarbonate 5 per cent.

Sphygmomanometer, 2 baby cuffs, stethoscope, strapping 2·5 cm.

Blood investigation tubes, Sequestrene, lithium heparin, fluoride oxalate, dry.

Record chart.

(Simpson Memorial Maternity Pavilion, Edinburgh.)

If 180 ml. of blood per kg. body-weight is given, 85 to 90 per cent of the baby's blood will be replaced. It should be noted that the baby is not only getting blood, the offending antibodies, hæmolysed red cells and bilirubin are also being withdrawn and anæmia corrected. This tides the infant over the first two weeks, until he can produce sufficient of his own Rh positive blood and get rid of the maternal antibodies. Giving the baby Rh negative blood does not alter his Rh factor, the baby will continue to produce Rh positive blood.

The blood must be fresh (not stored) and the same ABO group as the baby's. Blood is warmed by placing in water not above 40° C (104° F) tested by thermometer, or allowed to come to room temperature. To avoid hypothermia the temperature of the room should be 26·6° C (80° F).

The stomach is aspirated if a feed has been given within three hours, mechanical suction or mucus extractors should be at hand.

A sedative is not usually prescribed because sudden quietening of the baby which may indicate impending collapse, would not be readily noted when sedated.

An antibiotic, such as ampicillin and cloxacillin (Ampiclox), is administered routinely 6 hourly in most centres for three days.

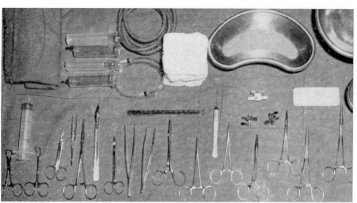

Fig. 381

STERILE EQUIPMENT FOR REPLACEMENT BLOOD TRANSFUSION.

LINEN

2 gowns: sheet with operating aperture.
gauze swabs 4 packs of 5.

EQUIPMENT

receiver; gallipot; bowl 25 cm.
metal ruler 15 cm.; 2 metal 3-way stopcocks.

DISPOSABLE

Umbilical cannulae F.G. 6 and 9.
syringes 20 ml.: eyeless needled suture with
3/0 silk: 3-way stopcock. Luer fitting
extension tubing, blood transfusion tubing.

INSTRUMENTS

2 small towel clips.
straight Mayo forceps 15 cm.
Bard Parker handle 4, blade 23.
small aneurysm needle: probe.
one dissecting forceps plain.
one dissecting forceps toothed.
3 straight mosquito forceps.
1 curved mosquito forceps.
3 fine Allis's forceps.
2 Spencer Wells forceps.
1 pair iris scissors.
1 pair stitch forceps.

(*Simpson Memorial Maternity Pavilion, Edinburgh.*)

OBSERVATION

The doctor is notified of :

1. Progressive increase, decrease or sudden drop in heart-beat rate. Cardiac arrest is usually heralded by bradycardia and may be caused by the use of unwarmed blood or by hypocalcæmia.

2. **Cyanosis, greyness, pallor.** 3. **Respiratory distress.**

4. **Tremors or twitching, which might indicate hypoglycæmia or hypocalcæmia.**

The midwife sits at the baby's head. The bell of the stethoscope is strapped to the baby's chest under the sterile drapes and the midwife records the apex beat every five minutes. If very anæmic, heart failure may occur.

A Midwife Records Intake and Output as follows:

Name				Date		Blood used	Baby No.
Time	Vol. out (ml.)	Vol. in (ml.)	Heart rate	Drugs		Clinical Comment	

AFTER CARE

The baby is placed in a warm cot, and " specialled " for six to eight hours; hæmorrhage from the umbilicus may occur; records of apex beat, temperature and respirations are made every hour. The serum bilirubin is estimated six hours after transfusion and subsequently as indicated.

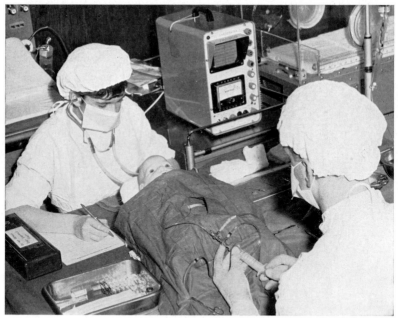

FIG. 382

PÆDIATRICIAN GIVING REPLACEMENT BLOOD TRANSFUSION.

Resuscitaire, heated Isolette in readiness. Cardiorater records the rate and rhythm of baby's heartbeat. Midwife records intake and output of blood, drugs, baby's condition.

(*Simpson Memorial Maternity Pavilion, Edinburgh.*)

All babies who have suffered from hæmolytic disease are prescribed iron and Abidec on discharge and attend a special " follow up " clinic for 2 months at weekly intervals for the detection of such conditions as anæmia, deafness, cerebral palsy and mental retardation.

PREVENTION OF Rh HÆMOLYTIC DISEASE

Because transplacental bleeding is likely to occur during (a) **termination of pregnancy,** (b) **Cæsarean section,** (c) **version** and (d) **manual removal of placenta,** due to disruption of the chorio-decidual area, **these procedures are avoided** if possible when Rh incompatibility is suspected. Abdominal palpation should be done gently. Transplacental bleeding occurs most commonly during the third stage of labour.

The Kleihauer technique is used to detect the fetal red cells present in post-delivery samples of maternal blood: a fetal cell score of 5 implies the presence of 0·2 ml. of fetal blood in the maternal circulation.

There is less hæmolytic disease when there is ABO incompatibility between the blood of an Rh negative woman and her Rh positive fetus. Any fetal blood cells entering the woman's circulation, as may occur during labour, will be immediately destroyed by anti-A and anti-B antibody in the woman's blood before Rh antibodies are produced.

PROTECTION BY INJECTION OF ANTI-D IMMUNOGLOBULIN

The idea was suggested, and much of the research done, in Liverpool. Results are most encouraging and give hope that Rh hæmolytic disease may in the future be preventable.

The Rh negative ABO compatible woman delivered of her first and every subsequent Rh positive baby is given within 48 hours an I.M. injection of anti Rh (D) gammaglobulin that coats the offending fetal Rh positive cells. These are then removed from the maternal circulation before the maternal reticulo-endothelial system is stimulated to produce anti-D antibodies. Some recommend giving anti-Rh (D) gammaglobulin to Rh negative women following abortion after 12 weeks.

KERNICTERUS

In this serious condition signs of cerebral irritation and deepening jaundice are manifested due to the effect of unconjugated bilirubin on the brain cells.

When the serum bilirubin, which is normally under 2 mg. per 100 ml. in the newborn, rises above 4 mg. jaundice becomes visible and when the indirect fraction reaches the critical level of 20 mg. kernicterus is liable to occur. Bile staining and necrosis of brain cells are present.

Kernicterus of prematurity occurs in the smaller premature baby who shows evidence of jaundice, no doubt due to the extreme immaturity of the liver. When a premature baby is jaundiced for over 36 hours the serum bilirubin is estimated.

Signs are manifest during the middle of the first week of life.

Jaundice becomes more intense. Disinclination for feeds and lethargy.

Cerebral signs such as head retraction, neck, back and limb rigidity, muscular twitching, high pitched cry, downward eye rolling are evident.

Grunting expiration, irregular breathing, apnœic spells.

Cyanotic attacks. Convulsions may occur.

Collapse may occur suddenly; a few of these infants recover but they may be mentally subnormal, deaf, or suffer from spastic paralysis.

MANAGEMENT

1. **Careful examination of babies for signs of increasing jaundice.**

2. **Serum bilirubin estimations are made twice daily** in cases where a high bilirubin level exists; if rising, every 6 hours.

3. **Replacement blood transfusion is given** and repeated if necessary to lower the high serum bilirubin level.

OTHER CAUSES OF JAUNDICE IN THE NEWBORN BABY

Jaundice of immaturity (formerly known as " physiological ") is due to immaturity of the liver which **is intensified in premature babies.** Phototherapy may be employed. If jaundice persists for over 36 hours serum bilirubin is estimated and when over 18 mg. per 100 ml. or rising, and clinical signs warrant it, a replacement transfusion is given.

2. SEPSIS

Umbilical infection may spread to the liver, and in some instances no external signs are apparent, the jaundice usually occurring towards the end of the first week.

In acute pyelonephritis and septicæmia jaundice may be manifest.

3. CONGENITAL OBLITERATION OF THE BILE DUCT

Jaundice appears after several days, deepens in colour until the skin has a greenish bronze hue, which persists for weeks. The stools are putty-coloured, the urine contains bile. Serious hæmorrhage may occur, and only a few of these babies survive the necessary operative treatment.

HÆMORRHAGIC STATES OF THE NEWBORN BABY

MELÆNA

This most commonly occurs at the meconium stage. Oozing of blood takes place from the intestinal mucous membrane and is usually slight, but a massive hæmorrhage may occur. **The baby is pale** and collapsed in such cases, sometimes prior to the passage of blood in the stools. Save napkins for inspection, notify the doctor, treat shock. Blood transfusion and vitamins K_1 (Konakion 1 mg.) and C may be administered.

It must be remembered that blood from a cracked nipple may be swallowed and give rise to melæna, but in such a case the baby is not pale and the melæna is slight. Inexperienced midwives sometimes confuse meconium with melæna; meconium is dark green, melæna is black. If there is a pink ring on the napkin surrounding the stool, or if, when the napkin is placed in water, pink staining occurs, blood is present.

HÆMATEMESIS

This is not usually severe, and may be due to the swallowing of blood during labour.

HYPOPROTHROMBINÆMIA

Which is almost invariably present during the first three days of life, signifies a lack of prothrombin in the blood, so its clotting power is diminished, and when bleeding occurs, no matter what the cause, it tends to persist. Vitamin K_1 (Konakion 1 mg.) is usually administered.

OTHER CAUSES OF BLEEDING IN THE NEWBORN

1. **The small blood vessels may be damaged,** as occurs in intracranial injury.

2. **In anoxia the blood vessels throughout the body become engorged with blood** and oozing may take place into the organs and tissues.

3. Œstrogen withdrawal causes slight uterine bleeding in female babies (see p. 503).

4. **Omphalorrhagia** (*bleeding from the umbilicus*) **is usually due to shrinking of the cord** or an ineffectively applied ligature, and in such cases re-ligature is indicated. Death has occurred in such cases. 30 ml. of a baby's blood is the equivalent of 600 ml. of an adult's.

When bleeding occurs after the cord is off, it is commonly due to umbilical sepsis. The administration of vitamin K_1 and the application of adrenaline and pressure, or, in rare cases, a pair of artery forceps, will control it.

QUESTIONS FOR REVISION

Explain in 10 lines how you would cope with each of the following: (1) a mildly asphyxiated baby; (2) administration of oxygen by: (*a*) mask, (*b*) nasal catheter, (*c*) positive pressure; (3) endotracheal intubation; (4) mouth to mouth breathing.

A hypothermic baby feels .... to the touch; has a .... cry; respirations are ....; he is .... to feed; temperature is below ....

ASPHYXIA NEONATORUM

C.M.B.(N. Ireland) paper.—Mention as many causes of asphyxia neonatorum as you can and describe in detail how you would deal with a baby suffering from " white asphyxia."

C.M.B.(Scot.) paper.—Discuss the causes, risks and treatment of asphyxia neonatorum.

C.M.B.(Eng.) paper.—How would you resuscitate a baby who fails to breathe at birth? Give your reasons for the treatment you would adopt.

C.M.B.(Eng.) paper.—What are the signs of fetal distress? How should a baby born in a state of severe asphyxia be treated?

C.M.B.(N. Ireland) paper.—A newborn infant fails to breathe. What may cause this, and what would you do?

C.M.B.(N. Ireland) paper, 1969.—List the causes of fetal anoxia. Give a brief account of the immediate steps to be taken in the resuscitation of the newborn.

C.M.B.(Eng.) paper, 1969.—List the reasons why a newborn baby may not start to breathe. What actions would you take?

C.M.B.(Eng.) paper, 1970.—100 word question.—Asphyxia neonatorum.

NEONATAL INFECTIONS

Amplify what is meant by " intelligent mask wearing ".

Define ophthalmia neonatorum (Eng. or Scot. as applicable). Give 4 prophylactic measures. What precautions are taken in bathing the eyes? Why is the gonococcus the most dreaded organism?

For what conditions might the following drugs be used in the treatment of neonatal infections: cloxacillin; neomycin bacitracin powder; Terramycin ointment; hibitane 0·5 per cent in spirit; soluble penicillin; Colomycin; dequalinium; neomycin and kaolin; Ampiclox; framycetin cream; ephedrine.

What early signs would suggest: oral thrush; urinary tract infection; epidemic gastroenteritis; omphalitis; pemphigus; pneumonia?

C.M.B.(Scot.) paper.—Name four common infections which may occur in a nursery and state how each of these may be prevented.

C.M.B.(Scot.) paper.—Discuss nursing technique with a view to preventing infection of the newborn.

C.M.B.(N. Ireland) paper.—Describe the care of the skin, the eyes and the umbilical cord of the newborn with particular reference to the prevention of infection.

C.M.B.(Eng.) paper.—Outline the care necessary to prevent infection in the newly born infant.

C.M.B.(N. Ireland) paper.—An infant of one week, who is in a ward with other babies, begins to vomit its feeds and have loose green motions. What measure should be taken to deal with this situation?

C.M.B.(N. Ireland) paper, 1969.—What is ophthalmia neonatorum? Describe the prevention and treatment of this condition.

C.M.B.(Eng.) paper, 1969.—What infections may arise in the newborn infant? What steps should be taken to prevent these?

C.M.B.(Scot.) paper, 1969.—What infections may occur in the first two weeks of life? How may these be prevented?

HÆMOLYTIC DISEASE OF THE NEWBORN BABY

How would you deal with the umbilical cord if the mother has Rh antibodies ? **Why might sonar be used** prior to amniocentesis ?

What precautions are taken when transporting the amniotic fluid to the laboratory ? **During replacement transfusion:** (*a*) what observations does the midwife make ? (*b*) how is the baby kept warm ? (*c*) why is no sedative administered ? (*d*) why is the stomach sometimes aspirated ?

Define: (1) transplacental bleeding and state how a midwife could try to prevent this; (2) kernicterus—give signs and treatment.

With what techniques do you associate the following names: Kleihauer; Coombs; Tuohy ?

C.M.B.(N. Ireland) paper.—What is hæmolytic disease of the newborn ? Describe briefly the clinical appearance and the methods of diagnosis.

C.M.B.(N. Ireland) paper.—Give an account of the clinical manifestations of Rhesus incompatibility in the newborn infant. Describe briefly how an exchange transfusion is performed.

C.M.B.(N. Ireland) paper.—What are the causes of jaundice in a baby in the first week of life ? Describe briefly the treatment of any one of them.

C.M.B.(Eng.) paper.—Describe the common causes and management of jaundice in he newborn child.

C.M.B.(Eng.) paper. 100 word question.—Amniocentesis.

C.M.B.(Eng.) paper. 100 word question.—Hæmolytic disease.

32

Birth Injuries—Malformations

INTRACRANIAL INJURY AND HÆMORRHAGE

A NUMBER of babies who are stillborn or who die during the first week are found at post-mortem examination to have intracranial injuries. Physical and mental impairment may ensue in the babies who survive, and some cases of spastic paralysis are due to this cause: midwives should be as much concerned with prevention as with treatment of this grave condition.

STRUCTURES INVOLVED

The falx cerebri, a fold of meninges (dura mater), which dips down between the two halves of the cerebrum, is liable to be torn due to excessive or rapid compression of the fetal head during labour.

The tentorium cerebelli, a fold of dura mater, continuous with, but at right angles to, the falx cerebri and lying between the cerebrum and cerebellum is also liable to be torn.

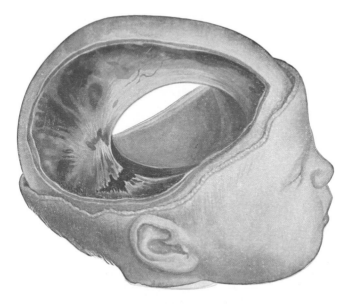

FIG. 383
Tearing of the tentorium cerebelli and hæmorrhage.

583

The vein of Galen, which is in close proximity to the tentorium, is the usual source of bleeding. The hæmorrhage is usually subdural and the presence of blood in the spinal fluid on subdural tap is diagnostic. Ultrasound has been used for diagnosis and a mid-line shift of the falx cerebri is manifest on the echo encephalogram.

Predisposing Causes

Premature babies, because of lack of protection by their soft skull bones and wide sutures as well as the delicacy of the cerebral vessels and tissues, are particularly prone to intracranial injury; the hæmorrhage is usually intraventricular.

CAUSES

1. ANOXIA

Profound venous engorgement of the cerebral vessels.

2. TRAUMA

Due to compression of the fetal head.

Excessive compression	Rapid compression	Upward moulding
(a) Contracted pelvis.	(a) Aftercoming head	(a) Aftercoming head
(b) Occipito-posterior.	in breech delivery.	in breech delivery
(c) Large baby.	(b) Precipitate labour.	(b) Face to pubes.
(d) Rigid pelvic floor.		

N.B.—The word " compression " is used as well as the word " moulding " to indicate how intracranial trauma occurs. If the compression is severe but of short duration as in the aftercoming head in a breech presentation no moulding is manifest, but nevertheless serious damage to the intracranial structures may have been inflicted.

PREVENTION

The midwife should try to recognize early, conditions in which the application of forceps or episiotomy might avert intracranial damage, and deliver with care and skill babies presenting by the breech or face to pubes.

In the following circumstances babies should be closely observed for signs of intracranial injury for at least 48 hours, even although these are not manifest at birth.

Prolonged labour.	Breech delivery.	Asphyxia.
Difficult labour.	Face to pubes.	Premature labour.

The indication for forceps rather than their application may necessitate intensive after care.

SIGNS

These depend on the severity of the condition, and all the signs are not necessarily manifest. In mild undiagnosed and untreated cases, signs, *e.g.* screaming, tenseness and rigidity may not be evident until the third or fourth day.

In severe cases at birth the infant is shocked, the eyes roll upwards or sideways (nystagmus) and twitching of the facial muscles may occur.

Difficult grunting expiration, often moist, due to excess of mucus; sometimes shallow, rapid and irregular with attacks of apnœa and cyanosis.

The sucking and swallowing reflexes are sometimes diminished; vomiting may occur.

Trunk and limbs may be rigid, the fists clenched; limpness is also common. Darting, adder-like movements of the tongue are seen

Worried and anxious expression: wrinkling of forehead; eyes wide open for long periods staring with a " knowing look." The infant is often pale or ashen grey with dark circles round the sunken eyes.

Twitching, convulsions, feeble murmuring cry or bouts of shrill shrieking, followed by limpness, due to exhaustion, and an ashen grey colour. Head retraction, rigid neck. Tense or spongy fontanelle.

The temperature is unstable.

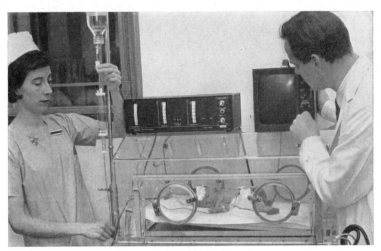

FIG. 384

MONITORING EQUIPMENT FOR NEONATAL INTENSIVE CARE.

Beckman vital signs monitor records pulse, temperature, respirations, blood pressure. Pædiatrician adjusting electrocardiograph tracing.

(*Neonatal Intensive Care Unit, Simpson Memorial Maternity Pavilion, Edinburgh.*)

Treatment

At birth, as for severe asphyxia. Some give vitamin K_1 (Konakion) 1 mg.

Place the baby in a quiet, warm room (intensive care unit).

The following should be at hand : oxygen, mechanical suction or mucus extractors; laryngoscope, endotracheal tube; diazepam (Valium); sodium phenobarbitone.

Handle the baby as little as possible. Do not weigh, measure or bath the baby. Handling provokes convulsions but the infant should be turned from side to side every hour or two. The baby should not be removed from his cot. Secretions that accumulate in the pharynx must be removed by suction.

SEDATION

The doctor will order a sedative such as diazepam (Valium). If the drug is not effective the midwife must notify the doctor for it is essential that the infant be relaxed and asleep. Sodium phenobarbitone, 15 mg. followed by 7·5 mg. is sometimes given six or eight hourly intramuscularly, Syrup of Luminal, 4 ml., contains 8 mg. phenobarbitone.

33

FEEDING

No food or fluid is given for 6 hours, to avoid aspiration of vomitus. The infant is fed in the cot, naso-gastric tube feeding often being advisable. Sufficient fluid must be given to maintain the fluid balance.

CONVULSIONS IN THE NEWBORN

These may be due to intracranial injury and severe infections, *e.g.* meningitis.

Biochemical imbalance, *e.g.*, hypoglycæmia and hypocalcæmia are important causes.

Premonitory signs such as twitching of the muscles of the face, hands and feet may be manifest.

Convulsions vary in length and severity and the stages may not be clearly defined.

Rigidity of the limbs and spine with head retraction usually occur; the eyes roll or stare and cyanosis rapidly deepens due to respiration being interrupted because of spasm of the diaphragm.

Generalized convulsive movements may follow; head, arms and legs jerking spasmodically, froth appears on the lips and strabismus may be present. The convulsion gradually subsides but slight twitching may persist.

Following the seizure the child is in a comatose state, limp and pale or ashen grey in colour.

Convulsion Chart (*Simpson Memorial Maternity Pavilion, Edinburgh*)						
Date	Time	Type (tonic, clonic)	Region(s) involved	Apnœa	Cyanosis	Duration

Treatment

The doctor is notified.

If regurgitating milk turn baby face downwards and clear the airway.

Mucus is removed from mouth and nose by mechanical suction or mucus extractors.

Baby is propped over on side to prevent the tongue from blocking the larynx.

Oxygen is administered. Warm blankets are applied.

Sedatives such as phenobarbitone 8 mg. or diazepam (Valium) 0·25 to 0·5 for initial control, maintenance dose 0·1 mg./kg. t.d.s.

The midwife should obtain blood by heel stab and do an immediate Dextrostix test for hypoglycæmia when a convulsion occurs during the first 48 hours of life.

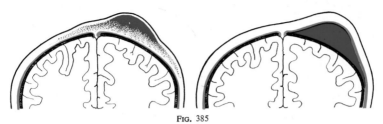

Fig. 385

Black line = skull bone.   *Faint blue line = pericranium.*   *Yellow line = scalp.*

CAPUT SUCCEDANEUM

A caput succedaneum is an œdematous swelling on the fetal skull, a serosanguineous (serum and blood) infiltration into the scalp tissue. Due to pressure by a " *girdle of contact* " which is usually the cervix; the venous blood supply is retarded, and the area lying over the os (*the presenting part*) becomes congested and œdematous.

A secondary caput may form:

(*a*) **In occipito-posterior positions** when the head rotates forwards.

(*b*) **In cases where the head is held up on the perineum.**

1. **Is present at birth.**
2. **May cross a suture.**
3. **Tends to grow less.**
4. **Disappears within 36 hours.**
5. **Is diffuse, pits on pressure.**
6. **A double caput is always unilateral.**

CEPHALHÆMATOMA

A cephalhæmatoma is a swelling on the fetal skull, an effusion of blood under the periosteum covering it, due to friction between the skull and pelvis. It occurs in cases of cephalopelvic disproportion and precipitate labour, when tearing of the periosteum from the bone causes bleeding.

As the pericranium (periosteum) is adherent to the edges of the skull bones, the swelling is confined to one bone.

No treatment is necessary, the blood is absorbed and the swelling subsides. After one week a ridge of bone may be felt round the periphery of the swelling, due to the accumulation of osteoblasts.

1. **Appears after 24 hours.**
2. **Never crosses a suture.**
3. **Tends to grow larger.**
4. **Persists for weeks.**
5. **Is circumscribed, does not pit.**
6. **A double cephalhæmatoma is usually bilateral** (Fig. 388).

CAPUT

CEPHALHÆMATOMA

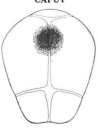
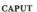
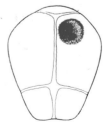

May cross a suture   Does not cross a suture

Fig. 386

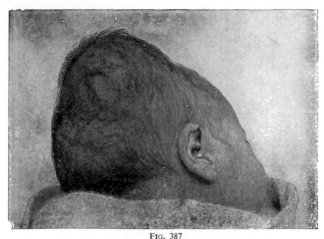

FIG. 387
Unilateral cephalhæmatoma.

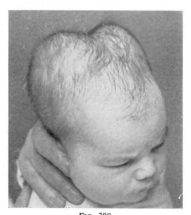

FIG. 388
Bilateral cephalhæmatoma.

MOULDING OF THE BABY'S HEAD
For definition see p. 51

Head moulding varies with presentation and position, and an experienced midwife can diagnose these by examining the shape of the head and position of the caput. The engaging diameter is always diminished.

When moulding is excessive, as occurs in cases where disproportion between the fetal head and the maternal pelvis exists, cranial compression occurs and serious intracranial injury may be inflicted. A large caput is usually present in such instances.

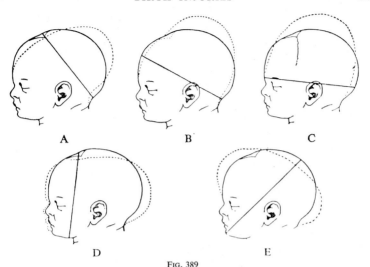

FIG. 389

TYPES OF MOULDING IN HEAD PRESENTATIONS SHOWN BY DOTTED LINE.

Top row.—A, Vertex presentation head well flexed. B, Vertex presentation, posterior position (note that the moulding is higher). C, Vertex presentation head deflexed (the sugar-loaf head). Bottom row.—D, Face presentation. E, Brow presentation.

FRACTURES

Fractures in the newborn are always complete, not greenstick, and because of rapid callus formation and bone growth permanent deformity is rare.

THE SKULL

Fractures are rare, but spoon-shaped indentations may occur, due to pressure from the promontory of the sacrum in the rare cases in which a woman with pelvic deformity is allowed to go into labour. If the baby survives, the depression gradually becomes rectified as growth proceeds.

THE SPINE

The spine is seldom fractured, unless by mismanagement in delivering the after-coming head in a breech presentation, *i.e.* by bending the cervical vertebræ acutely backwards. Stillbirth results.

THE HUMERUS

Fracture may occur in dealing with shoulder dystocia and in bringing down extended arms if the midwife does not " splint " the humerus while so doing. Deformity is evident and the infant does not move the arm freely.

Treatment

Medical aid is required. Attempts to elicit crepitus should not be made.

Adhesive strapping is applied to the upper arm, which is then placed alongside the trunk, with a pad of wool in the axilla. The forearm is flexed, with the fingers touching the clavicle on the opposite side, and a 10·2-cm. (4-inch) bandage used to bind the arm

33A

to the body, taking care not to impede respiration. Callus forms in about 10 days and the infant is then allowed free movement.

For a fractured clavicle most authorities consider no treatment is necessary.

INJURY TO MUSCLES AND NERVES

The sterno-mastoid muscle in the neck may be bruised and lacerated if the head is pulled sideways in delivering the anterior shoulder, or if the neck is twisted in rotating the shoulders during breech delivery. A small hæmatoma forms, and a swelling the size of a pigeon's egg appears one or two weeks after birth. Gentle massage and movement, with stretching of the neck muscles carried out after feeds are sufficient to cause regression of the tumour.

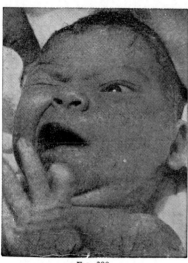

Fig. 390

Left-sided Facial Paralysis.

Note that the eye is open on the paralysed side, the mouth drawn over to the non-paralysed side.

FACIAL PARALYSIS

Facial paralysis occurs when the facial (seventh cranial) nerve is compressed unduly, as may be done with the forceps blade, or by hæmorrhage and œdema round the nerve. It may occur in a spontaneous delivery if, when grasping the head, undue pressure is applied on the mastoid process or over the ramus of the lower jaw where the facial nerve is very superficial.

Signs

The paralysed side is smooth; the corner of the mouth droops and milk dribbles out, but sucking is not interfered with; the eye usually remains open. In crying, the mouth is drawn over to the uninjured side of the face.

No treatment is required other than the application of an ophthalmic ointment dressing over the eye, if open, during sleep. The condition improves in one or two weeks; should paralysis persist, the damage is probably intracranial.

ERB'S PARALYSIS

The upper arm hangs limply, close to the body, and the infant cannot lift it although he can move the hand and fingers. The arm is inwardly rotated and the half-closed hand turned outwards (the waiter's tip).

Erb's paralysis is due to damage or stretching of the roots of the brachial plexus (a nerve junction at the side of the neck under the clavicle). This occurs when the neck is twisted or stretched, as might happen in delivering the aftercoming head of the breech, or in excessive lateral flexion of the neck when delivering the shoulders in a vertex presentation.

Treatment

Until a light metal splint is procured, a padded bandage is applied round the wrist and pinned to the pillow region of the cot, to maintain abduction and external rotation of the arm. The upper arm is kept at right-angles to the body, the forearm flexed, fingers pointing to the pillow and the palm facing the side of the head.

Massage and passive movement are usually ordered. The arm may recover in weeks, or it may be months. Severe damage may give rise to permanent " birth palsy," the arm being short and wasted.

INJURY TO ABDOMINAL ORGANS

Rupture of the liver, which is relatively very large in the newborn, may be caused by grasping the body during a breech delivery. The condition is usually diagnosed at post-mortem examination, but occasional survival has been recorded.

ALIMENTARY LESIONS

ŒSOPHAGEAL ATRESIA

This is associated with a fistula between the œsophagus and trachea in 90 per cent of cases due to faulty development of these structures. (Hydramnios is usually present, probably because the fetus is unable to swallow liquor amnii.)

Œsophageal atresia should be suspected prior to giving the first feed by the presence of fine frothy mucus in the mouth and nostrils and a history of hydramnios. An adult No. 8 Jaques catheter should be passed into the

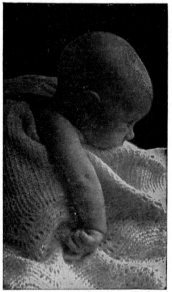

Fig. 391
Erb's paralysis.

œsophagus (a soft thin one may curl up); if obstructed at 5 to 7 cm. œsophageal atresia is suspected.

X-rays are used to confirm the diagnosis; a radio-opaque catheter being inserted into the œsophagus.

Treatment

On no account should the baby be given water or milk to drink; he is liable to inhale it, collapse of lung may occur, pneumonia ensue, and the success of the necessary surgical operation will be impaired. If fed the baby coughs, splutters and becomes cyanosed. **Suction ought to be used at once** or the baby held upside down to drain off the fluid. He is then kept in a semi-raised position to prevent gastric juice from entering the trachea through a fistula, any accumulation of secretion in the nose and throat being removed by suction. **Medical aid is summoned.** The pouch should be emptied prior to transporting the infant for chest surgery; the baby kept warm, propped up and suction used repeatedly.

INTESTINAL OBSTRUCTION

DUODENAL ATRESIA

This is the commonest cause; volvulus, fibrous bands or adhesions may also occlude the bowel. **Vomiting is persistent,** first milk then bile; green vomitus that stains what it falls on continues. The upper abdomen may be distended, and following the passage of meconium no further stools are passed.

Fluids and electrolytes must be replaced but nothing given by mouth. An immediate operation is often successful.

ANO-RECTAL ATRESIA

(Imperforate Anus)

The anal sphincter may be closed by a membrane, in which case it can be reconstructed operatively. In certain types operation is carried out immediately; a colostomy is sometimes performed.

On examining the infant and attempting to take the " first " temperature rectally, no anus is found to be present. A small amount of meconium may be passed, because frequently in such cases a fistula from the intestine opens between the fourchette and the vaginal orifice in girl babies, and on the perineum in boys.

PYLORIC STENOSIS

Pyloric stenosis is rare during the first week. The gastric contents are forcibly ejected. Waves of gastric peristalsis, running from left to right, are usually visible abdominally after feeds. The treatment of pyloric stenosis is mainly surgical.

Pyloric spasm gives rise to similar signs, but is less serious, and may start within three days of birth. The vomitus contains much mucus. The condition is amenable to medical treatment.

CONGENITAL ABNORMALITIES

Great concern is being felt regarding the number of congenital abnormalities that now occur; about 2 per cent of births. They may be physical or mental. The causes are not fully understood but are usually divided into two main groups :—

1. GENETIC OR INHERITED

The defect is transmitted via the genes in the ovum or spermatozoon.

MONGOLISM; ANENCEPHALY; CLEFT PALATE; CLEFT LIP; ACHONDROPLASIA.

2. ENVIRONMENTAL CAUSES

(*a*) ANOXIA.   (*b*) INFECTION.   (*c*) RADIATION.
(*d*) SEVERE MALNUTRITION.   (*e*) DRUGS.

In the early embryonic state tissues are particularly vulnerable to deprivation of vital substances, *i.e.* oxygen and nutrients, and this may impair their structure and impede function. The very small delicate organs have little resistance to infection or noxious substances and are readily damaged ; the placenta, never a perfect barrier, is less effective prior to the 12th week.

If the adverse factor is active during the time at which a particular tissue is being laid down or a special organ is being formed—*e.g.* heart, brain, limb, eye, ear—that organ is likely to be damaged. Cardiac defects, mental subnormality, absence of limbs, cataract and blindness or deafness, may result.

(*a*) ANOXIA

The embryo requires a constant supply of oxygen and lack of this may seriously affect the developing brain cells.

Oxygen lack may occur if:

(i) The mother's blood is deficient in oxygen due to conditions that produce cyanosis, *e.g.* serious cardiac or pulmonary disease, general anæsthesia inexpertly induced.

(ii) The placenta is partially separated as may occur during a threatened abortion.

(b) INFECTION

The infection rubella, occurring during the first 12 weeks of pregnancy, is the most outstanding example (see p. 200).

(c) RADIATION

Exposure to radioactive substances (used in industry) is dangerous in pregnancy.

Diagnostic (abdominal) radiology is avoided during the first 30 weeks of pregnancy.

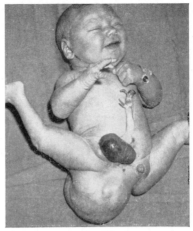

FIG. 392

Multiple malformation of pelvis and perineum, sacral meningocele, bladder normally situated.

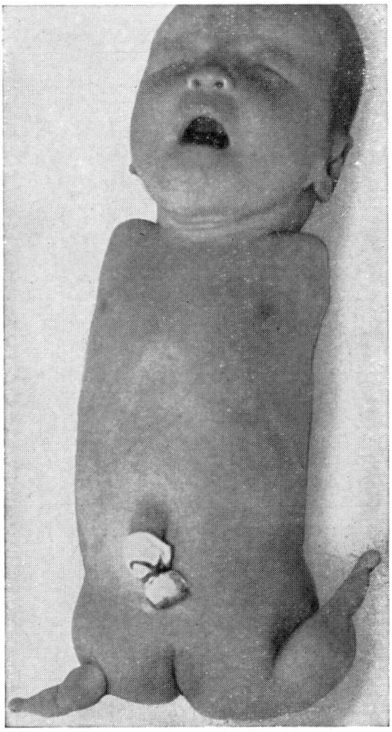

(d) DRUGS

Great caution is now being observed in prescribing drugs during the first 12 weeks of pregnancy when the developing embryo is at risk.

During 1960-62 in Great Britain 244 babies were born with phocomelia and/or amelia (see Fig. 393).

This grave tragedy is thought to be due to the action of the drug Thalidomide ingested by pregnant women during the fourth to eighth week of pregnancy as a sedative or as an anti-emetic for morning sickness.

Midwives should warn expectant mothers against taking drugs other than those prescribed by the doctor.

Progestogens and adrenal corticoid hormones administered in early pregnancy have produced male type genitalia in female babies. (Preparations now on the market do not have such side effects.)

HYDROCEPHALY

The hydrocephalic head is unusually big, the sutures and fontanelles are large and often full, the bones thinned out because of an excess of cerebro-spinal fluid in the

FIG. 393

Baby with amelia (no arms), phocomelia (long bones absent), due to Thalidomide.

ventricles of the brain. Hydrocephaly is mainly caused by some obstruction in the cerebro-spinal fluid pathway. The forehead is prominent.

EFFECT ON LABOUR

The fetus may present by the breech, and on abdominal palpation the large soft head in the fundus may be thought to be the buttocks.

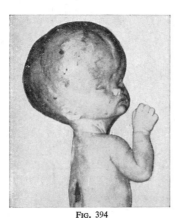

FIG. 394

HYDROCEPHALY.

Cerebro-spinal fluid, 2·1 litres withdrawn by Drew Smythe catheter via the spina-bifida.

(*Aberdeen Maternity Hospital.*)

In cases where the vertex presents, the head is high and feels large. But because the soft head is so compressible it may partly enter the brim, is not mobile, and may not on that account be recognized by the novice.

On vaginal examination, a wide fluctuant area is felt over the sutures and fontanelles. If undiagnosed, labour will be obstructed.

An inexperienced midwife may not detect hydrocephaly until a small fetus, presenting by the breech and born as far as the umbilicus, does not advance.

TREATMENT

In vertex presentation craniotomy and application of Briggs forceps is performed during the first stage of labour. In breech presentation the head is perforated (craniotomy) through the occiput or roof of the mouth; crushing is not always necessary as the head collapses when the fluid escapes. A long metal catheter is sometimes inserted into the spinal canal through an incision or spina-bifida and the fluid drained off. In a case at the Simpson Maternity Pavilion, 2·3 litres were withdrawn in this way.

Hydrocephaly may develop after birth, and if suspected by undue growth of the head, the occipito-frontal circumference should be measured daily, the normal increase being 1·25 cm. per month. Widening of the occipito-mastoid suture is almost diagnostic: ventriculography may be employed for confirmation of the diagnosis. The eyes point downwards giving the " setting sun " sign. Some hydrocephalic babies die, others live, but may be mentally sub-normal.

Good results have been obtained by draining the excess cerebro-spinal fluid from the lateral ventricle of the brain into the right atrium of the heart by using a Holter or a Pudenz Heyer valve.

ANENCEPHALY

This is a severe form of arrested development; the vault of the skull and cerebrum being absent. Frequently it is accompanied by an extensive spina-bifida. Because there is transudation of fluid from the exposed meninges, hydramnios is usually present; this makes palpation difficult, but as the abdomen is usually X-rayed in cases of hydramnios the malformation is detected during pregnancy.

Labour is induced prematurely, and the fetus commonly, but not invariably, presents by the face. The second stage may be somewhat prolonged, because the cervix must dilate further to allow passage of the shoulders, which are broad in comparison with the small head. Anencephalic fetuses live for only a few moments; 75 per cent are female.

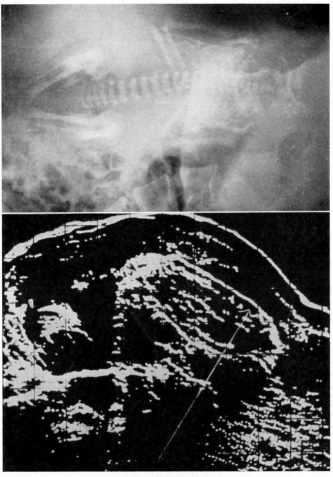

FIG. 395 (*Upper*)
X-RAY OF ANENCEPHALIC FETUS.

FIG. 396 (*Lower*)
ULTRASONOGRAM OF SAME FETUS.
(*Simpson Memorial Maternity Pavilion, Edinburgh.*)

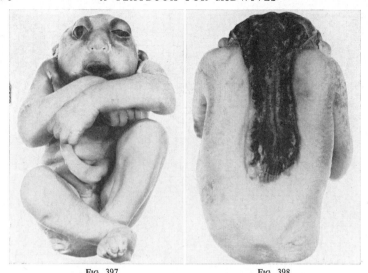

FIG. 397   FIG. 398

ANENCEPHALY WITH SPINA-BIFIDA (*Myelomeningocele*).

Fig. 397.—Anterior view.   Fig. 398.—Posterior view showing extensive spina-bifida.

ENCEPHALOCELE: MENINGOCELE

These tumours, on the fetal skull, covered with meninges, usually protrude through the lambdoidal suture. An encephalocele contains brain substance: it pulsates, is opaque, does not fluctuate, and usually has a pedicle. A large encephalocele may obstruct labour.

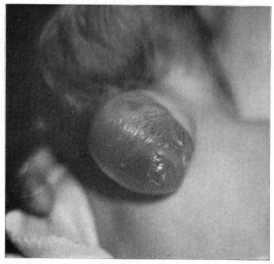

FIG. 399

MENINGOCELE (*cervical*).

A meningocele contains cerebro-spinal fluid, is fluctuant, does not pulsate, and becomes tense when the baby cries. A large meningocele usually ruptures during delivery; small ones have been dealt with successfully by aspiration or other surgical means.

The sac should be covered with a N.A. (non-adhering) dressing or sterile gauze moistened with isotonic saline, wrapped in cotton wool and bandaged pending the arrival of medical aid.

SPINA-BIFIDA

This fairly common defect is due to failure of the neural arches of the vertebræ to unite during embryonic life and permits the meninges, and sometimes the spinal cord to protrude through the gap. Several adjacent vertebræ may be involved.

3,000 *occur in Britain every year.*

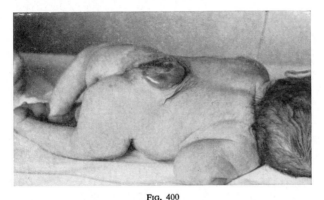

Fig. 400
Spina-bifida.
Note hair on skin surrounding tumour. The limbs are paralysed.

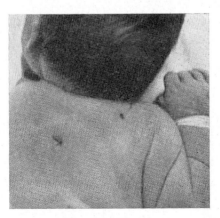

Fig. 401
Very slight spina-bifida; manifest by dimpling of the skin.

34

The commonest form is recognized by the presence of a reddish mass, soft and fluctuant, in the sacro-lumbar region. More serious cases have exposed nerve tissue= myelomeningocele.

The midwife should notify the doctor, apply a non-adhering dressing (non-oily) and isolate the baby.

In many centres operation is carried out immediately, day or night (or within 12 hours), and the incidence of meningitis and paralysis has been reduced by so doing, but some severe cases may not be suitable for surgery. Fifty per cent of babies develop hydrocephalus after operation. *The shunting of cerebro-spinal fluid as described (on p. 594) under hydrocephalus has improved the prognosis in cases of spina bifida.*

Spina bifida occulta may be manifest by mere dimpling of the skin or a patch of hair. The bony defect can be seen by radiography.

EXOMPHALOS

Exomphalos is a protrusion of the abdominal organs, contained within a sac of peritoneum, through a large umbilical opening, sometimes 7·6 cm. in diameter. A non-adherent dressing is applied and the infant transferred from the labour ward to the operating theatre; care being exercised to avoid rupturing the sac. Operative measures are usually successful, if carried out without delay, even when the sac has ruptured and the abdominal organs are exposed.

UMBILICAL HERNIA

Umbilical hernia consists of a small swelling which projects from the umbilicus, usually a few weeks after the cord has separated, seldom containing bowel or omentum and easily reducible. Medical advice is sought.

The modern view is that no treatment (not even a pad and binder) is indicated in the majority of cases, spontaneous cure taking place within 18 months, but if not, operative repair will be necessary, preferably at the age of 18 to 24 months. If large, operation may be considered at 9 months.

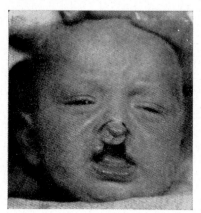

FIG. 402

Bilateral cleft lip and palate.

CLEFT LIP: CLEFT PALATE

Cleft lip and cleft palate can occur singly or together, and either may be unilateral or bilateral. The malformation is due to lack of union of the fronto-nasal palate, and may be slight or severe.

Every newborn baby's mouth should be inspected in a good light, as the soft palate only may be cleft.

In such a case choking and cyanotic attacks may occur at feeding time and milk is returned down the nose.

The cleft lip may be unilateral and very slight, or more extensive. The most severe form is manifest when bilateral (or double) cleft lip and cleft palate are both present. There is a wide gap between the nostrils, with a piece of bone projecting through it. Between the double cleft in the palate the vomer can be seen.

TREATMENT

The unilateral cleft lip may be repaired during the third to sixth weeks (some are done on the 10th day) to obtain a good cosmetic result; other surgeons prefer to wait until the infant weighs 4·5 kg. (10 lb.) with hæmoglobin over 11·8 G. (80 per cent) and no respiratory infection.

Bilateral cleft lip requires a more extensive surgical procedure and this is usually deferred until the infant is three months old.

Operation on the cleft palate is done when the child is about 18 months old; after then, the earlier the operation the better will the speech be.

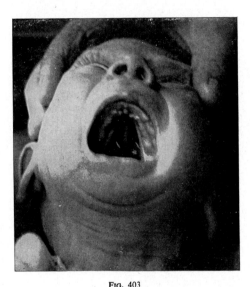

FIG. 403
Bilateral cleft palate.

To allay their disappointment mothers should be assured that the cosmetic results are now excellent, and they should be given ample experience while in hospital in feeding the baby (held in the upright position) and cleansing the mouth.

A large soft teat should be used to give the infant some of the satisfaction of sucking. Special teats with a flap to fill the gap in the palate are on the market.

DENTAL PLATES

For complete clefts of the lip and palate, dental plates are now being used to achieve the maximal degree of pre-surgical alignment of the segments of the maxilla prior to operation. They are applied during the first week of age, worn all the time, taken out and cleansed after feeds. Biting of the lower gums on the splint is an essential part of the treatment. The plates are remade every three or four weeks until the fourth month when the lip is repaired This succession of progressively smaller plates pulls the cleft segment and gum margins together. The babies do not resent them. With reasonable care there is no danger of choking or of swallowing the plates. It is important to keep the lips well lubricated with petroleum jelly.

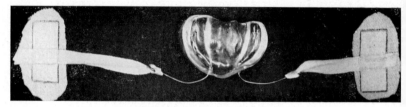

FIG. 404

DENTAL PLATE FOR NEWBORN.

The tapes fastened to the wire of the plate are held in position by a strip of adhesive which is attached to pieces of elastoplast on the cheeks. This avoids excoriating the skin during the frequent removals to cleanse the plate.

(*by courtesy of Orthodontic Department, School of Dental Surgery, Edinburgh.*)

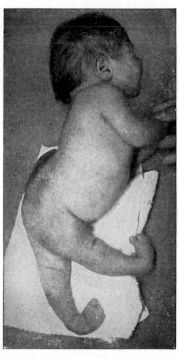

FIG. 405

Talipes equino varus.

Advantages:

(*a*) Bottle feeding is possible. (*b*) There is less risk of respiratory infection.

(*c*) Infection of the Eustachian tube with the risk of deafness is avoided.

(*d*) The teeth are likely to be less irregular.

(*e*) Repositioning helps the dentist and orthodontist in their care of the teeth.

CLUB-FOOT

TALIPES EQUINO VARUS

This deformity, in which the foot is bent downwards and inwards, may be unilateral or bilateral; the cause is not properly understood. There ought to be free movement of the normal foot in all directions and it should be possible to dorsiflex it until the small toe almost touches the leg.

TALIPES CALCANEO-VALGUS

The foot is turned upwards and bent outwards—the opposite of talipes varus

Treatment

Gentle but firm manipulation and splinting is commenced on the day of birth, and the deformity fully corrected as soon as possible even for prematures. Manipulation is carried out every four days and the foot maintained in the over-corrected position by adhesive strapping, Denis Browne's splints, or, in some centres, plaster fixation. Except when the deformity is excessive, complete correction is achieved at the age of 12 months.

CONGENITAL DISLOCATION OF THE HIP

This abnormality, which may be unilateral or bilateral, occurs in about 1 in 1,000 babies, and is five times more common in the female.

It has been suggested that laxity of the capsule of the hip joint may be due to the relaxing action of hormones affecting the fetus *in utero*. The condition is more common in lands where babies are bound to a " cradle board " with the thighs straight.

Orthopædic surgeons are eager that the condition be recognized during the first few days of life in order to achieve the most successful result and to avoid the necessity for operation.

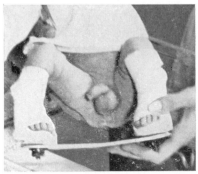

FIG. 406
DENIS BROWNE'S SPLINT.
Baby 30 days old, adhesive tape applied for 28 days.
(*Neonatal Intensive Care Unit, Aberdeen Maternity Hospital.*)

BARLOW'S TEST

This is a modification of Ortolani's test.

Each leg with hip and knee flexed is held in one of the examiner's hands with the middle fingers over the greater trochanter and the thumb on the inner side of the thigh approximately opposite the lesser trochanter. With the thighs held in mid-

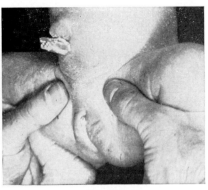

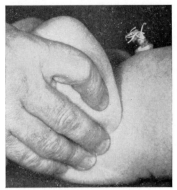

FIG. 407
Both thumbs applied to the inner aspects of the infant's thighs in front of the lesser trochanters.

FIG. 408
The middle fingers are placed over the greater trochanters.

Showing position of hands in carrying out Barlow's test for congenital dislocation of hip.
(*Courtesy of Zimmer Orthopædics Ltd., 176 Brompton Road, London, S.W.3.*)

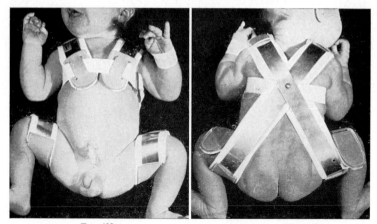

FIG. 409   FIG. 410

BARLOW SPLINT IN POSITION.

(Courtesy of Zimmer Orthopædics Ltd., 176 Brompton Road, London, S.W.3.)

abduction lifting with the middle finger will cause reduction of a dislocated hip, a movement that can be felt as a click or clunk.

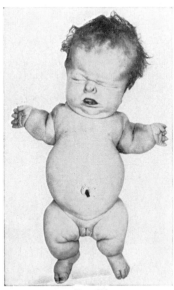

FIG. 411

Achondroplasia

If no such " click " occurs then the hip is not dislocated.

In cases of doubt, steadying the pelvis with one hand while the doubtful hip is examined with the other hand makes the test more sensitive.

Treatment

A Vynide covered Duralumin splint, such as the Barlow, is applied at birth and worn constantly during the first three months of life to maintain 90 degrees flexion and full abduction: the infant is seen at weekly intervals for adjustment of the splint.

ACHONDROPLASIA

In this rare condition the limbs are short due to failure in the ossification of the long bones during early fetal life. The body is of normal length. The majority of these babies survive and mental development is normal, but they remain permanently dwarfed.

BIRTH MARKS

Most birth marks consist of an abnormal collection of small blood vessels and are not due to the various experiences during pregnancy often quoted by mothers. Small flat pinkish red areas, commonly seen on the eyelids and nape of the neck, disappear in a few weeks.

Cavernous hæmangioma, known as " *strawberry marks*," are bright red in colour, slightly elevated and sharply defined. They appear during the first week of life, increase in size until six months and usually disappear before the 6th year.

The spider nævus, a common vascular blemish, has a centre with blood vessels radiating from it and can be treated with a diathermy needle.

Port wine stain (or capillary hæmangioma) is a deep purple discoloration, which is not raised and does not blanch on pressure, frequently seen on the face and sometimes extensive and very disfiguring. It is resistant to treatment but can be made paler by the repeated application of thorium X. Cosmetic disguise is usually necessary for lesions on the face and good proprietary preparations are available.

Pigmented nævi, or moles, vary in size and may be covered with fine hair; the author having seen cases of melanomata in which the lesions were 10·2 to 12·7 cm. (4 to 5 inches) in diameter. Some have a malignant tendency. Excision and radiotherapy are employed.

No treatment is given for congenital nævi during the neonatal period.

THE MENTALLY SUBNORMAL INFANT

DOWN'S SYNDROME (*The Mongol*)

This is one of the few types of mental subnormality recognizable at birth, probably because of the striking resemblance they bear to each other.

Mongols have an extra chromosome (trisomy 21)—47 instead of 46. **The cause is unknown.**

The condition is associated with ageing of the maternal ovaries; the incidence in age groups having been estimated as follows:

Mothers under 25	.	.	.	1 in 3,000
,, under 35	.	.	.	1 in 2,000
,, over 35	.	.	.	1 in 600
,, over 45	.	.	.	1 in 35

The head is small with a flat occiput; the slanting eyes, short upper lip and small mouth give the characteristic appearance which is said to resemble that of the Mongolian race. Rosy cheeks are present at birth, a feature which persists throughout life. The hands are short with crumpled palms: *significant differences in the dermal configuration of finger, palm and sole patterns have been observed.* A palmar crease unbroken from side to side (the simian crease) is present; the great toe is widely separated from the other toes: the baby when held in the arms feels soft and hypotonic.

40-50 per cent have congenital cardiac lesions from which a number die in infancy.

Leukæmia is 15 times more common than in normal babies.

DIAGNOSIS

A diagnosis of Down's syndrome should not be made until the facial appearance of both parents is studied.

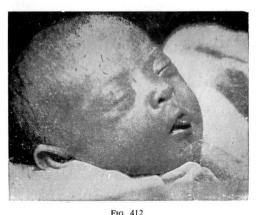

Fig. 412
Down's Syndrome.
(The mongol)

Should a skin biopsy be required for confirmation of the diagnosis permission must be obtained in writing. A venous blood sample for chromosome analysis is preferable.

Mongolism occurring when the maternal age is under 30 is fully investigated. Some of these are translocation mongols who have only 46 chromosomes and this may recur in 30 per cent of cases.

In a subsequent pregnancy amniotic fluid can be withdrawn on abdominal amniocentesis at 14 to 16 weeks and the exfoliated skin cells examined microscopically. Therapeutic abortion may be considered if the fetus carries a translocation chromosome.

The midwife should neither tell the mother nor imply that the child is mentally subnormal. Some think it is kinder to allow the fact to dawn gradually on her, but that decision rests with the doctor, who may prefer to inform both parents together at home after the first week and when the diagnosis is certain.

Mongol children learn to walk later than usual (2 to 3 years); their speech is usually poor: they are clean in their habits and happy children; some live to a ripe old age.

The policy of 1971 is to keep as many of these children out of hospital as is possible; the family environment being considered best for every child. Much depends on the parents' wishes. Local authorities are now providing day training centres for mentally handicapped children. Some can be gainfully employed as adults in industry at repetitive tasks in protected conditions.

THE MICROCEPHALIC INFANT

These infants have a small brain and miniature head of less than 27·9 cm. (11 inches) occipito-frontal circumference at birth. The forehead is shallow and receding, the fontanelles small or closed. All babies whose heads are less than normal in size are not necessarily microcephalic even although mentally retarded. Spasticity of the limbs is often present. The condition is estimated to occur in about 1 in 15,000 births.

EDUCATIONAL ROLE OF THE MIDWIFE

Many of the environmental causes of congenital abnormalities are preventable and the midwife must participate in the programme of health education that should be inaugurated to avoid these.

All women (and schoolgirls of 14 to 15 years) should be made aware of the importance of prenatal supervision. They must know that women should attend for advice as soon as they become pregnant, otherwise they will not obtain the necessary supervision and instruction at the vital early period when the embryo is at risk.

Advice should be given, without giving rise to alarm, about :

(*a*) **The danger of taking drugs** other than a mild aperient, unless prescribed by the doctor. Many common drugs found in the home have been found to be harmful.

(*b*) **The risk of contact with Rubella** and the importance of reporting such contact at once. The vaccination of girls before puberty with Cendevax vaccine.

(*c*) **The necessity for a wholesome diet** rich in body-building foods, iron, dairy products, fruit and vegetables: **the need for rest and obtaining medical advice** for bleeding in early pregnancy.

Dealing with Parents of the Handicapped Baby

The mother is likely to be profoundly distressed if her baby has some genetic physica deformity or mental subnormality and *may question the midwife regarding*:—the **cause; whether she or her husband is to blame; whether the condition could have been prevented.**

The mother should be assured that:—

neither she nor her husband is blameworthy: that the causes are not fully understood. Any further information or explanation will be given by the doctor in charge.

The midwife should give emotional support and help the mother to accept the situation. She should also assure her regarding facilities available.

It does not require much imagination to understand the mother's feelings and to appreciate the bitter disappointment both parents must face.

The woman needs mental comfort and assurance. On no account should the midwife register surprise or exhibit disapproval of the mother's immediate reaction which may, particularly in young mothers, be one of self-pity or rejection of the infant. Having recovered from the initial shock the majority of parents resolve to do what is best for their child and to give him the loving care he will need. In fact some are over-protective.

Parents need guidance in day to day management, for their attitude and co-operation affect the child's progress. They also need hope and encouragement to enable them to cope with continuing doubts and difficulties.

FACILITIES AVAILABLE

Mothers should be told of the excellent results achieved by surgeons in dealing with physical deformities, remedial and cosmetic.

Appliances are provided to correct disabilities and, when necessary, to replace undeveloped limbs. To further surgical correction and enable the child to lead a happy independent life physiotherapists, speech and occupational therapists are available. Local authorities provide day residential training centres for children severely handicapped (physically and mentally). **The help of social workers** should be elicited in order that arrangements for contact with exisiting associations and agencies can be made.

Parent clubs, at which experience in overcoming problems in home management of the child can be shared: giving the mother help and fellowship in what can be, as in cases of spina bifida, a most distressing situation. The child must be provided with special opportunities for development that come naturally to the active normal child.

GENETIC COUNSELLING

Genetic counselling clinics have been established in some centres in Britain: the geneticist explains and where possible reassures regarding the risk of certain hereditary abnormalities and diseases occurring or recurring. Guilt feelings are dispelled by such counselling.

About 2 per cent of babies are born with a congenital abnormality; not all are genetic.

Chromosomes

The 46 chromosomes in each cell of the body are of two types, sex determination and autosomal. The autosomes, the non-sex chromosomes, carry the genes that transmit the hereditary characteristics of the parents, *i.e.* blood group, Rh factor, colour of skin and eyes, stature, intelligence and so on. Some persons are genetically predisposed to diseases such as diabetes, cancer, hypertension. Sickle cell anæmia is due to an abnormal hæmoglobin gene. Phenylketonuria is a hereditary condition. Talipes, cleft lip and palate, anencephaly all have an inherited factor in their causation. Down's syndrome is caused by having an extra autosome (known as trisomy), 47 instead of 46.

Abnormalities in sex chromosomes can give rise to intersex states, disturbances in sexual function, male and female sterility; hermaphroditism being an abnormality the midwife may encounter.

Prenatal investigations by transabdominal amniocentesis are made to obtain embryonic cells which are examined to determine various factors: the sex of the embryo, chromosomal, metabolic and other inborn anomalies.

It may be possible in future to screen pregnant women over 40, prior to the 14th week, in an endeavour to reduce the number of babies born with Down's syndrome. On detecting the presence of the extra chromosome—trisomy 21—therapeutic abortion should be considered.

Chromosomal studies are sometimes made in cases of sterility and may also be requested by an adoption society if a parental disorder is suspected of being hereditary. Disputed paternity can be disproved (but not proved) if the child has a blood group substance not present in the putative father or lacks a blood group substance the father would have transmitted.

Genetic counselling is a highly specialized subject and midwives would be well advised not to express an opinion regarding the possible recurrence of some abnormality.

The medical geneticist explains the situation and the chances of recurrence; the parents decide whether to plan having any more children.

QUESTIONS FOR REVISION

BIRTH INJURIES

State how a midwife would (*a*) prevent; (*b*) recognize; (*c*) treat (*until the doctor's arrival*) a fractured humerus.

What is the cause of a sterno-mastoid hæmatoma ? How would you recognize facial paralysis ? **Describe** how a midwife might cause Erb's paralysis. What are the signs ? In what position will the doctor fix the arm temporarily ?

Explain in not more than 20 lines each, why intracranial injury is liable to occur in the following circumstances and state how the midwife could try to avoid this: the premature baby; breech delivery; face to pubes delivery; rigid pelvic floor.

What do you understand by the following: (1) diminished sucking and swallowing reflex; (2) grunting expirations; (3) apnœic episodes ?

What is: (*a*) moulding; (*b*) greenstick fracture; (*c*) Erb's paralysis; (*d*) duodenal atresia ? Where is the: (*a*) falx cerebri; (*b*) brachial plexus; (*c*) pericranium; (*d*) tentorium cerebelli; (*e*) sterno mastoid muscle; (*f*) vein of Galen ?

How would you deal with a baby in a convulsion ? What would you note and record ?

C.M.B.(Scot.) paper.—What is a caput succedaneum ? How is it formed and from what other swellings should it be differentiated ?

C.M.B.(N. Ireland) paper.—Describe the clinical appearance of convulsions in a newborn infant. Discuss briefly the treatment of the condition.

C.M.B.(Eng.) paper.—What are the causes of intracranial birth injury ? What is the clinical picture and how is the baby nursed ?

C.M.B.(Scot.) paper.—Describe the causes, signs and management of intracranial injury of the newborn.

C.M.B.(Scot.) paper.—What swellings may be found on a baby's head within a few days of birth ? How would you differentiate and treat the condition ?

C.M.B.(Scot.) paper.—What are the signs of intracranial trauma in a new-born infant? Describe the management.

C.M.B.(Eng.) paper.—What are the causes of intracranial birth injury? What is the clinical picture and how is the baby nursed?

CONGENITAL ABNORMALITIES

What precautions are taken when transferring a baby with œsophageal atresia to hospital ? How would you suspect hydrocephaly: (*a*) on abdominal palpation; (*b*) during delivery; (*c*) during first 2 weeks of life ?

A mother asks you whether she should keep her mongol baby at home: what would you say ?

Differentiate between œsophageal and duodenal atresia; meningocele and encephalocele; exomphalos and umbilical hernia; hydrocephaly and anencephaly.

For what reasons are the following appliances used: Denis Browne's splint; Barlow's splint; dental plates; Pudenz Heyer valve.

C.M.B.(Eng.) paper.—Give an account of the abnormalities of the alimentary tract of a baby which may reveal themselves in the first seven days of life.

C.M.B.(N. Ireland) paper.—Discuss the care of an infant who becomes cyanosed and breathless during its first feed. What important causes must be excluded ?

C.M.B.(Eng.) paper.—How would you examine a newborn baby in order to detect congenital abnormalities ?

C.M.B.(N. Ireland) paper.—A newborn infant is thought to be a mongol. What are the clinical features which may be present, and what is the basic cause of the condition?

C.M.B.(N. Ireland) paper.—Which congenital abnormalities should be diagnosed in the first week of life ? Describe briefly the treatment of any two of these.

C.M.B.(N. Ireland) paper.—Write short notes on *three* of the following: (*a*) meningomyelocele; (*b*) exomphalos; (*c*) cleft palate; (*d*) congenital dislocation of hips; (*e*) cold injury (cold syndrome).

C.M.B.(N. Ireland) paper.—Write short notes on the diagnosis and treatment of three of the following in the newborn: (*a*) anal atresia; (*b*) congenital dislocation of the hip; (*c*) club foot; (*d*) cleft palate; (*e*) œsophageal atresia.

33

Obstetric Operations

INDUCTION OF LABOUR

Labour may be induced when, in the interest of the life or health of mother or fetus, pregnancy should not be allowed to continue.

INDICATIONS FOR INDUCTION

(1) **True postmaturity** (see p. 655).   (2) **Severe pre-eclampsia.**

(3) **Placental dysfunction.**   (4) **Rh iso-immunization.**

(5) **To ensure a live child** in cases of previous intra-uterine death during the last month of pregnancy and in diabetes when Cæsarean section is not indicated.

METHODS OF INDUCTION

Intramuscular Injection

The administration of oxytocin by intramuscular injection is considered to be dangerous and is no longer employed.

Buccal Pitocin:—The administration of Pitocin by placing a series of tablets of Pitocin citrate between the upper gum and cheek is used with great caution. The dose has been reduced by some from 200 to 50 units because of strong contractions caused by its cumulative effect, and rupture of uterus occurring in a number of cases. Vigilant observation by midwives experienced in the technique is as necessary as when Pitocin is administered by intravenous drip.

The uterine contractions, being more painful, tend to prevent the woman from relaxing during labour. Pethidine 150 mg. is given within one hour of the onset of contraction. *The linguets are placed in alternate cheeks and dissolve in one hour. The woman is told not to suck, chew or swallow them. The linguets are removed and the mouth rinsed prior to ingestion of food or fluid.*

Buccal Pitocin is more succesful if the membranes are punctured first.

INTRAVENOUS OXYTOCIN DRIP
(Pitocin or Syntocinon)

Oxytocin given by intravenous drip is more easily controlled, less drastic in action and more reliable in effect.

Lie, presentation and fetal heart must be checked: cephalo-pelvic disproportion excluded before the induction is started.

The drip tends to ripen the cervix and stretch the lower uterine segment.

It is used to stimulate uterine action as follows :

1. **In some cases of therapeutic and missed abortion and for hydatidiform mole** (high dosage).

2. **To induce premature labour when pregnancy must be terminated in the interest of mother or child,** as in cases of severe pre-eclampsia, Rh iso-immunization.

3. **To avoid postmaturity** in conditions such as pre-eclampsia and essential hypertension in which fetal anoxia and intra-uterine death may occur.

4. **To stimulate uterine action in cases of hypotonic inertia.** In such circumstances the drip should be given with great caution = 0·5 units.

5. **Prevention of postpartum hæmorrhage.** When used to induce labour the drip is often continued during and for one hour after the third stage.

6. **Treatment of postpartum hæmorrhage.** Oxytocin drip is given to maintain good uterine contractions following the immediate control of bleeding.

CONTRA-INDICATIONS TO OXYTOCIN DRIP

Hypertonic uterine action. Fetal distress. Conditions that could obstruct labour.

Method

Prior to starting the drip an enema is given. If the membranes are punctured simultaneously with starting the drip, the induction-delivery interval is reduced by 50 per cent. Commonly it is 12 hours.

The two-bottle technique is employed in order that the oxytocin drip may be stopped and started as required and the vein kept patent. The second bottle with 5 per cent dextrose, being attached via a Baxter 3-way tap, allows the solution from either bottle to be given.

Dosage: Two units of Syntocinon are mixed thoroughly with 540 ml. of 5 per cent dextrose. A polythene cannula is introduced into the vein and the infusion given at 1·2 ml. (20 drops) per minute, increasing by 0·3 ml. (5 drops) every 15 minutes to a maximal rate of 2·4 ml. (40 drops). If labour does not start, a fresh bottle of dextrose containing twice the number of units of Syntocinon (*i.e.* 4) is prepared and the rate of flow started as previously at 1·2 ml. (20 drops) per minute and increased by 0·3 ml. (5 drops) every 15 minutes. Rarely is it necessary to increase the dose in a fresh bottle with 8 units.

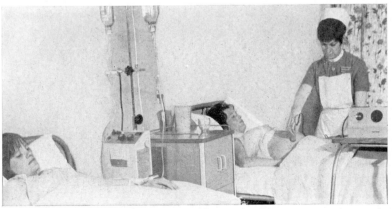

FIG. 413

AUTOMATED ELECTRONIC INFUSION UNIT.

Useful when the I.V. infusion is being administered slowly, *i.e.* o·3 ml. (5 drops) per minute. Dextrose and Syntocinon.

DOPTONE FETAL BLOOD FLOW DETECTOR in use to monitor fetal heart during labour.

(*Aberdeen Maternity Hospital.*)

Automatic oxytocin titration is used in some centres: a motor-driven pump controls the dosage which is very low to begin with and doubled every 12·5 minutes until the desired strength is reached.

In case of pre-eclampsia with œdema the rate of flow must be carefully regulated.

WHEN LABOUR STARTS

Instead of increasing the rate of flow every 15 minutes this is done every 30 minutes.   When labour is established no further increase in strength of solution or rate of flow is made.

Contractions lasting 45 seconds occurring every 2 or 3 minutes should be aimed at and maintained.   Sedatives and analgesics are administered as required.

To prevent post-partum hæmorrhage the drip should be continued slowly throughout labour, speeded up during the third stage if necessary, and gradually reduced one hour later.

INDICATIONS FOR A WEAK SOLUTION OF OXYTOCIN

When a woman has had a previous Cæsarean section or is a grande multipara or if she is on the verge of or in poorly established labour caution must be observed regarding dosage.

Initially, only 0·5 units of Syntocinon in 540 ml. dextrose 5 per cent is administered at 1·2 ml. (20 drops) per minute and increased every 30 minutes by 0·3 ml. (5 drops) to a maximal rate of 2·4 ml. (40 drops).   If labour does not become established, a fresh bottle of dextrose containing 1 unit of Syntocinon is given, the next bottle is increased to 2 units; some may require a further bottle with 4 units.   Each fresh bottle is given at 1·2 ml. (20 drops) and increased as previously by 0·3 ml. (5 drops) every 30 minutes to 2·4 ml. (40 drops) until labour is established.

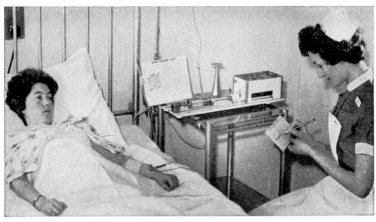

Fig. 414

PALMER INTRAVENOUS SYRINGE PUMP.

Slow-injection apparatus which accurately controls the rate of administration; it is particularly useful in cases of pre-eclampsia or essential hypertension.

(Aberdeen Maternity Hospital.)

OBSERVATION

Merely recording findings is not sufficient. The doctor must be notified when any sign of serious import develops, *e.g.* slowing of the fetal heart.

1. RATE OF FLOW

The drip must be started cautiously and the correct dosage adhered to.

2. UTERINE CONTRACTIONS

Within 10 minutes slight hardening of the uterus is felt on palpation. Constant supervision is essential until the maximal dosage is reached.

Each contraction—time, duration, strength—is recorded. If contractions do not start, that fact is recorded every half-hour.

As a precautionary measure ampoules of amyl nitrite should be at hand to damp down tetanic contractions should they occur.

3. FETAL CONDITION

The fetal heart-rate is recorded (in graph form) every five minutes during the first half-hour, then every 15 minutes. Some monitor the fetal heart, in high risk cases, with the cardiophone.

4. MATERNAL CONDITION

It is advisable to take the blood pressure every hour : the pulse should be taken at frequent intervals and recorded hourly.

The temperature is recorded every four hours and if raised a high vaginal swab is taken and an antibiotic given.

INDICATIONS FOR STOPPING THE OXYTOCIN

1. **Strong contractions** lasting over 60 seconds.

2. **Tumultuous contractions,** no relaxation between them.

3. **Fetal distress.** Slowing of the fetal heart, meconium-stained liquor.

4. **Any deterioration in the woman's general condition.**

These indications should be reported in their incipient stages.

SURGICAL INDUCTION

PUNCTURE OF THE MEMBRANES

This is the most certain method of induction; labour usually commencing within 24 hours. It is widely used in cases where immediate termination of pregnancy is imperative, *e.g.* postmaturity, pre-eclampsia and Rh iso-immunization.

In cases of postmaturity or pre-eclampsia in which placental dysfunction may be present it is an advantage to see whether the liquor is meconium stained or not.

If the fetus is dead this method is not used because of the danger of infection.

The possibility of prolapse of cord should be kept in mind when the presenting part is high and mobile.

Method

The patient is placed in the lithotomy position, the vulva cleansed thoroughly, the bladder emptied. A general anæsthetic is not usually required, except for an apprehensive primigravida.

Induction Pack: lithotomy sheet, gown, towel 91 ×91 cm., 2 sheets sterifield paper, polythene sheet. Tin foil bowl, wool balls, 5 swabs. Perineal pad.

Individually packed = Stiles, Allis's, Kochers forceps. Goodwin or Cresswell amniotomy forceps. Obstetric cream, Hibitane 1-2,000: caps, mask, gloves.

In some centres a high vaginal or cervical swab is taken after 24 hours and Ampicillin 500 mg. + 250 mg. given six-hourly when the membranes have been ruptured for 24 hours or if pyrexia, 37·5° C. (99·6° F.) is present.

If labour does not commence after 6 to 12 hours an oxytocin drip is usually given. (*Many start the drip simultaneously.*)

Version

The term " version " is applied when an alteration in the lie of the fetus *in utero* **is brought about** or the location of its upper and lower poles reversed. It may occur spontaneously or by manipulation.

The term " cephalic version " is used when the head of the fetus is made to present, and **" podalic version "** when the breech is made to present.

EXTERNAL VERSION

External version is carried out by abdominal manipulation. It is usually done to rectify a breech or shoulder presentation in the latter part of pregnancy, preferably between the 30th and 36th week, or at the beginning of labour if the membranes are intact. Version is performed by the doctor. A midwife should not attempt external version during pregnancy, but would be justified in doing so for shoulder presentation at the onset of labour or for the second twin if medical aid was not immediately obtainable.

The woman should be on a table or bed the head of which can be lowered quickly.

Mental and physical relaxation should be attained, and it is a good idea to divert the woman's attention by engaging her in conversation during the manœuvre; some give a sedative. She is more likely to tighten her abdominal muscles if she is told what is being done, or why. Warm hands and smooth gentle manipulation are essential. The fetal heart is checked afterwards, and it is usual to find some alteration in rate and rhythm for a few minutes.

When external version under general anæsthesia is to be perfomed, a laxative should be prescribed two days before to empty the lower bowel, and no food ought to be taken during the previous six hours. **The important factor in version is to get the fetus flexed into a ball** so that it can be turned more readily, and to ensure that a well-flexed head or the breech will present.

The head and back should be located and the fetus turned by using steady pressure, making it follow its nose if possible; otherwise the head may extend, resulting in a face or brow presentation. **The membranes are punctured** to permit the head or breech to engage.

After version the woman should remain in the recumbent position, under observation for three or four hours, and if there is no vaginal bleeding she is allowed to get up. A light meal should be given before she is discharged under the care of a relative or friend.

The woman is asked to report back in one week, to have the presentation checked. An unstable lie is investigated further, see p. 388.

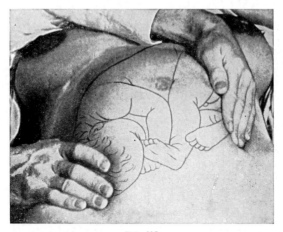

FIG. 415
External cephalic version. Head in right iliac fossa.

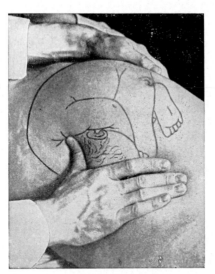

FIG. 416
External cephal version almost completed.

Some authorities do not employ anæsthesia, because they consider the force that might be used on an unconscious woman may be greater than is in the interest of mother or child.

If version fails radiological assessment of the pelvis may be considered.

THE MIDWIFE'S DUTY

The X-ray films should be at hand, also a fetal stethoscope. The bladder should be emptied. Some obstetricians want the foot of the bed to be raised 60 cm. on blocks for half an hour prior to version, to disengage the breech from the pelvic brim. Morphine 15 mg. may be prescribed by the doctor. Talcum powder is sprinkled on the skin to reduce friction.

CONTRAINDICATIONS

Previous classical Cæsarean section, antepartum hæmorrhage, hydrocephalus, Rh negative woman. Severe hypertension, twins.

BI-POLAR VERSION

Bi-polar version is rarely performed nowadays except in remote areas of developing countries; shoulder presentation being the most likely indication. This manœuvre is a combination of internal and external manipulation carried out during labour before engagement of the presenting part or rupture of the membranes and when the os is not sufficiently dilated to admit the hand. It necessitates a general anæsthetic and is difficult to perform.

Bi-polar version is always podalic: the whole hand is introduced into the vagina and two fingers, passed through the os, displace the shoulder. The external hand applies steady pressure abdominally over the breech and moves it down into the lower pole of the uterus: the membranes are then punctured and a foot brought through the os.

INTERNAL VERSION

The whole hand is introduced into the uterus so the os must be sufficiently dilated for its insertion: deep anæsthesia is necessary to relax the uterus and abdominal wall. Transverse lie is the main indication.

This operation must not be attempted when the liquor has drained away and the uterus is moulded round the fetus, nor in cases of prolonged labour in which the lower uterine segment is stretched and thin: to do so might cause rupture of the uterus. Some consider internal version should only be done for the second twin (if the need arises).

SHOULDER DYSTOCIA

Prophylaxis:—The midwife must avoid delivering the shoulders in all cephalic presentations until they have rotated internally into the antero-posterior diameter of the outlet. This will be evident by external rotation of the head which occurs after restitution. With restitution the shoulders are still in the oblique diameter of the outlet.

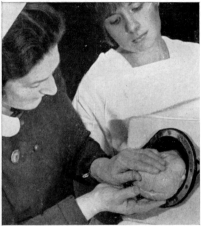

The head has rotated externally. The midwife uses downward traction (Fig. 417).

FIG. 417

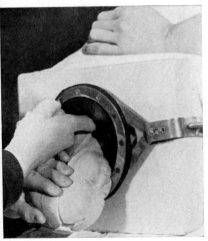

FIG. 418

If the shoulders are not in the antero-posterior diameter, hook two fingers into the anterior axilla, rotate the shoulder forwards and apply judicious traction to the head downwards and backwards. **Should this fail,** as it may do with a very large baby or when the anterior shoulder is caught on the pubic bone, an assistant tries to dislodge the anterior shoulder abdominally by pushing it towards the mid-line. At the same time an attempt is made to push the anterior shoulder forwards vaginally. Judicious traction is then applied to the head in a downward backward direction. (Fig. 418). (The neck must not be twisted.)

If this fails to bring down the anterior shoulder, deliver the posterior shoulder by drawing the head in an upward curving direction while the assistant uses supra-pubic

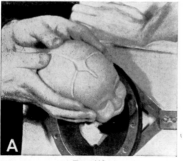

pressure on the anterior shoulder (see Fig. 419). The lithotomy position or raising the buttocks on a firm pillow and an episiotomy will facilitate matters.

Four fingers are inserted behind the posterior shoulder and an attempt is made to push it into the hollow of the sacrum. If this causes the anterior shoulder to be dislodged it can then be rotated forwards.

Fig. 419

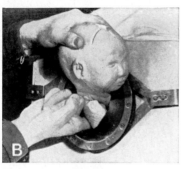

Fig. 420

Further traction can be applied by placing the fingers in the axilla of the posterior arm and if this does not succeed, an attempt is made to rotate the shoulders and make the posterior shoulder anterior (Fig. 420).

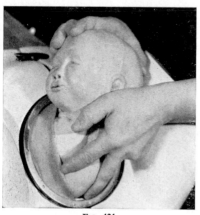

As a last resort the whole hand is inserted into the hollow of the sacrum, two fingers splint the humerus of the posterior arm, flex the elbow, sweep the forearm over the chest and bring the hand out—a very difficult manœuvre (Fig. 421).

N.B. Unfortunately the position of the doll in Figure 421 is the L.O.A. and in Figures 419 and 420 it is R.O.A. Figure 421 was photographed at a later date on a different model and to show splinting of the humerus L.O.A. gave the best photographic angle.

Fig. 421

The doll has been brought down to vulval level to demonstrate the various manœuvres.

EPISIOTOMY

The making of an incision into the perineum to enlarge the vulval orifice is known as an episiotomy. Such an incision is directed away from the anus to avoid a third-degree tear: the clean cut is more easily repaired and heals better than a ragged laceration.

INDICATIONS FOR EPISIOTOMY

1. **Delay due to:** rigid perineum; disproportion between fetus and vulval orifice.

2. **Fetal distress.**—To hasten the birth of the baby.

3. **To facilitate vaginal or intra-uterine manipulation,** *e.g.* forceps: breech delivery.

4. **Premature baby** under 2,268 G. to avoid intra-cranial damage.

5. **Severe pre-eclampsia or cardiac disease,** to reduce the effort bearing down entails.

6. **Previous third degree tear** which may occur again because of the scar tissue which does not stretch well.

TYPES OF EPISIOTOMY

(1) MEDIO-LATERAL *(Recommended for midwives)*

The incision is begun in the centre of the fourchette and directed postero-laterally, usually to the woman's right. It should be not more than 3 cm. long and is directed, diagonally in a straight line which runs 2·5 cm. distant from the anus. If the anus is considered to be 6 on the clock, the incision would be directed to 7 o'clock.

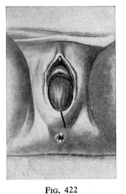

Fig. 422
Medio-lateral incision for episiotomy.
The right is usually preferred.

(2) MEDIAN

The incision, begun in the centre of the fourchette, is directed posteriorly for approximately 2·5 cm. in the mid-line of the perineum. It is favoured by, and is most success-ful in the hands of, the experienced obstetrician who will have absolute control of the fetal head: otherwise there is a risk that the incision will be extended during delivery and produce a third-degree tear. When vaginal manipulation is necessary or the baby large, the median incision does not provide as much space as the medio-lateral incision.

The advantages are (*a*) **less bleeding,** (*b*) **more easily and successfully repaired,** (*c*) **greater subsequent comfort for the woman.**

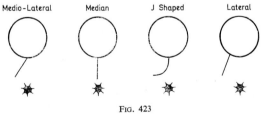

Medio-Lateral   Median   J Shaped   Lateral

Fig. 423
Types of Episiotomy.

(3) J-SHAPED

The incision is begun in the centre of the four-chette and directed pos-teriorly in the mid-line for about 1·8 cm. and then directed outwards to-wards 7 on the clock to avoid the anus. The suturing of this incision is difficult: shearing of the tissues occurs: the repaired wound tends to be puckered.

(4) LATERAL

This incision is begun one or more cm. distant from the centre of the fourchette and is condemned. Bartholin's duct may be severed: the levator ani muscle is weakened, bleeding is more profuse: suturing is more difficult and the woman experiences subsequent discomfort.

EPISIOTOMY BY MIDWIVES

The following statement was issued by the Central Midwives Board, England, June 1967.

" The necessity for the performance of episiotomy may become apparent late in labour when immediate action is required. Unless medical aid is immediately available the operation should be performed by the midwife, after infiltration of the perineum with local anæsthetic when time permits."

Student midwives should receive instruction on the indications for and technique of making an episiotomy during their period of training and if possible practical experience.

" A practising midwife should have available a supply of a local anæsthetic when in attendance on a woman in labour."

" 10 ml. of a 0·5 per cent solution or 5 ml. of a 1 per cent solution of lignocaine or similar agent should be sufficient to infiltrate the perineum before doing an episiotomy."

" Suture of the perineum should normally be referred to a registered medical practitioner."

(The Midwives Committee of the Joint Council for Northern Ireland permit midwives to use lignocaine (Xylocaine) 10 ml. of an 0·5 per cent solution and to make an episiotomy.)

The Central Midwives Board, Scotland, (1968) regard the administration of a local anæsthetic and making an episiotomy as treatment within a midwife's province.

LOCAL ANÆSTHESIA FOR EPISIOTOMY

Modern local anæsthetics are relatively safe.—Lignocaine (Duncaine ; Xylocaine) is safe and efficient: it takes effect rapidly (1 or 2 minutes).

TOXIC REACTIONS

All anæsthetic drugs are potentially toxic.—The midwife need not be unduly apprehensive: when adequately informed she will avoid such reactions: should they be caused inadvertently she will recognise and treat them promptly.

(1) **If the anæsthetic is injected into a blood vessel** the concentration in the blood stream could be dangerously high. Precautions must be taken prior to injection by withdrawing the piston and if no blood appears the needle has not entered a blood vessel : the injection should then be given while slowly withdrawing the needle.

(2) **Giving too high a concentration** of the drug or an excessive amount of a suitable concentration. The Central Midwives Board have limited the concentration and the amount to be given by midwives, *i.e.* 10 ml. of an 0·5 per cent solution, or 5 ml. of a 1 per cent solution. Both injections contain the same amount of lignocaine. Midwives will no doubt, for additional safety, carry and use one strength of solution.

TOXIC SIGNS

Drowsiness: twitching of face and limbs: convulsions: respiratory depression: circulatory collapse.

Treatment

Clear airway: lower head and raise legs: give oxygen.

INFILTRATION OF THE PERINEUM

10 ml. sterile syringe with no metal fittings. Ampoule 0·5 per cent lignocaine. needle 3·75 cm. (1½ inch) 21 G. Sterifield paper 60 cm. (24 inches). 5 gauze swabs.

(*a*) **The lithotomy or dorsal position is adopted in hospital:** at home the dorsal, with hips elevated on a firm pad.

(b) **Vulva** swabbed with Hibitane 1 in 2,000. Explanation and assurance are given as necessary.

INJECTION OF LOCAL ANÆSTHETIC

During the interval between contractions the first two fingers of the gloved left hand are inserted into the vagina, between the perineum and the fetal scalp, to ensure that the drug is not inadvertently injected into the fetus.

The needle is introduced in the midline of the inner edge of the fourchette and directed subcutaneously for a distance of 3 cm. (1¼ inch), usually to the woman's right side, along the line the episiotomy will follow, which should be 2·5 cm. distant from the anal sphincter.

Having introduced the needle for 3 cm. and prior to injecting lignocaine **the piston of the syringe is withdrawn** and, if no blood appears in the barrel, a blood vessel has not been entered so 3 ml. of lignocaine are injected while the needle is slowly withdrawn. Giving the injection while the needle is moving ensures that the drug does not enter a vein. (Some inject 0·5 ml. of analgesi as the needle is being inserted.)

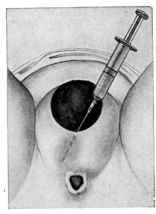

FIG. 424
Injection of local anæsthetic.

Without removing the needle, redirect it for 3 cm. (1¼ inch) so that the tip will be one cm. from the tip of the first injection, pull back piston and if no blood appears inject, while slowly withdrawing the needle, a further 3 ml. of analgesic. Redirect the needle on the other side of the first injection and proceed as previously to inject the last 3 ml. of analgesic. **The three injections will infiltrate over a fan-shaped area and the incision is made down the centre.**

(*Midwives not permitted to administer a local analgesic could use inhalational analgesia, e.g. Entonox, or Penthrane which will relieve, but not abolish, the pain of incision.*)

SUGGESTIONS FOR EPISIOTOMY BY MIDWIVES

There are so many different opinions regarding the various aspects of episiotomy that no one method will be acceptable to all midwives. The preferences of the medical practitioners who are likely to be called to repair the incisions should be known.

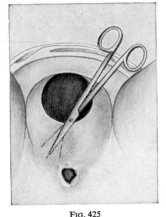

FIG. 425
Making the incision.

Timing the Incision

Judgment is needed, for the episiotomy must be made neither too soon nor too late: the head should be well down on the perineum, low enough to keep it stretched. Some consider that 4 to 5 cm. of scalp should be showing but the bulging thinned perineum is probably a better criterion. In breech presentation the posterior buttock would be distending the perineum.

If made too soon bleeding will be profuse from the thick vascular tissue: if the descending head has not displaced the levator ani muscle it will be damaged.

If made too late the supports of the neck of the bladder are weakened, the pelvic floor overstretched: bruised tissues do not heal well: mother and fetus are subjected to unnecessary stress and the purpose of the episiotomy is defeated.

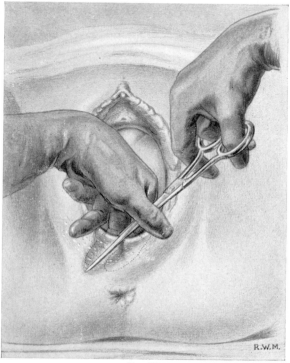

FIG. 426
FINGERS PROTECTING FETUS

Position of the Patient

In hospital the dorsal or lithotomy position is convenient: on district the dorsal position with the hips elevated on a firm pad. The left lateral position is not recommended because the scissors may slip sideways and incise the labium.

MAKING THE INCISION

The length of the incision made by midwives would be not more than 3 cm. (1¼ inch) on the stretched perineum.

The vulva is swabbed with Hibitane 1 in 2,000. After injecting the local anæsthetic and waiting for one or more minutes, two fingers are inserted between the perineum and the fetal scalp to protect it from injury by the scissors. During a uterine contraction would be a suitable time as it is easier to gauge the required length of the incision when the perineum is on the stretch.

One deliberate cut should be made beginning in the centre of the fourchette (edge of the perineum) 3 cm. (1¼ inch) in length and directed 2·5 cm. away from the anus. A tentative series of small snips will result in a ragged incision which is difficult to suture and slow to unite. The episiotomy ought to be adequate to remove any resistance to the fetal head. Mayo straight, blunt pointed, scissors 17·5 cm. (7 inches) are commonly used. They must be sharpened at frequent intervals: blunt scissors bruise the perineum.

Bleeding from the Episiotomy

Bleeding always occurs to some extent but it can be profuse when the incision is made too soon and the perineum is thick. The pressure exerted by the fetal head usually controls any bleeding: if not, direct pressure using a gauze swab can be applied. Should bleeding continue after the birth of the baby, which is not control-lable by firm pressure with a folded vulval pad,

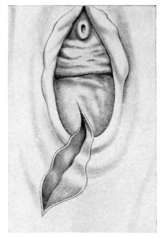

FIG. 427
Episiotomy wound.

two Spencer Wells forceps 12·7 cm. (5 inches) should be applied to the bleeding vessels.

The episiotomy should be repaired as soon as possible (delay may occur in district practice): union of tissues is better, with less risk of sepsis and a broken down wound; nor should the woman be subjected to the prolonged apprehension of " stitches ".

HINTS ON SUTURING THE EPISIOTOMY

(These are intended for Midwives in Remote Areas Overseas)

Published Statement—June 1970—by the Chairman of the Central Midwives Board, England. "It is the view of the Board that midwives who have been taught the technique of repairing the perineum, and are judged to be competent, may be authorised by the doctor concerned to carry out this procedure; the final responsibility will rest with the doctor."

If suturing is carried out without delay the local anæsthetic given for making the episiotomy should still be effective. Healing would take place if sutured within 12 hours: after 24 hours satis-factory union is unlikely.

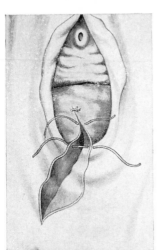

FIG. 428
First suture inserted in apex of wound.

Two helpers could support the thighs in the lithotomy position. The area is cleansed with antiseptic solution and blood clot removed from the vagina. Oozing from the uterus may obscure the field and, if so, one half of a perineal pad should be inserted into the vault of the vagina (subsequent removal of the pad is, of course, mandatory). A good light is essential.

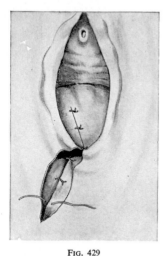

FIG. 429
Deep sutures inserted.

Some attach an Allis's tissue forceps on either side of the incision at the junction of perineal skin and vaginal epithelium, to facilitate adequate inspection of the wound in depth and, when suturing, to provide an aid to the accurate apposition of the incised edges of the fourchette. The full extent of the laceration is determined, including that the anal sphincter is intact.

An episiotomy, which is comparable with the wound of a second degree tear, must be repaired in three layers—

(1) **Vaginal wound:**
    (a) deep and superficial tissues,
    (b) vaginal mucosa.

(2) **Pelvic floor muscles and perineal body.**

(3) **Perineal skin** and subcutaneous tissue.

It is most important that the first stitch inserted is at the apex of the incision, the upper limit of the wound in the posterior vaginal wall. Some use three or four interrupted sutures of chromic catgut No. 1 on a round-bodied Mayo needle No. 2 for the deep tissues. Ethicon eyeless needled chromic suture W 579. If the deep structures are not properly sutured, lochial discharge may collect in the dead space and decompose; the epithelium breaks down exposing a gaping infected cavity.

To avoid injury to the rectum while inserting the deep sutures the forefinger of the left hand placed in the vagina can press the rectum downwards. Superficial sutures in the vaginal mucosa must be close enough (8 mm.) to prevent blood seeping into the deep tissues and forming a hæmatoma. Some authorities use a continuous suture to ensure against this, but too many stitches may cause puckering and shortening of the posterior vaginal wall.

EXTERNAL SUTURES

The future integrity of the pelvic floor depends on good union achieved by suturing the wound layer by layer: the muscles must be united, the perineal body reconstructed.

The practice of stitching the skin of the perineum by using a very large needle and taking a deep bite, embracing the perineal body, is now condemned; this provides no union of deeper structures and no support. Merely suturing the skin of the perineum is futile: the wound must be sutured in its entire depth.

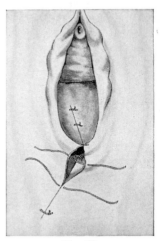

FIG. 430
External sutures.

The skin and subcutaneous tissues are carefully apposed and united with interrupted mersilk sutures No. 1 inserted not less than 0·5 cm. from the edge of the incision, otherwise when œdema occurs they may cut out. Ethicon W 562 on a curved cutting needle may be used. Allis's forceps previously applied facilitate good alignment of the perineal skin and vaginal epithelium at the fourchette. The edges of the incision should merely meet and must on no account be tied tightly or the wound is likely to break down.

Chromic catgut No. 0 or 1 with a half circle cutting needle No. 7 is favoured by many. A No. 2 Mayo needle is recommended for the inexperienced who may break the needle by attaching the needle-holder too near the eye; it should be 1 cm. distant. Others think that, with early bathing, catgut becomes soggy and they prefer fine silk (Mersilk) Ethicon W 562. Silk and catgut cause less pain for the woman than silkworm gut and nylon, which are now less frequently used. Leaving long strands that are knotted together exerts undue tension on the wound and is uncomfortable.

At the end of the procedure it would be a wise precaution to insert the gloved finger into the rectum in case a suture has been extended beyond the intended limit.

Repair of Perineal Lacerations

All perineal lacerations should be sutured and this the doctor will do as soon as possible. A good light is essential.

A general anæsthetic is necessary for the repair of a third degree tear.

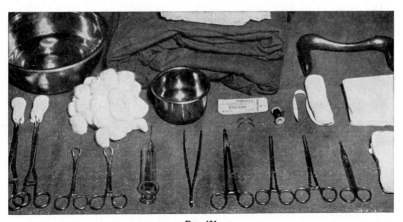

FIG. 431

PERINEAL SUTURE TROLLEY.
(*Simpson Memorial Maternity Pavilion, Edinburgh.*)

LINEN AND DRESSINGS

1 gown, cap, mask, gloves and hand towel.
1 lithotomy sheet, 2 towels, 91 cm. (36 × 36 inches).
10 gauze swabs; 20 wool swabs.
1 tampon with tape; 1 perineal pad.

METAL WARE

1 hand lotion bowl.
1 swabbing bowl; 1 gallipot.

Catgut, chromic, No. 1. Mersilk No. 1.
or Ethicon needled sutures W 759 W 562.

INSTRUMENTS

2 sponge-holding forceps, 2 Mayo towel clips.
1 × 20 ml. syringe, No. 12 needle.
1 toothed dissecting forceps.
1 Mayo needle-holder; 2 Allis's tissue forceps.
1 Mayo scissors; 1 Sims' speculum.
1 cutting needle, No. 7, half-circle.
1 round-bodied needle, No. 2 (Mayo).
or Ethicon W 562 No. 1 mersilk.

lignocaine (Duncaine), one per cent., 1 × 2ml. syringe.

TRANSVAGINAL PUDENDAL NERVE BLOCK

The use of pudendal nerve block has tended to replace all forms of general anæsthesia, unless the woman is grossly unco-operative, when operative procedures are required for vaginal delivery, *e.g.* rotation of head in occipito-lateral or occipito-posterior positions, forceps delivery, or breech extraction.

Local infiltration of the perineum is supplemented by pudendal block to anæsthetize the nerves supplying the pelvic floor, vagina and vulva.

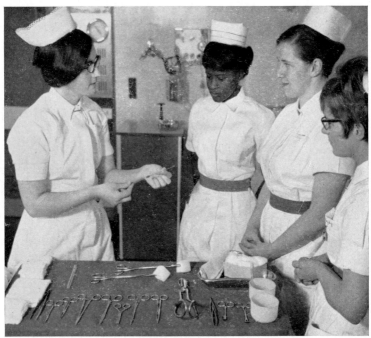

FIG. 432

FORCEPS DELIVERY UNDER PUDENDAL NERVE BLOCK.

Sister showing pudendal needle with guide and explaining midwife's duties before and during application of forceps under pudendal nerve block.

(*County Maternity Hospital, Bellshill, Lanarkshire.*)

Requirements as for perineal infiltration are needed, with additional lignocaine (Duncaine), 20 ml., 0·5 and 1 per cent.; 1 syringe, 20 ml.; 1 filling cannula, one 15 cm. 20 gauge pudendal needle, with guide. The ischial spines are located per vaginam and each pudendal nerve area is infiltrated with 10 ml. Duncaine, 1 per cent, by the doctor.

Some obstetricians infiltrate the vulval ring and perineum without pudendal nerve block for low forceps delivery.

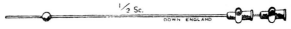

FIG. 433

Transvaginal pudendal needle with guide.

ADVANTAGES OF LOCAL ANÆSTHESIA

(*a*) **Reduction of the maternal mortality rate.**—There is no risk of inhalation of gastric contents as may occur during general anæsthesia.

(*b*) **Greater safety for the fetus.**—There is no depressant action on the fetal respiratory centre.

(*c*) **No interference with uterine activity**—less postpartum hæmorrhage.

(*d*) **Less trauma** because of the greater gentleness and manipulative skill required with a conscious patient.

PARACERVICAL NERVE BLOCK

To relieve pain and backache when the cervix is 5 or more cm. dilated, 10 ml. lignocaine (Duncaine) one per cent, is injected via the lateral vaginal fornices into the base of each broad ligament. The injection is given slowly with a two-minute interval between the two injections otherwise fetal bradycardia may occur. The needle ought to be directed away from the baby's head and the fetal heart should be monitored. Unfortunately the effect only lasts for 1 to $1\frac{1}{2}$ hours.

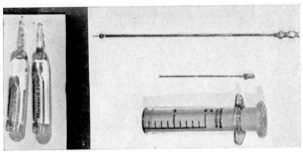

FIG. 434

REQUIREMENTS FOR PARACERVICAL BLOCK.

2 × 10 ml. ampoules bupivacaine (Marcain 0·25 per cent).
1 Oxford pattern paracervical needle.
1 Syringe 20 ml. 1 filling cannula.

(*Aberdeen Maternity Hospital.*)

The Oxford pattern needle and guard, 17·8 cm. (7 inches) long has been designed for the purpose.

Delivery of the Fetus by Forceps

Midwifery forceps consists of two blades, with a cephalic curve that accommodates the fetal head and a pelvic curve which conforms to the curve of the pelvic canal. Where the handle and shank unite, the two blades cross to form a lock.

LOW FORCEPS

In this case the largest presenting diameter is below the level of the ischial spines and the head distending the perineum; the more common indications being delay, physical or emotional fatigue. Haig Ferguson's, Bonney's or Wrigley's forceps are suitable for this purpose.

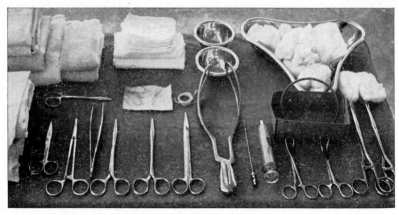

Fig. 435

Requirements for Forceps Delivery under Pudendal Nerve Block.
(*County Maternity Hospital, Bellshill, Lanarkshire.*)

This equipment is wrapped in : (1) balloon cloth ; (2) double twill cotton ; (3) polythene dust sheet.

LINEN
1 gown; lithotomy sheet; baby wrap.

DRESSINGS
10 gauze swabs.   20 wool swabs.
2 anal pads.   2 vulval pads.
cord ligatures.   1 vaginal tampon.

BOWL PACK
2 polypropylene basins.   1,200 ml. (two-pint)
  measuring jug.   Triangular placenta basin.
  2 gallipots.

SEPARATELY WRAPPED
Gloves ;   cap ;   mask ;   episiotomy scissors.
Local infiltration needles, gauge 20 to 22.
Mucus extractors.
Kiellands forceps.

INSTRUMENTS
2 pairs sponge-holding forceps.
2 pairs Mayo towel clips.
1 disposable catheter and dish.
1 20 ml. disposable syringe.
1 pudendal needle and guide.
1 pair Wrigley's midwifery forceps.
1 pair Mayo scissors.
1 pair scissors, 12·7 cm. (5 inch).
2 pair 17·6 cm. (7-inch) Spencer Wells forceps.
1 pair 12·7 cm. (5-inch) Spencer Wells forceps.
1 pair toothed dissecting forceps.
1 Mayo needle holder.
1 round-bodied needle ⎫
1 curved cutting needle ⎬ in rust-proof paper.
Mersilk No- 0 or No. 1 (catgut added later).

Ethicon eyeless sutured needle in foil pack W 759 No. 1 chromic, No. 2 round bodied half curved needle and W 562 curved cutting needle with No. 1 Mersilk.

MID-FORCEPS

In this case the head is engaged; the presenting part (not only the caput) is at the level of the ischial spines ; the most common indications being deep transverse arrest, occipito-posterior position of the vertex and fetal distress. Haig Ferguson's and Barnes Neville's forceps are generally used in Great Britain.

Kielland's forceps are straight and have a sliding lock. They are admirably suited for rotation of the fetal head in cases of deep transverse arrest or occipito-posterior position, particularly under pudendal nerve block.

INDICATIONS FOR FORCEPS

Forceps are applied during the second stage only.

Although it is not within the midwife's province to decide when forceps should be applied, she must be aware of the various indications for their use, in order that she may notify the doctor in time and have the necessary equipment at hand. (A pædiatrician is present in hospital.)

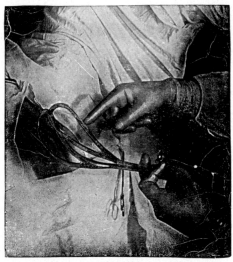

FIG. 436

SELECTING THE BLADE TO BE INSERTED FIRST.
With forceps held as shown, select the blade which will lie in the left side of the woman's pelvic canal, the handle of which is in the operator's left hand, the lower blade.

1. DELAY IN THE SECOND STAGE DUE TO
    (*a*) **Hypotonic uterine action.**   (*c*) **Deep transverse arrest.**
    (*b*) **Minor degrees of outlet contraction.**   (*d*) **Persistent occipito-posterior position.**

2. MATERNAL COMPLICATIONS :
    (*b*) **In cases of severe pre-eclampsia and eclampsia,** to eliminate strenuous pushing, which raises the blood pressure and is apt to provoke fits.
    (*b*) **Maternal distress,** incipient or established.
    (*c*) **In the more serious degrees of cardiac disease** or advanced pulmonary tuberculosis, forceps are sometimes, but not always, applied.

3. FETAL COMPLICATIONS :
    (*a*) **Fetal distress.**
    (*b*) **Prolapse of cord during second stage.**   (*c*) **The aftercoming head of the breech.**

The Midwife's Duties

Dentures and hairpins are removed; the signed permission slip for operation and anæsthesia attached to the patient's chart.

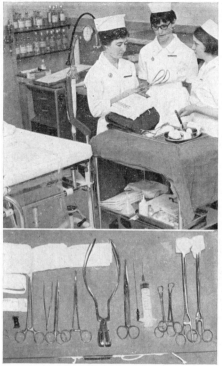

FIG. 437

LABOUR WARD SISTER GIVING CLINICAL INSTRUCTION

(non-sterile set-up) midwives' duties during forceps
delivery, including resuscitation of infant.

(*Simpson Memorial Maternity Pavilion, Edinburgh.*)

Requirements for catheterization, episiotomy and perineal suture are at hand.

Equipment must be in readiness to treat a shocked baby, control post-partum hæmorrhage and combat shock.

The woman is usually delivered in the lithotomy position, and both legs must be raised and lowered simultaneously to prevent injury to the sacro-iliac joints.

To avoid trauma of leg veins, care is taken by padding leg rests and preventing undue pressure by stirrup-rods. A polythene sheet is placed under the buttocks to direct fluid into the bucket.

The midwife washes pubes, groins and thighs with a perineal pad.

The doctor swabs the vulva and passes the catheter. A sterile towel is placed under the buttocks, lithotomy leggings or sheet is arranged in position.

The senior midwife listens to the fetal heart and notifies the doctor when the uterus contracts; assists with rotation of the anterior shoulder, as requested.

MALMSTROM VACUUM EXTRACTOR (*Ventouse*)

This apparatus is used to aid expulsion of the fetus. It consists of a metal cup (four sizes are provided) which is attached to the scalp by suction. Connected to

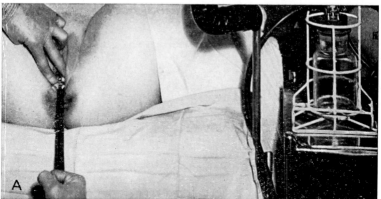

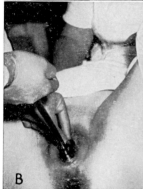

FIG. 438

MALMSTROM VACUUM EXTRACTOR (VENTOUSE).

(A) Showing (1) downward traction, (2) vacuum bottle.

(B) Baby's scalp appearing. Traction outwards and upwards.

(C) Showing (1) cup attached to scalp, (2) upward traction, (3) hand holding suction pump, (4) vacuum bottle and pressure gauge.

(*Simpson Memorial Maternity Pavilion, Edinburgh.*)

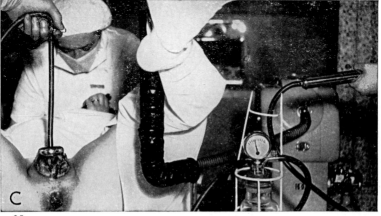

the cup is rubber tubing containing a metal chain that terminates in a traction handle; the rubber tubing extends through the handle and enters a glass container fitted with a pressure gauge. Leaving the glass container is a short piece of rubber tubing to which the hand pump that extracts the air is attached. An electric pump is now available.

APPLICATION OF THE CUP

Local infiltration of the perineum or pudendal nerve block is used; Pethilorfan may be given.

The cup is applied to the presenting part (the posterior area of the vertex and not over a fontanelle, to aid flexion) and a vacuum created by using the pump; the negative pressure being registered on the gauge.

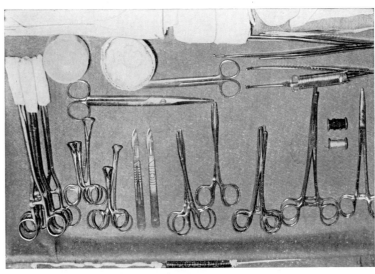

Fig. 439
Requirements for tubal ligation
(*Simpson Memorial Maternity Pavilion, Edinburgh.*)

INSTRUMENTS
3 or 4 Rampleys swab holders.
6 towel clips.
2 B.P. handles No. 4; blades No. 23.
6 Spencer Wells forceps.
3 Allis's tissue forceps.
1 dissecting forceps toothed.
2 dissecting forceps plain.
2 Mayo curved forceps.
2 Mayo scissors.
2 Mayo needle holders.
1 Michel clip holder.
1 Michel clip inserter.
2 gallipots, foil dish.

GOWN PACK
4 gowns, hand towels, caps, masks.

LINEN AND DRESSING PACK
1 laparotomy sheet.
4 dressing towels 91 × 91 cm.
2 packs (5) Raytec swabs 22 cm.
2 packs (5) Raytec swabs 10 cm.
1 gauze dressing for Mastisol.

SUTURES
Chromic catgut No. 2/0; No. 1.
Linen thread No. 60.
Mersilk No. 0.
For skin Ethicon W 793 or 775
No. 1 Mersilk on Colt's needle
or Ethicon W 759 or W 755
Chromic No. 1

Suction takes 5 to 10 minutes by hand pump, 4 minutes by electric pump and draws the scalp into the cup, to which it adheres.

Intermittent traction, synchronous with the uterine contractions, is applied. If the vacuum is excessive or the period of traction exceeds 45 minutes necrosis of the scalp will occur which may result in a bald patch.

The large caput succedaneum or chignon that forms on the scalp looks formidable but will disappear within a week.

INDICATIONS FOR USE

FIRST STAGE OF LABOUR (mainly)

Delay as in cases of hypotonic uterine action and deflexed occipito-posterior position. (The os should be half dilated): traction applied during 45 minutes of uterine contractions will, by bringing the head in close contact with the cervix, aid cervical dilatation and stimulate uterine action.

SECOND STAGE OF LABOUR (less commonly).

For delay as in occipito-posterior position of the vertex.

Some give the baby Konakion (vit. K_1) one mg. to counteract hæmorrhage into the scalp tissue.

TUBAL STERILIZATION

TUBAL LIGATION

Through a small abdominal incision the Fallopian tubes are ligated and a segment excised as a means of sterilization. The operation is performed within 48 hours after delivery; the tubes being readily accessible then.

The common indications are (1) medical conditions that would endanger life or health, (2) cases of high parity, *e.g.* with 4 live children. Husband and wife must state in writing that they consent and understand the nature and implications of the operation.

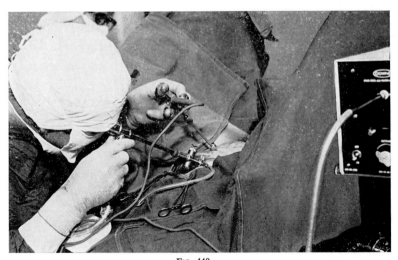

FIG. 440

STERILISATION BY LAPAROSCOPY.
(*Simpson Memorial Maternity Pavilion, Edinburgh.*)

LAPAROSCOPIC STERILIZATION

The laparoscopic technique is sometimes used. The bladder is emptied. Three to five litres of carbon dioxide gas is injected into the peritoneal cavity by means of a special trocar and cannula: the incision is enlarged to one cm. and the laparoscope inserted. A dilator is introduced via the cervix to manipulate the uterus. A second stab incision is made in the abdomen; the Palmer biopsy drill forceps introduced and a coagulation

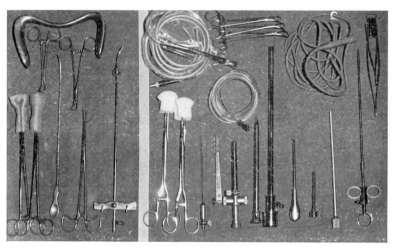

Fig. 441

Instruments for Tubal Sterilization by Laparoscopy.

Vaginal Instruments	Abdominal Instruments
2 Sponge holders.	2 Sponge holders.
1 Uterine sound.	1 Verres needle.
1 Volsellum forceps.	1 Bard Parker handle No. 3; blade No. 12.
1 Uterine cannula.	1 Laparoscopic trocar and cannula.
2 Towel clips.	1 Laparoscope.
1 Sims speculum.	1 Small trocar and cannula.
	1 Palmer biopsy forceps and insulated sheath.

Top of Fig. 441

Fibre light lead: tubing for carrying gas; 3 towel clips; diathermy cable; Michel clip holder and inserter; dissecting forceps.

(*Simpson Memorial Maternity Pavilion, Edinburgh.*)

current passed. The centre of the area of the Fallopian tube that has been coagulated is severed by means of the forceps drill. Through the same incision the other Fallopian tube is dealt with.

This operation is performed 6 weeks after confinement, but has been done earlier.

The women are discharged home in 9 hours if no condition exists warranting further hospital care.

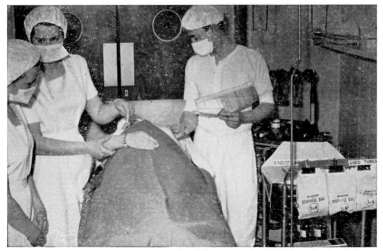

FIG. 442

Anæsthetist verifying identity of patient, medication, case notes. Sister stressing to student midwife the importance of checking identity wristband.

(*Aberdeen Maternity Hospital.*)

SAFEGUARDS AGAINST ERRORS IN OPERATING THEATRE

1. TO AVOID OPERATING ON WRONG PATIENT

(*a*) **An identity disc or band should be attached to the patient's wrist** by the ward sister and checked with the operation list by the theatre sister. Name, initials, hospital number and nature of operation should be stated.

(*b*) **The correct case notes, X-ray films, and signed " consent to operation and anæs-thetic " form should accompany the patient. The obstetrician identifies the patient.**

(*c*) **Pre-operative medication ordered and given should be recorded on the chart.** This is checked by the anæsthetist.

(*d*) **For the baby an identity wrist-band should be prepared** and applied in the theatre.

2. TO AVOID LEAVING ANY FOREIGN BODY WITHIN THE OPERATIVE AREA

An efficient system of counting and checking swabs, packs, instruments, needles, should be set out in writing and observed in practice.

Swabs

Swabs to be used within the body must be white and contain a radio-opaque substance. (Raytec swabs are on the market.) Such swabs must not be used as dressings.

Swabs should be in bundles of five (that number is recommended for universal use) and counted by the " scrubbed " nurse and the " unscrubbed " nurse together before the operation begins.

Swabs used in theatre for purposes other than within the body, *e.g.* by anæsthetist or pædiatrician, or for cleansing the skin, should have a distinctive colour (usually **green**) and should also have radio-opaque material incorporated in the meshes.

The " unscrubbed " nurse accounts for swabs discarded from the field of operation. A rack with hooks arranged in rows of five facilitates this.

The obstetrician is responsible that all swabs are removed from within the wound before closure of the incision. He will ascertain that the swab count is correct; " scrubbed " and " unscrubbed " nurses having accounted for recovery of the number of swabs issued.

Instruments and Needles

The number of instruments and needles used at each operation should be known. The " scrubbed " nurse counts hæmostats and needles prior to starting the operation and accounts for them before the wound is closed.

The number of non-absorbable sutures inserted should be recorded on the chart and checked when they are removed.

Vaginal tampons or packs are removed by the obstetrician. If left intentionally, the size, number and time of removal should be recorded on the chart.

The ward sister is responsible for their removal at the time stated.

Anæsthetic Requirements

The trolley for general anæsthesia must always be in readiness with cylinders of nitrous oxide (more rarely halothane, cyclopropane) and other gases ; oxygen cylinders must be checked and suction apparatus in readiness.

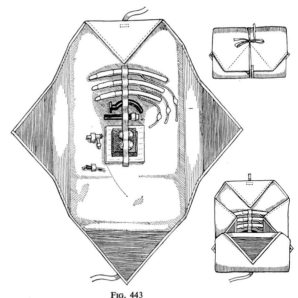

FIG. 443

AN.ÆSTHETIC PACK.

Three cuffed Magill endotracheal tubes, size 7, 8, 9.

Guedel airway, No. 3.	1 anæsthetic needle for sodium thio-
Catheter mount.	pentone (Pentothal) and relaxants
Cobb's connector.	2 green gauze swabs. 2 wool swabs.

Pre-sterilised disposal Graham's Venflon or Viggo cannula are also available.

(*Aberdeen Maternity Hospital.*)

Atropine and scopolomine should be available for intravenous use. Sodium thiopentone (Pentothal) and suxamethonium (Scoline), one of the shorter-acting muscle relaxants, may be administered.

Sterile packs should be at hand with the necessary equipment for the induction of general anæsthesia. *The anæsthetic pack shown on page 634 has proved its efficiency.*

THE FOLLOWING EQUIPMENT MAY BE REQUIRED

Stomach tube and Brunswick disposable syringe 50 ml. with catheter nozzle; vomit bowl; swab holders; green gauze swabs.

Airways ; mouth gags ; laryngoscope ; endotracheal tubes ; sphygmomanometer ; bin-aural and fetal stethoscopes ; oscillotonometer.

DRUGS FOR RESUSCITATION

Digoxin; nikethamide; hydrocortisone.

Vasopressor substances such as methylamphetamine (Methedrine).

MIDWIVES' DUTIES

The midwife keeps the equipment clean, trolleys tidy and provides an adequate supply of sterile syringes, needles, drugs and other necessary requirements.

A midwife stays with the woman from the time she is brought into the anæsthetic room until she is transferred to the theatre.

Absolute quietness should prevail and talking should be a mere whisper; the patient should not hear the rattling of instruments.

One midwife should be delegated to assist the anæsthetist as required, preparing injections and ensuring that the arms do not slip off the table.

DANGERS OF INHALATION OF GASTRIC CONTENTS

The stomach contents are highly acid and the anæsthetist endeavours to avoid inhalation of regurgitated fluid or food. Cricoid pressure (Sellick's manœuvre) is sometimes applied to compress the œsophagus and prevent regurgitation.

Some pass a large stomach tube, 34 FG and empty the stomach by suction or syphonage. Others pass a plastic tube size 14 FG intranasally and allow it to drain throughout the operative procedure.

A cuffed endotracheal tube is inserted by the anæsthetist to ensure a clear airway.

A tilting table or labour ward bed, *e.g.* Steel's, which is controlled by the anæsthetist who can rapidly lower or raise the head, has proved to be invaluable.

Suction apparatus, instantly ready, is imperative.

MENDELSON'S SYNDROME
(Pulmonary Acid Aspiration Syndrome)

This significant cause of obstetric anæsthetic deaths is due to the inhalation of vomited or regurgitated gastric juice. It can occur even when no food has been partaken for many hours: the acid gastric juice being highly irritant to the bronchial tree and the lungs produces broncho-spasm, dyspnœa, cyanosis and pulmonary œdema. Death may ensue in hours or days.

Prophylactic treatment. This consists in giving 10 ml. mist magnesium trisilicate, less than 30 minutes prior to a general obstetric anæsthetic, to reduce the acidity of the stomach contents.

The anæsthetist may use cricoid pressure during induction of the anæsthetic.

Active treatment. The bed is lowered at the head, airway cleared by suction: oxygen given: intermittent positive pressure ventilation may be necessary. Steroids and amino-phylline are administered for the relief of bronchospasm: dextrose is given intravenously: antibiotics are usually prescribed.

INTRAVENOUS ANÆSTHESIA

Sodium thiopentone (Pentothal) is given intravenously to induce anæsthesia.

No food should be taken for six hours prior to giving sodium thiopentone (Pentothal), because the barbiturates may cause the cardiac sphincter of the stomach to relax and the presence of vomitus in the pharynx may induce laryngeal spasm. Moreover vomitus may be inhaled and cause a degree of cyanosis which may be lethal to the fetus *in utero,* and may result in the death of the mother from asphyxia.

REQUIREMENTS FOR INTRAVENOUS ANÆSTHESIA

Ampoule sodium thiopentone, 0·5 G.

Ampoule of 20 ml. distilled water to make 2·5 per cent solution.

Rubber velcro arm band.

Green swabs (5); dressing towels.

Drawing-up needle.

Hypodermic needles, sizes 18 and 12.

Venflon self-retaining cannula.

20-ml. syringe, eccentric nozzle.

2-ml. syringe, central nozzle.

Gown, cap, mask, gloves and hand towel.
Hibitane in spirit for skin preparation.

SPINAL ANÆSTHESIA

REQUIREMENTS:

Two-ml. syringe and needle to raise skin-weal; Luer-lok 5-ml. syringe.

Rowbotham's introducer; fine spinal needles with stilettes; heavy cinchocaine (nupercaine) in ampoules, as prescribed; ampoules of methoxamine (Vasylox).

The equipment, including cinchocaine, must be autoclaved before use.

EPIDURAL ANÆSTHESIA

Epidural (extradural) anæsthesia is being used with increasing frequency in British obstetric centres to provide continuous analgesia and so abolish the pain of normal labour. It is particularly useful in cases where prolonged labour is anticipated, *e.g.* inco-ordinate uterine action, posterior vertex position. Cephalo-pelvic disproportion must be excluded. For severe pre-eclampsia epidural anæsthesia may be extended to produce a hypotensive effect.

Epidural anæsthesia is very successful when Cæsarean section is performed for complications such as respiratory or cardiac disease and diabetes.

The first injection is given when labour is well established with the cervix at least 4 cm. dilated and the woman in definite discomfort; the procedure being carried out and supervised by an obstetric anæsthetist. The system of topping up by the injection of more local anæsthetic via an indwelling plastic catheter is most effective.

Method

A Tuohy needle G. 16 is introduced into the epidural space in the lumbar region and a fine polyvinyl or nylon catheter inserted through the bore of the needle and left *in situ.* The site of the catheter insertion is covered with gauze swabs and sealed off to exclude infection from seepage of urine, fæces or amniotic fluid.

The catheter is taped up the woman's back to shoulder level. A plastic self-retaining cannula is introduced into a convenient vein in the hand or fore-arm, prior to injecting the anæsthetic (lignocaine or bupivacaine) so that ephedrine or other intravenous therapy may be administered without delay should the need arise.

Positive pressure respiratory apparatus must be in readiness and the sphygmomano-meter cuff in position for the frequent blood pressure readings that are necessary.

Specific posturing of the woman, *e.g.* head down and lying on one side for the first 10 minutes after injection may be necessary to achieve adequate dispersal of the local anæsthetic.

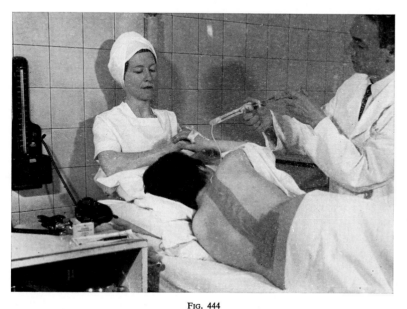

FIG. 444

EPIDURAL ANÆSTHETIC.

" Topping up " a continuous epidural anaesthetic; repeat dose of local anæsthetic being injected through a millipore bacterial filter.

The following measures must be taken to ensure prompt action in emergency.

(1) **An indwelling cannula** (Graham's Venflon) is introduced into a vein on the back of the hand, in order to administer any necessary drugs without delay.

(2) **On the bedside locker:**

(*a*) **Ampoules of ephedrine** and a sterile syringe.

(*b*) **Bag and mask for intermittent positive pressure ventilation (with Oxygen).**

(3) **The bed must be the type that can be put into the " head down " position rapidly.**

(4) **A vasopressor substance,** *i.e.* methylamphetamine (Methedrine), should be available for treatment of induced hypotension.

(*Aberdeen Maternity Hospital.*)

Accidental injection of the full dose of local anæsthetic into the spinal subarachnoid space (containing the cerebro-spinal fluid) will produce a " total " spinal anæsthetic. This will result in precipitate hypotension and respiratory arrest either of which lead to cardiac arrest if not treated promptly. Therefore every patient having epidural anæsthesia must: (1) be on a tilting bed; (2) have positive pressure oxygenation apparatus ready (at the head of the bed) plus pharyngeal suction apparatus; and (3) have an indwelling intravenous cannula and, beside the bed, ampoules of ephedrine.

MIDWIVES DUTIES

The most rigorous aseptic technique is necessary. Ampoules (or bottles) of local anæsthetic are autoclaved once only.

The patient should have an enema, bath, and her bladder emptied prior to the injection, as micturition is liable to be inhibited following administration of the epidural anæsthetic. It would be expedient to encourage her to pass urine just prior to each subsequent topping up injection, usually every 2 to 3 hours.

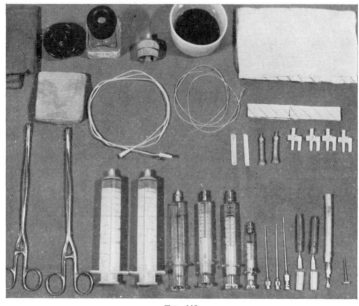

FIG. 445

EPIDURAL PACK.

1 gallipot for iodine.
2 sponge holding forceps.
10 green gauze swabs.
1 lumbar puncture towel.
2 disposable syringes 50 ml.
3 glass syringes 10 ml. luer lok tip.
1 glass syringe 2 ml. luer lok tip.
1 filling cannula.
1 spinal needle.

2 hypo needles No. 17.
1 Tuohy needle.
1 Sise introducer.
1 Portex epidural cannula.
1 × 164 cm manometer tubing.
4 stop-cocks 3 way.
2 MacIntosh balloons, luer adaptors.
1 Millipore bacterial filter.

Sterilized separately and added to pack

10 ml. lignocaine hydrochloride 1 per cent (Xylocaine).
60 ml. bupivacaine (Marcain) 0·25 per cent with adrenalin 1-400,000. Sterilized in Honeywell jar.

Cap, mask, gown, gloves.

(Aberdeen Maternity Hospital.)

Observation

The blood pressure is taken every 5 minutes during the half hour following the first injection and then every 30 minutes. When the drug is taking effect the woman experiences a sensation of heat and swelling in her legs and numbness in the buttocks: the lower limbs may have reduced motor function according to the strength of the local anæsthetic used.

Hypotension must be noted and dealt with. This may be due to the supine hypotensive syndrome because of the pressure of the uterus on the inferior vena cava. Turning the woman on her side usually relieves this and the nausea that accompanies hypotension. It may be necessary to raise the foot of the bed: the anæsthetist may give a vasopressor drug such as ephedrine 10 mg.

Should labour be prolonged over 12 hours pressure areas must be treated.

The contractions (frequency, length, strength) are noted by abdominal palpation as the woman is not always aware of these. The maternal pulse and fetal heart rate are both recorded every 15 minutes. Vaginal and rectal examinations are essential to determine the onset of the second stage as the woman has no urge to push if the anæsthetic extends to affect sacral segments. In the majority of cases outlet forceps are necessary.

Ergometrine or Syntometrine are liable to cause headache and hypertension if given when a vasopressor drug has been administered; oxytocin is preferred.

Full muscle tone in the lower limbs returns in 3 to 4 hours after delivery but not until sensation returns is the woman allowed out of bed.

Cæsarean Section

The operation to remove the fetus through an incision in the abdominal wall and uterus is known as " hysterotomy," and when performed after the 28th week of pregnancy the term " Cæsarean section " is used. It was first employed in Roman times to remove the child after the death of the mother.

MAIN INDICATIONS

CONTRACTED PELVIS	DISORDERED UTERINE ACTION
CEPHALO-PELVIC DISPROPORTION	SEVERE PRE-ECLAMPSIA
PLACENTA PRÆVIA FETAL DISTRESS	DIABETES PROLAPSE OF CORD
FAILED SURGICAL INDUCTION	PREVIOUS CÆSAREAN SECTION

Other factors are also taken into consideration, such as bad obstetric history, the older primigravida.

The tendency to treat breech, shoulder and posterior face presentations by Cæsarean section in the interest of the fetus is increasing.

Some authorities advocate radiological examination prior to Cæsarean section to exclude fetal abnormalities.

BRIEF DESCRIPTION OF CÆSAREAN SECTION

ELECTIVE CÆSAREAN SECTION

This is one which is planned because the need is apparent prior to labour. The woman is admitted to hospital after the 38th week for one or two days prior to operation, which is usually performed on the approximate day of delivery or sooner if the membranes rupture.

LOWER SEGMENT CÆSAREAN SECTION

The abdomen is opened through a vertical paramedian or midline incision, below the umbilicus. The Pfannenstiel incision which is transverse is preferred by some because it heals well and with good cosmetic result. The peritoneum is incised transversely at the utero-vesical junction, where it is loosely attached, and the bladder gently pushed down.

The lower segment is incised transversely. It may be necessary to use one or two blades of obstetric forceps to extract the head. The mouth is cleared of mucus, the body extracted and the baby held upside down for a few seconds. The cord is clamped and cut.

The edges of the uterine wound are defined with Green-Armytage or Allis's forceps and sutured with catgut in three layers. The abdomen is closed in the usual manner.

CLASSICAL CÆSAREAN SECTION

A paramedian incision is made 16 cm. (6 to 7 inches) long and extending slightly above the umbilicus: the uterine incision is also longitudinal, and involves the upper segment. The membranes are pierced, the child and placenta extracted.

The contractions of the upper segment during the post-operative period militate against good healing of the uterine scar, and rupture takes place during a subsequent pregnancy in about 4 per cent of cases.

PRE-OPERATIVE PREPARATION

ON ADMISSION (*a few days before the expected date of delivery*)

Routine examination of blood and urine is carried out, with the exception of certain tests previously made on booked patients. The vulva is shaved, the bowels kept regular without using purgatives which might start labour.

On the previous day skin and bowel preparation are similar to what is given for any abdominal operation. A sedative is administered to ensure sound sleep during the night; no food or fluid is given for 6 hours prior to operation.

Premedication does not include a narcotic drug when a general anæsthetic is to be employed, because of the depressant effect on the fetal respiratory centre.

Some give Mist. Mag. Trisilicate 10 ml. within half an hour prior to a general anæsthetic being given.

The patient, her charts, permission slip and X-ray films are taken to the anæsthetic room : an identification band having been applied to her wrist.

If the woman has been in labour a plastic No. 14 FG catheter is inserted intranasally, gastric contents removed by a Brunswick syringe and left draining throughout the operation.

A catheter is introduced and the bladder emptied: the urine drains into a plastic bag or perineal pad throughout the operation.

SET-UP OF THEATRE FOR CÆSAREAN SECTION

The set-up and instruments required are very similar to what are needed for an abdominal section, with the addition of midwifery forceps, hypodermic syringes, ergometrine and requirements for the reception and resuscitation of the baby.

PACKS FOR CÆSAREAN SECTION

All packs are wrapped in double twill and one layer green cotton, which act as covering drapes for tables and basin stands. (*An outer paper dust wrapper is applied.*)

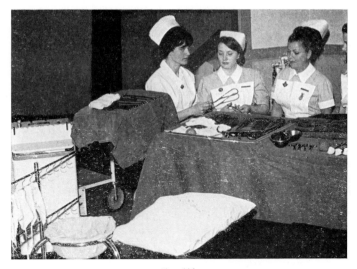

FIG. 446

PRE-SET TRAYS FOR CÆSAREAN SECTION.

Labour Ward Sister giving clinical instruction using non-sterile equipment.

(*Simpson Memorial Maternity Pavilion, Edinburgh.*)

1. LINEN AND DRESSING PACK

1 **Laparotomy sheet,** 210 cm. (84 × 84 inches).
2 **draping sheets,** 158 cm. (54 × 54 inches).
2 **dressing towels,** 91 × 100 cm. (36 × 40 inches).
1 **moisture repellent cotton square,** 91 × 100 cm. (36 × 40 inches.)
3 **packets × 5 Raytec swabs.**
3 **packets × 5 Raytec abdominal swabs,** 30 cm. (12 × 12 inches), with tapes.
1 **perineal pad.**
1 **gauze dressing for Mastisol.**

3 **gallipots for Hibitane,** 0·5 per cent in spirit, Merthiolate, Mastisol.
1 **kidney basin for soiled scalpel.**
1 **tray for sutures,** 15 × 20 cm. (6 × 8 inches).
1 **green towel folded for sutures.**
Michel clips, holder and inserter.
Paper bag with clips for broken glass.

2. PACK 4 sets of GOWN, CAP, MASK, HAND TOWEL.
one 1-basin for hand lotion.

3. BOWL PACKS. Two 2-basin

4. BABY PACK

1 cellular cotton baby blanket; 1 Turkish towel wrap; 5 green gauze swabs.
3 mucus extractors; 2 rubber bands on Spencer Wells forceps to ligate cord—autoclaved once only.
No. 8 Jaques catheter. (1 × 10-ml. syringe to extract gastric fluid.)

See immediate care of baby, p. 645.

5. ADDITIONAL PACKS

(*a*) For removal of previous scar:

    1 Bard Parker handle and blade;
    2 dissecting forceps; 1 pair scissors.

(*b*) 2 ml. syringes and needles No. 12.
(*c*) Disposable catheters.　　　(*d*) Gloves.

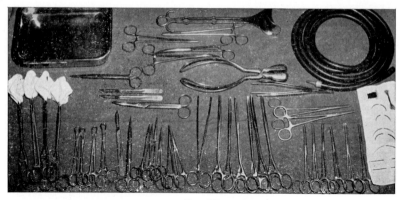

FIG. 447

Instruments for Cæsarean Section.

(*Simpson Memorial Maternity Pavilion, Edinburgh.*)

6. INSTRUMENT PACK

8 swab-holding forceps.

6 towel clips.

3 Bard Parker handles No. 4 ; blades No. 23.

8 Spencer Wells forceps.

4 Criles forceps.

6 curved Mayo artery forceps.

2 pairs toothed dissecting forceps.

1 pair plain dissecting forceps.

1 abdominal retractor.

1 pair Wrigley's midwifery forceps.

1 pair curved Mayo scissors.

2 pairs straight Mayo scissors.

6 Green Armytage tissue forceps.

6 Allis's tissue forceps.

2 Mayo needle-holders.

Argyle plastic disposable suction tubing 183 cm. and nozzle.

Needles and Sutures (*see p.* 644.)

1,200 ml. (two pints) of crossmatched blood and giving set are in readiness. A dextrose drip may be set up at the beginning of the operation and this facilitates the giving of blood or oxytocin should the need arise. To women " at risk " of deep vein thrombosis some give Macrodex 0·5 litre I.V. during and following operation.

Oxytocic and other drugs with the requisite syringes are on the anæsthetist's tray.

Digoxin, nikethamide, methylamphetamine (Methedrine), hydrocortisone, should be at hand.

Hibitane, 0·5 per cent in 70 per cent spirit, for skin. Mastisol or adhesive plaster. Elastoplast Airstrip dressing, or Steristrip skin closure.

MIDWIVES' DUTIES DURING CÆSAREAN SECTION

The " scrubbed " nurse counts the swabs in the presence of the " non-scrubbed " nurse. The anæsthetised patient is brought in and the " non-scrubbed " nurse applies pressure on the suprapubic region to empty the bladder.

THE STERILE OR " SCRUBBED " NURSE

Hands to obstetrician holder with swab or polyester foam sponge soaked in Hibitane, 0·5 per cent in spirit, and another with skin paint. Places moisture repellent cotton or surgical sheet, 91 × 100 cm. (36 × 40 inches), over patient's thighs ; hands four towel clips and drapes to surround incision area. Helps to apply laparotomy sheet.

SKIN INCISION

Places instrument table over thighs. Hands scalpel and three swabs; places kidney-basin on table to receive discarded scalpel. Places dissecting forceps, scissors and Crile's forceps on table. Hands short lengths of catgut No. 2/0 or linen No. 60 to ligate vessels.

PERITONEAL INCISION

Lays two artery forceps, two Allis's tissue forceps, clean scalpel and scissors on table. Hands two dry packs with forceps attached to each tape (used to pack off intestines). Hands abdominal retractor.

UTERINE INCISION

Places clean scalpel, dissecting forceps and curved scissors on table. Gives dry, taped swab for mopping wound. Places midwifery forceps on table in readiness. Hands suction-nozzle as membranes of the fetal sac are being punctured.

EXTRACTION OF BABY

Clears all instruments from the table on which the baby will be laid. The obstetrician will hold the baby upside down to facilitate pulmonary drainage. Time of birth noted. Mechanical suction to clear the airway may be used. Hands swabs to wipe nose and mouth, two Kocher's forceps and scissors for cord.

The anæsthetist gives ergometrine intravenously as the baby's body is being extracted.

(The infant wrapped in a cellular cotton blanket is taken by the pædiatrician to the recovery room where mechanical suction, oxygen and other resuscitative equipment are available.)

Hands six Green-Armytage forceps to pick up edges of wound. Hands basin for placenta and Mayo forceps to detach membranes.

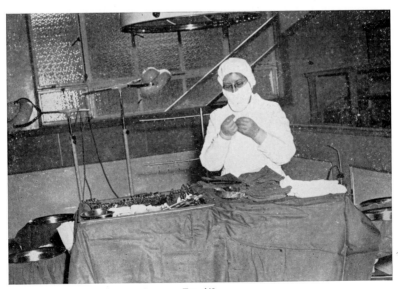

FIG. 448
Edinburgh Trolley-Top Trays in use.
(*Simpson Memorial Maternity Pavilion, Edinburgh.*)

SUTURES

Ethicon needled sutures (eyeless needles) sealed in foil packets are now widely used. Obstetricians have individual preferences, a selection is given here.

SUTURE OF UTERUS

Places clean towel on instrument table with needle-holders and dissecting forceps. Hands catgut No. 1, chromic, on round-bodied needle for three layers of sutures. Ethicon W 759 or W 727. Hands taped swab to mop uterine wound.

Swabs are now counted and checked by obstetrician, scrubbed and non-scrubbed **nurses, a swab rack with hooks in rows of 5 facilitates this.**

SUTURE OF PERITONEUM

Hands four Allis's forceps and a round-bodied needle with catgut No. 1 plain, and needle-holder. Obstetrician wipes wound with Hibitane, 0·5 per cent in 70 per cent spirit.

SUTURE OF SUPERFICIAL MUSCLE

Ethicon 770 No. 2 chromic catgut on No. 2 half-circle cutting needle.

SUTURE OF FAT

Ethicon W 734 on medium curve taper point needle No. 0 plain catgut.

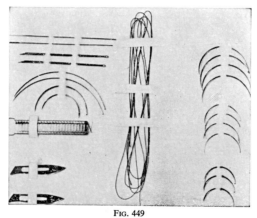

Fig. 449

Cæsarean Section Suture Pack
(*Aberdeen Maternity Hospital*)

2 Sims' straight cutting needles.	2 × 23 Bard Parker blades.
2 Hagedorn needles.	4 No. 2 half-circle round body.
2 Colt's needles.	4 No. 7 half-circle round body.
1 No. 2 half-circle cutting.	3 No. 2 Mayo round body.
1 No. 7 half-circle cutting.	4 × 25·4 cm. (10 inch) lengths Mersilk
Michel clips.	Size 0.

Added to Trolley

A	B
Chromic catgut No. 1 × 4.	No. 2 × 4.
Plain catgut No. 2/0 × 1.	No. 2/0 × 1.

From this selection of needles and sutures the needs of obstetricians who do not use Ethicon needled sutures can be met.

SUTURE OF THE SKIN

Hands four Allis's forceps, Michel clips with holder and inserter, or Mersilk No. 2/0 or No. 1 on Sims' straight needle or Ethicon W 562. Obstetrician wipes wound with antiseptic, applies gauze dressing on which Mastisol is painted or steri-strip dressing applied; removes laparotomy sheet.

The obstetrician expresses clots from the uterus: catheter removed: the vulva is swabbed and a pad placed in position.

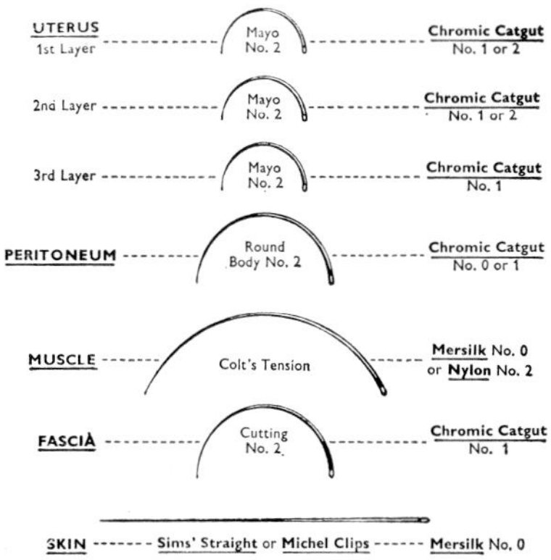

IMMEDIATE CARE OF THE BABY

A resuscitaire with suction, oxygen, drugs, laryngoscope, endotracheal tubes, Apgar score board, blood sample tubes, ampoules of soda bicarb. and fructose should be provided; cord ligatures, elastic bands or clamps, 10 ml. syringe and catheter. Newborn baby chart. Means of identification.

Some use a No. 8 Jaques catheter and 10-ml. syringe to aspirate the gastric fluid and prevent regurgitation and inhalation of the stomach contents.

UTERUS 1st Layer	Mayo No. 2	Chromic Catgut No. 1 or 2
2nd Layer	Mayo No. 2	Chromic Catgut No. 1 or 2
3rd Layer	Mayo No. 2	Chromic Catgut No. 1
PERITONEUM	Round Body No. 2	Chromic Catgut No. 0 or 1
MUSCLE	Colt's Tension	Mersilk No. 0 or Nylon No. 2
FASCIA	Cutting No. 2	Chromic Catgut No. 1
SKIN	Sims' Straight or Michel Clips	Mersilk No. 0

FIG. 450

Needles for Cæsarean Section.

(*County Maternity Hospital, Bellshill, Lanarkshire.*)

Cæsarean babies tend to become limp within a few moments, even when they have cried vigorously at birth; adequate pulmonary drainage, oxygen and warmth are usually sufficient to restore the infant's colour and muscle tone.

The cord is ligatured and clamp removed; means of identification applied, sex and time of birth recorded and the baby transferred to the nursery.

POST-OPERATIVE CARE

The patient is placed on her side, with a pillow behind her shoulders until conscious.

The midwife records the pulse every 15 minutes for at least three hours, and watches for any sign of wound or vaginal hæmorrhage.

As soon as consciousness is regained a sedative such as papaveretum (Omnopon) 20 mg. is administered, the midwife remaining with the patient until the drug has taken effect.

The blood pressure is taken on return to the ward and every two hours: if shocked or having blood, every half-hour for three hours, then four-hourly for 24 hours.

DURING THE EVENING

The patient is sponged, vulva swabbed, mouth and back attended to. Tea (and, if desired, toast) is served. Papaveretum (Omnopon) 20 mg., is administered and to ensure a comfortable night it is repeated at midnight and at 4 a.m. if necessary.

The woman may not void urine on the day of operation as she is taking very little fluid and it may be 24 hours before a catheter need be passed unless she is very uncomfortable.

Temperature, pulse and respirations are recorded every four hours. The patient is turned on alternate sides every two hours until ambulant.

SECOND DAY

Papaveretum, 20 mg., is given six-hourly. Vulval swabbing is carried out and a daily sponge bath given. The physiotherapist inaugurates deep breathing and leg exercises. If the patient is in good condition, she is allowed out of bed. **The legs are examined, groins palpated for tenderness every day.**

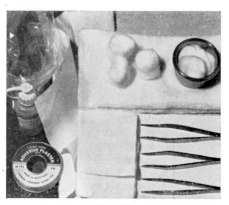

FIG. 451

Cæsarean Dressing Pack—Non-touch Technique.

3 disposable dressing forceps.	1 wound dressing.
2 gauze swabs.	2 Sterifield paper.
6 wool balls.	Hibitane, 0·5 per cent in spirit.
	Elastoplast.

(*Aberdeen Maternity Hospital.*)

THIRD DAY

Promethazine (Phenergan) or Ponstan may be given instead of papaveretum.

A laxative, such as Senokot is given; a prepacked enema or a Dulcolax suppository may be necessary if the bowels do not move within 12 hours.

One-half of the clips are removed on the sixth day, the remainder on the eighth day. The woman is discharged on the 10th to 12th day. The Health visitor is notified and help in the home arranged for.

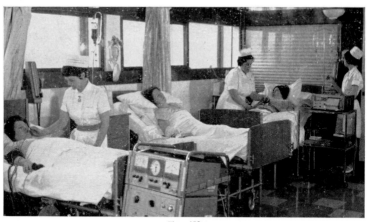

FIG. 452

INTENSIVE CARE UNIT.

"**Bed Monitor**," (*in foreground*)—which records vital signs: temperature, pulse, respirations, blood pressure.

Cardiotocograph (*in background*)—which gives continuous electronic monitoring of the fetal heart and the strength and frequency of uterine contractions.

(*County Maternity Hospital, Bellshill, Lanarkshire.*)

The dangers of Cæsarean Section:
To the mother:—Hæmorrhage, paralytic ileus, vein thrombosis, sepsis.
To the infant:—Respiratory distress syndrome is the main danger.

SUBSEQUENT PREGNANCIES

All women having had Cæsarean sections ought to be booked for hospital confinement and admitted 2 or 3 days prior to the expected date of delivery. Under no circumstances should any subsequent confinement be booked to take place at home. The woman should be instructed to report any abdominal pain during the last month and to come to hospital at once should any sign of labour occur.

SYMPHYSIOTOMY

This operation used to be performed prior to the Cæsarean section era. It is not popular in Britain today but is employed in some African countries where the women are unlikely to return for a repeat Cæsarean section.

The fibro-cartilage of the symphysis pubis is incised during labour when cephalo-pelvic disproportion exists. The ventouse vacuum extractor may be used in conjunction, to facilitate delivery. Following symphysiotomy some women suffer permanent backache; others may have disability in walking. During subsequent labours the pubic joint gives sufficiently to permit vaginal birth.

EMBRYOTOMY

All operative procedures involving " cutting into " and destruction of the fetus to diminish its bulk are included under the term " embryotomy."

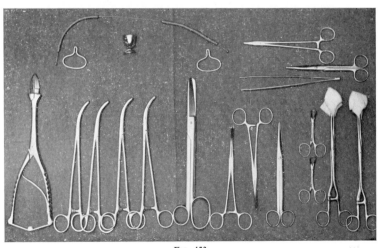

Fig. 453
INSTRUMENTS FOR EMBRYOTOMY.

2 sponge holders; 2 towel clips.	1 Blond Heidler decapitating wire saw.
1 Mayo scissors 20 cm.	1 needle holder.
2 Mayo forceps; 4 Briggs forceps.	1 Mayo scissors 15 cm.
1 embryotomy scissors.	1 dissecting forceps.
	1 Simpson perforator.

(Simpson Memorial Maternity Pavilion, Edinburgh.)

The four operations are :

CRANIOTOMY, CLEIDOTOMY, DECAPITATION, EVISCERATION.

They are usually, but not invariably, carried out on the dead fetus, in order to terminate labour which will obstruct or has obstructed.

The need for embryotomy should not arise except in cases of hydrocephaly or other gross fetal malformation, for, with good prenatal care, conditions liable to obstruct labour can be diagnosed during pregnancy. With competent supervision during labour, factors which cause obstruction can be detected and rectified early, or dealt with by lower segment Cæsarean section.

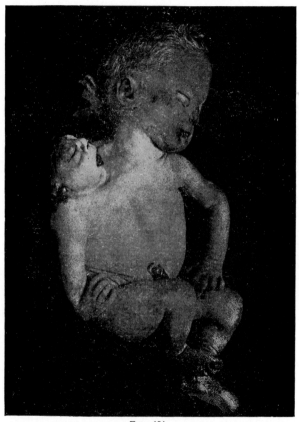

FIG. 454
Double-headed monster.

CRANIOTOMY

The indications are hydrocephaly, large baby, contracted pelvis, impacted brow and face presentations.

If necessary dehydration and ketosis are combated: cross-matched blood should be available; catheter passed; episiotomy made.

INSTRUMENTS

Skull perforator (Oldham's or Simpson's); midwifery forceps. A blunt hook and crotchet may be required to extract the aftercoming head of the breech. The " set up " is similar to that described for forceps delivery. (*The use of the cranioclast and cephalotribe is no longer advocated.*)

Procedure (For midwives in remote areas of developing countries)

After making an episiotomy midwifery forceps are applied to steady the head during perforation. The point of the perforator, which should be sharp and kept under control so that it does not slip off the skull and lacerate maternal tissues, is inserted. The point of insertion in a vertex presentation would be the parietal bone; in a face the orbit or roof of mouth; the aftercoming head of the breech presentation, sub-occipital region or behind the ear.

Having perforated the skull the blades of the perforator are opened to make a cruciform incision in the skull bone; then closed and passed into the cranium, opened widely and rotated to fragment the brain tissue; the perforator is withdrawn. Traction on the midwifery forceps is applied to extract the head.

If unsuccessful or if the cervix is not fully dilated 4 pairs of Briggs forceps (which resemble but are larger than curved Mayo forceps) are attached to the edges of the perforated bone, a bandage is threaded through the handles and a 907 G. weight attached and allowed to hang over the foot of the bed. This method facilitates dilatation of the cervix and accomplishes extraction slowly.

CLEIDOTOMY

This operation consists in the cutting of one or both clavicles, to reduce the width of the shoulders in cases such as a contracted pelvis or an excessively large baby, when craniotomy has been performed and the shoulders also are too large. Embryotomy scissors are used.

DECAPITATION

Decapitation, as the name implies, is severing of the head from the trunk; the indications being :

(*a*) An impacted shoulder presentation; (*b*) locked twins; (*c*) double-headed monster.

INSTRUMENTS

Blond Heidler decapitator; or sharp and serrated decapitation hooks; embryotomy blunt-pointed scissors; blunt hook and crotchet; heavy volsellum.

This operation would only be necessary for a neglected shoulder presentation; one that had become impacted. If an obstetrician was available Cæsarean section would be done, if not, to avoid uterine rupture or to terminate a dangerously long labour, decapitation would be necessary.

On no account should version be attempted by the midwife. Because of excessive retraction of the upper segment this would be difficult to do. Because of the extreme thinning and overstretching of the lower uterine segment, by the fetus lying transversely, the risk of ruptured uterus would be very great indeed.

Ketosis and dehydration must first be combated by I.V. dextrose 5 per cent prior to administering a general anæsthetic; a catheter is passed; a liberal episiotomy performed. The arm is brought down and pulled on firmly to bring the neck within reach.

The best decapitating instrument is the Blond Heidler wire saw. The thimble introducer is attached to one end of the wire and passed round the baby's neck. The handles are attached to both ends and by pulling on alternate handles the neck is severed. The body is delivered by traction on the arm; caution being exercised to avoid lacerating the maternal tissues by the sharp spikes of bone.

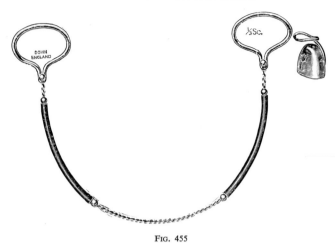

Fig. 455

Blond Heidler Wire Saw Decapitator.
(*By courtesy of Down Bros. and Mayer and Phelps Ltd., Mitcham, Surrey.*)

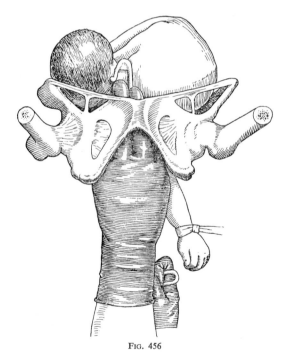

Fig. 456

Decapitating hook (Jardine's) is passed round neck of fetus.
Traction is made on arm to bring the neck within easier
reach and to fix the head and trunk.

The decapitated head is then fixed at the brim by suprapubic pressure and extracted by inserting a finger in the mouth or foramen magnum, aided by the use of a crotchet or heavy volsellum forceps. Midwifery forceps could be applied; the head may have to be perforated if difficulty is encountered.

A sharp decapitating hook can be used if the wire saw is not available. The hook is passed along the palmar surface of the fingers of the midwife's left hand, over the baby's shoulder and round the neck. The hook is manipulated until it grasps the neck securely. Backward and forward movement of the handle will sever the neck. Embryotomy scissors could be used to complete the decapitation.

EVISCERATION

The operation consists in making an opening in the fetal abdomen with embryotomy scissors for the removal of the contents of the abdominal cavity. It is performed when, because of excessive distension by a fetal tumour or ascites, labour is obstructed. Occasionally evisceration may be carried out in cases of impacted shoulder presentation to reduce the bulk of the fetus when the neck is inaccessible for the operation of decapitation.

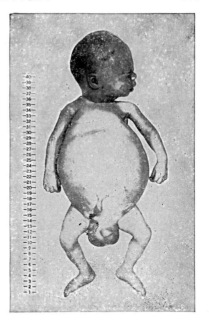

Fig. 457
Fetal ascites.

QUESTIONS FOR REVISION

How would you try to prevent shoulder dystocia ? How would you deal with it ?

INDUCTION OF LABOUR

Give 4 reasons why labour may be induced. What do you mean by induction delivery interval ? How long is it usually ? **Describe in not more than 10 lines:** (*a*) your duties regarding the administration of buccal pitocin; (*b*) observation of a woman having puncture of membranes and oxytocin drip.

What are the dangers in giving an intravenous oxytocin drip: mention the observations you would make when giving it. State what you would set out in readiness for surgical induction of labour. Prolapse of cord may occur, what is the midwife's responsibility ?

C.M.B.(Scot.) paper.—Give an account of (*a*) the indications, and (*b*) the methods available, for the induction of labour.

C.M.B.(N. Ireland) paper, 1969.—What are the main indications for induction of labour ? What are the responsibilities of the midwife in: (*a*) induction of labour by oxytocin " drip "; (*b*) surgical induction of labour ?

C.M.B.(Eng.) paper, 1969.—To what particular points would you pay attention in the management of labour in the following patients: (*a*) a primigravida with an intravenous infusion of oxytocin in progress; (*b*) a multiparous patient who has had a previous Cæsarean section.

EPISIOTOMY

Differentiate between a median, medio-lateral and J-shaped episiotomy and state advantages and disadvantages of each. **What are the C.M.B. rules regarding:** (*a*) making an episiotomy; (*b*) administering a local anæsthetic ? **What are the toxic reactions of local anæsthetics ?** How could these be averted ?

Why: (*a*) should the piston of the syringe be withdrawn prior to injecting the local anæsthetic ? (*b*) is injecting the drug while the needle is being withdrawn a wise precautionary measure ? (*c*) should an episiotomy not be made too soon ? **How long is the incision ?** How far distant should the incision be from the lateral border of the anus ? How would you control bleeding from the incision ?

C.M.B.(Eng.) paper.—What are the indications for episiotomy? When should a midwife undertake this procedure? Describe the technique employed.

C.M.B.(Eng.) paper. 100 word question.—Episiotomy.

VERSION

Define the following types of version : external; cephalic; internal; podalic; and state when and why they are employed. Under what circumstances would a midwife be justified in performing external version ? Describe the procedure.

FORCEPS DELIVERY

In what instances would a midwife anticipate the application of forceps ? What preparations are made regarding (*a*) pudendal nerve block ; (*b*) vulval toilet ; (*c*) the baby ?

C.M.B.(Eng.) paper.—What circumstances occurring during labour might necessitate the use of obstetric forceps ? How would you prepare the patient for the operation of forceps delivery ?

C.M.B.(N. Ireland) paper.—Enumerate the articles set out for a forceps delivery, mentioning the purpose of each one.

C.M.B.(N. Ireland) paper, 1969.—What are the indications for forceps delivery ? Describe, in detail, the preparations necessary for such a delivery.

C.M.B.(Eng.) paper, 1970.—Give an account of the reasons for which obstetric forceps may be used in the second stage of labour.

CÆSAREAN SECTION

Describe the immediate pre-operative care of the patient. What are the duties of the non-scrubbed nurse ? Why should swabs be in packs of 5 ? How would you prepare to receive the baby in the theatre ? Outline the post-operative care during the first three days.

C.M.B.(N. Ireland) paper.—How would you nurse a mother during the first two weeks following a Cæsarean section ?

C.M.B.(Eng.) paper.—Describe the nursing care of a patient who has had a Cæsarean section, from the immediate post-operative period to the 7th day.

C.M.B.(Scot.) paper.—Give the nursing care of a patient following Cæsarean section.

For what purpose are the following instruments used: Simpson's perforator; Brigg's forceps; Blond Heidler wire saw; embryotomy scissors ? Why are destructive procedures rarely carried out on the fetus now ? Under what circumstances might they have to be undertaken by a midwife ?

ANÆSTHESIA

What is Mendelson's syndrome? How could the midwife try to prevent this?

Why is the bladder emptied prior to each injection of epidural anæsthetic ? How often is the blood pressure taken after the first injection ? Why must the uterine contractions be carefully noted by the midwife ? **What would you do,** in the absence of the anæsthetist, for hypotension ? **Why are outlet forceps usually necessary ?**

For what reasons are the following used : Venflon cannula, Brunswick syringe, Tuohy needle, Rowbotham's introducer?

Give the pharmaceutical names for the following : Nupercaine, Marcain, Xylocaine, Methedrine, Scoline, Pentothal, Vasylox.

Differentiate between : Anæsthesia and analgesia,; spinal and epidural anæsthesia; paracervical and pudendal block.

34

Intra-uterine Death: Placental Dysfunction: Postmaturity: Babies at Risk

Prior to the 28th week intra-uterine death of the fetus would be termed an abortion: after the 28th week and during labour the term stillbirth is used.

PRENATAL DEATH OF THE FETUS

(1) *Early in Pregnancy*:—Abortion threatens but does not take place spontaneously (see missed abortion, p. 143, for signs, risk of blood coagulation disorders and treatment).

(2) *After mid-term*:—Fetal death is ultimately due to anoxia and the majority of cases are associated with diseases such as pre-eclampsia, diabetes; Rh hæmolytic disease, gross fetal malformations.

(3) *Signs:*

(*a*) The fetal heart beat is not heard on successive examinations.

(*b*) Fetal movement ceases and is no longer felt by the mother.

(*c*) The uterus is " small for dates " and there is cessation of uterine growth.

(*d*) Œstriol excretion is markedly reduced.

(*e*) No vascular pulsation by ultrasonic fetal pulse detector.

RADIOLOGICAL EVIDENCE
Because of radiation hazards radiology is not used by all obstetricians to diagnose fetal death

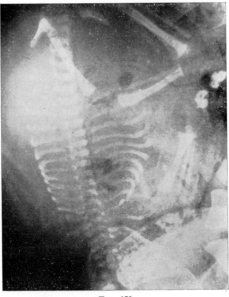

FIG. 458

SIGN OF FETAL DEATH.

The presence of intra-fetal gas in the blood vessels of the umbilical cord and in the chambers of the heart.

(*Simpson Memorial Maternity Pavilion, Edinburgh.*)

653

SPALDING'S SIGN

There is gross overlapping of the bones of the vault of the skull due to disintegration of the brain substance. It is rarely seen less than seven days after intra-uterine death. Slight overlapping is not diagnostic as this may occur at the onset of, or during, labour with a live fetus.

INTRA-FETAL GAS

This is the earliest conclusive sign observed one week earlier than Spalding's sign. Bubbles of gas form in the heart and large blood vessels: more rarely are they seen in the umbilical cord vessels (see fig. 458); they have been observed as early as 12 hours after fetal death.

The following are suggestive but not diagnostic radiographic signs:—

The thoracic cage collapses and the ribs fall together.

Hyperflexion of the spine with bizarre fetal attitudes.

Transverse lie with the fetus slumped in the lower pole of the uterus.

The treatment *is to induce abortion or labour by I.V. oxytocin drip.* Surgical induction is never employed because of the risk of intra-uterine sepsis from anaerobic organisms.

Maceration occurs when the fetus *in utero* has been dead for 12 to 24 hours, and is brought about by aseptic autolysis. Large blebs containing dark coloured fluid appear on the skin: later extensive denuded areas showing the shiny fascia are manifest. The tissues are soft, discoloured and œdematous with a tendency to disintegrate. Maceration usually indicates that death occurred in pregnancy rather than during labour: pre-eclampsia, diabetes, Rh hæmolytic disease being possible causes. In 25 per cent of cases no cause is obvious.

INTRA-NATAL FETAL DEATH

Adverse conditions existing during pregnancy may persist and, combined with the stresses imposed by labour, may prove fatal to the fetus. Oxygen deprivation may be the result of (*a*) placental dysfunction, (*b*) interference with the circulation in the umbilical cord, (*c*) premature separation of the placenta. For the premature baby anoxia is lethal.

The term "fresh stillbirth" is used when death occurs during labour; there is no maceration.

Consideration for the Mother

Student midwives should be reminded that the loss of a baby at birth is a bitter disappointment to the mother: one of the joys of womanhood has been snatched from her grasp. She feels frustrated, after all the anticipation and preparation. Kindly understanding and sympathy are needed.

The mother should not be subjected to the anguish of seeing other mothers handling their babies: nor should she be within sight or sound of the nursery. Most hospitals permit the husband or a relative to visit as soon as possible. Early discharge should be arranged.

PLACENTAL DYSFUNCTION

The normal placenta undergoes some degenerative processes at the end of pregnancy; it becomes senile but still maintains an adequate reserve to meet fetal needs during labour.

Conditions associated with Dysfunction
PRE-ECLAMPSIA   ESSENTIAL HYPERTENSION   DIABETES

Premature degenerative processes occur, probably due to adverse changes in the chorionic villi and placental blood vessels: these result in reduced blood flow in the choriodecidual space.

The efficiency of the placenta as an organ of transport becomes markedly decreased; the fetus is deprived of an adequate supply of oxygen and nutrients, growth is inhibited, and on occasions intra-uterine death occurs.

Clinical Features of Placental Dysfunction

1. **Small baby syndrome.** The size of the fetus increases slowly after the 30th week. There is no increase in maternal girth and weight.

2. **The amount of liquor amnii is found to be reduced** on abdominal palpation from about the 34th week onwards.

3. **Diminished secretion of urinary œstriol** occurs and when, after the 34th week, the level is from 3 to 5 mg. per 24 hours the fetus is at risk. Levels below 2 mg. per 24 hours are indicative of fetal death. The absolutely accurate collection of the 24-hour specimen of urine is necessary. Unless urgent this is done on two consecutive days. The urine should be kept in the " Frig " at 4° C.

URINARY ŒSTRIOL
Klopper.

Weeks of Pregnancy	20	24	28	32	36	40	
Range (mg.)/24 hrs	2–8	6–13	8–18	11–24	17–30	20–49	

Some authorities do not consider the œstriol test to be of value except in conjunction with other signs of placental dysfunction.

Serial ultrasonic measurements of the fetal bi-parietal diameter growth are made: if adequate the feto-placental unit is likely to be satisfactory.

MANAGEMENT IN CASES OF PLACENTAL DYSFUNCTION

1. **Additional rest in bed is prescribed** to increase uterine blood flow.

2. **The woman is not subjected to conditions that would diminish her oxygen intake:**
   e.g. Air-travel is contraindicated.

3. **Labour is induced prematurely** by puncture of the membranes and oxytocin drip if necessary.

4. **Postmaturity is not permitted to occur.**

5. **Prolonged labour is avoided.**

Supervision during labour

The midwife must supervise the fetal condition with assiduous care. Monitoring the fetal heart with the cardiophone gives a more reliable and complete assessment. Fetal scalp blood sampling may be employed.

Should fetal distress be manifest the doctor is notified immediately. Cæsarean section may be necessary and with the pack system preparations can be made in 6 to 7 minutes.

POSTMATURITY

After the 41st week of pregnancy the fetus is said to be postmature. The perinatal mortality rate is doubled at 42 weeks and trebled at 43 weeks: stillbirth being more common than neonatal death. The high death rate in postmaturity is associated with conditions that cause placental dysfunction, a combination that is particularly lethal to the fetus. (*Authorities are not agreed as to whether postmaturity causes anoxia.*)

Labour is likely to be prolonged due to inco-ordinate uterine action and because the hard head does not mould well: forceps delivery is usually necessary.

DIAGNOSIS

Unfortunately conclusive evidence of postmaturity is not available when the decision has to be made whether the woman has gone beyond the calculated date of confinement or not. She may, of course, be in error regarding the date of her last menstrual period.

1. **A bimanual examination, at the 6th to 12th week of pregnancy,** is made by some as a means of establishing the period of gestation.

2. **Recording the date of quickening would be helpful.**

3. **When the cervix is long, hard and closed,** it is commonly accepted that the onset of labour is not imminent.

MANAGEMENT OF POSTMATURITY

Some allow the woman to go into labour spontaneously and perform Cæsarean section if fetal distress is manifest.

1. **Induction of labour is carried out in the majority of cases** at the 42nd week, the same vigilant care being exercised as in placental dysfunction.

2. **If placental dysfunction is present, as might occur in pre-eclampsia, essential hypertension, diabetes,** the woman would not be permitted to go beyond term, in fact labour would be induced before then. In cases where premature separation of placenta had occurred, i.e. threatened abortion or antepartum hæmorrhage, induction of labour at or prior to term would be advocated.

3. **Older primigravidæ are not usually permitted to go beyond the 40th week.** Difficulties may arise, necessitating forceps delivery and, although pudendal nerve block has eliminated the hazards of a general anæsthetic, the fetus is at risk. Cæsarean section is likely.

4. **Puncture of membranes is carried out followed by oxytocin drip, immediately or within 6 to 12 hours.** The risk of prolapse of cord demands vigilant supervision.

Cæsarean section will be performed:—

(a) **Should labour not start 18 hours after puncture of membranes and oxytocin drip.**

(b) **If fetal distress occurs during labour.**

THE POSTMATURE BABY

There are no absolute criteria of postmaturity

1. **Hard skull bones,** small fontanelles and narrow sutures are suggestive, but not conclusive.

2. **Excessive weight is not decisive:** babies at term may weigh 4,536 G (10 lbs.)

3. **The baby's skin is loose,** due to loss of subcutaneous fat, and may be dry, cracked, and desquamating: nails long; but these are sometimes seen in babies who are not postmature.

The placenta gives no reliable clue. The calcareous particles, often so abundant as to give the appearance of coarse sandpaper, have not been found in particular association with postmaturity.

BABIES AT RISK

All physical and mental handicaps are not obvious at birth. Certain conditions—inherited, present during pregnancy, labour or the first week of life, may predispose the infant to some incapacitating disability.

Local authorities have introduced an "at risk" register so that they will be informed by hospital and domiciliary midwifery staff regarding the babies who have been subjected to these conditions. The doctor and the Health Visitor will thus be enabled to detect the handicap early and arrange for the appropriate treatment. Midwives may be required to state on " notification of birth " or discharge forms any " at risk " conditions, to which the baby was exposed, or is afflicted by.

The criteria of " at risk " conditions are so comprehensive in some areas that 60-70 per cent of their new born babies are on the register : some consider that 10-20 per cent would be a reasonable number.

The following are examples of " at risk " conditions:—

FAMILIAL:—Deafness: blindness.

PRENATAL:—Rubella: pre-eclampsia : diabetes: pyelonephritis: antepartum hæmorrhage.

LABOUR:—prolonged: difficult: malpresentation.

FIRST WEEK OF LIFE:—Severe asphyxia: low birth-weight: intra-cranial injury: hæmolytic disease: light for dates: twins: congenital abnormalities: failure to thrive.

QUESTIONS FOR REVISION

Oral Questions

In what conditions would you suspect placental dysfunction ? What are the signs of intra-uterine death ? How would you collect urine for œstriol assay ? What precautions are taken when placental dysfunction exists ? (*a*) during pregnancy; (*b*) during labour.

Define the following: maceration; intra-uterine growth retardation; Spalding's sign; œstriol assay; small baby syndrome.

C.M.B.(Eng.) paper.—Describe the functions of the placenta. How may the efficiency of the placenta be impaired ?

C.M.B.(Scot.) paper.—Give the causes of intra-uterine death and indicate how this diagnosis might be established.

C.M.B.(Scot.) paper.—Describe the subsequent care of a patient delivered of a still-born baby.

C.M.B.(Eng.) paper, 1970.—50 word question.—What is an " at risk " register ? What is the purpose of such a register and what are the main groups of infants included in this register ?

C.M.B.(Eng.) paper, 1970.—50 word question.—What points concerning a mother should be brought to a health visitor's notice before transfer to her care ?

35

Aids to Diagnosis during Pregnancy

RADIOLOGY: ULTRASONOGRAPHY: BLOOD TESTS: URINE ANALYSIS

Radiology is one of the aids to diagnosis in obstetrics, used mainly to supplement and confirm findings which have been made on clinical examination during pregnancy.

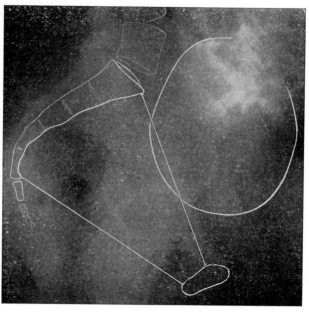

FIG. 459

Lateral radiograph (retouched), showing the antero-posterior diameters of the brim and outlet.

RADIATION HAZARDS

Certain risks may be involved in the use of X-rays, but these must be balanced against the advantages in the saving of maternal and infant life.

1. A slight increase in the number of cases of leukæmia and other forms of cancer in children was suspected but some question this.

2. An increased mutation rate in the germ cells of mother and child which may affect future generations by causing congenital disease and abnormalities.

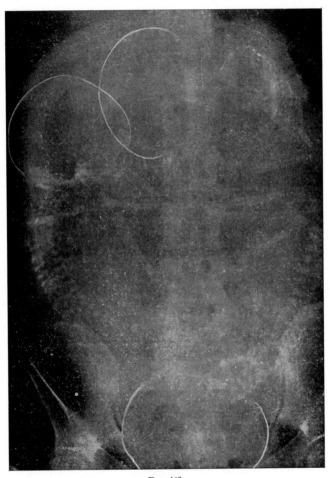

Fig. 460

Triplets (retouched).

Attempts to prevent these dangers are being made by the use of modern radiological techniques; shielding of fetal and maternal gonads, shorter exposures, smaller doses and shorter wave lengths. The number of films taken is now limited to the minimum required to obtain the necessary information and these are taken in later pregnancy.

PELVIC SIZE AND SHAPE

Radiography to determine pelvic size and shape might be indicated (*after the 32nd week*) in the following circumstances:—

1. **When there is a history of injury or disease of the pelvis or spine,** or of a previous difficult labour.

2. **In cases of limp or deformity,** cephalo-pelvic disproportion, persistent breech or shoulder presentation.

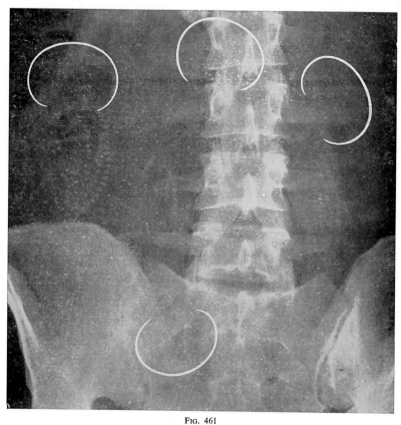

FIG. 461

QUADRUPLETS (RETOUCHED)

All four babies (*born* 1963) survived and were discharged weighing over 2,495 G. (5½ lb.). The mother had two sets of twins, aged 6 and 2 years.

(*Aberdeen Maternity Hospital.*)

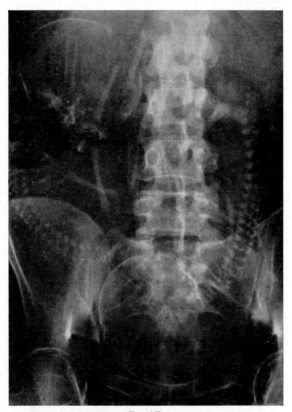

FIG. 462
TWINS, ONE VERTEX ONE BREECH.
(*Simpson Memorial Maternity Pavilion, Edinburgh.*)

FETAL ABNORMALITIES

Malformations, such as anencephaly and hydrocephaly, achondroplasia, conjoined twins, spina-bifida, may be diagnosed.

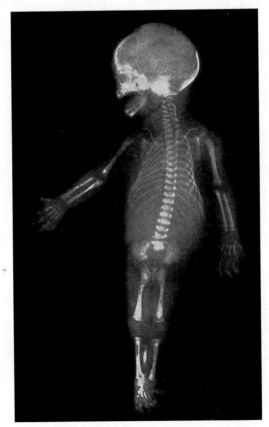

Fig. 463

SYMPODIA (MERMAID-LIKE FETUS).

The lower limbs are fused to form a tail-like structure with one foot, eight toes; no uterus, external genitalia, urethral or anal orifices; no sex identified; weight 1,531 G. (3 lb. 6 oz.); stillborn.

The fetus was the second of dizygotic (binovular) twins; the first, born alive, weighed 3,374 G. (7 lb. 7 oz.).

(Maternity Hospital, Motherwell.)

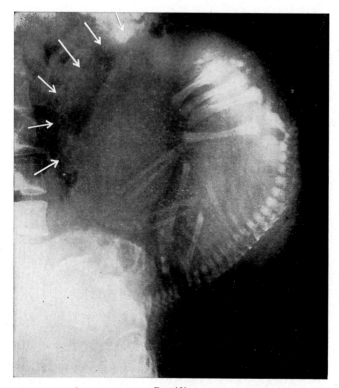

FIG. 464

Soft tissue X-ray showing placental area which is indicated by arrows (lateral view).

UTERINE RADIOGRAPHY

Localisation of placenta.—By soft tissue X-ray (*placentography*) it is possible in about 90 per cent of cases to diagnose placenta prævia by the absence of placental shadow in the upper uterine segment. Arteriography is also used.

In cases of infertility, opaque substances injected into the uterus and Fallopian tubes produce a shadow on an X-ray film which demonstrates the patency or non-patency of the tubes.

THE USE OF ULTRASONOGRAPHY IN OBSTETRICS

Ultrasonography is a means of diagnosing the presence, size, and position of a mass from the sound echo evoked by the density of the mass. In the 1914-1918 war ultrasound was used in submarine warfare (known as Asdic). If the presence of a submarine was suspected, a beam of ultrasonic energy was projected and the echo received would depend on the resistance of the mass, *e.g.* a rock, shoal of fish or a submarine. Ultrasound was first employed in obstetrics by Professor Ian Donald, Queen Mother's Hospital, Glasgow, and is now a successful diagnostic technique with none of the radiation hazards of radiography.

The woman lies on a couch and a probe connected to the diasonograph is "run over" her abdomen which has been smeared with olive oil to obtain acoustic coupling.

The apparatus used, the Diasonograph, transmits a beam of ultrasonic energy (sound waves far above the range of human hearing) generated by an electric current causing a small crystal in the probe to vibrate. When this beam strikes objects of differing resistance, fetal limbs, skull, or placenta, the echo is amplified and displayed on an oscilloscope screen. Two cathode ray tubes are used and a polaroid camera records the echoes as dots of light. The image so produced is an ultrasonogram, an echo picture. The examination takes only a few minutes, the results are immediately available.

The A scan is a one-dimension picture useful when measuring a diameter as in fetal cephalometry.

The B scan gives a composite two-dimensional picture.

The full bladder technique. The bladder containing urine shows up as a well defined black area on the oscilloscope or on the photograph. This is an aid to delineating the gestation sac in early pregnancy, as well as fetal parts and placenta later.

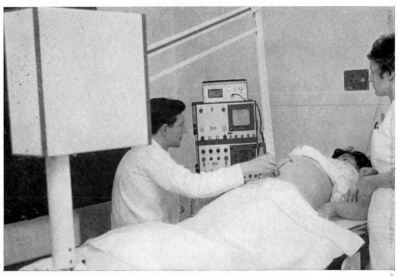

FIG. 465

DIASONOGRAPH APPARATUS.

Doctor applying probe to skin of abdominal wall.

(*Simpson Memorial Maternity Pavilion, Edinburgh.*)

ULTRASOUND AS A DIAGNOSTIC AID

Diagnosis of pregnancy. An early gestation sac, after 6 weeks amenorrhœa, shows up as a very small white ring with black centre. (*The quintuplets at Queen Charlotte's Hospital 1969 were diagnosed at 9 weeks.*)

Hydatidiform Mole shows as a white speckled area: Sonar is being relied on with great certainty in the diagnosis of this condition.

Twins are diagnosed in mid-pregnancy by the identification of two separate heads.

Hydramnios is shown by large clear areas of fluid. Blobs which appear to be floating in the fluid are limbs: when no fetal head is obvious anencephaly is suspected.

Placental Localization. In cases of antepartum hæmorrhage this technique is invaluable; the placenta being localized with greater accuracy than by soft tissue radiography.

Prior to amniocentesis localization of the placenta will minimize the risk of transplacental bleeding and the subsequent production of Rh antibodies.

Fetal cephalometry. The bi-parietal diameter of the fetal head is measured after the 30th week by ultrasound at weekly intervals to determine the growth rate in cases of suspected placental dysfunction. Normal growth of the bi-parietal diameter after the 30th week is 0·15 to 0·2 cm. per week. Serial cephalometry is less time consuming than serial urinary œstriol estimations and is equally reliable.

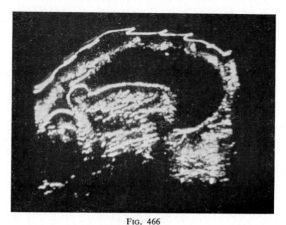

FIG. 466
ULTRASONOGRAM OF ANENCEPHALY AND HYDRAMNIOS.
(*Aberdeen Maternity Hospital.*)

THE ULTRASONIC FETAL PULSE DETECTOR
(*Ultrasound cardioscope*)

The Sonicaid and the Doptone, portable battery run machines, are in common use today. By utilizing ultrasound and the Doppler effect, blood pulsation can be heard. The sounds are not these of the fetal heart beat but the pulsations in the blood vessels. Olive oil is smeared on to the skin before the transducer is applied in order to obtain good acoustic coupling.

The apparatus is employed as follows:

1. **To detect the presence of a living fetus:** (*a*) pregnancy diagnosis (from 12 weeks); (*b*) threatened abortion; (*c*) missed abortion; (*d*) hydatidiform mole; (*e*) **intrauterine death.**

2. **To localize the placental site:** (*a*) in cases of antepartum hæmorrhage (*to a limited degree*); (*b*) prior to abdominal amniocentesis.

3. **To confirm the diagnosis of thrombosis in** major leg veins. If the vein is occluded by a thrombus no pulsation is detected (for method see p. 482).

BLOOD TESTS

GROUPING

Blood of different individuals belongs to one of four groups, classified under the ABO system. The patient should be given blood of her own particular group if possible, but in an acute emergency, when there are neither facilities nor time for ascertaining this, Group O blood, being compatible with all four groups, may be given.

DIRECT CROSS-MATCHING

As an additional precaution against giving incompatible blood, the serum from the recipient's clotted blood is mixed with blood from the " pilot tube " which is attached to the bottle of donor blood. If agglutination of red cells is manifest, the donor blood is not compatible.

RHESUS FACTOR GROUPING

The Rh factor of every pregnant woman should be ascertained early in pregnancy because of the grave risks in giving Rh positive blood to an Rh negative woman. In an emergency Rh negative Group O blood may be given, but as only 5 per cent of all donors are Rh negative Group O, the indiscriminate use of this blood would severely tax the resources of the blood bank.

RH ANTIBODIES

Rh antibodies.—Tests for the presence of antibodies are carried out on Rh negative women: Coombs' indirect anti-globulin test (I.A.G.T.). Coombs' direct anti-globulin test (D.A.G.T.) is used when examining the baby's blood if hæmolytic disease is suspected.

WEINER CLOT OBSERVATION TEST

Blood is withdrawn into a plain test tube. If the fibrinogen concentration of the blood has decreased to a critical level (100 mg. per 100 ml.), coagulation may be delayed. If the fibrinogen has fallen to a lesser degree clotting will be delayed beyond the normal maximum of 10 minutes; the clot will be small, unstable, and may fragment, depending on the fibrinolytic activity, and dissolve when kept at 36·9° C. (98·4° F.) for one hour.

HÆMOGLOBIN

Hæmoglobin is often expressed in percentage of the normal which is taken to be 100. A more accurate method of estimating the amount of hæmoglobin is in G. per 100 ml. of blood, 14·8 G. being considered 100 per cent.

Midwives can roughly estimate the percentage of hæmoglobin by multiplying the result in grammes by 7, i.e. 10 G. = 70 per cent.

The baby at term has a hæmoglobin of 13·6 to 19·6 G.

Grammes per 100 ml.		Per cent	Grammes per 100 ml.		Per cent
14·8	=	100	9·6	=	65
14·1	=	95	8·9	=	60
13·3	=	90	8·1	=	55
12·6	=	85	7·4	=	50
11·8	=	80	6·6	=	45
11·1	=	75	5·9	=	40
10·3	=	70	5·2	=	35

BLOOD REQUIRED FOR LABORATORY TESTS

TEST	Test Tube	Amount of Blood	Normal Result
RHESUS FACTOR / ABO GROUP . . .	Plain	5 ml.	
ANTIBODIES	Plain	10 ml.	
WASSERMANN	Plain	5 ml.	
SERUM BILIRUBIN . . .	Plain	3 ml.	below 1 mg. per 100 ml.
COOMBS'	Plain	5 ml.	
BLOOD UREA	Lithium heparin	3 ml.	15 to 40 mg. per 100 ml.
FASTING BLOOD GLUCOSE .	oxalated fluoride	2 ml.	65 to 105 mg. per 100 ml.
ERYTHROCYTE SEDIMENTATION RATE (E.S.R.)	Sequestrene	5 ml.	From 2 to 5 mm. in first hour.
BLOOD CULTURE . . .	Bacteriological broth, 50 ml.	5 ml.	
WHITE CELL COUNT . . .	Sequestrene	2·5 ml.	5,000 to 10,000.
RED CELL COUNT . . .	Sequestrene	2·5 ml.	5,000,000.
COAGULATION TIME . . .	Plain	1 ml.	5 to 8 minutes.
PROTHROMBIN TIME . .	Sodium citrate or sodium oxalate	2·5 ml.	
HÆMOGLOBIN	Sequestrene	2·5 ml.	14·8 G. (100 per cent) per 100 ml. blood.
PLASMA FIBRINOGEN . .	sodium citrate	5 ml.	300 to 400 mg. per 100 ml.

URINE ANALYSIS

In Pregnancy

Note the appearance.—Crystal clear urine may contain protein; blood gives a red or dark brown colour; bile produces a greenish-gold or greenish-brown colour.

Odour.—An offensive odour may be due to pus; an odour of stale fish is associated with an *E. coli* infection. A fruity odour, or one of violets, is due to ketones.

Reaction.—Freshly voided urine is usually slightly acid and turns blue litmus-paper red; alkaline urine turns red litmus-paper blue.

The specific gravity is taken by means of a urinometer and normally ranges from 1,010 to 1,025.

PROTEINURIA (Albuminuria)

Proteinuria may be present in the following conditions in obstetrics: pre-eclampsia, eclampsia, serious hyperemesis, cardiac decompensation and pyelonephritis. A trace is also found in urine which contains blood, pus, vaginal discharge or liquor amnii.

Tests for Protein

ALBUSTIX REAGENT STRIPS test for protein. If positive, further tests are made.

URISTIX REAGENT STRIPS detect proteinuria and glycosuria simultaneously.

HEAT COAGULATION TEST

Filter the urine if not clear: fill a test tube three-quarters full of urine. If alkaline, add a few drops of dilute acetic acid, otherwise the protein will not coagulate and will therefore not be detected. Heat the upper part to boiling point. (*Heating the urine will cause urates to disappear*; *the addition of acetic acid will cause phosphates to disappear.*)

THE SALICYL-SULPHONIC ACID TEST

This is a cold test which is rapid and sensitive. With a pipette add a few drops of 20 per cent salicyl-sulphonic acid to half a test tube of urine, and a turbid streak will appear if protein is present. If the urine is alkaline, a few extra drops of salicyl-sulphonic acid are needed.

ESBACH'S QUANTITATIVE TEST FOR PROTEIN

The vulva is swabbed with water and a midstream specimen of urine obtained.

The urine must be filtered unless clear, and acidified if alkaline. If the specific gravity is over 1,010 the urine must be diluted with an equal volume of water, because the protein precipitate does not settle properly if the specific gravity is over 1,010.

The graduated tube is filled to the mark " U " with urine and to the mark " R " with reagent. The tube is stoppered, then inverted two or three times without shaking and allowed to stand undisturbed for 24 hours. The height of the precipitate in the tube is read and recorded in grammes per litre, the result being doubled if the urine is diluted.

The patient's name, time when set up, and whether the urine is diluted must be clearly marked.

GLYCOSURIA

A trace of glucose is found in the urine of about 10 per cent of pregnant women (see p. 62), and when diabetes is present.

CLINITEST REAGENT TABLETS estimate glucose in urine.

CLINISTIX REAGENT STRIPS are specific for glucose and exclude lactose.

URISTIX REAGENT STRIPS now commonly used detect glucose and protein simultaneously. If glucose is detected by Clinistix or Uristix reagent strips Clinitest tablets are used to estimate quantitatively.

LABSTIX TESTS simultaneously for pH, protein, glucose, ketones and blood in urine.

KETONURIA (acetonuria)

Ketones are found in the urine of obstetric patients who are diabetic or have any condition in which the carbohydrate intake is diminished, such as hyperemesis gravidarum.

During prolonged labour, with or without vomiting, acidosis will occur unless the carbohydrate intake is adequate.

ACETEST REAGENT TABLETS are used in some clinics.

KETOSTIX REAGENT STRIPS detect the presence of ketones and are more rapid in action.

BLOOD IN THE URINE

In obstetric practice blood in the urine is most commonly due to vaginal bleeding. Very occasionally it may be due to nephritis, and is then bright red; in cases of eclampsia the urine may be dark brownish-red, almost chocolate colour, due to the presence of blood in highly concentrated urine.

HEMASTIX REAGENT STRIPS test for blood in urine.

BILE IN THE URINE

Bile is found in the urine when jaundice is present, in cases such as severe hyperemesis gravidarum, and puerperal sepsis due to the *Clostridium welchii.*

ICTOTEST REAGENT TABLETS detect the presence of bilirubin in urine.

PUS IN THE URINE

Pus is found in cases of urinary tract infection. The only reliable test is by microscopic examination.

CHLORIDES IN THE URINE

Midwives may occasionally be required to test for urinary chlorides, mainly sodium chloride, particularly in hyperemesis gravidarum.

When chlorides are absent or less than 3 G. (some say 5) per litre, a state of chloride deficiency exists, and the intravenous infusion of isotonic saline solution is indicated.

FANTUS QUANTITATIVE TEST

In a small test tube place 0·6 ml. (10 drops) of urine and 0·06 ml. (1 drop) of 20 per cent potassium chromate. With a Pasteur pipette add drops of 2·9 per cent silver nitrate. The number of drops required to produce a slight reddish coloration in the precipitate indicates the number of grammes of chloride per litre of urine.

The normal 24-hour excretion is 9·5 to 14·5 G. (Harrison).

Uricult: dip slide system for urine culture suitable for large scale screening. A slide with MacConkey's medium on one side, nutrient agar on the other is dipped into urine and placed in a plastic container; incubated or kept at room temperature; sent for identification and sensitivity test. Used for asymptomatic bacteriuria.

QUESTIONS FOR REVISION

URINE ANALYSIS

For what reason should urine (*a*) be acidified when examined for protein ? (*b*) be diluted when setting up an Esbach test ? Why do normal pregnant women have glycosuria? Which is the most reliable test for pus ?

C.M.B.(Scot.) paper.—What abnormal constituents are present in the urine in a case of (*a*) pre-eclampsia; (*b*) hyperemesis gravidarum; (*c*) pyelonephritis of pregnancy ? Describe the tests for these.

C.M.B.(N. Ireland) paper.—Enumerate the abnormal constituents which may be found in the urine of a patient 28 weeks pregnant. Describe their significance.

C.M.B.(Scot.) paper—Discuss the importance of urine testing during pregnancy.

C.M.B.(Eng.) paper.—What abnormal constituents of the urine may be found in pregnancy? What may be their significance?

36

The Administration of Some Drugs used by Midwives

The number of drugs used in obstetric practice is very great and only some of those commonly prescribed are mentioned below. A midwife requires to use certain of these in the course of her work; some must be prescribed by the doctor, others she is permitted to give on her own authority. The majority are mentioned throughout the text.

WARNING REGARDING DRUGS IN PREGNANCY

Great caution is now being observed by doctors in prescribing drugs during pregnancy, and particularly during the first trimester. Some drugs that can be bought by the public as anti-emetics are believed to be harmful to the fetus.

The midwife must warn pregnant women regarding these and refrain from recommending any drug, however innocuous it is thought to be, until further research proves it to be harmless to the growing embryo.

The midwife's need for giving drugs is concerned mainly with:

1. **Relief of pain during labour.** 2. **Resuscitation of the newborn.**

3. **Prevention and treatment of hæmorrhage.**

Very rarely does the occasion arise for midwives to administer other drugs without medical sanction. In hospital, standing or written orders are issued and in an emergency medical aid is readily available.

Domiciliary midwives carry drugs as approved by the Central Midwives Boards and their employers, usually the Local Authority.

DANGEROUS DRUGS REGULATIONS 1964

Midwives are not permitted to give on their own authority narcotic and sedative drugs other than pethidine, medicinal opium and tincture of opium. *Opium is now rarely used.*

Midwives must observe the requirements of the Dangerous Drugs Regulations which include the following:

" (a) A certified midwife, who has in accordance with the provisions of the Midwives Act, 1951(k), or the Midwives (Scotland) Act, 1951(l), notified to the Local Supervising Authority within the meaning of those Acts her intention to practise, is hereby authorized, so far as necessary for the practice of her profession or employment as a midwife, to be in possession of medicinal opium, tincture of opium and pethidine which she has procured upon furnishing to the supplier thereof a midwife's supply order, and to administer those drugs or preparations so far as is necessary as aforesaid, subject to the following conditions, that is to say:

    (i) she shall not procure from a person supplying it an amount of a drug or preparation, greater than that specified in the midwife's supply order which she furnishes to him;

    (ii) she shall on each occasion on which a supply of the drug or preparation is procured enter in the drugs book (being a book kept by her and used solely for the purposes of this paragraph) the name of the drug or preparation obtained, the date, the name and address of the person supplying it, the amount supplied and the form in which it was obtained;

    (iii) she shall, on administering a drug or preparation to any woman, as soon as practicable enter in the drugs book the name of the drug or preparation administered, the name and address of the woman to whom it was administered, the amount administered and the form in which it was administered, and the entry so made shall, notwithstanding any other requirement of these Regulations, be a sufficient record of the administration;

    (iv) she shall, except when the necessities of the practice of her profession or employment as a midwife otherwise require, keep every drug or preparation in her possession in a locked receptacle which can be opened only by her."

Examples of narcotic, analgesic and hypnotic drugs that the midwife is not authorized to give and cannot procure without a doctor's prescription:

Morphine ; papaveretum (Omnopon) ; barbiturates such as amylobarbitone (Amytal) ; pentobarbitone (Nembutal) ; butobarbitone (Soneryl) ; tranquillizers such as chlorpromazine (Largactil) ; promazine (Sparine) ; perphenazine (Fentazin) ; prochlorperazine (Stemetil).

Sedative drugs that midwives may prescribe are set out on page 252 under "Relief of Pain in Labour." Local anæsthetics for episiotomy see p. 618.

Panasorb, pentazocine and Codis tablets do not require a doctor's prescription.

Quotation from Central Midwives Board rules

" A practising midwife must not on her own responsibility use any drug, including an analgesic, unless in the course of her training, whether before or after enrolment, she has been thoroughly instructed in its use and is familiar with its dosage and methods of administration or application." Also

" When a midwife administers or applies in any way any drug other than an aperient, she must forthwith make a proper record of the name and dose of the drug and the date and time of its administration or application."

ADMINISTRATION OF DRUGS
INTRAMUSCULAR INJECTION

When giving drugs to babies intramuscularly the needle must be inserted on the slant and not at right angles; the tissues are shallow and bone may be penetrated.

To avoid injury to the sciatic nerve or hip joint the upper outer quadrant of the buttock is preferred. The anterior area of the thigh may be used but the needle must point towards the knee.

Injections should not be given into the arm of a baby.

INTRAVENOUS INJECTION
Technique
APPLICATION OF TOURNIQUET

A piece of soft rubber tubing or Velcro arm band is applied to the extended arm tightly enough to distend the veins without obliterating the arterial pulse (*at the wrist*). A simple knot that can be released instantly by pulling on one end of the tubing should be used. Velcro can be released easily.

Clasping and unclasping the fist helps to make the veins stand out.

SYRINGE AND NEEDLE

The syringe should be of the disposable or all-glass type with an eccentric nozzle to allow the barrel to rest closely on the forearm so that if the woman moves her arm the relation of needle to vein will not be disturbed. Number 12 needle is the smallest suitable size.

INSERTION OF THE NEEDLE

The skin is cleansed. Air must be expelled from the syringe prior to venepuncture.

Penetration of the skin is made with the needle almost parallel to the vein, bevel downwards; while doing so the vein is steadied in position by stretching the skin that lies over it with the thumb of the left hand which is grasping the patient's arm below the elbow.

The skin is pierced a little to one side of the vein, and the needle advanced alongside it for about 3 mm. (⅛ inch) before being inclined sufficiently to be introduced into the vein. This minimizes the risk of penetrating both walls of the vein. A slight sensation of " give " is detected as the vein is entered by those experienced in the technique.

Successful penetration of the vein is confirmed by raising the syringe and needle slightly with the right hand and gently withdrawing the plunger with the left, when dark venous blood will be aspirated into the syringe. **No injection is made unless blood appears in the syringe.**

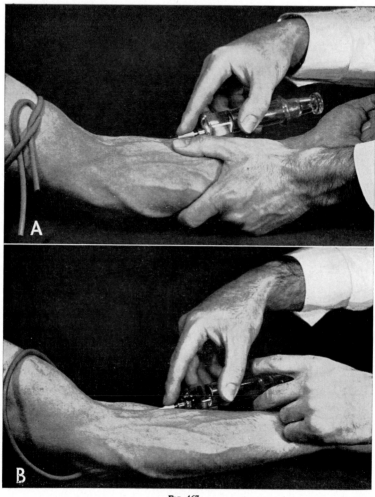

FIG. 467

INTRAVENOUS INJECTION.

Note that the position of the right hand remains unchanged throughout the procedure.

A, Penetration of skin with needle held almost parallel to vein : left thumb fixes vein by stretching the skin over it.

B, Tourniquet released to restore venous circulation after aspiration of blood into syringe confirms successful penetration of vein.

(Aberdeen Royal Infirmary, Department of Anæsthetics.)

The venous circulation is restored by releasing the tourniquet, *i.e.* pulling the end of the rubber tubing, using the finger and thumb of the left hand.

Pressure on the plunger by the thumb of the left hand is applied to give the injection.

It should be noted that the grip of the syringe by the right hand remains unaltered throughout the procedure.

COMPARISON OF IMPERIAL AND METRIC SYSTEMS OF WEIGHTS AND MEASURES

The abbreviation G. for gramme and mg. for milligram should be placed after the number to which they apply, *e.g.* 100 mg.

UNIT OF WEIGHT, THE GRAMME

1 KILOGRAM (kg.)   = 1,000 grammes (G.) or 2·2 lb. (35 oz.).
1 GRAMME (G.)   = 1,000 milligrams (mg.) or gr. 15·4.
1 MILLIGRAM(mg.)   = 1,000 micrograms or gr. 1/64th.
1 MICROGRAM (µg.)

CONVERSION CHART—WEIGHT
AVOIRDUPOIS—METRIC

lb.	oz.	Gramme	Kilo	lb.	oz.	Gramme	Kilo
—	1	28	0·028	4	12	2,155	2·155
—	2	57	0·057	5	—	2,268	2·268
—	3	85	0·085	5	4	2,381	2·381
—	4	113	0·113	5	8	2,495	2·495
—	5	142	0·142	5	12	2,608	2·608
—	6	170	0·170	6	—	2,722	2·722
—	7	198	0·198	6	4	2,835	2·835
—	8	227	0·227	6	8	2,948	2·948
—	9	255	0·255	6	12	3,062	3·062
—	10	283	0·283	7	—	3,175	3·175
—	11	312	0·312	7	4	3,289	3·289
—	12	340	0·340	7	8	3,402	3·402
—	13	369	0·369	7	12	3,515	3·515
—	14	397	0·397	8	—	3,629	3·629
—	15	425	0·425	8	4	3,742	3·742
1	—	454	0·454	8	8	3,856	3·856
1	4	567	0·567	8	12	3,969	3·969
1	8	680	0·680	9	—	4,082	4·082
1	12	794	0·794	9	4	4,196	4·196
2	—	907	0·907	9	8	4,309	4·309
2	4	1,021	1·021	9	12	4,423	4·423
2	8	1,134	1·134	10	—	4,536	4·536
2	12	1,247	1·247	10	4	4,649	4·649
3	—	1,361	1·361	10	8	4,763	4·763
3	4	1,474	1·474	10	12	4,876	4·876
3	8	1,588	1·588	11	—	4,990	4·990
3	12	1,701	1·701	11	4	5,103	5·103
4	—	1,814	1·814	11	8	5,216	5·216
4	4	1,928	1·928	11	12	5,330	5·330
4	8	2,041	2·041	12	—	5,443	5·443

APPROXIMATE APOTHECARIES AND METRIC EQUIVALENTS

APOTHECARIES GRAINS (gr.)		METRIC MILLIGRAMS (mg.)		GRAMME (G.)
$\frac{1}{300}, \frac{1}{320}$	=	0·2		—
$\frac{1}{240}$	=	0·25		—
$\frac{1}{200}$	=	0·3		—
$\frac{1}{150}, \frac{1}{160}$	=	0·4		—
$\frac{1}{120}, \frac{1}{130}$	=	0·5		—
$\frac{1}{100}$	=	0·6		—
$\frac{1}{80}$	=	0·8		—
$\frac{1}{60}$	=	1		—
$\frac{1}{50}$	=	1·25		—
$\frac{1}{40}$	=	1·5		—
$\frac{1}{30}$	=	2		—
$\frac{1}{25}$	=	2·5		—
$\frac{1}{20}$	=	3		—
$\frac{1}{15}$	=	4		—
$\frac{1}{12}$	=	5		—
$\frac{1}{10}$	=	6		—
$\frac{1}{8}$	=	7·5		—
$\frac{1}{6}$	=	10		—
$\frac{1}{5}$	=	12		—
$\frac{1}{4}$	=	15		—
$\frac{1}{3}$	=	20		—
$\frac{1}{2}$	=	30		—
$\frac{3}{4}$	=	50		—
1	=	60		—
$1\frac{1}{2}$	=	100	=	0·1
2	=	125	=	0·125
$2\frac{1}{2}$	=	150	=	0·15
3	=	200	=	0·2
4	=	250	=	0·25
5	=	300	=	0·3
$7\frac{1}{2}$	=	450	=	0·45
10	=	600	=	0·6
15·4	=	1000	=	0·87
20			=	1·2
30			=	1·75
40			=	2·4
50			=	3
60			=	3·5
120			=	7
240	($\frac{1}{2}$ oz.)		=	14
480	(1 oz.)		=	28

APPROXIMATE FLUID MEASURE EQUIVALENTS

METRIC		IMPERIAL			METRIC		IMPERIAL	
1,000 millilitres (1 *litre*)=		35 fl. ounces			4 millilitres =		60 minims	
600	,,	= 20	,,		3	,,	= 45	,,
500	,,	= 17	,,		2	,,	= 30	,,
400	,,	= 14	,,		1	,,	= 15	,,
360	,,	= 12	,,		0·8	,,	= 12	,,
300	,,	= 10	,,		0·6	,,	= 10	,,
250	,,	= $8\frac{1}{2}$	,,		0·5	,,	= 8	,,
100	,,	= $3\frac{1}{2}$	,,		0·4	,,	= 6	,,
30	,,	= 1	,, (8 *fl. drachms*)		0·3	,,	= 5	,,
15	,,	= $\frac{1}{2}$	,, (4 ,,)		0·25	,,	= 4	,,
8	,,	= $\frac{1}{4}$	,, (2 ,,)		0·2	,,	= 3	,,
4	,,	= $\frac{1}{8}$	,, (1 ,,)		0·1	,,	= $1\frac{1}{2}$	,,

COMPARISON OF METRIC AND BRITISH LINEAR MEASURES (APPROX.)
THE METRE IS THE UNIT OF LENGTH

METRE		CENTIMETRE		MILLIMETRE		INCHES
1	=	100	=	1,000	=	$39\frac{3}{10}$
$\frac{1}{10}$	=	10	=	100	=	4
$\frac{1}{40}$	=	2·5	=	25	=	1
$\frac{1}{100}$	=	1	=	10	=	$\frac{2}{5}$
$\frac{1}{1000}$	=	0·1	=	1	=	$\frac{1}{25}$

CENTIMETRES TO INCHES 1 inch −2·5 cm. approx. (actually 2·54 cm.)

CENTIMETRES	INCHES	CENTIMETRES	INCHES	CENTIMETRES	INCHES
2·5	1	14	$5\frac{1}{2}$	30·5	12
3·8	$1\frac{1}{2}$	15·2	6	31·8	$12\frac{1}{2}$
5·1	2	16·5	$6\frac{1}{2}$	33	13
6·4	$2\frac{1}{2}$	17·8	7	34·3	$13\frac{1}{2}$
7·6	3	19	$7\frac{1}{2}$	35·6	14
8·3	$3\frac{1}{4}$	20·3	8	36·8	$14\frac{1}{2}$
8·9	$3\frac{1}{2}$	21·6	$8\frac{1}{2}$	38·1	15
10·2	4	22·9	9	39·4	$15\frac{1}{2}$
10·8	$4\frac{1}{4}$	24	$9\frac{1}{2}$	40·6	16
11·4	$4\frac{1}{2}$	25·4	10	41·9	$16\frac{1}{2}$
12·1	$4\frac{3}{4}$	26·7	$10\frac{1}{4}$	43·2	17
12·7	5	27·9	11	44·4	$17\frac{1}{2}$
13·3	$5\frac{1}{4}$	29·2	$11\frac{1}{2}$	45·7	18

91 cm.=1 yard;   68·25 cm.=$\frac{3}{4}$ yard;   45·5 cm.=$\frac{1}{2}$ yard;   22·75 cm.=$\frac{1}{4}$ yard

MILLIMETRES TO INCHES

MILLIMETRES . .	1·5	3·1	6·2	12·5	18·7	25
INCHES	$\frac{1}{16}$	$\frac{1}{8}$	$\frac{1}{4}$	$\frac{1}{2}$	$\frac{3}{4}$	1

CENTIGRADE TO FAHRENHEIT CONVERSION TABLE

To convert Centigrade to Fahrenheit, multiply by 9, divide by 5, add 32.
To convert Fahrenheit to Centigrade, subtract 32, multiply by 5 and divide by 9

CENTIGRADE	FAHRENHEIT	CENTIGRADE	FAHRENHEIT	CENTIGRADE	FAHRENHEIT
Freezing	Freezing				
0	32	30	86	36·6	98
1·6	35	30·5	87	36·9	98·4
4·4	40	31·1	88	37·2	99
7·2	45	31·6	89	37·7	100
10	50	32·2	90	38·3	101
12·7	55	32·7	91	38·8	102
15·5	60	33·3	92	39·4	103
18·3	65	33·8	93	40	104
21·1	70	34·4	94	40·5	105
23·8	75	35	95	41·1	106
26·6	80	35·5	96	48·8	120
29·4	85	36·1	97	100	212
				Boiling	Boiling

AVERAGE BODY TEMPERATURE RANGE

Centigrade	Fahrenheit	Centigrade	Fahrenheit	Centigrade	Fahrenheit
34·4	94·0	36·6	98·0	38·8	102·0
34·5	94·2	36·7	98·2	39·0	102·2
34·6	94·4	36·8	98·4	39·1	102·4
34·7	94·6	37·0	98·6	39·2	102·6
34·8	94·8	37·1	98·8	39·3	102·8
35·0	95·0	37·2	99·0	39·4	103·0
35·1	95·2	37·3	99·2	39·5	103·2
35·2	95·4	37·4	99·4	39·6	103·4
35·3	95·6	37·5	99·6	39·7	103·6
35·4	95·8	37·6	99·8	39·8	103·8
35·5	96·0	37·7	100·0	40·0	104·0
35·6	96·2	37·8	100·2	40·1	104·2
35·7	96·4	38·0	100·4	40·2	104·4
35·8	96·6	38·1	100·6	40·3	104·6
36·0	96·8	38·2	100·8	40·4	104·8
36·1	97·0	38·3	101·0	40·5	105·0
36·2	97·2	38·4	101·2	40·6	105·2
36·3	97·4	38·5	101·4	40·7	105·4
36·4	97·6	38·6	101·6	40·8	105·6
36·5	97·8	38·7	101·8	41·0	105·8

QUESTIONS FOR REVISION

C.M.B.(Eng.) paper.—Name the drugs you may have to use in your midwifery practice, and give the indications for the use of each. What rule relating to the use of drugs does the Central Midwives Board lay down ?

C.M.B.(Scot.) paper.—What drugs may a midwife employ on her own responsibility ? Describe their use.

C.M.B.(Eng.) paper.—What drugs may a midwife use during the course of labour ? Give the (*a*) indications, (*b*) dosage, (*c*) method of administration in respect of each drug.

C.M.B.(Eng.) paper, 1970.—50 word question.—How may a domiciliary midwife obtain a supply of dangerous drugs for use in her practice ?

C.M.B.(Eng.) paper, 1970.—50 word question.—Outline the procedure whereby the domiciliary midwife is authorized to possess and administer dangerous drugs.

37

Confinement in the Home

There are many instances in which the midwife should not undertake the management of labour at home. In a number of cases some obstetrical or medical abnormality exists which necessitates supervision by specialists and the provision of facilities for operative procedure. Hospitalization is then essential.

WOMEN "AT RISK"

Obstetric patients "at risk" can be detected by "screening" during the prenatal period. Important points are: high parity, age, height: medical and obstetrical histories; findings in the present pregnancy poor socio-economic conditions.

CONDITIONS IN WHICH HOME CONFINEMENT IS CONTRAINDICATED
Either mother or baby is "at risk"

THE HOME	THE MOTHER		THE BABY
	OBSTETRICAL	MEDICAL	
Overcrowding.	Cephalo-pelvic disproportion.	Cardiac disease.	History of previ stillbirths, neon: deaths, or no liv child.
Infectious disease present.	Pre-eclampsia: eclampsia.	Tuberculosis.	
Destitution.	Multiple pregnancy.	Diabetes.	Breech presentation.
Insanitary conditions.	Antepartum hæmorrhage.		
	Hydramnios.	Venereal disease.	Gestation period than 36 weeks.
	Rh iso-immunization.	Essential hypertension.	Rh. haemolytic dise
	Previous; Cæsarean section, difficult forceps delivery; postpartum hæmorrhage or adherent placenta.	Subfertiliity	Fetal abnormalities
	Primigravida over 30 yrs.	Severe anaemia.	True postmaturity.
	Multigravida 4+ ,, over 35 yrs.		Small baby syndrom

PREPARATIONS FOR CONFINEMENT

The midwife must visit the home before confinement to see whether it is suitable and to give the necessary advice. The mother should be told what to do, and what she should provide. It is a good plan to give her a leaflet of printed instructions.

C.M.B.(Eng.) code of practice.—*A midwife must, if the confinement is to be a domiciliary one, visit, by arrangement with the patient the house in which it is proposed the confinement shall take place.* Where the midwife considers the accommodation or facilities are unsuitable *she should notify the Medical Officer of Health of the Local Supervising Authority.*

C.M.B.(Scot.) rule.—*A midwife must, as soon as practicable, visit the patient and inquire into the suitability of the accommodation and of the equipment, and* where these are not suitable she must notify the fact to the Local Supervising Authority.

A midwife should be competent to advise mothers of all classes in regard to what they will need for their confinement and baby.

CLEANLINESS AND ARRANGEMENT OF THE ROOM

In most cases the mother is confined in her own bedroom. If a choice of room is available, the ideal would be a bright, quiet one, conveniently near the bathroom and certainly on the same floor. Some form of heating must be provided by day and night in cold weather to prevent neonatal hypothermia.

The bedroom should not have been recently occupied by anyone suffering from a contagious disease or septic condition, as it has been proved that organisms can survive in dust for a considerable time.

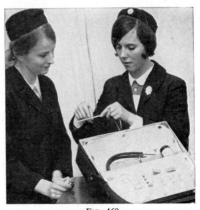

Fig. 468

PRENATAL DISTRICT BAG.

Staff Midwife shows student midwife how to obtain blood for hb test.

Mediswabs, sterile disposable blood lancets, pipette with rubber tubing and mouthpiece. Screw-topped bottle containing 4 ml. of Drabkin's solution. Sphygmomanometer and stethoscope. Fetal stethoscope. Labstix.

(*Simpson Memorial Maternity Pavilion, Edinburgh.*)

The room should, of course, be clean, but there is little value in clean walls, fresh curtains and a scrubbed floor if the blankets and quilt are dirty. It is what the woman in bed comes in contact with that matters most. The carpet can be cleaned with a

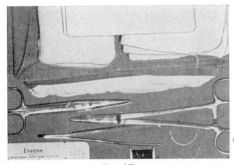

Fig. 469

REQUIREMENTS FOR PERINEAL REPAIR (*on District*).
(*Simpson Memorial Maternity Pavilion, Edinburgh.*)

1 Mayo needle holder: Mayo scissors.
1 toothed dissecting forceps.
No. 1 chromic catgut: Ethicon W 759 with half circle round bodied needle.
For skin No. 1 Mersilk: Ethicon W 562 with curved cutting needles.
1 dressing towel: water repellant paper sheet.
10 gauze swabs: perineal pad: gown: gloves.

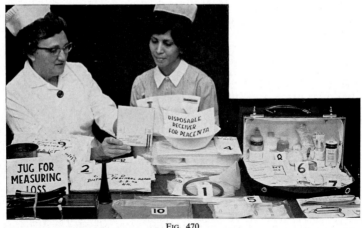

FIG. 470

EQUIPMENT FOR HOME CONFINEMENT.

1. **Enema tubing and funnel; K.Y. Jelly; disposable rectal catheter; Dulcolax suppositories; disposable razor.**
2. **Perineal repair pack:**—1 tinfoil tray; 1 scissors; 1 dissecting forceps; 1 needleholder; Ethicon foil packed eyeless needled and No. 1 chromic sutures W 759 and Mersilk on cutting needle W 562; 1 perineal pad; 10 gauze swabs; 1 paper hand towel; 1 paper dressing-towel. *(All wrapped in sterifield paper and disposal bag.)*
3. **T.P.R. chart; low reading thermometer; weighing scales; metric tape measure.**
4. **Pack for vulval toilet; Vaginal examination pack; Catheter pack.**
5. **Disposable mucus extractors.**
6. **Drugs:**—Syntometrine, ergometrine, Konakion, nikethamide, neonatal nalorphine (lethidrone), Lignocaine 5 ml. one per cent. solution. Fortral. *(N.B.—Midwife carries Pethidine.)*
7. **Syringes and needles, disposable.**
8. **Lotions:** Hibitane, PHisoHex, Hibitane in spirit, obstetric cream, mediswabs.
9. **Delivery pack:**—2 tinfoil bowls; |2 cord forceps; 2 scissors (1 for episiotomy); 1 Spencer Wells forceps with elastic band for ligating cord; 2 perineal pads; 3 paper dressing towels; cotton-wool balls; 1 gown; 1 turkish wrap (for baby); 1 disposable bowl for placenta. *(All wrapped in sterifield paper, green dressing towel and in a disposable bag).* Allis's forceps to puncture membranes, if necessary, packed separately. Jug for measuring blood loss.
10. **Plastic apron;** nail brush; eye dropper; torch; disposable gloves; disposa glove; Labstix for urine testing; Dextrostix reagent strips.

Entonox, Blease Samson neonatal resuscitator. Vicker's resuscitation kit.

Maternity set supplied by local authority:—1 lb. cotton wool. 2 dozen perineal pads (wrapped separately), cord ligatures, dressings, powder, accouchement pad, polythene draw sheet.

(Simpson Memorial Maternity Pavilion, Edinburgh.)

vacuum cleaner or washed with soap and water and protected with a piece of linoleum, canvas or mackintosh, but not paper which only gets ruffled. There is no reason why a modern bedroom need be stripped so bare of furnishings as to be unattractive. The thorough cleaning should be completed at least one month before the date of confinement, the mother obtaining assistance for this strenuous task.

On no account should any sweeping or dusting be done when labour is in progress. Dirty surfaces can be wiped with a cloth wrung out of antiseptic lotion.

THE BED

Blankets and quilt should be clean. The bed should be placed so that it is accessible from both sides and conveniently situated in regard to light. A single bed is ideal, but, of course, this is not always available. Sagging springs make delivery awkward; they cause blood to collect in the vault of the vagina during the third stage. Two or three 25-cm. (10-inch) boards under the mattress will remedy the sagging; book-shelves could be used in an emergency.

FURNISHING

Two tables will be necessary; a card table and a strong kitchen chair would do. The possibility of spoiling furniture should be kept in mind, and an inverted kitchen tray placed under jugs and kettles will prevent such damage.

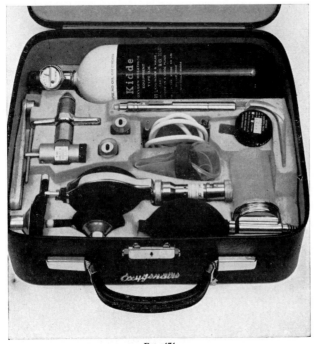

FIG. 471

INFANT RESUSCITATION KIT.

A portable kit suitable for domiciliary resuscitative procedures. The insufflator can be connected to the oxygen cylinder and the instrument has a blow-off fitted to prevent intermittent positive pressure ventilation being given at pressures greater than 30 cm. water. Nose and pharynx must first be cleared, an airway inserted. Angle of jaw held forwards.

(*Vickers Ltd., Basingstoke, Hampshire.*)

LINEN

The linen to be used during confinement should be boiled and ironed. The amount required varies, depending on whether the membranes rupture early or not; four sheets being considered the minimum for labour and immediately afterwards. Pieces of old folded sheeting are useful to lay under the patient and reduce the amount of " washing." Six towels are needed to cover tables and jugs as well as for the hands.

REQUIREMENTS PROVIDED BY PATIENT

For the Confinement

2 large basins: 1 for the mother, 1 for midwife s hands. 1 bed-pan. Slop-pail; box for soiled dressings..

2 kettles; 1 jug (1,200 ml.).

Plastic sheet, 2×1 metres (2×1 yards).

Hibitane or Savlon.

1 new nailbrush, boiled and kept in jar of antiseptic solution.

Large pieces of clean, strong brown paper, or newspapers, to protect the mattress.

1 or 2 hot-water bottles with covers.

PERSONAL BELONGINGS

2 old nightdresses for labour.

1 clean washable dressing-gown.

2 pairs clean stockings, slippers, usual toilet articles, soap, etc.

2 bath, 2 face towels: 2 face cloths.

2 firm uplift brassières. Sanitary belt.

Nightdresses.

FOR THE BABY'S IMMEDIATE NEEDS

A soft bath towel to wrap baby in when born. A baby bath or large wash-hand basin; soft bath towel and face towel. Face cloth, and one of different colour for buttocks; cake of good soap.

Bathing aprons, one plastic, and one made from a bath towel. Baby clothes. Safety-pins.

Cot and bedding (a drawer can be used in an emergency). Stool or low chair.

A full list of baby's requirements is given in the Baby Care section.

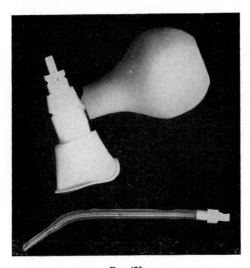

Fig. 472
BLEASE SAMSON NEONATAL RESUSCITATOR.

This apparatus could be employed in domiciliary practice in preference to mouth to mouth breathing. It may be used with mask or endotracheal tube. The pharynx and nostrils must be cleared first: the lower jaw held up.

(Hutchinson Blease Ltd., Deansway, Chesham, Bucks.)

IMMEDIATE PREPARATIONS FOR LABOUR

The woman will have been told the signs of labour and what to do pending the midwife's arrival, *i.e.* she will see that the room is warm, boil two kettles and set one apart to cool and have the clean bed linen and baby clothes sought out.

On arrival the midwife notes whether delivery is imminent, takes a history of the labour and examines and prepares the woman as in hospital.

The mattress is protected with layers of brown paper or newspaper, especially in the middle, and laid over these is the large plastic sheet.

If basins are not sterile and there are no means of boiling them, they can be scoured, rinsed, smeared with Hibitane and scalded by pouring boiling water over them.

The management of labour is similar to that in hospital. The placenta must be burned or otherwise disposed of by the midwife.

POSTNATAL VISITS

The midwife greets the woman by asking her how she feels, removes outdoor uniform, washes her hands and puts on cap, mask and gown. While unwrapping bowls and preparing solution she questions the woman about her well-being and the baby's behaviour.

DAILY OBSERVATIONS

Temperature, pulse, respirations are taken; breasts and nipples examined; bladder palpated; fundal height measured; perineal pad inspected. The woman is questioned regarding her appetite, sleep, bowels. Any untoward signs and symptoms are reported to the doctor.

The mother is asked if the baby feeds well and is contented, and should be told to keep one napkin for inspection of stool every day. The baby is examined as in hospital; the midwife watches the baby being fed, at least once daily, during the first few days.

ROUTINE CARE

After taking the woman's temperature and pulse, the baby clothes are arranged in proper order on the back of a chair by the fire; the bed-pan is cleansed and warmed.

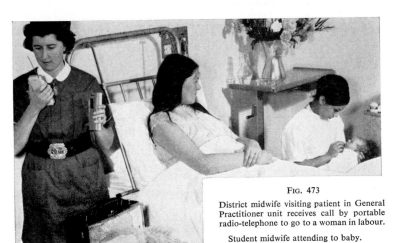

Fig. 473

District midwife visiting patient in General Practitioner unit receives call by portable radio-telephone to go to a woman in labour.

Student midwife attending to baby.

(Courtesy of Portsmouth Group Hospital Management Committee.)

Preparations are made to wash the woman's thighs, lower abdomen and buttocks, care being taken not to shake the blankets and disseminate dust and organisms. Breast, and swabbing technique are carried out as in hospital.

TEACHING THE MOTHER

When the infant is being bathed, the mother should be allowed to watch the procedure, and if this is her first baby each step should be carefully explained. As well as giving any necessary advice, a daily lesson in baby care should be taught, applying it to the woman and her own baby and covering subjects such as the prevention of cracked nipples, increasing the milk supply, why babies cry and what to do about it, prevention and treatment of sore buttocks.

To avoid neonatal hypothermia the bedroom temperature should be maintained at 18·3° to 21·1° C. (65° to 70° F.) (see p. 560).

Inexperienced mothers should be helped and supervised two or three times while changing napkins, bathing or dressing their babies. All this takes time but it is well spent, and one and a quarter hours should be allotted for a post-natal visit if everything is to be done properly, mother and child both being left clean, comfortable and contented.

If bottle fed, the baby should be properly established on a suitable formula and the mother instructed on how to make up the feeds and on the necessity for further supervision and advice at the child health clinic.

Any necessary instruction is given to the home-help regarding the comfort and care of the woman. Bowls are destroyed if disposable, otherwise wiped with Hibitane and scalded; her gown and cap wrapped in clean paper and laid in a drawer or cupboard. The cold sterile water-jug is filled with boiling water, all soiled dressings and papers burned and the room left tidy. The midwife should write her report before leaving the house.

The Guthrie test is carried out after the 6th day (see p. 799).

The question of family planning is discussed.

CENTRAL MIDWIVES BOARD RULES

According to the Central Midwives Boards a midwife must visit her patients daily for not less than 10 days after the end of labour, *i.e.* the early postnatal period. In England she is expected to, in Scotland she must visit morning and evening for the first three days. If a rise in temperature (or any other condition requiring close supervision), be found at the morning visit, an evening visit must be paid unless the midwife is relieved from the obligation by the Local Supervising Authority.

QUESTIONS FOR REVISION

C.M.B.(Eng.) paper.—Write not more than five lines on the importance of each of the following in deciding where a mother should have her third baby:

1. Her husband's occupation.
2. Her age.
3. Her past obstetric history.
4. Her blood group.

C.M.B.(Scot.) paper.—Why should a patient having her fifth (or subsequent) child be advised to be delivered in hospital?

C.M.B.(Eng.) paper.—Before an expectant mother is booked for a home confinement what factors must be considered?

C.M.B.(Eng.) paper, 1970.—50 word question.—What are the social criteria to be met in selection for home confinement?

C.M.B.(Eng.) paper.—Discuss the conditions which should be fulfilled to allow home confinements.

C.M.B.(Eng.) paper.—Why should you persuade a gravida-7, aged 36, who wants to have her baby at home, that she should be delivered in hospital?

38

Infertility

All midwives should have some knowledge of what is done at the infertility clinic, so that they may encourage infertile women to seek advice, and comprehend the patient's version of the investigations made.

The majority of women become pregnant within the first year of married life unless contraceptive methods are used, and a marriage is not considered sterile until two years have elapsed. The woman who marries nearer the age of 40 than 20 is less likely to conceive, and should probably be referred for special advice after one year.

The causes of infertility may be medical, gynæcological, endocrinological, psychological, social, or a combination of these. In about 40 per cent of cases the husband is partially and in 15 per cent completely responsible for infertility. Investigations therefore cover all of these fields, and the woman will have to attend the infertility clinic on several occasions.

INVESTIGATION

The following facts should be ascertained: the age of husband and wife, their occupation, especially if in contact with certain metals and radio-active substances, the number of years married and whether contraception has been practised.

A diet history is taken and in many cases the diet is found to be low in first-class proteins, whole grain foods, fresh fruit and vegetables. The woman's family history and her own previous medical history are taken; tuberculosis, mumps, pelvic infection being significant.

The menstrual history is studied. When the woman has previously given birth to a child her obstetric history must be reviewed; miscarriages and uterine infection are important: immunological causes are now under consideration. Excessive smoking or alcoholism may be contributory factors to infertility.

General development is noted. Height, weight and blood pressure are taken, heart and lungs examined.

The vulva is inspected, and a bimanual and speculum examination made to detect any gross pelvic pathology, trichomoniasis or moniliasis; a Papanicolaou smear is taken (see p. 783).

Blood is examined for Wassermann, grouping, hæmoglobin, Rh factor; the erythrocyte sedimentation rate taken if pelvic infection is suspected. Urine is tested for protein and glucose.

For conditions such as tuberculosis, diabetes, renal or venereal disease, the woman is referred to a medical specialist.

Further detailed investigations will be made regarding the functional activity of the ovaries, tubes and cervix, to find out (*a*) whether ovulation takes place; (*b*) whether there is any barrier to fertilization of the ovum.

Is the Woman Ovulating ?

Regular normal menstruation is a suggestive but inconclusive sign that ovulation is taking place. An endometrial biopsy (section of endometrium for microscopic examination), taken about six days previous to a menstrual period, will show the premenstrual changes due to the action of the corpus luteum which can only be present following ovulation. (The biopsy also shows whether the endometrium is healthy and contains sufficient glycogen for the successful embedding of the fertilized ovum.)

A drop in temperature, followed by a rise, occurs at the time of ovulation, so the woman may be asked to take and chart her temperature every morning from one menstrual period to the next. This information is also useful in order to ensure that coitus may take place at about the time of ovulation as the ovum only lives unfertilized for about 36 hours. The spermatozoon may live for 5 to 7 days.

INFERTILITY IN THE HUSBAND

If the seminal fluid does not contain at least 50 per cent of normal active spermatozoa, the husband is infertile. (*In cases of high fertility about* 200 *million spermatozoa are deposited in the vagina during coitus.*) There are other causes of male infertility, therefore it is important that the husband attend for examination and investigation.

Instruments for tubal insufflation.

2 cannulæ.
1 uterine sound.
1 teneculum forceps.
1 Sims' speculum.
2 sponge-holding forceps.

Instruments for endometrial biopsy.

2 sponge-holding forceps.
1 Sims' speculum.
1 teneculum forceps.
1 uterine sound.
2 endometrial biopsy curettes.
1 dissecting forceps.

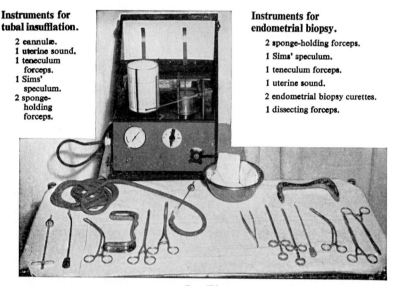

Fig. 474

Apparatus for Testing and Recording Tubal Patency and Functional Activity.

Is there any Barrier to Fertilization?

The cervical secretion during the period of ovulation alters in character and becomes thin in consistency to provide a medium in which the spermatozoa will survive. **An apparatus known as a consistometer is used** to determine the viscosity of the mucus. **Huhner's** test, in which the cervical mucus is examined after coitus, will show if sufficient healthy spermatozoa are present in the mucus.

Cervical infections are treated, and if the os is unduly small it is dilated. Fibroids are present in about 10 per cent of infertile women who are over 30 years of age, and may have to be removed.

The Fallopian tubes may be wholly or partly occluded, due to previous infection, and only in a minority of cases is this due to gonorrhœa; tubercular salpingitis is not rare; some infections are due to septic abortion. Adhesions from a suppurating appendix or pelvic infection may cause occlusion or kinking. It has been estimated that in 30 per cent of cases the cause of infertility is in the Fallopian tubes.

Insufflation of the tubes is carried out to test their patency, and in some cases pregnancy follows this test, probably because of the removal of a mucus plug or by rectifying kinks or spasm of the tubes. Hystero-salpingography is performed in some cases by injecting an opaque substance, Urografin 76 per cent into the uterus and tubes. On an X-ray film the blocked or narrowed part of the tube can be detected.

Laparoscopy may be employed (see p. 632). If the tubes are patent, dye (20 ml. aqueous methylene blue 0·5 per cent), introduced through the cervix, is seen traversing the tubes.

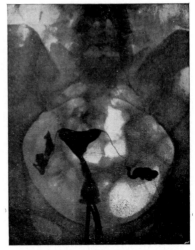

Fig. 475

Hystero-salpingography, showing normal bilateral tubal patency.

ENDOCRINE IMBALANCE

Lack of pituitary gonadotrophic hormone inhibits the production of œstrogen and reduces the likelihood of ovulation. Insufficiency of œstrogen may affect the cervical and vaginal secretions and also reduce the contractions of the Fallopian tubes. Uterine hypoplasia (under-development) is probably due to lack of the ovarian hormone, œstrogen.

The psychological aspect is a contributory one.—Over-anxiety to conceive may, by stimulating the sympathetic nervous system, produce spasm in the Fallopian tube. The fact that some women become pregnant after giving up hope of doing so and adopting a child is suggestive of this.

TREATMENT

The treatment of infertility is directed towards the alleviation or adjustment of whatever is preventing conception, and about 40 per cent of the patients attending infertility clinics become pregnant. Coitus is advised during the period of ovulation. A good nourishing diet is needed to ensure a virile ovum and spermatozoon that will survive.

In the treatment of infertility due to ovarian dysfunction and failure of ovulation it is now possible in a limited field to attempt to induce ovulation by one of two methods.

(1) **Gonadotrophin** obtained either from pituitary or urinary extractions can be given as a follicle stimulating and luteinizing hormone. Weekly determination of pregnanediol excretion is made to ascertain whether ovulation occurs.

(2) **Clomiphene citrate,** a new orally-administered non-steroidal agent can be used to stimulate ovarian function and to bring about ovulation in certain infertile women.

Up-to-date successful reports have been published concerning the occurrence of ovulation and pregnancy following the use of both methods.

39

Vital Statistics

REGISTRATION OF BIRTHS AND STILLBIRTHS

Under the Registration of Births Act information regarding a birth or stillbirth must be given by one of the parents. The majority of parents fulfil this req uirement of the law, but should they neglect to do so the duty falls on the occupier of the house or any person present at the birth, including the midwife.

In the case of an illegitimate child the information must be given by the mother. The child is registered under the mother's surname and can only be given the father's name if he attends personally along with her and the entry is made at the joint request of both. The father of an illegitimate child cannot register the birth in the absence of the mother.

ENGLAND

The birth is registered within 42 days of birth by the Registrar of the district in which the child is born. A short cerificate giving name, sex, date and place of birth is issued free at the time of registration: a full copy at this time costs 15p.; later the fee will be 65p.

SCOTLAND

The birth is registered within 21 days of birth by the Registrar of the district in which the child is born, or, if preferred, the district of the parents' home address. An abbreviated certificate is issued free. If the parents ask for a full certificate it costs 20p. (if ordered at a later date, 50p.).

THREE CLASSES CONCERNED WITH REGISTRATION

1. **An infant born at any stage of pregnancy who breathes or shows other signs of life after complete expulsion from its mother is born alive.** If such an infant dies after birth, both the birth and the death must be registered.

2. **An infant who has issued forth from its mother after the 28th week of pregnancy and has not at any time after being completely expelled from its mother breathed or shown any other signs of life is a stillborn infant** and must be registered.

3. **The birth before the 28th week of pregnancy of an infant who did not breathe or show signs of life after complete expulsion from its mother is neither a live birth nor a stillbirth** and need not be registered.

NOTIFICATION OF BIRTHS AND STILLBIRTHS

The Public Health Act, 1936 (England) and the Notification of Births Acts, 1907 and 1915 (Scotland) make it obligatory for the father of the child or any person in attendance on the mother at the time of birth to give notice in writing to the Medical Officer of Health of the area **within 36 hours,** under a penalty of £1.

Local Health Authorities supply doctors and midwives with prepaid addressed envelopes together with the forms of notification of birth.

The purpose of notification of births is that the Medical Officer of Health may arrange for the health visitor to call at the home as soon as the midwife ceases to visit or the woman returns home from hospital.

Doctor or midwife is required to record on the Notification of Birth's card any malformation discovered in the child whether live or stillborn (in order to compile statistical data).

STILLBIRTHS

A stillbirth is (as defined on p. 688) a birth after the 28th week of pregnancy in which the baby does not breathe or show any other signs of life after being completely expelled from the mother. It is conceivable that in delivering a baby presenting by the breech the cord may be pulsating when the baby is born as far as the umbilicus, but if after delivering the head the baby does not breathe or show any other signs of life it is stillborn.

Stillbirths must be registered; they must also be notified to the Medical Officer of Health.

The stillbirth rate is the number of stillbirths registered during the year per 1,000 registered total (*live and still*) births in the year. During 1970, England, 13. Scotland, 13·9.

Midwives' Duties Regarding Stillbirths (imposed by Statute)

1. REGISTRATION OF STILLBIRTHS

" When a registered medical practitioner is present at a stillbirth or examines the body, it is his statutory duty to give the qualified informant (usually the father or mother) a certificate of stillbirth. If a registered medical practitioner is not present at a stillbirth but arrangements for maternity care have been made with one, the midwife should inform him and ask him to examine the body and complete the certificate of stillbirth. Otherwise the midwife should give the certificate if she was present at the stillbirth or examined the body."

Under the Population (Statistics) Act, England and Scotland, 1960, *the stillbirth certificate requires a statement of the duration of pregnancy, weight of the fetus and cause or probable cause of death.*

2. NOTIFICATION OF STILLBIRTHS

This information will enable the Medical Officer of Health to inquire into the causes of stillbirths and to ensure that the woman takes advantage in a subsequent pregnancy of the resources provided for her by the State.

3. The Local Supervising Authority must be notified in all cases of stillbirth, whether or not a medical practitioner was present, using for the purpose the prescribed form (*C.M.B. rule*).

4. DISPOSAL OF A STILLBORN BABY

A stillborn baby must not be disposed of until the necessary legal requirements have been met.

The certificate of stillbirth issued by the doctor is taken to the Registrar of births and deaths. He will issue a certificate for disposal of stillbirth which must be presented to an undertaker. In certain cases the coroner will issue an order for burial. Arrangements can then be made for cremation or interment in a burial ground.

No death grant is paid for a stillborn baby.

Causes and Prevention (p. 691).

MATERNAL MORTALITY

The maternal mortality rate is the number of deaths registered during the year of women dying from causes attributed to pregnancy and childbirth per 1,000 registered total (*live and still*) births in the year. During 1970 the maternal mortality rate was: England—total deaths 146 or 0·18 per 1,000. Excluding abortion, 114 or 0·14 per 1,000, (deaths due to abortion 32 or 0·04 per 1,000). Scotland—Total deaths 17 or 0·19 per 1,000.

In England the Registrar-General excludes in his maternal mortality rate deaths due to abortion; the Chief Medical Officer to the Department of Health and Social Security and the Registrar-General for Scotland include these.

The Prevention of Maternal Mortality

A maternal death is a tragedy. The childbearing woman is probably the most important person in the community, for the baby, husband and family all depend for their health and happiness on the mother's care. A maternal death also does harm indirectly by creating fear of childbirth in the minds of relatives and neighbours. Midwives must therefore do all in their power to prevent maternal deaths.

THE DECLINE IN MATERNAL MORTALITY

Childbirth is safer now than at any period in history. During this century until 1935 the maternal death rate had remained between 4 and 5 per 1,000. The main causes of death in England in 1969 were: abortion 35; toxæmia 24; thrombosis and embolism 16: hæmorrhage 6. The reduction in the maternal mortality rate can be attributed in large measure to advances in the knowledge, prevention and treatment of these main causes.

Mortality is lowest in the second pregnancy, and rises steeply after the third.

The following factors have contributed to the decline in maternal mortality:

1. **Early recognition and improved treatment of pre-eclampsia.** With efficient management, eclampsia can now usually be averted.

2. **The increased use of blood transfusion and the "Flying Squad."** Along with preventive measures and improved methods of treating postabortum, antepartum and postpartum hæmorrhages, the blood bank and "Flying Squad" have done much to prevent loss of maternal life.

3. **Bacteriological advances.** The classification of hæmolytic streptococci, bacteriophage typing of staphylococci, the testing of the sensitivity of organisms to the sulphadrugs and antibiotics have lowered the maternal mortality rate still further.

4. **The introduction first of sulphonamides,** then of antibiotics, has progressively lowered the number of deaths from sepsis.

5. **Improved standards in the Maternity Services including more intensive prenatal care** and the greater willingness of women to take advantage of such care.

6. **Earlier hospitalization for complications** of pregnancy and labour; better selection of cases for hospital confinement and more prenatal beds available.

7. **Better social conditions,** including nutrition, have improved health and physique; family planning has reduced the number of children a woman bears; fewer children now are born to overworked, malnourished multigravidae. The National Health Service has improved the well-being of British childbearing women.

8. **Improved anæsthetic techniques** and the skill of obstetric anæsthetists.

9. **Closer co-operation** with diabetic, renal, cardiology, hæmatology and chest physicians.

How the Midwife can help to Prevent Maternal Deaths

1. **By co-operating with all branches of the Health Service** to ensure that the mother is receiving the necessary advice, health education, close supervision and care.

2. **By maintaining high standards** of prenatal, intranatal and postnatal care, paying special attention to the prevention of hæmorrhage, embolism and eclampsia.

INFANT MORTALITY RATE

The infant mortality rate is the number of deaths registered during the year of infants dying under one year of age per 1,000 registered live births in the year.

During 1970 the infant mortality rate was England, 18·2 ; Scotland, 19·6. These figures show a marked reduction from the rate of 140 to 150 which obtained at the beginning of this century.

Such an improvement may be attributed to two main factors:

1. PREVENTIVE MEDICINE

(a) The passing of the Notification of Births (Extension) Act, 1915 (Scotland), and the Maternity and Child Welfare Act, 1918 (England), placed the responsibility on the Local Authority for providing infant welfare clinics and health visitors.

(b) Improvements in housing and sanitary conditions, with a higher standard of living; immunisation of infants against infectious diseases; more rigid observance of methods to prevent cross-infection among babies in maternity and children's hospitals.

(c) Education of the public and their increased interest in nutrition, the care of babies and parentcraft teaching.

2. MEDICAL ADVANCES

The appointment of pædiatricians to supervise the health of all newborn babies in maternity hospitals. More effective methods of resuscitation ; biochemical studies of the newborn.

Increased knowledge in treating premature and sick babies, especially the use of chemotherapeutic agents, antibiotics and mechanical monitoring devices.

NEONATAL MORTALITY RATE

The neonatal mortality rate is the number of deaths registered during the year of infants dying under the age of 1 month (28 days) per 1,000 registered live births in the year. During 1970, England, 12·3 ; Scotland, 12·8.

The neonatal mortality rate has great obstetrical significance, for the majority of these babies die during the first 48 hours of life.

A death grant of £9.00 under the National Insurance Scheme is paid on the death of a child under 3 years, if contribution conditions are fully satisfied.

The Prevention of Stillbirths and Neonatal Deaths

Stillbirths and early neonatal deaths are very closely related, the same obstetrical causes giving rise to both. The midwife must therefore share the responsibility for a proportion of these deaths.

Preventive medicine has played some part, in that the improved nutrition and health of childbearing women have resulted in more vigorous babies who can withstand the trauma of birth and survive the critical first few days of life.

The midwife should ensure that the mothers under her care are having a nourishing diet and are taking the food supplements made available by the State.

PERINATAL MORTALITY RATE

This term is applied to stillbirths and to neonatal deaths during the first week of life per 1,000 live and stillbirths in the year. During 1970, England, 23·5; Scotland, 24·8.

In Britain about 21,000 perinatal deaths occur every year. Midwives must make an effort to reduce this serious loss of infant life.

CAUSES

1. PREMATURITY

Prevention is the best treatment and includes:

(*a*) **Good prenatal care.** (*a*) Education of the mother regarding health, diet, rest; (*b*) expert supervision to detect and treat conditions such as pre-eclampsia, ante-partum hæmorrhage, multiple pregnancy.

(*b*) **Good intranatal care.** As premature babies do not stand up well to labour, the woman in labour should be transferred to hospital. Constant vigilance of the fetal condition during labour is essential. Episiotomy is performed when the baby is expected to weigh under 2,268 G. (5 lb.).

(*c*) **Good neonatal care.** This embraces efficient transport of the infant to hospital and expert nursing by midwives under the supervision of a pædiatrician.

2. ANOXIA

This is a high cause of stillbirth; neonatal asphyxia and respiratory distress syndrome often associated with pneumonia occur following prolonged labour and early rupture of membranes, therefore conditions giving rise to these should be avoided if possible.

3. INTRACRANIAL INJURY

This serious condition can sometimes be averted by (*a*) seeking medical assistance for delay during the second stage before fetal distress is manifest; (*b*) slow, skilful delivery of the aftercoming head of the breech baby.

The treatment of the foregoing conditions has been given in detail under their respective headings.

4. CONGENITAL MALFORMATIONS

Severe spina-bifida and the gross abnormalities such as anencephaly cause a number of deaths which, so far, cannot be prevented.

Predisposing Causes

Pre-eclampsia.—Early recognition and treatment will help to reduce the 10 per cent loss of babies who are either stillborn or too puny to survive.

Eclampsia.—By treating pre-eclampsia the serious condition of eclampsia with a perinatal mortality rate of 10 to 30 per cent can usually be prevented.

Multiple pregnancy.—The death rate in the case of twins is almost three times as great as in single births. Midwives should encourage those pregnant women to take advantage of the opportunity to enter hospital for rest during the 30th to 36th week and to be delivered in hospital.

Antepartum hæmorrhage.—Early and more prolonged hospitalisation, expectant treatment, blood transfusion and Cæsarean section will save many babies.

Breech presentation.—By careful abdominal palpation the midwife will detect a higher number of breech presentations. She should not undertake to deliver the woman at home, nevertheless, she must be qualified to deal competently with cases not previously diagnosed.

Immunization of Infants

Midwives should be aware of the protective measures available whereby babies can be inoculated against diseases such as whooping cough, diphtheria, poliomyelitis and measles. They can inform mothers regarding the need for this as well as assuring and persuading those who are apprehensive or reluctant regarding inoculation.

Immunization is provided free by the family doctor and at child health clinics.

SMALLPOX

The routine vaccination of babies is no longer recommended by the Department of Health and Social Security—(July 1971). Smallpox vaccination is a prerequisite for travellers to countries where the disease remains prevalent.

POLIOMYELITIS

This disease rarely occurs during the first six months of life.

The Sabin type vaccine is the method of choice; three oral doses are given, and a booster dose at school entrance.

WHOOPING COUGH (*Pertussis*)

The risks associated with whooping cough, and the mortality rate, are greatest during the first year of life.

Three injections for a primary course are required, given at intervals of 6 to 8 weeks between first and second doses and 6 months between second and third (see Schedule).

DIPHTHERIA

About 50 per cent of mothers have no immunity to diphtheria so their babies are susceptible from birth.

Triple antigens are given to avoid giving multiple injections; combined pertussis, diphtheria and tetanus antigens are given. (Quadruple vaccines for diphtheria, pertussis, poliomyelitis and tetanus are sometimes used.)

MEASLES

A live modified measles virus vaccine is now available for protection against this disease. One injection only is given, not before 9 months of age and preferably soon after first birthday and before smallpox vaccination. Immunity seems to be fairly prolonged.

Disposable needles and syringes are now used for each injection ; otherwise they must be autoclaved. The skin is cleansed with alcohol and the injection given subcutaneously.

Ampoules and bottles should be well shaken to get uniform suspension, otherwise the dose may be inadequate.

Lymph and antigens should be stored in a cold room and not exposed to sunlight.

37

SCHEDULE OF IMMUNIZATION PROCEDURES

Recommended by the Ministry of Health (Nov. 1968)

Age	Prophylactic	Interval	Notes
During the first year of life	Diph./Tet./Pert. and oral polio vaccine. (First dose) Diph./Tet./Pert. and oral polio vaccine. (Second dose) Diph./Tet./Pert. and oral polio vaccine. (Third dose)	Preferably after an interval of 6-8 weeks. Preferably after an interval of 6 months.	The earliest age at which the first dose should be given is 3 months, but a better general immunological response can be expected if the first dose is delayed to 6 months of age.
During the second year of life	Measles vaccination	After an interval of not less than 3-4 weeks	

Additional Notes

1. The basic course of immunization against diphtheria, pertussis, tetanus and poliomyelitis should be completed at as early an age as possible consistent with the likelihood of a good immunological response. Live measles vaccine should not be given to children below the age of nine months, since it usually fails to immunize such children owing to the presence of maternally transmitted antibodies.

2. Examples of timing of basic course of immunization:

Age	*1st dose*	*2nd dose*	*3rd dose*
	3 months	5 months	9-12 months
	4 months	6 months	10-12 months
	5 months	7 months	about 12 months
	6 months	8 months	about 12-14 months

Interval	Interval
6-8 weeks	Preferably 6, and not less than 4, months

3. The desirable commencing age for immunization is six months of age because: (*a*) before this age the antibody response may be reduced by the presence of maternal antibody; (*b*) the child's antibody-forming mechanism is immature in the early months of life; and (*c*) severe reactions to pertussis vaccine are less common in children over six months old than at three months of age.

QUESTIONS FOR REVISION

VITAL STATISTICS

What advice would you give to the parents regarding registration of births ? **Define the following mortality rates: infant, neonatal, perinatal, stillbirth, maternal. State the obstetrical causes** of stillbirths and neonatal deaths. **Name the factors** which have helped to reduce these death rates.

C.M.B.(Eng.) paper. 50 word question.—What is meant by the term " vital statistics " ?

C.M.B.(Eng.) paper.—What is a stillbirth ? To what may it be due ? What are the midwife's duties if she delivers a stillborn child ?

C.M.B.(N. Ireland) paper.—How can good antenatal care prevent stillbirths ? Describe in what way the midwife can help to reduce stillbirths during labour.

C.M.B.(Eng.) paper.—What is meant by the term " neonatal death " ? What are the chief causes ? Indicate what preventative measures may be taken to avoid neonatal deaths.

C.M.B.(Eng.) paper.—In 1900 the maternal mortality rate was over 4 per 1,000 ; today it is less than 1 per 1,000. How has this improvement been made ?

C.M.B.(Eng.) paper.—Explain how antenatal care helps to reduce the perinatal mortality rate.

What are the three classes under which live and stillborn babies are registered?

In which district is a baby registered, and by whom ?

To whom are births notified ? Why ? What is the duty of the midwife *re* notification of births ?

An unwed mother asks you: (*a*) regarding registration of the birth of her baby, to the man she is co-habiting with; (*b*) if the fact that the baby is illegitimate will be recorded on the birth certificate; (*c*) if the father can register the birth ?

A birth is registered in England within .... days: in Scotland within .... days: **a birth must be notified within** ....

Differentiate between: (*a*) notification and registration of births; (*b*) neonatal and infant deaths; (*c*) stillbirth and perinatal death.

Discuss the midwife's role in the prevention of: stillbirths; maternal deaths; perinatal deaths.

Preventive medicine has reduced the infant mortality rate. Write 10 lines elaborating this statement.

C.M.B.(Eng.) paper. 50 word question.—Maternal mortality.

C.M.B.(Eng.) paper. 50 word question.—Define the maternal mortality rate. List the main causes of maternal death.

C.M.B.(Eng.) paper. 50 word question.—Perinatal mortality.

C.M.B.(Eng.) paper. 50 word question.—Define perinatal mortality and give its rate in England and Wales.

C.M.B.(Eng.) paper. 50 word question.—Discuss the value of vital statistics in obstetrics.

C.M.B.(Eng.) paper.—More babies die in the first week of life than at any other time. Briefly describe the causes of this high mortality.

C.M.B.(Eng.) paper.—What advice would you give to a mother concerning protection of her baby against infectious disease ?

C.M.B.(Eng.) paper. 50 word question.—What is meant by the perinatal mortality rate ? Give the main causes of perinatal death.

C.M.B.(Eng.) paper. 50 word question.—What is meant by notification of birth ?

C.M.B.(Eng.) paper. 50 word question.—What is meant by registration of birth ?

C.M.B.(Eng.) paper.—Birth notification and registration.

C.M.B.(Eng.) paper. 50 word question.—Describe the notification, registration and disposal of a stillborn child.

C.M.B.(Eng.) paper.—What are the duties of the midwife when a stillbirth occurs in her practice ?

C.M.B.(Eng.) paper.—Outline the immunization procedures in infancy which are at present in common use.

C.M.B.(Scot.) paper.—Define perinatal mortality. How may the perinatal mortality rate be reduced ?

A mother is reluctant to have her baby immunized: how would you assure and persuade her ? When is smallpox vaccination usually carried out ? **A mother asks** how and when vaccination will affect her baby ? (*a*) will the arm be sore ? (*b*) will the baby be upset ? **What is special about the Sabin type poliomyelitis vaccine ?**

40

History of Midwifery

With Emphasis on the Part Played by Midwives

PRE-HISTORIC TIMES

Although one might surmise that in the remote ages the first woman who helped another in childbirth was a midwife, this is probably not quite correct, for only a husband or a female relative was permitted to attend the woman in labour. Later, women outside the family circle earned their livelihood in this way and became known as midwives.

Tribal customs during labour were based on belief in magic; charms and incantations being used to ward off demons. Practices during prolonged labour were crude, even cruel, for the midwives had no understanding of the process of birth.

Models are in existence (5000 B.C.) of the woman squatting during childbirth, supported behind by another woman in a similar attitude. Birth stools were a later development and are mentioned in the Old Testament.

The healing of the sick was in the hands of witch doctors and medicine men, and although priests and other men of learning took over the practice of medicine, midwifery remained in the hands of uneducated midwives, so progress did not take place.

BIBLICAL TIMES

Midwives are mentioned in the Old Testament, Genesis xxxv. 17, and xxxviii. 28, also in Exodus i. 15-21, when Pharaoh, King of Egypt, commands the midwives to slay all the Jewish infants of the male sex. The midwives feared God so they disobeyed this order, saying unto Pharaoh, " Because the Hebrew women are not as the Egyptian women ; for they are lively, and are delivered ere the midwives come in unto them." And so the story of Moses, hidden in the cradle of bulrushes came to be told.

THE HIPPOCRATIC ERA (470 to 370 B.C.)

In ancient Greece, Hippocrates, the Father of Medicine, inaugurated the scientific approach to the healing of the sick. He believed that disease was due to natural causes, so he discarded practices based on superstition or magic, as well as on religious rites and priestcraft.

Midwifery still remained in the hands of midwives who sought the advice, but not the help, of physicians in difficult cases only. Hippocrates took some part in the management of childbirth, and the midwives contemptuously called him a " he-grandmother."

THE FIRST TO THE FOURTH CENTURY, A.D.

Soranus of Ephesus, who lived during the second century, studied and taught midwifery and the treatise he wrote became the basis of various books on the subject. During the third and fourth centuries midwifery was ignored by physicians, and by custom and law they were prohibited from attending women in labour.

THE FIFTH TO THE FIFTEENTH CENTURY

One Thousand Years of Darkness

With the decline of the Roman Empire the teaching of Hippocrates and Soranus fell into disuse. During this period of intellectual stagnation, herbs, potions and incantations were again used in healing the sick, and superstitious untrained midwives had complete control of midwifery. The assistance they gave during labour was in dilating the os manually, massaging the abdomen, and supporting the perineum with a linen cloth. Pulling on the cord and manual removal of the placenta were also practised.

In the fifteenth century it was the established continental practice for midwives to be examined by members of the medical profession regarding their methods of procedure.

THE SIXTEENTH CENTURY

The invention of printing gave great impetus to learning, and in Germany, in 1513, the first book on midwifery was printed. This book, based on Soranus's teaching, was, in 1540, translated into English as *Ye Byrth of Mankynde,* and for a century and a half was the only book on midwifery printed in English. Few midwives could read, so their abysmal ignorance persisted.

Doctors were rigidly excluded from the birth chamber, and a physician in Hamburg in 1522, who dressed as a woman in order to witness the birth of a baby, was punished by being burned to death. In 1580 a law was passed in Germany preventing swineherds and shepherds from attending women in labour.

Although some progress was being made in medicine and surgery, knowledge of obstetrics lagged far behind. Childbearing women were therefore deprived of the benefits which could only accrue if the physicians, with their education and access to further learning, were permitted to enter the field.

The Dawn of Progress—Ambroise Paré (1510 to 1590)

This celebrated French surgeon laid the foundation of the modern art of obstetrics. He advocated the operation of podalic version (mainly for shoulder presentation), and his skill in delivering the child alive enhanced his prestige with the midwives. He was the first to deliver women in bed instead of on the birth stool ; he also sutured the perineum.

Paré founded a school for midwives at the Hotel Dieu in Paris, and those trained there were able to recognize abnormalities and were willing to seek the help of the surgeons who had taught them.

Louise Bourgeois, a midwife of outstanding character and ability, was trained under Paré and attended the ladies of the French court. Her writings on obstetrics were quoted in many subsequent publications.

THE SEVENTEENTH CENTURY

William Harvey (1578 to 1657), who discovered the circulation of the blood, drew attention to the deplorable ignorance of midwives and to the multitudes of women who had perished because of this.

The reluctance of women to be delivered by men continued. In 1658 a practising midwife, the daughter of Dr Willughby, a Middlesex physician, was perturbed because of a breech presentation. She requested her father to creep into the birth chamber on his hands and knees, unknown to her patient, and persuaded him to remain and assist her with the delivery.

Gross pelvic deformity caused by rickets, which was first described in the seventeenth century, necessitated the assistance of a physician or surgeon to deliver the woman. Midwives did not usually seek medical aid until labour was hopelessly obstructed, and the ensuing death of mother or child gave physicians unwarrantably bad reputations.

During 1663 Louis XIV employed a surgeon from Paris to attend one of his mistresses, in preference to the gossiping midwives. He was pleased with the decorous conduct of the man-midwife and honoured him with the more dignified title of accoucheur. The fashion spread amongst the ladies of the court and was followed by the women of France. The French accoucheurs, therefore, gained vast experience and built up a school of midwifery which attracted doctors from all over Europe to study there. Mauriceau published in 1668 a treatise on midwifery, far ahead of any other book on the subject, which was translated into English in 1672 by Hugh Chamberlen, of forceps family fame, and greatly assisted the progress of midwifery in Britain.

THE EIGHTEENTH CENTURY

Midwifery forceps to deliver a live child were invented by one of the Chamberlens, a Huguenot family of whom four generations practised medicine in England from 1569 to

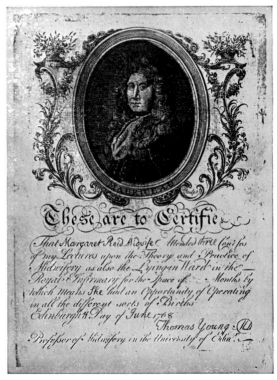

FIG. 476

Certificate awarded to Margaret Reid, midwife, in 1768; signed by Thomas Young, Professor of Midwifery in the University of Edinburgh.

1683. They went to great lengths to keep their instrument a secret, but knowledge of it leaked out and in 1733 Edmund Chapman, an English obstetrician, gave the first description of the Chamberlen forceps.

In 1813 the Chamberlen forceps were found under the floor of an attic in a house near Malden, Essex, where they were hidden in 1683 on the death of Dr Peter Chamberlen because he had no son to succeed him.

The First School of Midwifery in England

Dr John Maubray in 1725 started the first school of midwifery in England, giving lectures twice weekly. He pleaded for the building of a lying-in hospital in London.

Queen Charlotte's was the first maternity hospital in Britain. It was founded in 1739 by Sir Richard Manningham. In 1752 it became the General Lying-in Hospital, and later (1791) the name was changed when Queen Charlotte became its patron. Three other London maternity hospitals were opened in 1747 to 1750.

The Edinburgh Royal Infirmary allocated four beds for midwifery in 1752 and medical students were permitted to attend, but not until 1833 in Scotland and 1886 in England did the subject of midwifery become compulsory for medical students.

Introduction of the Left-Lateral Position for Delivery

This position is peculiar to Great Britain, being introduced by Burton of York, who practised there in 1733. The French said this was British prudery, making the woman turn her back on the doctor.

WILLIAM SMELLIE, 1697 to 1763

William Smellie, the Master of British Obstetrics, gained his knowledge of medicine as an apprentice and began his career as a doctor in Lanark, Scotland, in 1720. At this time midwives sought the help of doctors only for preternatural labours (not head first), and Smellie was perturbed over the loss of so many babies. Wishing to study normal labour and to learn more about the application of forceps, he travelled to London, a journey which took 13 days, and to Paris.

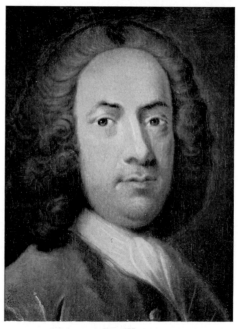

FIG. 477

WILLIAM SMELLIE.

(From a painting by himself at 22 years of age.)

In 1739 he set up in practice in London, where he taught midwifery in the homes of the poor to classes of 4 to 12 doctors. During a period of 10 years over 1,000 doctors attended his courses of lectures and clinical demonstrations, some coming from the Continent and America, such was his fame.

With no university education and no research facilities, his achievements were remarkable. He discarded the superstitious notions regarding childbirth and laid the foundation of the art and science of obstetrics as we know it today.

Smellie described the pelvis and fetal skull and their measurements, and demonstrated how to diagnose the positions of the vertex vaginally by the sutures and fontanelles. It was he who explained the mechanism of labour.

He also devised a lock for midwifery forceps, which permitted each blade to be inserted separately.

The midwives bitterly resented this man-midwife who was invading their field by delivering cases of normal labour. But it was mainly he, by his professional skill and gentle, tactful manner, who did so much to overcome their obstinate prejudice against men-practitioners. Unfortunately the malicious statement of a particularly vituperative midwife, Mrs Nihell, that he was " a great horse godmother of a he-midwife " is frequently quoted and remembered regarding him, but is far from being a just assessment of this great and good man.

Smellie's influence on obstetrics was profound, and it has been said that he accomplished for midwifery in his lifetime more than any individual before or since. His volumes on midwifery are full of obstetrical wisdom which is still valid.

The contributions of Sir J. Y. Simpson and Dr J. W. Ballantyne to obstetrics have been considered on pages 251 and 82 respectively.

HISTORY OF PUERPERAL SEPSIS

Puerperal sepsis was known at the time of Hippocrates, but epidemics of the disease coincided with the establishment of lying-in hospitals.

Charles White of Manchester (1773) and Alexander Gordon of Aberdeen (1795) were the first to state that puerperal fever was infectious and could be carried from patient to patient. Oliver Wendell Holmes in the United States of America (1843) maintained that epidemic fever in the puerperium was due to lack of cleanliness.

Semmelweis of Vienna (1844) noticed that the death rate in the wards where medical students and doctors delivered the women was three times greater than in the midwives' wards. During 1847 one of his colleagues died after cutting his finger during a post-mortem examination, and the symptoms were similar to those of puerperal sepsis. He concluded that puerperal sepsis was due to the matter carried on medical students' hands from the post-mortem room. His suggestion was ridiculed by his colleagues, and not for a further 30 years was it accepted.

The invention of the microscope and the work of Pasteur and Lister led to the recognition of the causative organisms and the employment of methods of combating them. Improved technique, the avoidance of unnecessary interference and the introduction of chemo-therapeutic agents and antibiotics have reduced still further the incidence of puerperal sepsis.

THE BRITISH MIDWIFE

Sixteenth to Twentieth Century

Few records are available regarding the practice of midwifery in Britain until the 16th century. Following the Reformation, the Church of England accepted responsibility for the issuing, by the Bishops, of licences for midwives to practise. Midwifery was practised entirely by midwives, who were completely ignorant of the most elementary facts of anatomy and obstetrics, and in 1616 a petition was made unsuccessfully to James I by Peter Chamberlen, " That some order may be settled by the State for the instruction and civil government of midwives." A second petition, submitted in 1687 by a midwife, suggested the establishment of a corporation of midwives, but the College of Physicians of London opposed it.

The first chair of midwifery, anywhere, was created in Edinburgh during 1726 for the purpose of giving instruction to midwives. (Later, medical students were permitted to attend the lectures given by the Professor.) The magistrates of Edinburgh insisted upon the production of certificates from a physician or surgeon testifying that the midwives had received instruction prior to practising their profession. Courses of instruction were given to midwives in various centres throughout Britain during the 18th century, and a few hospitals issued certificates.

In 1756 Dr John Douglas wrote a pamphlet, deploring the lamentable state of midwifery practice in London and suggesting (1) proper courses of instruction for midwives ; (2) the establishment of training schools in maternity hospitals, and (3) an examination before a certificate to practise was granted. The pamphlet was a fertile seed which eventually bore fruit.

In 1813 the Society of Apothecaries tried to persuade Parliament to pass a law forbidding women to practise as midwives for gain without having undergone an examination and obtaining a certificate of their ability to practise as midwives. The Committee of the House of Commons would not permit any mention of midwives, who at that time were of the lowest strata of society, unable to read or write, the gin-drinking type, later immortalized by Dickens as Sairey Gamp.

The Ladies' Obstetrical College, London, was founded in 1864, and the daughters of professional men attended lectures and became midwives. Florence Nightingale in 1867 organized a small training school for midwives in King's College Hospital, but, due to an epidemic of puerperal sepsis originating in a woman who was delivered while suffering from erysipelas, the scheme was abandoned. Miss Nightingale concluded that small separate rooms would reduce the high maternal mortality rate—a prophetic observation at a time when the nature of infection was not understood.

In 1872 the Obstetrical Society of London proceeded to constitute an examining Board, which awarded certificates to successful candidates, testifying to their competence to attend normal confinements. During 33 years, until 1905, when its function was taken over by the Central Midwives Board, 6,174 certificates were awarded.

In the matter of State registration of midwives, Britain lagged behind continental countries by a hundred years. Austria, Norway, Sweden and France adopted regulations governing the training and control of midwives during the first three years of the 19th century; Holland and Russia during 1865.

THE ROYAL COLLEGE OF MIDWIVES

This body was set up in 1881 as The Midwives Institute, for the main purpose of gaining recognition and registration of midwives. It was responsible for the promotion of the first Midwives' Bill, which was introduced into the House of Commons in 1890, but the Bill was bitterly opposed by untrained midwives as well as the medical profession and failed to pass into legislation. A further seven Bills were introduced between 1891 and 1900, but were unsuccessful.

At last, in 1902, the first English Midwives Act was passed, and State registration of midwives became compulsory by law. Scotland followed in 1915 with a similar Act.

The Midwives Institute celebrated its 60th anniversary in 1941, and the title was changed to The College of Midwives. In 1947 the Royal prefix was granted.

The aim of The Royal College of Midwives is to further the education and efficiency of midwives, in order to provide the best possible service to mothers and babies. It is a negotiating body, representing the midwives' interests, and has been the chief instrument in promoting progress in the practice of midwifery by midwives and the means of improving their conditions of service, salary and status.

THE CENTRAL MIDWIVES BOARD

The Midwives Act of 1902 (Eng.) sanctioned the setting up of the Central Midwives Board, prescribed its constitution and laid down its duties and powers. The Board was authorized to frame rules regulating the training and practice of midwives, to conduct examinations and maintain a roll of persons who had been awarded its certificate. The Board also organizes examinations for the Midwife Teacher's Diploma.

The primary function of the Central Midwives Board is to protect the public by providing well-trained midwives who must carry out a code of practice as laid down by the Board. The actual duty of supervising the midwife in practice is the responsibility of the Local Supervising Authority.

The training period for midwives has gradually been lengthened to meet advances in knowledge and improved methods of practice. From the year 1902 to 1916 the training period lasted three months; since 1938 it has been one year for trained and two years for untrained nurses. In Scotland only nurses who are State Registered or State Enrolled are eligible for training.

The Board now consists of 17 members, six of whom are midwives, two appointed by the Department of Health and Social Security and four by the Royal College of Midwives The Department of Health also appoints three doctors, one administrator (an Assistant Secretary of the Department of Health and Social Security) and one Senior Administrative Medical Officer of a Regional Hospital Board. One doctor is appointed by the Royal College of Obstetricians, the Royal College of Physicians, the Royal College of Surgeons, the Society of Medical Officers of Health, County Councils Association and the Association of Municipal Corporations.

The Central Midwives Board for Scotland was set up in 1915. Seven of the 16 members are midwives. Its functions are similar to those of the English Board.

ADDRESSES OF CENTRAL MIDWIVES BOARDS

ENGLAND	N. IRELAND	SCOTLAND
Iolanthe House, 39 Harrington Gardens, South Kensington, London, S.W.7.	5 Annadale Avenue, Belfast 7.	24 Dublin Street, Edinburgh, EH1 3PU

The Midwives Acts

The Midwives Act of 1902 (Scotland, 1915), gave protection to the title ' 'Midwife " and made it a legal offence for any woman to use the title when not certified as such. It also made it illegal for an unqualified woman, habitually and for gain, to attend women in childbirth except under the direction of a doctor. The Act required all practising midwives to notify the Local Supervising Authority in January every year of their intention to practise and to notify the Central Midwives Board of any change of name or address.

The Midwives Acts of 1902, 1918, 1926 and 1936 are now consolidated in the Act of 1951 and a similar consolidating Act of the same year applied to Scotland.

THE LOCAL SUPERVISING AUTHORITY

The Local Supervising Authority is the Local Health Authority, *i.e.* the Council of a county or county borough; the administrative officer is the Medical Officer of Health. The Local Supervising Authority was set up under the Midwives Act, 1902 (Scotland, 1915), to exercise general supervision over all midwives practising in their area, in accordance with the rules of the Central Midwives Board. The Local Supervising Authority also investigates charges of malpractice or misconduct and reports on these to the Central Midwives Board.

The midwife sends an official notification to the Local Supervising Authority in the following circumstances.

In the case of:

1. Intention to practise.
2. Change of name or address.
3. Stillbirth or death of mother or child.
4. Laying out a dead body.
5. When liable to be a source of infection.
6. If the patient refuses to seek medical advice. (Scotland.)
7. When the patient's accommodation and equipment are not suitable for confinement (*recommendation in England, compulsory in Scotland*).

The supervisor of midwives who may be a Registered Medical Practitioner or a senior midwife with administrative ability assists the Medical Officer of Health in the actual duty of supervising midwives in the area.

Domiciliary Service of Midwives

The Midwives Act, 1936, and the Maternity Services (Scotland) Act, 1937, made it compulsory for every Local Authority to employ sufficient midwives for attendance on women confined at home in their area. The status of district midwives was much improved by their employment on a salaried basis.

Under the Health Services and Public Health Act, 1968 the services of a domiciliary midwife employed by the local authority can be made available to a management committee controlling the hospital.

REFRESHER COURSES

These must, according to the Central Midwives Boards, be provided or arranged for by the Local Supervising Authority. Practising midwives are required to attend such a course in England and Scotland within five years of having passed the C.M.B. examination or having attended such a course.

The free midwifery service provided under the National Health Service Act which came into force in 1948 has been referred to on page 82.

PROGRESS IN OBSTETRICS

Not until the medical profession entered the field of obstetrics was any real progress made. Only then did childbearing women derive any benefit from the advances made in medicine and surgery which could be applied to obstetrics.

The invention of midwifery forceps gave men practitioners a great advantage. The introduction of anæsthetics, as well as the knowledge of antisepsis and asepsis, made obstetrical operations possible. Advances in physiology, biochemistry, bacteriology, hæmatology, radiology, ultrasonography, endocrinology and pharmacology have brought obstetrics to a level which could never have been attained by midwives alone.

Both doctor and midwife are essential, even for normal cases, if the woman is to receive the maximal benefit of all modern investigations and treatment during pregnancy and labour.

The proficient midwife of today is an expert in the care of women in normal pregnancy, labour and the puerperium, as well as a helpful collaborator with the obstetrician when dealing with abnormal or operative obstetrics.

She is also a teacher of health, preparation for childbirth and early parenthood.

TEAM WORK

The midwife co-operates as one of a team, which includes:

OBSTETRICIANS, PHYSICIANS, PÆDIATRICIANS, ANÆSTHETISTS, GENERAL PRACTITIONERS, BACTERIOLOGISTS, RADIOLOGISTS, HÆMATOLOGISTS

aided by:

HEALTH VISITORS; DIETITIANS; SOCIAL WORKERS and PHYSIOTHERAPISTS

all of whom are concerned with the welfare of mothers and babies.

QUESTIONS FOR REVISION

C.M.B.(Eng.) paper. 50 word question.—What is a " Local Supervising Authority " ?

C.M.B.(Eng.) paper. 50 word question.—The Central Midwives Board.

C.M.B.(Eng.) paper. 50 word question.—What is a medical aid form and when is it used ?

41

Preparation for Childbirth and Early Parenthood

by EXPERIENCED MIDWIVES

Expectant mothers today, having been subjected to mass media of communication on the subject of health education, including human reproduction, expect to receive information and advice that will equip them to approach and participate in the childbearing and rearing process happily and successfully. Their need is urgent. Many are aware of their inadequacy as future parents and are eager to attend courses of instruction: emotional problems and fears disturb their peace of mind; these should be clarified or dispersed.

Prospective parents are entitled to receive the necessary education from the professional groups best qualified to provide this.

THE MIDWIFE A TEACHER

Midwives are licensed to give obstetric care to women during normal pregnancy, labour and the puerperium: teaching is an integral part of that care. Their expert knowledge of midwifery and vast experience in dealing with women during pregnancy and labour qualify them as unrivalled teachers of expectant mothers. Midwives must therefore be given, and accept, responsibility for this duty.

The midwife understands the mothers' needs, obstetrical, educational, social and psychological. To meet these needs she will arrange a balanced programme, no more time than is justified being devoted to any particular aspect. Although the subject of labour looms large on the woman's horizon and she has an insatiable desire to hear or talk about it, the wellbeing of the unborn and the newly born child is equally important.

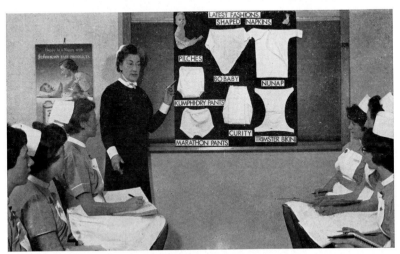

FIG. 478

Student midwives being shown how to teach expectant mothers
(*Royal Maternity Hospital, Rottenrow, Glasgow.*)

705

Midwives have always given individual instruction to their patients at prenatal clinics, in hospital and in the home; they should continue to do so. But individual teaching, although useful, is limited in scope and often confined to prescribing the remedy for some minor ailment. Organised group teaching is modern and preventive in outlook; it covers a more comprehensive field and is economical in teaching time.

Certain aspects in preparation for childbirth and early parenthood the midwife may delegate to other members of a team who are qualified to contribute to the welfare of mother and child but she must assume team leadership: hers is the key role: arranging and organizing the course of instruction, teaching the obstetric subjects and applying the subsidiary instruction given by other groups to the obstetric situation.

PSYCHOLOGICAL METHODS OF PREPARATION

The demand by expectant mothers for instruction in psychological methods of preparation for labour is so great that non-professional persons have undertaken such teaching. But the enthusiasm of unqualified people is no substitute for the expert knowledge and authoritative experience of midwives. The dissemination of information and advice that is physiologically unsound and obstetrically unsafe is to be deprecated and should stimulate midwives to undertake the professional responsibility which is theirs.

Midwives have in the past, by their kindly manner and understanding care, unknowingly employed psychological techniques, giving the woman sympathetic support and enabling her to achieve satisfaction in coping with the stresses of labour in a serene and dignified manner. They have, however, tended to rely to a greater extent on the pharmacological method for relief of pain but the midwife with vision will realize that she must actively participate in the prenatal teaching of psychological techniques if women in labour are to achieve emotional satisfaction and adequate pain-relief.

There is no mystique or miraculous element in any of the methods of preparation, including psychoprophylaxis, nor is there any justification for adopting a fanatical degree of fervour which demands absolute adherence to the minute details of the procedures taught. The methods now in vogue are based on psychological principles and the fact that they all succeed to a greater or lesser degree indicates that there is some underlying factor common to all. By studying these principles midwives will understand how they function and will be enabled to select the technique they prefer when preparing women for childbirth.

The psychological principles are:—

(1) SUGGESTION (2) DISTRACTION (3) CONCENTRATION
(4) CONFIDENCE AND ASSURANCE based on knowledge

(1) Suggestion

This is extensively used in hypnosis, 'which is a trance-like state: but suggestion could be used by midwives without carrying it to the stage of hypnosis. The hypnotized woman feels no pain when her hand is pricked with a needle, because it has been suggested to her that her hand is numb. This proves the influence of the mind over the body. If the midwife uses a persuasive manner and a pleasant tone of voice the expectant mother becomes more receptive to the teacher and to what she is being taught.

During pregnancy the midwife's attitude influences the expectant mother's approach to childbirth and when labour-ward midwives have the opportunity to meet the women whom they will eventually be looking after, their competent bearing and proficiency in describing the management of labour gives assurance and suggests that all will be well.

During labour, the friendly welcome, the calm unhurried manner suggest kindliness and competence; encouraging remarks re progress suggest a successful labour. Midwives are well aware of the power of suggestion; hypnotic drugs having no analgesic effect are alleged by patients to relieve pain.

(2) Distraction

This is probably the most powerful and the most widely used factor. Awareness of pain is reduced when attention is diverted by listening to an engrossing radio programme, by looking at some interesting performance or by doing something, *i.e.* house-work, knitting.

In psychoprophylaxis much use is made of distraction; the cortex of the brain is bombarded with so many distracting activities during a uterine contraction that the woman has little opportunity to be aware of pain.   She is required to breathe at four different rates and levels (now condemned), to hum or drum a tune, to use effleurage (stroking the skin), to keep alert and awake using muscle release (active relaxation).

Distracting activity should never be carried to excess as, when women are required to remain awake for over 12 hours using physical and mental energy to the stage of exhaustion. Women, when required to pant for long periods, are using tracheal breathing which causes hypoventilation that in cases of placental dysfunction or incipient fetal distress may have serious consequences.

Midwives will utilize harmless distracting activities, *e.g.* the radio, television, companionship.   **Controlled breathing with a sighing expiration** is one of the most helpful distracting activities used in labour today (see p. 715).

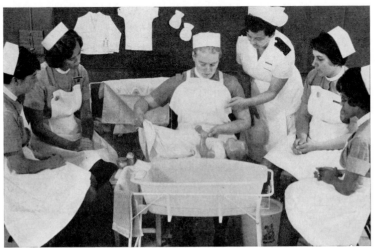

Fig. 479
Parentcraft sister teaching student midwives how to demonstrate
baby-bathing to expectant mothers.
(*Aberdeen Maternity Hospital.*)

(3) Concentration

This is closely allied to distraction for unless the woman concentrates on the diverting activity it will not be effective.   When concentrating on some engrossing subject a person can be oblivious to physical discomfort or the passage of time.

(4) Confidence

This is a psychological state stemming from knowledge and experience and is an excellent antidote to fear.   **Every method of preparation for childbirth makes use of giving instruction** that will enable the woman to comprehend the processes of pregnancy and labour in so far as they will affect her.   When a woman knows what to expect and realizes that labour is pursuing a normal course she is more likely to cope with any stress successfully.   Giving assurance is a means of instilling confidence.

THE WOMAN'S EMOTIONAL REACTION TO LABOUR

Every woman is entitled to approach the emotional aspect of childbirth in her own way: no person has the right to pontificate to another individual as to how she ought to feel or behave during labour. How a woman reacts to the pain of labour or feels towards her new born baby depends on the type of person she is, her attitude to love, marriage, motherhood and to life in general. Not all have the emotional endowment to glorify the pain of labour and to interpret it as being pleasurable, nor to find enrichment in the process.

ATTITUDE TO PAIN

The majority of women describe what they feel during a uterine contraction as pain. The use of the word " contraction " for " pain " does not lessen the sensation the woman experiences as pain. If she is led to expect a painless labour she reacts very badly when she feels pain whether it has been described as tightening, hardening or discomfort. The modern idea is to use the word " pain ". Everything possible should be done to enable women to have as comfortable a labour as is possible, and to achieve emotional satisfaction.

Coping with Pain

None of the exponents of psychological methods today promise a painless labour but women can be helped to cope with pain. Many of the techniques employed are designed to lower the receptivity of the cortex of the brain to painful stimuli: they raise the pain threshold. Persons with a low pain threshold would feel acute pain from a pin prick; those with a high pain threshold would scarcely notice it. Some interpret pain more acutely than others.

We are all aware that the mind affects the body: a revolting sight produces nausea; bad news causes fainting. Cultural factors may determine the woman's response to pain; some races scream with each labour pain, others are silent and withdrawn.

Analgesic drugs blur or cloud the consciousness of pain but they do have certain detrimental side effects.

PLANNING A COURSE OF INSTRUCTION

AIMS OF THE COURSE

(1) Physical Health Education

To give instruction on how to achieve the physical fitness, by healthy living and good nutrition, to produce a well-formed, mature vigorous child without depleting the mother's vital body-substances.

(2) Mental Health Education

(a) **To provide sympathetic assurance and understanding,** aiding the woman in the enjoyment of a serene outlook during pregnancy, in labour and in caring for her child.

(b) **To give suitable advice regarding the fears and anxieties** that disturb prospective parents, often due to lack of knowledge.

(3) Preparation for Childbirth

(a) **To employ modern means of communication in presenting the new psychological methods** of coping with the stress of labour: providing practice class demonstrations of exercises, relaxation, rhythmic breathing and labour positions.

(b) **To inform regarding the elementary processes of childbearing,** giving also a brief explanation of some common deviations from normal to enable the woman to approach labour in an enlightened, confident manner.

(c) **To assure regarding the provision of emotional support,** kindly professional companionship and supervision and the use of modern means of pain relief during labour.

(d) **To integrate the instruction given during pregnancy** with the realities of labour by permitting labour ward midwives to participate actively in the teaching programme.

(4) To arrange for and give instruction in Baby Care (see p. 736)

(5) To discuss subjects that concern inexperienced parents, e.g.

State benefits, budgeting for baby, family planning, family relationships and responsibilities.

TEAMWORK AND CONTINUITY

To ensure integration and continuity between what is taught during pregnancy and practised during labour it is imperative that instruction regarding childbirth should be given by midwives.

Labour ward midwives only, should apply relaxation techniques concerning labour because they understand the physiology and management of labour and can speak from the authority of sound knowledge and practical experience.

Without continuity in teaching the woman in labour cannot effectively carry out the instruction she has been given at prenatal classes. The labour ward midwives are deprived of the opportunity to give the necessary emotional support and physical relief.

10 CLASSES OF 2 HOURS

MEMBER OF TEAM	NO. OF CLASSES	LENGTH OF CLASS
Obstetrician	2	30-40 minutes
Organizing Sister	10	30-40 ,,
Labour Ward Sister	4	30 ,,
Nursery Sister	4	30 ,,
Post-natal Sister	2	30 ,,
Health Visitor	2	30 ,,
Physiotherapist	4	30 ,,
Dietitian	1	30 ,,
Social Worker	1	30 ,,
(Discussion and Tea)	10	20 ,,
		20 hours

An obstetrician would be present at the first class to explain:—

(*a*) **physical and emotional changes during pregnancy,**

(*b*) **what is done at the prenatal clinic,** (*c*) **avoiding drugs and infections.**

Following the tea break he could talk to husbands while Sister demonstrated a model layette.

Ten classes, each lasting 2 hours with a 20 minute discussion and tea break, would be ideal. Four subjects could be taught at one session by different people. Demonstrations of baby-care, exercises, relaxation, require little mental effort; if the talks are short and given in a bright, chatty style, interspersed with opportunities for comments and questions, the mothers-to-be should not suffer mental fatigue.

If a film depicting baby's birth is shown it should be the culmination of visual teaching during which parents are gradually introduced to and prepared for viewing a photographic presentation of the birth process. To some women this may be an emotionally traumatizing experience when they personally are approaching a similar event. Married couples are sometimes so distressed that they leave the room. A permissive attitude regarding attendance should be adopted.

A tour of the labour wards and nurseries is usually enjoyed and the staff on duty should be prepared to talk to the mothers-to-be and show the facilities available, *e.g.* admission room, analgesic gas machines, labour rooms, nurseries, incubators.

TIMING THE CLASSES

The need for one class, not later than the 8th week of pregnancy, is urgent in order to warn expectant mothers of the dangers in taking drugs not prescribed by the doctor. They must also be told to **avoid contact with certain infectious diseases such as German measles,** and could be advised regarding good food and the prevention of anæmia; minor disorders, **and baby's layette.** This early class could be held in the evening once every month and husbands invited to attend. The other nine classes could start at the 20th week, and in order that they are not completed too soon, they can be given every two weeks until the 36th week. **Special evening classes should be arranged** between the 20th and 28th weeks for those who go out to work. Duplication of classes will be necessary. A number of maternity hospitals in Great Britain give classes, 12 times per week. Expectant mothers will undoubtedly attend if the talks are enjoyable and instructive.

PROGRAMME OF 10 TWO-HOUR CLASSES WITH DISCUSSION DURING 20-MIN. TEA BREAK

Subjects	Minutes	Lecturer
1. At 6 Weeks		
What happens at the clinic and during labour: avoiding drugs and infections.	40	Obstetrician
Keeping fit: minor ailments: the expectant father.	40	Sister in Charge
Baby's layette.	20	Nursery Sister
2. At 20 Weeks		
Childbirth never so good: the womb and baby growing inside it: maternity clothes.	40	Sister in Charge
Waiting for the stork: how we will help you: controlled breathing.	20	Labour W. Sister
Limbering up: posture, relaxation.	30	Physiotherapist
3. At 22 Weeks		
Baby's outward journey: false and true labour.	30	Sister in Charge
Comfortable baby clothes: nappies new and old: handling and dressing baby.	30	Nursery Sister
Good food: food supplements.	20	Dietitian
Exercises: posture: relaxation.	20	Physiotherapist
4. At 24 Weeks		
Budgeting for baby: equipment needed: words heard at the clinic.	30	Sister in Charge
What to expect during and after labour.	30	Obstetrician
Stork on the way: coping with pain : relaxation and controlled breathing.	20	Labour W. Sister
Exercises: posture: relaxation.	20	Physiotherapist
5. At 26 Weeks		
The transitional and second stages: positions for backache.	20	Sister in Charge
Equipment and positions for bathing: why baby cries.	30	Nursery Sister
Family relationships and responsibilities: safety in the home.	30	Health Visitor
Posture: lifting: relaxation.	20	Physiotherapist
6. At 28 Weeks		
Induction of labour: stitches: forceps: relaxation: controlled breathing.	40	Sister in Charge
Labour positions: baby's birth: analgesic gas.	30	Labour W. Sister
Maternity benefits: State help.	20	Social Worker
7. At 30 Weeks		
Twins: breech: Cæsarean birth: relaxation: controlled breathing: the new father.	40	Sister in Charge
Demonstration of bathing baby: baby care.	40	Nursery Sister
Baby and you in hospital: reasons for routine.	20	Post-natal Sister
8. At 32 Weeks		
Planning baby's day: registering the birth.	30	Sister in Charge
Rehearsal for labour: why be afraid?	30	Labour W. Sister
Health visitor will call: attending baby clinic: immunization: vaccination	30	Health Visitor

Subjects	Minutes	Lecturer
9. At 34 Weeks		
Family planning.	10	Sister in Charge
Tour of hospital.	40	Sister in Charge
Breast and bottle feeding.	30	Nursery Sister
Taking things easy at home: attending for post-natal examination.	20	Post-natal Sister
10. At 36 Weeks		
Film of labour.	30	Sister in Charge
Your views aired.	30 ⎫	Two of the
Your questions answered.	30 ⎭	Lecturers.

Fathers are invited to attend: evening classes will be held.

SCHEME FOR TEACHING EXPECTANT MOTHERS

In the following scheme, drawn up for practising midwives, a number of procedures are incorporated which have been used in other methods of preparation for childbirth, including psychoprophylaxis. Only techniques that are obstetrically safe and psychologically and physiologically beneficial have been selected.

Experienced midwives are perfectly capable of instructing expectant mothers in the simple procedures necessary in preparation for childbirth.

The procedures are:

(1) **EXERCISES**   (2) **ACTIVE RELAXATION**   (3) **CONTROLLED BREATHING**
(4) **POSITIONS FOR LABOUR**

(1) EXERCISES FOR EXPECTANT MOTHERS

In the past a great deal of time and energy has been expended carrying out exercises in preparation for labour. They may have some psychological value in that the woman is doing something that she expects will help her. As a means for limbering up and keeping fit during pregnancy they are admirable but there is no proof that they have any beneficial effect on the course or the outcome of labour.

Midwives are aware that the pelvic joints are in a relaxed state due to endocrine action during pregnancy; strenuous pelvic rocking could therefore overstretch relaxed ligaments: hyperextension of the spine is not advocated. Pelvic floor exercises will not prevent lacerations nor improve the performance of the pelvic floor during labour; they are beneficial in the postnatal period to tone up a relaxed pelvic floor.

The Talk as given to Expectant Mothers

" You will want to look and feel fit for baby's birthday" so we will show you a few simple exercises to limber up your joints and muscles, improve your circulation, and give you a feeling of wellbeing.

" Good posture enables you to cope with the discomforts that occur in pregnancy due to alterations in your balance: as your abdomen grows larger and heavier you will tend to lean back too far and to walk in a slouching fashion, even to waddle, instead of carrying your baby with poise and grace. **Bad posture gives rise to low backache,** aching limbs and feet as well as general fatigue. You must first of all think " good posture ", walk tall, feel tall, hold your head high and show you are proud to be pregnant. . . . Relax your shoulders, hold them back and downwards, not stiffly. You will of course, have to hold your shoulders back to maintain your balance but don't overdo this. Gently straighten your knees. . . . Stand with your feet 22·9 cm. (9 inches) apart, toes pointing straight forwards; don't lean back on your heels, rest your weight on the outer arches and the balls of your feet. . . . Take in a few deep breaths now, expanding your ribs sideways without raising your shoulders. . . .

" Will you now take a dozen steps? Swing your legs from the hips, lean slightly forwards and propel your weight from your heels on to the balls of the feet and tips of the toes. Don't clamp each foot down as a solid mass: walk with a lilt in your step."

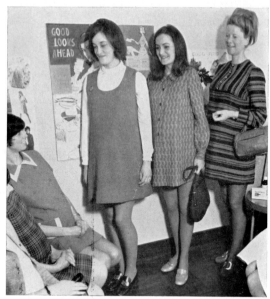

Fig. 480

THREE ATTRACTIVE LADIES-IN-WAITING ATTENDING MOTHERCRAFT CLASSES
AT ROYAL MATERNITY PRENATAL CLINIC, ROTTENROW, GLASGOW.

LIMBERING UP STIFF JOINTS

Feet.—" Sit down and take off your shoes. Let the outer edges of the feet rest on the floor, curl your feet and toes; relax—repeat 6 times."

Ankles.—" Stretch your leg forwards and rotate the foot in an inward direction six times, then with the other foot. Repeat exercise by rotating each foot in an outward direction—6 times. Stand tall, rise on tiptoes and lower six times: then raise and lower alternate heels. This exercise will strengthen your arches for the extra load you are carrying."

Arm Swinging.—" Stand tall, stretch your arms forwards and upwards while raising yourself on tiptoe: lower arms in a backward direction, lower heels—repeat 6 times."

Shoulder Rolling.—" Stand upright, finger tips on shoulders. Raise and swing shoulders backwards with a circular movement slowly; reverse movement in forward direction—repeat 6 times."

Spine Rotation.—" Stand properly, head high: arms outstretched at shoulder level: turn head and body to left, keeping the knees pointing forwards."

(2) RELAXATION

Relaxation as taught during the nineteen-thirties was passive; the woman being required to relax physically and mentally. Such a procedure is excellent to produce serenity and conserve energy during pregnancy and the early first stage of labour but is not so effective when the uterine contractions become strong and painful.

Active relaxation is used today: the woman remaining mentally alert in order to concentrate on physical relaxation and distracting activities, such as controlled breathing. The terms " muscle release " or " muscle decontrol " are sometimes used instead of " active relaxation " which could be described as mental activity with physical passivity.

It is easy to relax on a comfortable bed in a quiet, warm room, but very difficult when suffering pain or discomfort combined with fear of the unknown or the known experience in strange, sometimes noisy, surroundings. Active relaxation enables the woman to cope more successfully with pain and to be in control of the normal reaction to stress.

(The physiotherapist can be invited to teach the basic principles of relaxation.)

NEURO-MUSCULAR CONTROL

The usual response to a painful sensory stimulus is physical and mental tension, but the pregnant woman can be taught and by practice, achieve physical relaxation instead of tension in a situation that will be painful. This is done by neuro-muscular control. All purposeful movement is activated by a sensory stimulus to the brain, which responds by sending out a motor (nerve) response to the muscles concerned. Every muscular skill, such as walking, playing tennis or golf, has to be learned by neuro-muscular control: a conscious effort being made until, with practice, the movements become automatic.

The expectant mother can practice active relaxation by which she learns to be mentally alert attending to a distracting activity while also maintaining her voluntary muscles in a relaxed state. By instruction regarding the process of labour and how this will affect her; by the use of suggestion, concentration and distraction, the woman becomes assured and confident in her ability to cope during labour.

DEMONSTRATION OF PASSIVE RELAXATION

A friendly welcome creates an informal relaxed atmosphere. The room should be comfortably warm with firm mattresses 1.8×0.6 metres (6×2 ft.) each having two or more pillows; shoes off; roll-on belts removed (stretch nylon tights are ideal)—bladder empty.

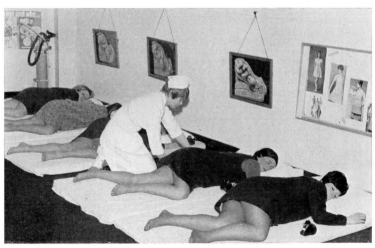

FIG. 481

LABOUR WARD SISTER WITH RELAXATION CLASS.
(Simpson Memorial Maternity Pavilion, Edinburgh.)

The Talk as to Expectant Mothers

The midwife speaks quietly using a low pitch and soothing tone:—

"Today we will consider how to relax your body and your mind. Later you will learn about, and practise active relaxation, the new method used in psychoprophylaxis in which your mind remains alert.

" **First let me tell you how relaxation will be useful to you** during pregnancy and in the early stage of labour. If you have difficulty in falling asleep at night relaxation will help you to drift into a sound sleep more quickly and to awake refreshed. In the later weeks you will need more rest during the day and this will be twice as beneficial if you can relax properly: you will learn to banish tension and enjoy a tranquil happy pregnancy.

" **When the doctor at the clinic or the midwife during labour makes an internal examination** it will be more comfortable for you and easier for them if you can relax. In labour you will get more relief from the sedative drugs given to you and you will have more energy to push when that time comes.

" **To recognize the difference between relaxed and tense muscles** clench your fist tightly, unclench it, then allow the hand to go limp. . . . Tighten your calf muscles then let go. . . . Wrinkle your forehead in a frown then relax the muscles concerned. . . . Purse your mouth as when tense, smile as when relaxed.

" **Will you lie down now on your left side,** the position you may use during the first stage of labour. . . . Place one pillow for your right knee and ankle to rest on: pull the end of the head pillow down and forwards. . . . Bring your under arm in front with forearm across the chest: you may put this arm behind if you like but if you do, it will be more difficult to turn on to your back during labour while Sister listens to baby's heart-beat every few minutes. Bend your right leg at the knee and place knee and ankle on the pillow."

" **Get yourself into a really comfortable position:** we will begin relaxing at the head and work downwards. Close your eyes gently, smooth all the wrinkles from your brow, . . . allow your lower jaw to sag but keep your lips closed lightly, let your tongue be limp. . . . Loosen the muscles of your neck and let your shoulders droop, at ease. . . . Allow your back to sink into the mattress, . . . relax the muscles of your abdomen. This is important as it will play some part in lessening labour pain. Slacken the muscles of your buttocks and thighs. . . . Let your knees and ankles go limp as they sink into the mattress, wriggle your toes then think of them as being lax and floppy.

" **Breathe quietly and you will soon feel drowsy."** (The midwife should silently pass from one to the other testing for tension by gently lifting elbow or fingers. . . .) " Sit up slowly because when you are so completely relaxed you might feel faint if you jumped up quickly. . . . Will you practise relaxing like this at home ? And do concentrate on relaxing the abdominal muscles. At the next class we will practise active relaxation and the positions for the late first and the second stage of labour."

ACTIVE RELAXATION

The method of active relaxation requires that the woman shall be mentally alert during labour, usually concentrating on some distracting activity such as controlled breathing.

Active relaxation must never be carried to excess or the woman in labour becomes exhausted, as has occurred when women under psychoprophylaxis have used forced breathing for 24 hours, refusing sedation and remaining awake during that time. Sedative and analgesic drugs should be administered as required. It is quite unnecessary to insist on the woman remaining alert between contractions: there is no reason why she may not close her eyes and relax. The midwife will rouse the woman when she feels the uterus contracting, in time for her to relax actively before she experiences pain.

Dissociation Drill (this is only carried out during pregnancy and not during labour). The procedure is utilized as a means of rehearsing active relaxation of groups of muscles while others are tensed. The purpose is to accustom the woman to relaxing physically in the presence of painful uterine contractions. To simulate a uterine contraction the expectant mother grasps and squeezes a tennis ball (or ball of newspaper) with her arm extended.

The teacher times the starting and ending of the imaginary uterine contraction, each woman increasing the intensity of squeezing the ball, then gradually lessening the grip. During this 60 seconds she concentrates on maintaining all other voluntary muscles in a relaxed state. (In psychoprophylaxis a leg or arm is raised to simulate a uterine contraction.)

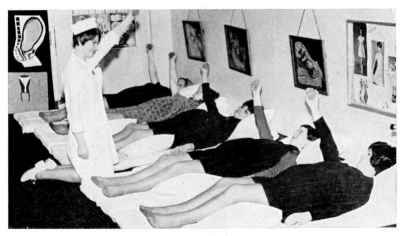

FIG. 482

LABOUR WARD SISTER DEMONSTRATES SQUEEZING A TENNIS BALL TO SIMULATE THE CONTRACTING UTERUS
(IN PREGNANCY) WHILE RELAXING VOLUNTARY MUSCLES.
(*Simpson Memorial Maternity Pavilion, Edinburgh.*)

(3) RHYTHMIC BREATHING

When a woman in labour concentrates on the rhythm of her breathing, which should be at her own normal rate, it becomes a distracting activity which helps to take her mind off the pain she experiences. Many women have stated that " The Breathing " was the most helpful agent in relieving pain. To make rhythmic breathing more purposeful to the woman it is described to her in detail. She is asked to breathe in through her mouth and to accentuate the expiration which should be audible like a sigh with a " pooh " sound, made by the lips. This soothing sound seems to have a calming effect and is a psychological, harmless, distracting activity.

Natural rhythmic breathing must not be confused with the type of breathing at abnormal levels and rates advocated by certain groups: research has proved these to be harmful to both mother and fetus, *i.e.*:—

Slow deep breathing can, by hyperventilation, induce alkalosis with an increase in the pH of maternal blood and a lowered serum calcium. Tingling of fingers occurs which may proceed to carpopedal spasm and even tetany.

Rapid shallow breathing or panting is only tracheal and, as very little air reaches the lungs, hypoventilation occurs and the fetus may be deprived of oxygen. In cases of placental dysfunction or incipient fetal distress the effect of panting could be harmful.

Panting is not now practised. To counteract any contraindicated expulsive effort, *e.g.* at the transitional stage, instead of panting, the woman can be taught to open her mouth and throat (*to avoid closing the glottis*) and to accentuate inspiration rather than expiration. This type of breathing can also be used during the actual expulsion of the baby's head.

" **Women in labour frequently breathe more rapidly at the acme of a contraction** but should be advised not to do so. Persistent rapid breathing or breath-holding is usually a sign of panic.

ACTIVE RELAXATION—WITH RHYTHMIC BREATHING

Talk as given to Mothers

" First we will repeat the method of physical and mental relaxation you learned at the previous class, using the tennis ball for an imaginary contraction of the womb. . . .

" Now we will practise active relaxation during which you will remain mentally alert, concentrating on rhythmic breathing. This type of relaxation is very good when the labour contractions are strong. . . .

" Will you all lie on your backs now with a wedge, or two pillows, to prop up your head and shoulders, and one pillow under your knees. Have your feet about 22·9 cm. (9 inches) apart, toes pointing outwards, all muscles relaxed. . . .

" Let us now practise the special type of controlled or rhythmic breathing.—Breathe in naturally through your nose and mouth . . . you will relax better by breathing with an open mouth. Concentrate on the rising of your relaxed abdominal muscles as you breathe in and the falling of them as you sigh your breath out with a soft soothing ' pooh ' sound made with your lips like this. . . . I will time your breathing at an average rate of about 18 per minute—in—out, in—out. . . .

" We will now practise breathing during a labour contraction while holding the tennis ball . . . squeezing the ball gently at first then harder and harder. A contraction is starting now! Breathe steadily in and out; let me hear the ' pooh ' sound. Relax all your muscles except the arm that is holding the ball. Gradually reduce your grip. . . . We will repeat that."

The transitional stage should be mentioned and the type of breathing as described for extension of the head (see below) recommended to counteract the tendency to premature pushing that frequently occurs at this time.

(4) POSITIONS IN LABOUR

" Let us now rehearse the positions you will adopt during the first stage." (See p. 714.)

" In the second stage you will be lying on your back using rhythmic breathing during contractions; resting and relaxing between them. The midwife will tell you when a contraction is starting so that you can be alert and ready to cope with it."

Position for Pushing

" When the time for pushing arrives you will be lying propped up on two pillows: you will then adopt a special position at the beginning of each contraction; flex your legs at the hips and knees, widely separate them and with your hands grasping the thighs under the knees, raise your legs; at the same time bend your spine forwards, chin on chest. Take one or two deep breaths, close your mouth firmly, tighten the throat muscles (close the glottis) hold your breath and push (bear down). You will be inhaling gas and oxygen and you may take another quick breath of gas and push again so long as the uterus is still contracted. . . . One sustained push is more effective than a series of short ones.

" Towards the end of the second stage you will have a very strong urge to ' push ' when baby's head descends on to the pelvic floor: but you must not bear down until the midwife tells you to do so. To counteract this desire to push open your mouth and your throat, relax the muscles of your neck: concentrate on ' breathing in ' deliberately, rather than on ' breathing out ', do not use the ' pooh ' sound.

" The second stage of labour is not as painful as you might expect: with every contraction baby descends a little farther until he is ready to be born.

" We will practise the second stage position now using the tennis ball and the analgesic gas mask. . . ."

BIRTH OF BABY'S HEAD

" To enable baby's head to be born easily you must relax your pelvic floor at the time the head is actually being born. The perineum will be fully stretched, but don't worry, it will have a numb feeling. You will have a tremendous urge to push but this is where your training in relaxation enables you to be in control and to refrain from pushing. Keep your mouth and throat open and breathe as described previously. If you pushed baby's head out quickly your perineum might tear and stitches would be needed.

HYPNOSIS

This is a trance-like state produced in the person who is willing to co-operate with the hypnotist. Through the power of suggestion the threshold for the perception of pain is raised; the degree of hypnosis used in obstetrics does not place the woman under the complete dominance of the hypnotist; she is rendered more responsive to suggestion and co-operates more willingly.

Midwives could use suggestion without carrying it to the hypnotic state. During pregnancy the woman can be told: (*a*) that the instructions she is given will enable her to control her reaction to pain; (*b*) that uterine contractions have a beneficial function, each one bringing the baby nearer to being born.

A soothing and pleasantly monotonous tone of voice and a persuasive manner are necessary to induce a tranquil frame of mind and engender a receptive attitude. The midwife's attitude during pregnancy should be optimistic, suggesting that all is well, instilling confidence without being assertive.

During labour the midwife's calm, competent bearing radiates confidence, encouraging remarks *re* progress suggest a successful outcome. Midwives are well aware of the power of suggestion, e.g. that a placebo relieves pain as do hypnotic drugs that have no analgesic properties.

PSYCHOPROPHYLAXIS

Handling Women trained under the British Method

Midwives should handle these women during labour with the utmost tact and encourage them to carry out the techniques they have been taught. To exhibit understanding of the method the midwife should mention muscle release or decontrol, effleurage (skin stroking) and ask what tune she hums; how she has been taught to deal with strong contractions. Extra pillows should be provided for the semi-sitting position some adopt.

The doctor should be requested to deal with those who persist with forced breathing when advised to desist or who refuse to accept sedative or analgesic drugs when the need is apparent. After 12 hours of excessive distraction and concentration the mental effort causes exhaustion; forced breathing may produce hyperventilation or hypoventilation (see p. 715).

Psychoprophylactically prepared women expect to participate actively in the processes of labour and to have all stages and procedures explained to them in detail.

Much encouragement and assurance regarding their progress and performance should be given: they wish to be reminded when and how to carry out the techniques they have been taught.

Some have been encouraged to believe that they are in control during labour and may refuse sedatives or advice. They have been conditioned to expect to enjoy labour as an enriching and ennobling experience. Lack of success may be attributed to the attendants; the method given credit for success.

These women do not expect to be left alone at any time and much of the alleged success of psychoprophylaxis stems from the constant supervision and professional companionship they receive from midwives during labour.

Midwives should apply any of the beneficial psychoprophylaxis principles when caring for all women during labour.

Unfortunately some women experience acute feelings of failure when anæsthesia or operative procedures are necessary or when they do not cope well with, or enjoy, labour: a number having suffered severe depression. This new phenomenon, resulting from psychoprophylactic teaching, is to obstetricians and midwives a very disturbing element.

KEEPING FIT DURING PREGNANCY

A woman ought to look after her health during pregnancy for her own sake, but she is much more likely to do so for the sake of her baby. In order to appeal to expectant mothers the subject should be presented in such a way that the welfare of the baby predominates.

In a very elementary manner a few facts regarding the embedding and development of the

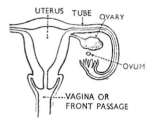

ovum could be taught. Simple illustrations showing how the baby is sheltered and nourished for nine months will interest the woman of average intelligence; such information being given only to stress the fact that the growing baby is dependent on the mother's food, on the fresh air she breathes and on her good general health.

The Talk as given

" Everyone knows that babies need good food and fresh air after they are born, but do you realize that babies need these before they are born as well ? Babies get milk, orange juice and cod-liver oil to make them healthy and strong, so if you take these foods now, the baby growing inside your body will also get the benefit of them.

" **We see babies out in their prams, getting fresh air,** but baby needs oxygen before he is born, too, so take him out for an airing every day, rain or shine. On sunny days sit in the garden or go to the park.

" **The baby inside the womb gets all the substances he needs for growth and good health from his mother's blood,** and these substances in her blood come from the food she eats. If your meals contain the necessary body-builders, calcium, iron and vitamins, baby will get them too and he will be strong and vigorous.

" **Just think of the gardener for a moment.** To ensure hardy plants he sows the seeds in well-prepared soil in a sunny garden. He tends the growing plants by watering them and keeping the weeds in check. He knows he won't get a good harvest otherwise."

HOW YOUR BABY GROWS

" **Your baby grows from two tiny cells,** no larger than the point of a fine needle, until he weighs about 3·1 kg. (7 lb.) on the day he is born. He obtains his food during this time without having to swallow or digest it, and gets oxygen without having to breathe. Both food and oxygen pass from mother to baby along the umbilical cord, which you see in this diagram is attached to baby's navel at one end and to the afterbirth at the other.

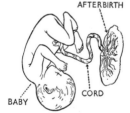

" **The afterbirth or placenta, is a mass of tissue which can be likened to the roots of a plant.** These roots are embedded in the wall of the womb, and by penetrating the small blood-vessels of that organ they absorb from the mother's blood the necessary food and oxygen."

THE NEED FOR BODY-BUILDING FOOD

" **Body-building foods are needed for baby's growth** and they include meat, fish, eggs, cheese and milk. You should have one of these at each of the three main meals. To give baby strong white teeth and straight limbs drink 1,200 ml. (2 pints) of milk every day. If you want your infant to have rosy cheeks when he is three months old, **give him** iron now ; take the iron tablets we have given you and eat foods such as liver, wholemeal bread and green vegetables."

" **But we must think of you as well as baby.** If you don't replace what baby is taking from your blood, you will become weak, easily tired and breathless, with no energy for housework. shopping and recreation.

" **An expectant mother should feel better than usual,** except for the little ailments such as morning sickness and heartburn; pregnancy isn't an illness, and life shouldn't become drab and the carrying of a baby a burden.

" **Plan your work so that you have time to rest and to go out.** Get yourself maternity clothes, so that you will enjoy walking out of doors, even during the last month. Wear sensible shoes to prevent backache, and I would recommend a maternity belt or corset during the last three months to give extra support.

" **Be sure that your bowels move every day.** Drink plenty of water and eat fruit and vegetables. If you are constipated, take a mild laxative, such as Senokot.

" **Go to bed early,** so that you will have nine hours sleep. During the last three months you will get tired towards the end of the day, so lie down for an hour after the midday meal."

SEE THE DOCTOR REGULARLY

" **There are early signs by which the doctor can tell that things are not as they should be** although you may feel perfectly well. Notify the doctor or clinic if you are ill and cannot attend. Do what the doctor advises. If he suggests more rest there is a reason why you should have it. If you are told to come into hospital but you feel you are needed at home, remember that this advice is in the interests of your baby and your family as well as yourself.

" **We want you to bloom with good health in readiness for your baby's birthday.** If you do, you won't get so tired during labour; you will have a better supply of breast milk; on getting up, you will feel stronger, ready to enjoy looking after your baby, family and home."

NUTRITION

The teaching of nutrition to expectant mothers is an essential part of prenatal care. Many pregnant women are malnourished although few are underfed; they are anæmic and flabby, some overfed with the wrong kinds of food.

From the nutritional point of view pregnancy and the first year of life are said to be the most important. It would therefore seem that maternal clinics at which health and nutrition could be supervised and taught during pregnancy are as necessary as child health clinics.

Many women have no knowledge of the foods that are beneficial or even necessary for the pregnant woman. Although the midwife may be aware of what constitutes a well-balanced diet and has scientific reasons for advocating certain foods, the factors that influence people in their choice of food and methods of cooking must be kept in mind, otherwise she is less likely to persuade expectant mothers to improve their dietary habits.

The food eaten in different countries varies according to climate, foods available, and custom. But even in a land such as Great Britain where a variety of foods is available, factors such as tradition, geographical location, religion, race, intelligence, education, social and economic status may influence the choice of food.

Married women in industry have increased the demand for processed, tinned and quickly prepared articles of food. All women should be taught more about what constitutes an adequate diet and how to plan and cook nutritious appetizing meals.

Functions of Food

The midwife is well aware of the functions of food and a few facts could be passed on to mothers, *e.g.* body-builders such as meat, fish, eggs, milk, cheese are needed for the health and growth of all the tissues of the body including the ovum and sperm from which the baby develops.

During pregnancy body-builders are needed for the growth of baby, the mother's womb. blood, and breasts

Food is eaten to allay hunger and carbohydrates such as bread and potatoes are reasonably cheap, readily available and satisfying, but they contain very little of the vital body-building food factors. Savoury foods are mostly proteins and although they are preferred because they appeal to the palate, unfortunately, they are expensive and that fact cannot be ignored. (*The midwife resident in hospital may have little idea of the cost of food.*) Vegetables contain the essential minerals but are not so appetizing but women must be persuaded to eat them because of their beneficial action. Fortunately, many body-building foods are also rich in minerals and vitamins, *e.g.* liver, eggs, milk, cheese.

Although the midwife knows the components of a well-balanced diet (see p. 63) she need not teach the details of this for if the amount of protein (90 *to* 100 *G. daily*) is adequate it is almost certain that the diet will be a well-balanced one.

Proteins, minerals and vitamins are the important constituents of food for the pregnant woman and she must be convinced of the need for these.

HINTS ON TEACHING NUTRITION

1. ADVICE SHOULD BE DEFINITE AND SPECIFIC

Telling a woman to take a nourishing diet has little educational value for each woman will have a different conception of what constitutes a nourishing diet. She may consider macaroni, ice-cream, cakes with cream filling to be highly nutritious, yet they contain no protein. Ambiguous terms such as "good", or "plenty", ought to be avoided.

2. SIMPLE DOMESTIC LANGUAGE SHOULD BE USED

Food should be discussed in terms of meals rather than protein, carbohydrate, fat and calories. The women can visualize and understand food values better when the food under discussion is what is served at meal times. The statement " three cooked meals a day " conveys immediately the idea of the body-building foods we advocate. Breakfast should be discussed, and kidney, eggs, bacon (not salty), fish, high quality sausages can be recommended. (*Many packaged cereals have little food value other than the sugar and milk added to them.*)

The need for a daily helping of meat, liver, chicken or fish at least 113 G. (4 oz.) at the main meal should be stressed. Vitamins and minerals will be contained in the potatoes and green vegetables served with the meat. Raw or stewed fruit should be advocated in preference to greasy suet puddings or very sweet desserts. Suitable supper dishes can be suggested which incorporate eggs, cheese or fish and salad.

3. THE NEED FOR IRON

This should be introduced on every possible occasion and by giving talks on subjects such as :—

FEED BABY BEFORE BIRTH.	BEAUTY HINTS FOR MOTHERS-TO-BE.
WHY MOTHERS ARE ANÆMIC.	EAT WISELY FOR BABY'S SAKE.
MEALS FOR LADIES-IN-WAITING.	KEEP FIT DURING PREGNANCY.

Merely giving a list of foods to be taken or avoided does not constitute a well-rounded lesson.

TEACHING AIDS

A cooking demonstration would be appreciated by the primigravid women who have limited experience in housewifery.

Dainty coloured china is a great asset when setting up trays with diets for expectant mothers.

Fresh foods should be displayed in preference to models which tend to look drab. Salads are always colourful, attractive, and give vitality to the demonstration ; new salad recipes are badly needed in Britain.

A bottle of milk should be on display as a constant reminder of the baby's need for calcium.

Posters are valuable visual aids. Cut-outs from the glossy magazines can be used as flannelgraphs to lend a gay tint of colour to the talk-demonstration.

Trays can be set with:

1. An ideal breakfast, lunch, dinner or supper. (*It is better to depict what s good rather than what is bad.*) 2. Body-building foods for one day. 3. Foods rich in iron. 4. Foods that keep weight under control.

The harmful effect of excessive salt in the diet should be explained and foods moderate in salt shown; those high in salt mentioned and condemned.

EAT THE FOODS THAT KEEP BABY AND YOU FIT

The Talk as given to Multigravid Women

" It is always mother who ' does without,' whether it is food, clothes or leisure. She is so busy providing father with good meals because he works hard; giving the children her share because they are growing fast and always hungry.

" But the expectant mother is the most important member of the family.

" Baby depends on you for the food he gets before birth. He grows from a speck the size of the point of a needle until he is a sturdy infant weighing 3·1 kg. (7 lb.). If you don't take in your diet the foods baby requires, he will rob your body of the substances he needs, and you will become anæmic and tired. Baby gets his rosy cheeks at your expense so try to provide the food needed to keep baby and you strong and healthy.

" Baby requires, most of all, body-building foods, iron and calcium (*lime*). Body-builders are foods such as meat, chicken, liver, eggs, milk and cheese, and one of these you should have three times every day. They are the only foods that build tissue (*or flesh*). Starchy foods and fats produce heat and energy and when taken in excess make you fat.

	Grams Protein.
Milk, 1,200 ml. .	40
Meat, 113 G. . .	20
White fish, 113 G. .	18
One egg . .	
Cheese, 15 G. . .	4
Whole-wheat bread, 150 G.	15
Total	103

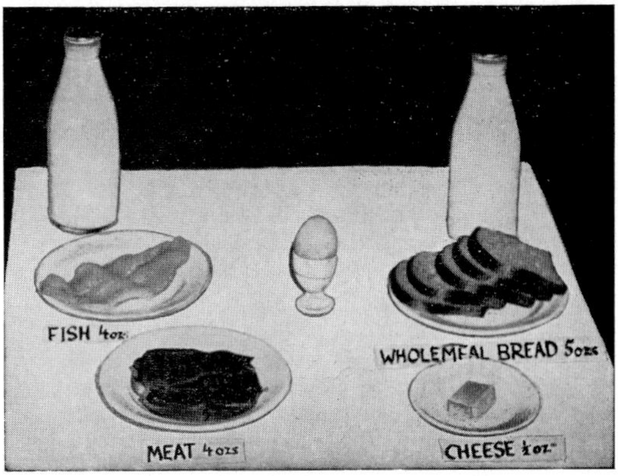

Fig. 483

One day's supply of body-building foods (proteins).

"IN YOUR DIET HAVE THREE COOKED MEALS EVERY DAY

"FOR BREAKFAST

" Bacon (not salty), egg, fish, or high grade sausages. If you can take porridge and milk also, so much the better; the crisp cereals contain less body-building substance.

"FOR THE MAIN MEAL

" Have 113 G. (4 oz.) of meat, liver, chicken or fish every day without fail. You won't take too much: few people could afford to eat more than they need of body-builders, as these valuable foods are expensive.

" AT SUPPER TIME

" Take another egg, fish, cheese or blood sausage.

" 600 ml. of milk contains one fifth of your needs in body builders; 1,200 ml. are better still. If you are overweight skim off the cream which is only fat and is not a body-builder.'

THE NEED FOR IRON

" Iron is the next most important substance needed by the mother-to-be. So many women are anæmic (bloodless) and this makes them feel tired and breathless. You need extra iron during pregnancy to supply iron for baby and for the additional blood you have to make for yourself at this time.

" During the years that you are having your babies you are very liable to become anæmic. That is why the doctor gives you iron tablets, but foods rich in iron are needed too.

" 1. You lose blood during menstruation and there is always the unavoidable loss of blood at childbirth.

" 2. Baby takes iron from you for his own blood and he also stores up a supply for the first three months of life for the milk he will get has no iron in it. Having three or four babies quickly, especially twins, is a terrific drain on the mother's supply of iron.

" 3. Many expectant mothers pay no attention to the kinds of food they eat and they become anæmic from lack of body-building foods and iron. Six slices of wholemeal bread gives you half of your day's supply of iron. Liver is best of all, but red meat, blood sausage, green vegetables, prunes and raisins are very good."

Good Food gives Good Health

" Of course you want a healthy strong baby : then eat the foods we recommend. If baby and you are well nourished you will both stand up to labour better and you will be ready sooner to look after baby, your family and home afterwards.

" Fruit and vegetables have important minerals and vitamins that are good for baby and you. Be sure you have an orange every day and other fruit if you can afford it.

" Remember too that baby is getting the benefit of these essential foods I have mentioned. We want you to come into labour looking the picture of health, feeling fit and full of vitality.

" Be careful with salt. You really should not eat salty foods and ought to add very little to your food at table. Too much may make your ankles swell.

" The doctors are concerned about a too rapid gain in weight during and after the fourth month. That is why you are always weighed at each prenatal visit. The foods that make your weight go up are the ones high in starch, sugar and fat. Bread, butter and jam is a fattening combination. Cakes and buns with whipped cream, ice-cream, chocolate and sweets should be very severely rationed.

" Give body-building foods to your husband and children to keep them healthy too.

" Suitable food isn't just a fad ; good health depends more on food than on anything else."

BEAUTY HINTS FOR LADIES-IN-WAITING

The title of this talk will no doubt appeal to the younger group of expectant mothers, but its real purpose is to stress health rather than beauty, with emphasis on nutrition. The midwife will find it well worth while going to some trouble in order to demonstrate the foods that are of value to pregnant women.

Young inexperienced housewives will appreciate being shown new ways of preparing meals, and the aid of a dietitian would be invaluable : cookery classes could be arranged.

The parentcraft teacher should stress that green vegetables and citrus fruits aid the absorption of iron.

TEACHING AIDS

Posters of sturdy babies should be on view, and will enable the midwife to correlate the mother's health and the baby's welfare.

The colourful salad mentioned in the talk should be freshly prepared and exhibited, as well as a tray of foods rich in iron and a bottle of milk, vitamin and iron tablets. These are shown to the class as they are mentioned.

The Talk as given

" Of course you are thrilled to be one of the fortunate ' ladies-in-waiting.' Let me assure you that the expectant mother can be more beautiful than ever, so banish the thought that you will be less attractive just because you are going to have a baby.

" **There is something radiant in the glowing cheeks, sparkling eyes, and natural red lips of the healthy, happy mother-to-be.** Remember too that if you are blooming with good health, you will feel fit and enjoy your pregnancy. Don't forget that **the baby you are carrying also gets the advantages of your aids to beauty ;** the nourishing food, the vitamin tablets, the fresh air and sunshine.

" **Motherhood is the crowning glory of a woman's life,** and your body at this time does its utmost to help you to produce a sturdy infant, so if you do your part you will be amply repaid in every way."

NATURE'S ROUGE

" **I'd like to recommend nature's rouge.** You get it in foods that are rich in iron, such as liver, meat, eggs, wholewheat bread and green vegetables ; the tablets the doctor orders for you are a great help, but the iron in food is better still. Fresh air and sunshine are also needed to make the red blood which gives that rosy glow to your cheeks.

" **Iron is a substance you must take a great deal of** when you are pregnant, because your baby removes a tremendous amount of it from your blood during the last three months. The reason for this is that baby's food after he is born, whether it is your milk or cow's milk, contains very little iron ; baby therefore stores the iron that he takes from you and uses it during the first four months of life, until he is given foods rich in iron, such as egg yolk. **Your supply must therefore be sufficient for baby's needs as well as your own."**

CLEAR SKIN AND BRIGHT EYES

" **If you would have a clear skin** drink at least two glasses of water daily ; flavour it with fruit juice for a change. Your complexion will be dull and pasty if you become constipated, but if you take plenty of fresh vegetables and fruit, as well as the water I have already mentioned, your bowels should move every day.

" **For bright eyes we recommend fresh fruit and vegetables** with their health-giving vitamins and minerals. Have you ever tried vegetable salad during the winter months ? Raw carrot, turnip and beetroot are delicious when grated ; add raisins to the carrot if you like, and arrange each vegetable separately in the salad bowl. Finely shredded raw cabbage is excellent if you add sufficient salad dressing to it. Chopped apple, with a sprinkling of crushed walnuts, well mixed with mayonnaise makes a very special salad, and if you add a little celery the flavour is quite delightful. Try it sometime. These foods are excellent for baby and you.

" **Your nails may tend to break off at the tips ;** this may well be because baby is taking a big share of the calcium (or lime) from your body to build for himself strong, straight limbs and a fine set of teeth. Milk is a rich source of calcium.

" **Do drink 1,200 ml. (2 pints) of milk every day;** use it for puddings ; add cocoa, Ovaltine or any flavour you choose if raw milk doesn't appeal to you. Cheese is also a rich source of calcium.

" **Tone up your hair by five minutes** of scalp massage and 100 brush-strokes at night. Many expectant mothers complain that their hair is dull and lifeless, but this occurs because they are not replacing, by taking nourishing food, the substances baby is taking from their bodies. A permanent wave doesn't always 'take' well during pregnancy, so it might be better to wait until baby is three months old."

Good Posture

" The biggest change is, of course, in your figure, but there is no reason why you cannot carry your precious burden with grace and dignity. **Good posture is the first essential;** head erect, chest raised, shoulders well back without lifting them, and the lower abdomen drawn in. An uplift brassière will support the breasts which become so much heavier and have a tendency to sag.

" A maternity ' roll on ' makes the pregnancy less noticeable, and the support it gives during the later months prevents backache and the tired feeling some women complain of. Do wear sensible shoes with a moderately low heel; extra support is required because the arches of your feet are carrying an additional load.

" Looking lovely and at your elegant best depends greatly on the clothes you choose, but good posture enables you to wear them with poise and style. Simple uncluttered lines are best.

ATTRACTIVE CLOTHES

" **Don't grudge yourself suitable maternity garments;** they are a necessity, not a luxury, and should be comfortable as well as becoming. When suitably dressed you can enjoy the same outdoor recreation as any other woman, so long as the games are not too exciting or strenuous.

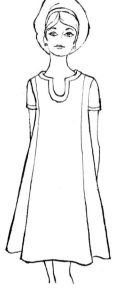

FIG. 484
VOGUE PATTERN.

" Sleekline washable neonspun dresses are flattering to the figure; a bright coloured silk scarf tied in a pirate knot gives individuality. Dicel crease resistant dresses are practical for housework, gay coloured floral ones you can wear at parties.

" **For wear in the mornings** tapered two-way stretch nylon or whipcord slacks with a U cut-out, worn with matching or contrasting satinized cotton tops, are popular with the trim, young mothers-to-be. **The simple flared pinafore dress** in charcoal grey coordinated with a gay contrasting jumper or check blouse is excellent from the fourth to the seventh month.

" Straight shift dresses are splendid for the tall girl but they are very revealing after the sixth month. Avoid front button-up dresses; they tend to gape later on. A Crimplene machine-washable non-iron dress with mandarin collar is a useful standby.

" Long-sleeved blouses team-up well with acrylic wool mixture pinafore dresses. Black stretch slacks with tapered leg line and elasticated nylon are ideal for the expanding waist-line. Kayser maternity tights with adjustable waistband can be worn with short dresses.

" **For simple social occasions** a brocade jacket is most flattering. Stoles help to keep secrets when worn elegantly.

" **You need not wear maternity clothes until the fifth month.** If you put them on too soon, you will be tired of them before the end of the ninth month, when you can't wear anything else.

" **Pregnancy itself is an aid to beauty,** for this new experience enriches your personality and gives to your face an expression of tranquillity and happiness. The understanding and tenderness shown by your husband helps to produce the serenity of mind which is so essential at this time, and which enhances the natural beauty of the lady-in-waiting."

BREAST FEEDING

The Talk as Given

" Everyone agrees that breast milk is the best food for babies; there is, however, no denying that many babies thrive on the bottle. But an infant gets more than food at the breast.

" The baby snuggled at the breast enjoys the warmth, the cuddling, the physical nearness of his mother. This induces a contented frame of mind, which, if it becomes a habit, may lay the foundation of a happy disposition.

"And what satisfaction it gives a mother to be aware that she is so necessary to her infant, for one of the joys of motherhood is to become. She sees her baby thriving on food she has produced, and knows she is giving her child a good start in life.

" From your point of view it is more convenient, for there are no bottles and pans to wash and no feeds to be heated at 06.00 hours in the morning. Breast feeding completes the process of childbirth and helps to restore your figure to what it was before you became pregnant."

DIFFICULTIES CAN BE OVERCOME

" There may be a few difficulties to overcome during the first few days, but you will be helped over these when the need arises. Hardly ever does the breast-milk upset baby, any difficulty that occurs is due to the method of feeding : it is possible that baby may take the milk too quickly or take too much. On the other hand, you may not have enough at first, but all of these things can be put right. To prevent your nipples from getting sore, we will show you how to look after them before baby is born.

" You may imagine that you will have to curtail your interests and pleasures outside the home if you breast feed your baby, but that really isn't so. During the first six weeks you will be resting more anyhow, and by that time baby will be on four-hourly feeding, and you can enjoy a visit to friends or the theatre within that time."

GOOD FOOD IS ESSENTIAL

" To ensure that you will have plenty of milk for your baby, start now. During these waiting months you should be having body-building foods, such as milk, eggs, fish, poultry and meat. They are the foods that help to produce milk.

"After baby is born you need the same good diet, but two other things are then important in helping to keep up a good supply of milk. These are calmness and sufficient rest. Make up your mind to take life easily for a week or two until baby and you have got the food question nicely settled. Shut your eyes to all the things that need polishing, and enjoy being lazy for a week or two.

" If he is your first baby, you may feel a little flustered with the responsibility of looking after your precious infant. Learn all you can about babies, but don't worry whatever you do. The health visitor will advise you and you can also attend the child health clinic.

" Persevere and you will succeed in giving your baby the food nature intended for him, as well as the contentment he enjoys when cuddled at his mother's breast."

STORK ON THE WAY

The Talk as given

" You are looking forward to the important day that lies ahead, your baby's birthday. It is true that for you it is a day of labour, but how hard and how long the labour will be depends to a great extent on yourself.

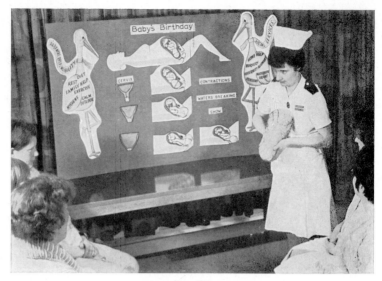

FIG. 485

TALK DEMONSTRATION ON LABOUR.
(*Aberdeen Maternity Hospital.*)

"Here is a drawing of the womb; this is the baby, lying head downwards in the bag of water which has protected him during pregnancy. You can see baby's cord attached to the afterbirth. The neck of the womb protrudes down for about 2·5 cm. (1 inch) into the vagina or front passage. Note that the opening into the womb is closed and sealed with a plug of mucus.

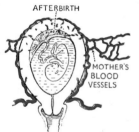

"When labour starts, the neck of the womb opens up and the plug of mucus escapes, with a slight staining of blood. That blood-stained mucus we call the 'show,' and you will see it a few hours before or after labour begins; it is one of the signs of labour."

HOW TO KNOW LABOUR HAS BEGUN

"There are three signs that labour has started, but don't wait for all three before sending for the midwife or coming to the hospital. We want to be with you from the beginning of labour, to help you as much as we can.

"1. SHOW

"This we have already mentioned.

"2. BREAKING OF THE BAG OF WATERS

"The bag of waters usually breaks some hours after labour has begun, but it may do so earlier. There is no pain when this happens, and perhaps only a slight trickle of water will come away.

" 3. CONTRACTIONS OF THE WOMB

" **This is a hardening of the womb,** which you can feel by placing your hand on your abdomen, and is accompanied by a feeling of abdominal discomfort. The contractions begin so gently that you won't realize you are in labour until you notice that they are coming regularly, probably every 15 minutes. Often there is backache as well, but not always.

" **These contractions stretch and open up the neck of the womb** until it is large enough to allow the baby's head to pass through it. This stretching or dilating period is known as the first stage, and occupies the whole of labour, except for the last hour or two. If the contractions are weak, labour will be slow, and you would, of course, expect a big baby to take longer to be born than a small one."

False Labour

" **You may be wondering about false labour,** which is fairly common during the last weeks. In that case you won't have any show ; the contractions are irregular and longer than true labour contractions which seldom last more than one minute.

" **False pains may be due to colic,** so make sure that you have a daily bowel movement during the later weeks of pregnancy, even if it means taking a mild laxative.

" **If you are in doubt or think you have started labour, come to the hospital,** especially if it is not your first baby. Certainly come if the contractions are strong, or if they are returning every 10 minutes or more often. And don't forget that **you may start labour before your expected date,** or you may go a week or more beyond that day."

MANAGEMENT OF LABOUR

'When labour starts, your external parts are washed and shaved by the midwife. Then you will be given a suppository or a small enema and a shower or bath. We shall ask you to take small light meals during the early part of labour to keep up your strength and so that you can help to push out your baby. **Remember that baby needs food** too so you should try to eat what we serve.

" **You will be given something to ease the discomfort** as soon as you really feel the need of it, but even the best drugs for this purpose slow down labour a little, so you should not clamour for them until you must. If you attend the " preparation for childbirth " classes you will probably require fewer sedative drugs.

" **Tell your husband or any near relative that they may come and sit with you,** if you wish, during the first part of labour ; bring a magazine and your knitting to pass the time or you can listen to the radio if you feel like it.

" **One thing you should not do is to ' bear down '** until we have told you to do so. If you look at this diagram (p. 726) you will see that baby cannot get through the neck of the womb until it is opened up sufficiently to allow him to pass. If you push too soon, the neck of the womb hardens and won't stretch, causing you unnecessary pain and a longer labour. It is bad for baby, too.

" **Towards the end of the second stage we shall ask you to hold your breath and push down,** but only while the womb is contracting. The muscles below (the pelvic floor) should be relaxed to make it easier for baby to be born, and you will be shown how to do this at the relaxation classes. Strangely enough, mothers usually complain less at this stage, and some prefer not to use the analgesia machine. But when you are drowsy from inhaling the analgesic gas you will experience very little discomfort and will certainly hear baby's first cry.

" **Baby usually announces his arrival by a lusty yell,** and you will experience a feeling of relief and great joy. He no longer needs oxygen and food through the umbilical cord ; so it is tied and cut ; now he will breathe and suck. Baby is wrapped in a warm bath towel and laid in a heated cot to rest after his strenuous journey. You may see him either before or after he is bathed, as you wish.

" **The after-birth comes away in about 5 to 10 minutes,** then you are tidied up and given some food. You may feel tired but elated, so to make sure that you will have a sound sleep we usually give you a sedative.

38A

" Baby's birthday is over : the little bundle is sleeping in his cot, and the majority of mothers say ' it was well worth it ' and ' wasn't nearly as bad as I expected.' "

REHEARSAL OF USE OF ANALGESIA MACHINES

ENTONOX, TRILENE, PENTHRANE

The demonstration should be preceded by :

(1) A talk on " What happens during labour." (2) A course in relaxation. (3) A tour round the labour and puerperal wards, and a glimpse of the babies.

The purpose of this rehearsal is :

1. To give the necessary tuition at a time when the woman is not distracted with pain or stupefied by drugs.

2. To reassure her regarding the safety and simplicity of the machine.

3. To make her familiar with the use of the mask.

4. To practise the various types of inhalation.

5. To gain her confidence and arouse enthusiasm for the analgesic gas.

Only the practical aspect of the subject should be taught and the mother's part in administration of the analgesic stressed. Much repetition will be necessary. Questions ought to be encouraged, but the midwife should tactfully keep them to the subject being taught.

TEACHING AIDS

A copy of the birth atlas, suitable illustrations of the birth canal. A machine similar to the one to be used during labour; extra masks for practice. Attractive pictures of babies and posters on health.

The Demonstration as given

" You all want your labour to be as comfortable as possible, and we are eager to do what we can to help you. To-day I am going to show you how you will use the apparatus during labour to relieve the sensation that some of you will call discomfort and others pain.

" Thousands of women all over Britain are grateful for the relief they got during labour from such a machine as this. It is perfectly safe for you and for baby. Not only is it simple to use, it is foolproof. The midwife is responsible for the working of the machine ; all you have to do is to breathe in the analgesic gas."

ANALGESIC GAS AND ITS EFFECT

" The gas is easy and pleasant to take ; it will make you feel calm and rather drowsy. It is not an anæsthetic, which is a substance that puts people to sleep and makes them unconscious. This gas is an analgesic, and an analgesic relieves pain without producing unconsciousness.

" If you decide that you don't want the gas, no one will force you to take it ; it is there for your benefit, and doctors and midwives are only too willing that you should have it.

" Some mothers are very keen to be awake in order to hear their baby's first cry. I can assure you that under this gas you will certainly hear it, a sound that will fill your heart with joy. You won't miss anything at all ; you will hear the midwife telling you when to inhale and when to stop, you will feel baby slipping out into the world, but it will be almost painless, so you can look forward to baby's birthday with pleasure.

" Gas will not be administered until you have been in labour for some little time. We start off by getting you to relax, and then when you need some relief we will give you a sedative which will probably make you sleep. Later on you will, if you require it, be given a second dose of the sedative, and when the effect of it is wearing off, the midwife will give you the analgesic gas.

" Here is the cylinder that contains the gas and oxygen; this piece of corrugated rubber tubing conveys the gas to the mask from which you will inhale. (During labour take care that you don't rest your arm on this tubing when you are inhaling gas or you won't get enough to be of any help.) We turn on the gas with this key, and it flows into the mask but it doesn't stream out as it does in your kitchen stove when you turn the gas on.

" You only get this gas when you actually inhale it (breathe it in)."

THE USE OF THE MASK

" The mask you are holding is similar to the one you will use during labour; it has a broad and a narrow end. Place the mask on your face like this ; the broad end is resting on my chin, the narrow end is on the bridge of my nose. Press the mask on firmly so that the rubber is in close contact with your face. Unless you do that, some of the gas will escape and you won't get the full benefit of it.

" If you have false teeth you should remove them before you start inhaling the gas.

"As far as you are concerned all you have to do is to breathe in and out with the mask on your face. The midwife will know when a contraction is coming by the hardening of the womb and she will tell you to inhale from the mask as soon as the womb contracts, and that will be before you feel any pain. The contractions will not last longer than one minute, but it takes about 20 seconds, or eight deep breaths of gas before you get relief; that is why you must start inhaling before you feel the pain. Stop inhaling when the pain goes.

" You may be wondering what would happen if you kept on inhaling after the contraction had ceased, or for longer than one minute. You would become sleepy and drop the mask, so, you see, you cannot take too much gas."

" During the first stage of labour you can inhale the gas lying on your side or your back, whichever is the more comfortable. During the second stage, the midwife will tell you which of the two positions she prefers for baby's birth. Between contractions you will relax but keep your mask beside you so that you can apply it again without delay."

Practice

" Will you lie down comfortably now, and practise using the mask without gas ? One inhalation includes breathing out as well as breathing in.

" Breathe through your nose and mouth, and use your abdominal as well as your chest muscles.

" Take full, regular breaths. (The midwife sets the pace at 18 to 22 breaths per minute.)

" Put on your masks now, and when I say ' Begin,' start inhaling; keep time with me as I say, ' In . . . out . . . in . . . out,' When I say ' Stop,' remove your mask and relax."

SECOND STAGE (PUSHING) INHALATIONS

" When baby's head is just showing, the time has come when you can assist by pushing. You will know then that it won't be long until your baby is born. The neck of the womb will have opened sufficiently to have permitted baby's head to pass through it, and the second stage will be well established.

" It is most important that you do not start pushing until the doctor or midwife tells you to do so. Pushing too soon will hinder rather than hasten baby's arrival, cause unnecessary pain, and may, later on, lead to falling of the womb.

" The contractions will be coming every two or three minutes now. The midwife will ' time ' them and tell you to start inhaling about 20 seconds before the next contraction is due, in order that you will have enough gas in your body to relieve the pain while you are holding your breath and pushing baby downwards."

Practice

" When I say, ' Begin,' put on your masks quickly and start inhaling; keep it up until I say ' Now.' You will then take a quick breath, hold it, but with lips tightly closed. Don't push here and now you must only push when you are actually in the second stage of labour. At that time you will keep pushing without taking a breath for as long as you can, then you will take another quick breath of gas, and again push for as long as you can.

" When I say ' Stop, remove your masks. During labour you may repeat the push twice ; it all depends on how long you can hold your breath, but a long sustained push is more effective than a number of short ones.

" It may be necessary for you to push with each succeeding contraction for a period extending to half an hour with your first baby ; then when baby's head is just about to be born the midwife will ask you to stop pushing and to breathe very deliberately.

DELIBERATE INHALATIONS FOR BIRTH OF BABY'S HEAD

" This type of breathing is only used for a matter of minutes, immediately before and during the birth of baby's head ; the purpose being to prevent you from pushing, so that baby's head will emerge slowly and gently. If you pushed at this time, as you will feel very much like doing, the skin at the opening of the birth passage would tear, and stitches would be necessary. So, to avoid this, stop pushing and breathe deliberately with your mouth and throat open concentrating on breathing in rather than breathing out immediately your midwife tells you to do so. At the same time try to relax your pelvic floor muscles to allow baby to be born easily.

" There must be no lull between in and out or out and in, because if you breathe steadily without hesitating for one instant you will not push, and that is what we want.

" This is the time when you need the greatest amount of gas, and as you may be inhaling constantly, you will get the maximal relief. Another midwife usually helps you to hold the mask in position to make sure you are getting as much gas as possible.

"As soon as baby's head is born the mask is removed, but you will be deliciously drowsy. You will feel baby's body slipping out quite painlessly. Very soon he will announce his arrival lustily, and you will be asking, ' Is it a boy or a girl ' ?

" This for you is a very precious moment. You may see baby before or after he is bathed, as you wish, and when baby and you are both tidied up, your husband and you can admire him together."

A DATE WITH THE STORK

In preparing this talk, the instructions given should coincide with the requirements of the local maternity home or hospital. For those who are to be confined at home a demonstration of equipment needed should be arranged later.

TEACHING AIDS

Posters of attractive babies, fruit and vegetables, bottle of milk, iron tablets, nightdress for breast feeding.

The Talk as given

"As baby's birthday draws near you may be surprised to find that you are eagerly looking forward to the big day that lies ahead ; in fact, you can hardly wait to find out whether your infant is boy or girl, dark or fair.

" Do try to keep your thoughts on baby rather than on yourself. If you begin to think about your own labour, switch off immediately and dwell on the fact that thousands of babies are born, simply and easily, every day, and that having a baby is a natural event in a woman's life. Picture yourself tucking baby into his cot or wheeling the pram ; happier thoughts. You will, of course, have been busy knitting, making or buying tiny garments for baby's arrival, and no doubt your husband and you have built many castles in the air regarding baby's future.

" But of all the preparations an expectant mother can make, none is more important than those for her own abundant good health.

THE LAST FEW WEEKS

"As your burden grows heavier you will feel cumbersome and become more tired towards the end of the day; so do take things easily, get off your feet as much as you can, and go to bed early. You don't need to coddle yourself, for the woman who carries on with her housework has an easier and shorter labour than the pampered type of woman who treats herself as an invalid.

" During the last weeks the slight abdominal discomfort you may feel, cramp in your leg or a desire to pass water frequently, may be a bit tiresome, but they will soon pass. Keep your heart light, for it won't be long until baby is here; you will regain your slim lines and enjoy wearing your favourite frocks once again.

" Do make sure that your bowels move every day, even if it means taking a mild aperient. We will, of course, give you a suppository or a small enema when labour starts, but it is better for you to have a regular motion every day until then.

" You have, I hope, been taking the diet we recommended, one which includes 1,200 ml. (2 pints) of milk, meat, fish, fruit and vegetables every day. Be sure to take your iron tablets, too, for baby and you both need a lot of iron during the last months.

" Go out every day even if it is wet or cold, so long as you are suitably clad. You need a change of scene as well as fresh air; the sight of other women wheeling their prams will remind you that very soon you will be doing the same."

MAKE PLANS EARLY

" Make an effort to have all your arrangements completed before the end of the seventh month, for, as you know babies do sometimes come too soon. Pack a small suitcase with the things you will need in hospital, or make out a list, for it isn't easy to think of what to take with you when labour starts at 02.00 hours. Your own dressing-gown, night dresses and slippers are always nicer than those the hospital can provide. Have two face cloths, so that one can be used for your face and breasts.

" Baby's clothes won't be needed until you are going home, but pack the case before you leave so that your husband won't have to search for them on that thrilling day when you are allowed to take your baby home.

" By all means take cosmetics with you for afterwards, but for your own sake you should not apply rouge, lipstick, or nail-paint until labour is over. Your natural colour is a guide to the doctor or midwife as to how you are faring during labour.

" Your watch will be handy at feeding times when the midwife tells you to feed baby for 5, 10 or 15 minutes. Take your purse and a little money with you for newspapers, telephone calls, or some item you may have forgotten to bring. Writing-paper and stamps you will almost certainly need."

STORK LATE IN ARRIVING

" Mothers often worry when the expected date arrives and the stork fails to appear. Don't let that disturb you, for babies rarely come on the exact date on which they are expected, in fact, half of the babies are a week late in arriving. It is, of course, possible that you have made a mistake in your dates. Attend the clinic or your own doctor or midwife every week as usual; they will keep a watchful eye on your progress.

" Let this, your first date with the stork, be a happy one. Look forward to it calmly with a glow of anticipation in your heart, and when baby's birthday is over and he lies cuddled in your arms it will be one of your most treasured memories."

REHEARSAL OF LABOUR

This class should be a very practical one and not merely a recapitulation of all that has previously been taught on the physiology of labour. As far as is possible the woman's part in the procedure of labour should be rehearsed or explained; an effort being made by vivid word pictures—positions and practice-breathing to set the scene. The rehearsal should be patient-centred not procedure-centred. Likely happenings during the pre-labour days can be narrated, lightening and passing urine frequently being mentioned as a sign that baby is settling down into the pelvis in readiness for his outward journey. Advice can be given regarding the need for additional rest and how to avoid constipation.

Signs of false and true labour should be related to the woman as a person and what she ought to do ; " show " and breaking of the waters being described once more. They could be told about women inadvisedly waiting for the waters to break before leaving home, with resultant anxiety, or even birth in the ambulance. A reminder to have a case packed with toilet articles, etc., for hospital ready to avoid fluster should the call come suddenly during the night. What to do and when to come to hospital should be clearly explained, and time allowed for questions. Assurance should be given about the stork sometimes being late in arriving and the need to continue attending the clinic.

They are advised not to start rhythmic breathing at home: women become parched and tired when this is carried on too long. They should come to hospital in time to use rhythmic breathing under supervision. A brief résumé of what happens on arrival at the hospital is given: if husbands are to be present this aspect will be discussed. A reminder is given about the need for sleep, light food and passing urine frequently and that relaxation with sedative drugs is all that is usually necessary during the first half of labour.

All the labour positions, passive and active relaxation, controlled breathing, holding the mask and using the tennis ball should be rehearsed. Relaxing the pelvic floor and the special breathing to counteract pushing during the perineal phase is practised. The gas and oxygen cylinder is put on view and a mask rehearsal given.

They can be shown how to relax when up and about during labour. If the woman is on her feet when a contraction comes on she should lean over the back of a chair, head resting on her arms, feet apart. If sitting in an easy chair she leans back, head lolling to one side, arms relaxed resting on chair arms, legs apart and relaxed.

The midwife rounds out the lesson with additional comments and advice particularly concerning the actual birth. The third stage needs little description. To enlarge on the moment of joyous relief when baby is born and the thankfulness experienced when baby lies asleep in his cot is a happy note on which to end.

CLASSES FOR HUSBANDS

Too often the expectant father is made to play a minor or supporting rôle. His feelings deserve greater consideration: he may be dubious as to how he will respond to the duties and responsibilities of fatherhood. He needs advice and encouragement.

The average husband has little idea of what is required of him as an expectant father, but it is only reasonable that he should take an active interest in the subject of childbearing and have some knowledge of the physical and emotional demands it makes on his wife.

During this century, men have been taking an increasing interest in the subject of child-bearing and rearing. Mothers in the past may have been too possessive, but they should be advised to allow the father to participate in baby care from the very first weeks.

Midwives should arrange evening classes to which husbands are invited with their wives, teaching subjects such as :

" KEEPING FIT DURING PREGNANCY," " THE DEVELOPMENT OF THE BABY BEFORE BIRTH," " WHAT HAPPENS DURING LABOUR."

They should not be encouraged to think of themselves as a small unique group but as modern sensible men.

Some hospitals have classes for husbands after the evening visiting hour in pre- and post-natal wards.

A WORD TO THE EXPECTANT FATHER

The Talk as given

" The fact that you are attending these classes shows that you have an up-to-date outlook and are willing to share with your wife some of the responsibilities as well as the joys of parenthood.

" Women should not be expected to bear the whole burden of childbearing and rearing alone; your wife needs your help, encouragement and understanding.

ENCOURAGE YOUR WIFE TO KEEP FIT

" If your wife is healthy and properly nourished she will feel well and enjoy her pregnancy; a good diet is most important and it is quality rather than quantity that matters. During pregnancy the baby deprives a woman's body of vital substances, for a baby grows at his mother's expense. Unless your wife replaces these substances by having nourishing food her body will suffer.

" Mothers are apt to neglect themselves, and to take what food is left after father and the children have been served, so you must see that she gets her fair share of body-building foods such as meat, fish, eggs and liver."

IRON IS VERY NECESSARY

" Baby, before birth, takes a great deal of iron from his mother's blood and unless your wife has a diet that is rich in iron she will become anæmic, feel breathless and tired; and pregnancy will be blamed for what is really due to anæmia.

" Liver is an excellent blood-forming food; encourage your wife to have it at least once a week. No doubt the doctor has prescribed tablets containing some form of iron, remind her to take them regularly every day.

"A well nourished woman stands up better to the stress of labour and has more energy to look after baby and the home afterwards. Baby also benefits; he will be more vigorous when born, and will have fewer illnesses during the first year of life."

OUTDOOR RECREATION

" Both baby and mother-to-be will profit from a daily outing; the change of scene will keep your wife more cheerful, she will enjoy her food, and sleep better. Of course she must have maternity garments in which she will feel less conspicuous; they are a necessity so do not grudge the money spent on them, for an expectant mother ought to enjoy a normal social life up to the last month."

Help as much as you can

"As the months wear on, your wife will be less able for the more strenuous household tasks. Assist her in turning heavy mattresses. If you already have an infant under 18 months old he will be heavy for your wife to lift, so do take care of him for a spell occasionally.

" See that your wife gets sufficient rest by lending a hand with the housework if extra domestic help is not available; otherwise you should not expect all the comforts and luxuries you usually enjoy at home."

THE EMOTIONAL ASPECT

" There is no doubt that the nervous system is more sensitive during pregnancy, and especially with the first baby. Moods of depression may overwhelm your wife for no reason; she doesn't know why she is depressed, and on these occasions tears flow on the slightest provocation. There is no need to be dismayed at the prospect of such episodes, for they only arise very occasionally. It is simply futile to tell her to ' snap out of it,' and to ignore these moods is a subtle form of cruelty.

" The pregnant woman may seem unreasonable, and won't appreciate logical argument; she will more likely respond to tenderness and understanding. Help her to look on the bright side; planning some small treat or an outing will direct her thoughts into happier channels. The man who willingly and pleasantly gives his wife a cup of tea in bed during the miserable time of morning sickness is providing the best medical and psychological treatment for that condition.

" **Every pregnant woman has vague fears**—fear of pain, fear of the process of birth, fear of the unknown. Many of these fears are groundless, but to her they are none the less real. Her judgment is all tangled up in the web of her emotions, and she needs the stabilizing influence of her husband's sound, well-balanced outlook."

CO-OPERATE WITH THE DOCTOR

" **See that your wife attends the clinic or her doctor regularly and always uphold the advice she has been given**; never suggest that it is unnecessary or that you do not approve. If, for example, your wife has been told to take extra rest, this may mean that her blood pressure is higher than it ought to be; **it is most important that she carries out the doctor's instructions** and I'm sure you will help her to do so. Your encouragement and sympathetic understanding at this time mean a great deal to her and will help to weld, even more securely, the marriage bond.

" **Take an interest in the various activities arranged for expectant mothers at the clinic** and encourage your wife to participate in them. The ' Preparation for Childbirth ' classes will help her to have an easier labour; at the course on baby-care she will be given advice on how to look after baby, and as you would expect, there is much to learn on that subject."

Learn about Babies

" **It isn't fair to learn about babies by experience.** When studying baby care for the welfare of your own infant you will find this interesting subject absolutely fascinating. The information so gained will help to keep your child healthy and happy and the confidence such knowledge gives will enable your wife and you to enjoy your baby instead of worrying over your lack of experience.

"**A little knowledge and a lot of common sense will solve most of the simple baby problems,** and a man is not as liable to panic over minor ailments as is the over-anxious mother. Take an interest in the preparations for the coming baby. Study catalogues of various makes of prams and learn about the good points to look for. It doesn't take much skill or ingenuity to make or remodel a few pieces of furniture and paint them in pastel shades. That is the sort of thing women appreciate."

WHEN LABOUR STARTS

" **Don't expect your wife to go into labour on the exact day ;** baby may arrive, one week, before or after the date given. There may be a few false alarms so I'll tell you the signs of true labour so that you can help to reassure your wife if she is in doubt. (These signs are well known to midwives and need not be repeated here.)

" **Keep calm and help your wife to carry out the instructions she has been given** at the clinic or by her doctor or midwife. As a rule there is no immediate urgency with first babies, but don't delay with subsequent ones as they sometimes arrive very quickly."

Should the Husband be Present at the Birth ?

" **There is no valid objection if he can be of any assistance to his wife ;** the British husband usually prefers to remain in the background even when the confinement takes place at home, but some husbands wish to be present.

" **Husbands are allowed to be present in certain countries;** in some hospitals in Great Britain, and in selected cases, they are permitted to be in the labour ward while the baby is being born. They should not be made to feel that they ought to be present.

" **Watching the birth of a baby is an experience which may emotionally upset those who are closely related to the mother** and husbands have been known to faint. The midwife's attention is concentrated on the two lives under her care at this critical moment and should not be diverted. The husband who intends to be present should attend classes so that he knows what to expect. He is there to give emotional support not as an observer.

" It is, however, a matter of tradition as well as of personal opinion, and though the wishes of the parents ought to be given due consideration, the immediate safety of mother and baby should be the deciding factor."

QUESTIONS FOR REVISION

C.M.B.(Eng.) paper.—Outline a talk to expectant mothers on the importance of nutrition in pregnancy.

C.M.B.(Eng.) paper.—What is the value of classes for preparation for childbirth and mothercraft ? What subjects should be included in a series of such classes ?

42

After Baby Comes

BUDGETING FOR BABY

The midwife ought to have some comprehension of housekeeping and budgeting and know the cost of equipment, such as prams, cots, baths, as well as the advantages and disadvantages of the various types, so that she is in a position to recommend articles at a suitable price to meet the needs of the different groups.

Expectant mothers may have been told what is required by neighbours or friends and be familiar with certain garments or articles; the teacher should not underestimate their knowledge and common sense. The intelligence and social background of groups may differ widely and the advice given must suit their mode of life. Teenage mothers may have difficulty in budgeting their weekly domestic allowance and on receiving the Maternity Grant may spend it unwisely. The midwife who is teaching expectant mothers needs understanding of such problems.

The market is flooded with a profusion of articles that attract the mother-to-be: but some are neither essential, serviceable nor commendable. The midwife must of course make allowance for the mother's youth, inexperience and desire to buy attractive items for her baby. It is always worth while visiting the baby equipment shops, or to send for catalogues to keep in touch with modern trends.

THE PRAM

Not all mothers can afford the well sprung coach-built type of pram nor can these be negotiated in lifts or stored in multi-storied flats; the chrome folding chassis with folding body is reasonable in price. A thick mattress and extra blankets are necessary in winter: foam-padded sides are needed when the carry-cot transporter is used. Mothers should be advised not to use a push chair for babies during the first year of life; their spines need the support of a firm mattress.

A WORD TO THE NEW FATHER

"**Around the fourth day after confinement** and on occasions, later, your wife may feel slightly depressed and dissolve into tears for no apparent reason. Be encouraging, because she may feel overwhelmed with her new responsibilities. Assure her of your assistance in the home, see that she gets good nourishing meals and sufficient sleep. This phase will pass when the glands in her body adjust to the post-natal state that follows childbirth.

"**After baby is born your wife may feel weak and be unable to cope with her daily housework,** so don't grumble if meals are late and the standard of housekeeping is not up to the usual level. A baby creates about three hours extra work daily and an inexperienced mother may take longer than that; lend a hand, this is only a temporary phase which will soon pass.

Above all, try not to feel neglected and resentful; the maternal instinct is very strong at this time and the mother's whole attention is centred on her baby almost to the exclusion of everything else. Be unselfish, remember that your wife has endured all the discomforts of pregnancy and labour, allow her to enjoy the pleasant task of looking after her baby.'

WHEN BABY CRIES AT NIGHT

When baby cries at night, as he may well do during the first week after going home from hospital, until he settles into a regular sleeping and feeding routine, **be patient.** A crying baby upsets the mother far more than the father, for the maternal instinct makes her unduly protective and overanxious. If you become irritable this only adds to the nervous tension your wife is experiencing.

LEARN TO ATTEND TO BABY

" **Why not help with some of the little jobs for baby,** many fathers enjoy doing them. If there are other children take over the care of the youngest one, toddlers are very liable to feel jealous and should be handled with patience, given a new toy and extra affection until they accept the new baby.

" **Very soon baby will recognize you and give you a beaming smile of welcome,** then you will appreciate the real joy of fatherhood.

" **The expectant father has a very important part to play** at this time, and will reap great satisfaction by sharing the load of parenthood. Babies are a source of constant delight, and it is worth while studying how to handle them physically and psychologically, in order that they may develop into healthy happy persons."

BABY'S LAYETTE

The mother-to-be gets great pleasure in buying or making baby's layette, for this provides an outlet for her urge to do something for her coming infant. It is understandable that her thoughts should turn to appearance, for she anticipates the joy of seeing her infant clothed in lovely garments. Without damping her enthusiasm, for we want to encourage her to take pride in her baby's clothes, she should be persuaded that **baby's health and comfort depend to a great extent on how he is clothed;** the question of cost, wearing and washing qualities must be considered, but there is no reason why suitable garments cannot also be attractive.

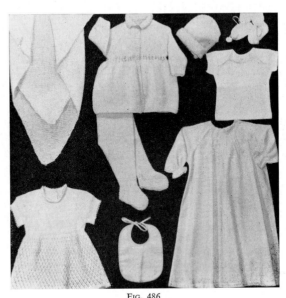

FIG. 486

SUGGESTIONS FOR BABY'S LAYETTE.
(*Royal Maternity Hospital, Rottenrow, Glasgow.*)

What the Midwife should know about Baby Clothes

The midwife should be conversant with the requirements of baby clothes, the cost, advantages and disadvantages of various fabrics including those that are flame-proof, *i.e.* Proban. Brushed nylon does not catch alight but it may melt and burn the skin. Regulations (1964) banning the sale of inflammable night wear do not apply to garments for babies under one year. The teacher ought to know the good points of the various styles and be able to recommend the newer designs. Such information can be drawn on when necessary to strengthen the argument for, or against, some particular material or pattern. **When fortified with such knowledge,** the midwife can talk with greater confidence and conviction.

WARMTH

Baby must be kept warm without causing undue perspiration, irritating his skin or inhibiting movement.

Babies are usually grossly overclad in summer, and sun and air, with their health-giving properties, never reach their skins. Excessive heat causes baby to lose his appetite, and constant profuse perspiration is weakening; the moist skin being prone to chafing and infection. Baby catches one cold after another. The garments worn should vary, just as with adults, according to the temperature of the room or, if out of doors, the weather.

COMFORT

This is essential for sound sleep, and to avoid the irritation that leads to persistent crying. Fabrics ought to be soft, light in weight, and smooth in texture. Designs should be roomy with no tight bands or other restrictions.

STYLE

Simplicity and comfort are the keynote of good style. Clothing should not interfere with baby's natural desire to wriggle and kick. Movement stimulates the circulation of blood and the absorption of food, as well as developing the muscles in readiness for sitting, standing and walking.

Fabrics

Wool is expensive, irritating to some skins, and when badly washed the garment shrinks, becoming hard, tight and short. **Pure wool in vests is irritating to some babies' skins;** in pilches and stockings it shrinks with the constant wetting. A mixture of silk or cotton and wool is better for these garments.

Wool and cotton mixtures, such as Osmalane, Viyella and the less expensive Clydella, are excellent for nightgowns and dresses. Proban flame-proof fabrics are now on the market. **Orlon** shawls and other garments should not be washed in very hot water; the fibres twist and the garment loses shape which cannot be rectified. Acrilan double knitting fibre is suitable for shawls and pram suits, it is soft and doesn't shrink.

HOW TO GIVE THE TALK-DEMONSTRATION

Showing a layette to a group of women is comparatively easy, but the educational value of such a demonstration is extremely limited unless each garment is used as a pivot round which much good advice is concentrated.

The garments should be immaculate, either freshly laundered or pressed for the occasion; a few of the more attractive items could be displayed on hangers, but it is probably better to exhibit each garment when describing it.

Have an intriguing opening sentence, such as: " One of the joys of the Lady-in-waiting is planning her baby's wardrobe." " Nothing gives the mother-to-be greater pleasure than sewing and knitting for the coming baby." " Who would think that fashions would change in the tiny garments babies wear; let me show you some of the latest models."

Arrange the clothes in the order in which you will show them, *e.g.* begin at the skin and work outwards. It is advisable to have a plain, dark surface behind you, such as a blackboard, against which you hold the garments to show up the detail.

Introduce the various articles in a different way to avoid monotony.

Exhibit each garment sufficiently long for the group to study the detail ; a glimpse is not sufficient. You, the teacher, must only glance at the garment, your eyes should be on the audience. It is better not to pass the garments round until the end of the demonstration, or the attention of the audience will be distracted from the garment you are describing.

Be prepared to answer questions as to the approximate cost, and have a general idea regarding the amount of material and wool required.

Hand out a typed list of garments to those who wish to have it.

N.B.—No two people would agree on the number of garments they consider to be essential ; mothers and midwives both have their personal preferences. Climate and financial status must be taken into account.

The Talk as given

" I know you all want your babies to look adorable, for every mother pictures her beautifully dressed infant lying asleep in his cot. There is no reason why baby clothes can't be lovely, but we must consider other things besides appearance, for baby must be kept warm and comfortable, sweet and clean.

The modern lady-in-waiting considers health and comfort before appearance when planning baby's wardrobe.

" Comfort is the important thing in baby's life, and as far as clothes are concerned it means freedom to wriggle and kick in garments made, in a roomy style, of fabrics that are smooth and soft. A comfortable baby is more likely to be contented during the day and to sleep soundly at night.

" Baby will be sleeping most of the time during the first three months, so the nightgown is most important. Day-gowns aren't really necessary ; in fact, a touch of embroidery on the nightgown and a dainty matinée jacket will make him quite presentable for visitors.

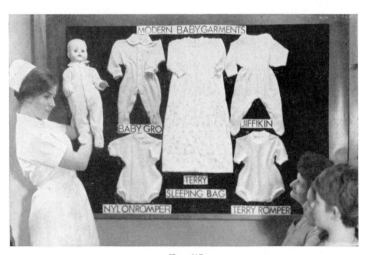

FIG. 487

Some modern baby garments.

(*Mothercraft Department, Royal Maternity Hospital, Rottenrow, Glasgow.*)

" **Baby must be kept warm in the cold winter months;** there is a danger of chilling him at night so get a wall thermometer and keep the bedroom temperature at about 18·3° C. (65° F.).

Don't keep him too warm in summer; if you keep him bundled in layers of wool he will become like a hothouse plant. It is weakening for baby to perspire all the time, and whenever a breath of cool air reaches him, he catches cold."

BABY GARMENTS

" *I will now show you the baby clothes.*

VESTS (3 or 4)

" **Bought vests are beautifully soft and kind to baby's skin.** This one of wool and silk has a splendid overlap, and is long enough. A wool and cotton mixture is also suitable.

" **Do remember how quickly baby grows;** your infant may weigh as much as 5·4 kg. (12 lb.) at three months, so select a roomy make of vest.

" **The modern envelope neck slips easily over baby's head,** yet it fits cosily round the neck with no draw-string for baby to pull tight.

" **In winter you may wish to have a hand-knitted one** like this to wear over the bought vest. It is made of non-shrink wool, and the rib pattern clings to baby and makes the vest stay in place better. Three tiny buttons in front give an ample opening to go over baby's head easily. " I'd like to warn you about draw-strings at the neck which baby might pull tight: don't use them.

" **Sew on a tab like this to pin baby's napkin to.**

" GOWNS (4)

" **The nightgown is the all purpose garment for the new baby,** who should not be lifted from cot or pram to be handled by relatives and friends.

" **Here is a model garment designed for the modern baby.** It is made from 1·3 metres (1½ yards) of Osmalane or Clydella and is 0·6 metres (27 inches) long with a deep hem; the draw-string at the bottom makes it into a cosy sleeping-bag, with plenty of kicking-space. Notice the front fastening with three buttons; there are no fastenings at the back to hurt baby's neck. **If you want to be up to date do not have a waistband.** It is of no use whatsoever, and only hampers baby's breathing and makes uncomfortable wrinkles to lie on.

" **The Babygro sleeping suit** with feet, stretches and will fit baby from birth to 12 months. The press stud fastenings down the inside of the legs are convenient for nappy changing. The ' Baby Chic ' Coverall or baby stretch of bri-nylon cotton terry is a similar garment.

" SHAWLS (2)

" **The best pattern in shawls has a plain centre and a closely knitted border.** The Shetland or lacy patterns are not now recommended as they aren't really warm, and baby's fingers get entangled in the meshes. These two shawls are 1·3 metres (1½ yards) square. This one is of three-ply wool and has a 30 cm. (12-inch) border of moss stitch (1 plain, 1 purl, reversed each row); this other one is made of two-ply wool and has a border of 4 plain 4 purl blocks.

" **Let me give you a special word of advice. A knitted shawl is not warm enough out of doors to carry baby in during cold weather, for it isn't windproof.** You need a large enveloping blanket as well. Neither is a knitted suit warm enough; many babies are not properly clad for out of doors in winter time.

"SNUGGLING BLANKETS (2)

" **I would like to recommend, very strongly, this blanket which is made from 0·9 metres** (one yard) **of fine flannel.** You can bind it with 3·8 cm. (1½ inch) ribbon like this, or buttonhole it with fine pastel-coloured wool. It is useful for everyday wear, is cosy at night, less expensive, and does not require to be stretched, when being dried, like a shawl.

"DRESSES (4)

" **Dresses are not really necessary during the first three months.** On chilly days this cream Osmalane or Clydella one would be very suitable. See how wide it is between the shoulders for that is where baby will need the width later on.

" **After the four-month milestone is passed** the dainty Tricel or Bri-nylon dresses that are so easy to launder may be worn when showing baby at her adorable best. The ready-made ones are extremely attractive; ask to see some of the dainty fabric dresses.

"MATINÉE JACKETS (3)

" **Baby need only wear these on cold days.** As they are a favourite gift to the new baby, I wouldn't make more than one. They are often knitted too loosely to have any warmth; but the cardigan-style buttons up to the neck and is really cosy. Don't you agree that this lemon-yellow one of baby nylon yarn is dainty, beautifully warm and a welcome change from pink or blue.

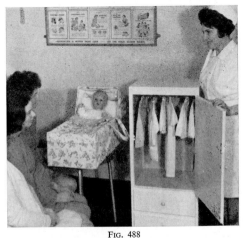

Fig. 488

BABY'S WARDROBE.
(*Mothercraft Department, Royal Maternity Hospital, Rottenrow, Glasgow.*)

"LEGGINGS

"**Along with the cardigan the leggings make a useful outfit to keep baby as warm as toast in the pram.** Some mothers like them instead of dresses, but wool leggings shrink with constant wetting and washing. Tights in red, blue or white bri-nylon, with matching Toppers make an attractive ultra-modern outfit.

"NYLON KNITTED HOODS (2)

" **On fine days baby's head should be bare,** but on cold windy days his ears should be kept warm, especially at teething time. This one is lined with silk for additional warmth.

" **Some mothers find little use for hoods, stockings and gloves,** but they are a necessity during winter in the northern counties of England and in Scotland.

" MITTS (2 pairs)

" These are useful if baby scratches his face or sucks his fingers, as well as for keeping tiny fingers warm in wintry weather. Wool ones can be dangerous if baby sucks them and chews the knots that form. Chilprufe mitts do not form knots and have a shirred elastic wristband. Sea island cotton mitts are excellent. **Mothers should be warned that loose** threads from the inside seam may wind around and severely damage tiny fingers. Seams should be oversewn securely.

"BIBS (6)

"Any soft material will do : these are made of four-fold butter muslin. If worn at feeding time they keep baby's gown sweet and clean ; later on they are necessary when baby starts dribbling. **Beware of the plastic ones.** They have been known to blow over baby's face, and he can't breathe through plastic ; he will suffocate.

" **There is a bewildering range of fabrics and styles in baby clothes,** but if you remember that baby must be kept warm, clean and comfortable, and that the garments should wash and wear well, the layette you select is almost certain to be a good one."

NAPKINS

" **Baby will need about 12 napkins every day,** so you require three dozen in order that you need only wash napkins once daily.

You may be interested to see the various ways of putting on the napkin

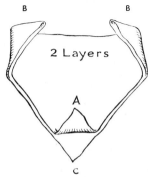

THE TRIANGULAR FOLD

" THE TRIANGULAR FOLD

" **There are different ways of using the triangular fold.**

" **1. Lay a medium-sized napkin folded corner-wise under the buttocks ; bring the corner A, single fold, well up between baby's legs** before wrapping the corners B around the inside of the thighs : this prevents soiling of B corners with stool. In this way all the ends are utilized to soak up urine.

" **2. A large napkin may be folded twice corner-wise, giving four layers ;** the three corners are pinned in front.

"THE PILCH METHOD

" **Fold the napkin like this.** Lay the broad end below the buttocks, and bring the narrower end up between the legs : the fold from behind lapping over the one in front, and the safety pins being inserted horizontally and nearer the front so that baby won't have to lie on them.

" **Try these methods and use the one you like best ;** experience will help you to decide.

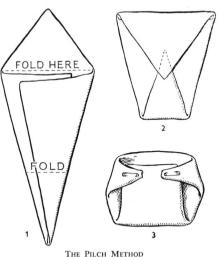

THE PILCH METHOD

FIG. 489

" **Turkish towelling ones** should be 0·6 metres (24 inches) square ; you will need two dozen. If two napkins are worn one should be laid under or wrapped round the buttocks :

two being too bulky to bring between the legs during the first two months. They absorb the quantities of urine baby passes as he grows older. Maws disposable nappy liner is placed in the centre of the terry napkin.

" **One-way napkin liners.** 'Marathon' or Johnson's disposable liners or Harrington's disposable nappy roll liner all permit urine to pass through to the outer napkin while keeping the buttocks dry. 4 are needed.

" **Disposable napkins such as the Paddi-pads are useful on occasions;** nappy rolls are also available. If plastic pants are used they should be washed daily to avoid an unpleasant odour, and napkins changed when wet, or sore buttocks will occur."

The new " **shaped** " napkins are not bulky and look neat but do not soak up as much urine as the triangular fold.

HOW TO HANDLE AND DRESS BABY

Many mothers would benefit from instruction on how to handle and dress their babies. It is evident that they do not realize how weak baby's spine is, for we see them unfastening the back of the dress of a three-weeks-old baby while they hold him in a sitting posture.

They also carry very young infants in an upright position and sometimes neglect to support the head and spine properly.

The Talk as given

" **Have you noticed how a crying baby is soothed and quietened in the arms of an experienced person:** this is because of the smooth firm way he is handled. A baby likes to feel supported and secure when he is lifted from his cot, so you must handle your baby deliberately yet gently, for quick jerking movements jolt and irritate him."

SUPPORT BABY'S HEAD AND SPINE

"**Always support the head of a baby until he is over three months old,** because his neck muscles are so weak. Watch while I show you how he should be lifted out of his cot.

" **Slip your left hand under his shoulders and support his head on your arm like this.** Slide your arm along his back to support the whole length of the spine; his head is now nestled

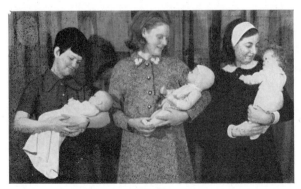

FIG. 490

STUDENT MIDWIVES DEMONSTRATING HOW TO HOLD A BABY.

(*a*) First three months; (*b*) second three months; (*c*) third three months.

(*Aberdeen Maternity Hospital.*)

in the crook of your elbow. At the same time put your right arm over and under the baby's buttocks. To lay him down continue to support his head and spine, then slip your hand out. I'll do that again.

" **The bones in a baby's spine are not properly hardened**; the muscles of the back are weak, so you should carry him like this. Don't sit him up when you are unfastening his clothes at the back. Turn him over and lay him face down on your knee. If you want your baby to have a nice straight back, let him lie flat in his cot or pram. Not until the fourth month should baby be propped up on pillows.

" **Let me show you how to handle baby on your lap.** Sit on a low chair and separate your knees slightly to make a lap.

" **To turn baby, grasp him by the body**; lift and roll him towards you, on to his face. To turn him back, roll him in the same direction—towards you.

" *Now, I shall let you see the different positions we use when bathing a baby* and in the next class you will see them again when I show you how to bath baby."

DRESSING BABY

" **If you plan baby's layette so that the clothes all fasten at the front or back,** the business of dressing will be much easier. Try to undress him without turning him oftener than is necessary. Undo all the available fastenings first, and you can slip loose garments, such as matinée jackets, off without moving baby very much.

" **Babies don't like clothes being pulled on over their heads,** so put them off and on from below if you can. Remember, too, that babies don't like being bundled up tightly; they love freedom to wriggle and kick even during the very first weeks, so wrap his shawl loosely round his arms.

" **This is the method of putting on a vest fastening at the front.** The far-away arm goes in first. Slip your fingers into the wrist-end of the sleeve and draw his hand through it to prevent tiny fingers or nails catching in the sleeve. Slip the vest behind his shoulders without raising him. Draw the arm nearest you into the sleeve in the same way, like this."

BATHING BABY

This is the most popular of all the talk-demonstrations, but one which demands greater teaching skill than the midwife might realize. The procedure embraces more than the woman can comprehend in one session, and demands the repetition which is so essential for good teaching.

A lesson on handling, dressing and undressing baby should have been given at the preceding class, to allow more time for the actual bathing procedure and to avoid blurring the demonstration with too much detail.

The following are eight ways in which repetition is employed in demonstrating how to bath a baby.

1. **The positions in which the baby is held are taught** at the previous class.

(*a*) While washing the hair. (*b*) Lowering the baby into the water.

(*c*) Turning baby over to wash the back. (*d*) Lifting baby out of the bath.

2. **Each piece of equipment is discussed,** before actually starting to bath the doll, stating why it has been selected and how it is used.

3. **The complete bathing procedure is demonstrated on a doll.**

4. **Any difficult manœuvre,** such as in (1) and the grip used while holding the baby in the water, should be repeated.

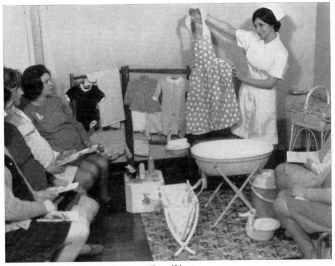

FIG. 491

DEMONSTRATION OF BATHING EQUIPMENT—SISTER SHOWING BATHING APRON.
(*Mothercraft Department, Royal Maternity Hospital, Rottenrow, Glasgow.*)

5. One of the expectant mothers (*less than six months pregnant*) **should be asked to bath the doll under the midwife's guidance.** The audience are so intrigued watching her performance that they do not realize the process has been repeated.

6. A printed copy of the demonstration may be distributed, so that the woman can study the procedure at her leisure and refresh her memory if necessary.

7. Later, she will be shown how to bath her own baby, whether born at home or in hospital.

8. She is given the opportunity to do it herself under supervision before being discharged.

The Bathing Demonstration as given

" INTRODUCTION

" **Bathing time should be one of the happiest hours of the day.** Baby loves stretching and splashing in the nice warm water, and what is more adorable than a newly bathed baby ? Bathing isn't just a job of work to be done as quickly as possible ; it is one of the mothering times, an occasion when baby and mother get to know each other better. By the gentle way she handles her baby and the caressing tone of her voice a mother expresses her love.

" **MORNING OR EVENING**

"Although many babies are bathed in the

39

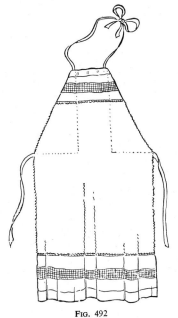

FIG. 492

Bathing apron made from a bath towel.

morning, there is no special reason why it should be so. **Choose the time that suits you best; baby** won't mind. Before the 18.00 hours feed is a good time; baby usually sleeps well after his bath, and night is the best time for sound sleep.

" **The house is warmer in the evening,** and when baby comes to the crawling stage he will need a bath at bedtime. We mustn't forget father, he may like to watch or to help. Allow yourself an hour at first, including preparation and clearing up; speed comes with experience."

ON TABLE OR KNEE

In hospital babies are usually bathed in their cots or on a table for convenience and speed. The table in many homes is in front of the window.

In the home the knee is to be preferred : baby feels loved and secure being in such close contact with his mother.

DISCUSSION OF EQUIPMENT

" Here we have everything set out that you are likely to need. This plastic baby bath is light in weight and does not get hot. (An oval washing-up bowl would do for the first three months.) Notice that the bath is placed on a strong stool to bring the edge of it to knee-level and so prevent backache from bending. This low chair without arms is similar to the one you will use when feeding baby.

"A tray is handy to hold baby's toilet articles which are few and simple. On this one there is a soap dish and cake of good face soap. **Note the two wash cloths,** a butter muslin one for the face and body; the Turkish one for the buttocks is washed with the napkins (some prefer disposable tissues). These cotton-wool balls in the glass jar are needed to clean baby's nose, but only to remove the smudges that can be seen. Here is a jar of cream for his buttocks, and a hairbrush. Talcum powder should be used sparingly if at all.

" **His night-clothes, as you see, are warming on a screen by the fire,** arranged, vest on top, in the order in which they will be put on. Baby's own soft face-towel and bath-towel are warming too.

" **Have a pail like this beside you,** to soak baby's napkins in until you are ready to wash them. Get a tiny chamber, if you like, to ' catch what comes,' but don't be too hopeful. We do not now recommend starting to train a baby until he is over eight months old ; you only upset him by your over-anxiety, and he will gain control sooner if you begin training when he understands what you mean (see p. 768).

" **This big jug is used to fill the bath.** You will all want to have a bathing-apron like this one (see p. 745), which is made from a bath towel and you would be wise to wear a plastic one underneath it to keep your lap dry, in case baby wets when his napkin is off."

PREPARATION

" **Have the room warm,** windows and doors closed and everything ready before you start.

" **Always put the cold water into the bath first;** toddlers have been known to fall in while mother was away getting the cold water.

" **Test the temperature of the water with a bath thermometer ;** it should be $37.7°$ C. ($100°$ F.). If you haven't a thermometer, use your elbow ; the water should feel gently warm, not hot. Don't use your hand, which could tolerate water that would burn baby's skin. **Never add hot water while baby is in the bath, because of the risk of scalding him.**

" **Notice that the chair you will sit on is at the right-hand side of the fire,** so that baby's head is cool, his feet warm. Have the toilet articles at your right side, to save stretching over baby to reach them. Wash your hands and put on the bathing apron."

The Actual Bath

" **Baby is already undressed, all but his vest and napkin.** Remove these and let him kick for a moment; he loves the freedom and it is good to let his skin become accustomed to the air. If his buttocks are dirty use the Turkish face cloth or disposable tissues.

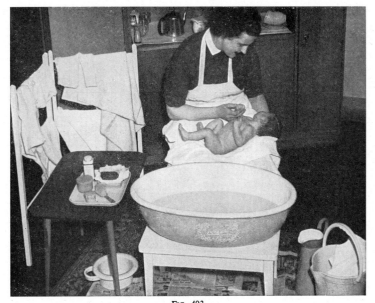

Fig. 493

Allowing baby to kick with clothes off prior to bath.
(*Simpson Memorial Maternity Pavilion, Edinburgh.*)

" **Wrap the bath towel round his arms and chest** and wash his face with the butter muslin cloth, without soap. Do one side at a time so that you don't cover his nose and mouth with the face cloth. Dry his face gently and very thoroughly.

"**Watch how his body is being held** with my left elbow, while his head, grasped in my left hand, is brought to the edge of the bath. Wet and soap the hair properly, **don't be afraid of the soft spot** on the top of the head, if you don't keep it clean, scurf will form. Dry his hair thoroughly, and be sure to dry the creases behind the ears or they will become sore.

" **Wet his body and legs with the face cloth,** then soap both your hands and wash him like this; first neck, arms and hands, roll him towards you and soap his back, then do his body and legs and be sure to go into all the creases.

" **We will now put him into the water.**

" **He is very slippery, so he must be held securely.** Place your left hand under his shoulders and grasp the left upper arm; his head will rest on your wrist. Put your right hand under his buttocks and grasp the left thigh. Lower him into the bath, keeping his head well out of the water. Rinse off the soap. When baby is a month old, turn him over and wash his back like this.

" **To lift him out of the bath grasp him in the same way, holding the ' far away ' arm and leg.** Lay him face down on your lap and dry him carefully. Use a gentle mopping movement, don't rub briskly, his skin is very delicate; dry all the folds of skin thoroughly and be careful with his finger-nails, they are easily torn.

" **Shake a little talcum on your hand,** and rub it into the dry creases, smear some cream on his buttocks. Put on his vest, and remember to put your fingers into the sleeve and draw his hand through it as I showed you last week. Put on his napkin, wrap a second folded one round his buttocks."

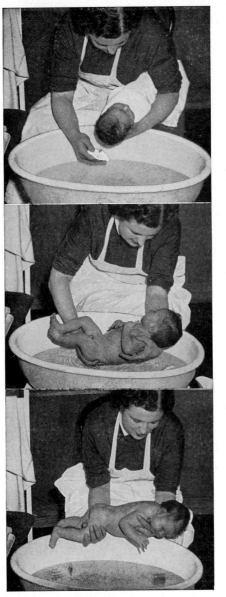

WASHING BABY'S HAIR
Note—
    Edge of bath at knee level.
    Body held securely with elbow.
    Head supported.

LOWERING BABY INTO BATH
Note—
    Head supported on wrist.
    Baby's left arm (*the far away one*) grasped securely.
    Left thigh being held and buttocks supported.

BABY BEING LIFTED OUT
face downwards.
    Baby's right arm and right thigh (*the far away ones*) are grasped securely.

Fig. 494
Demonstration of bathing baby as in the home.

The midwife should either dress the doll in night clothes or wrap the snuggling blanket over vest and napkin, and brush the hair. *She then stands up to face the audience with an appropriate closing sentence, such as,* " Baby is now ready for his feed, then he will be drowsy, and when tucked into his cot will soon be fast asleep. Father and mother will enjoy a quiet evening."

HEALTH EDUCATION

POSTNATAL EXERCISES; GOOD POSTURE; ADVICE
TO THE AMBULANT WOMAN

This talk could be given prior to exercise No. 1 (p. 751) on the third postpartum day or divided and given with the exercises on the third, fourth and fifth days.

The Talk as given

" I'm sure you are all eager to look and feel as well as you did a year ago and, of course you want to reduce your waistline and slim your hips. It takes six to eight weeks, or even longer, for your overstretched muscles to return to normal and we will show you how to assist nature in doing this so that you can regain your trim figure.

" We hope that your childbearing organs and tissues have healed and are going back to their normal state. But we also want you to be full of energy—not tired and listless—and within the next few weeks ready and eager to resume your household duties."

GOOD WHOLESOME FOOD

" In order to be fit and well you must have nourishing meals with plenty of body-building foods such as meat, fish, eggs, milk and cheese, as well as fruit and green vegetables that contain valuable minerals and vitamins. You need three cooked meals every day to build up your strength, foods rich in iron such as meat, liver, blood sausage, whole-wheat bread, and green vegetables will help to replace the blood you have recently lost.

" Good food helps to provide the energy you need in looking after your family and your home."

REST AND RECREATION

" Do ensure that you get sufficient sleep and rest after you go home. Go to bed at a reasonable hour so that you have at least nine hours' sleep; lie down during the afternoon if only for an hour.

" Get your husband to help you with any heavy work; it is very bad for you to lift heavy weights for at least six weeks, until your womb and birth passage are back to their normal state. If you have to move something heavy, such as a big arm-chair, push, don't lift it.

" We will show you how to avoid straining your back if in the course of your daily house-work you must lift something fairly heavy.

" Try to continue with some of your hobbies or social activities outside the home in order that you will be a cheerful companion for your husband and a good-natured mother to your children."

MAINTAINING GOOD POSTURE

" You will all admit that since baby was born you are tending to stand in a slovenly fashion and to walk in an ungainly manner; shoulders slumped forwards, abdomen bulging. This is because your muscles have lost the power to hold you erect and to enable you to walk gracefully.

" Try to be very figure conscious and cultivate the habit of good posture until your muscles and ligaments are restored to their natural strength again. We will help you, and we hope you will continue with good posture after you leave hospital.

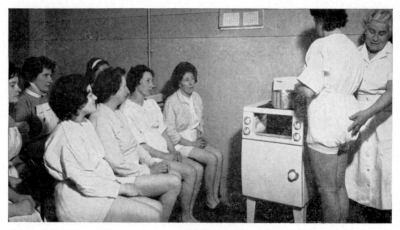

Fig. 495

Physiotherapist showing puerperal women how to maintain good posture while standing at kitchen stove.
(*Royal Maternity Hospital, Rottenrow, Glasgow.*)

" **You must get rid of the backward-leaning stance you adopted during pregnancy** or it will become an established habit. During the last months of pregnancy you had to lean backwards to counterbalance the size and weight of baby in your womb. You held your shoulders back and increased the hollow in the small of your back (*demonstrate this*): your weight was carried on your heels and your step lost its lithe spring.

" **Make a conscious effort to stand erect and walk with a graceful carriage.**

" **Bad posture gives rise to low backache :** it also induces a despondent outlook on life. **If you hold yourself in a trim and confident manner** your feelings and actions are more likely to be confident.

" **A woman should maintain pride in her** appearance even if she is a busy mother, and although she may have an excellent figure her appearance can be ruined by faulty posture."

REDUCING THE WAIST LINE

" **The abdominal wall muscles were grossly overstretched during the last three months of pregnancy.** These muscles also worked hard during labour pushing baby out into the world ; they are therefore lax or flabby and do not hold your abdominal organs snug in place as they ought to.

" **We will teach you exercises that will tone up these muscles** and help to flatten the bulging waistline."

WEAK PELVIC FLOOR MUSCLES

" **While baby was actually being born the outlet of the birth passage was dilated or opened to a very great extent;** the muscles of the pelvic floor were greatly overstretched and bruised : in fact, some of you required stitches. These pelvic floor muscles are meant to support and maintain the bladder and womb in their natural places, but if they remain lax you will have difficulty in holding urine in your bladder for as long as you did previously. You may have heard of ' falling of the womb '; this also is due to lax or slack pelvic floor muscles.

" **We will teach you exercises that will strengthen the pelvic floor muscles.**"

POSTNATAL EXERCISE NO. 1 (*third day*)

All or part of the preceding talk is given

Purpose

A. ADOPTING A GOOD SITTING POSTURE.
B. STRENGTHENING THE ABDOMINAL MUSCLES.
C. EXERCISING THE PELVIC FLOOR MUSCLES.

(Low chairs with reasonably firm seats, straight backs and no arms are provided.)

The women are seated throughout the lesson.
Outdoor shoes are worn not soft bedroom slippers.
The women wear tights into which their nightdresses are tucked.

A. GOOD SITTING POSTURE

(*a*) The mothers are asked to sit well back in the chairs.
(*b*) Feet are placed on floor directly under the knees.
(*c*) Hips and shoulders are pressed against the back of the chair.
(*d*) The hollow of the back is flattened out.
(*e*) The head is held erect.

Hold position and
> *Count five slowly—Relax. Repeat six times.*

B. STRENGTHENING THE ABDOMINAL MUSCLES

Draw the lower abdominal muscles inwards and upwards. Pull your " tummy " in.
> *Count five slowly—Relax. Repeat six times.*

C. EXERCISING PELVIC FLOOR MUSCLES

(*a*) Contract (*tighten*) the buttocks, hold thighs close together.
(*b*) Contract (*draw up*) the pelvic floor muscles as you would when urgently requiring to pass urine at a time when it is not convenient to do so.
> *Count five slowly—Relax. Repeat six times.*

Repeat (*b*) but concentrate on tightening the muscles that control the bowel (back passage) instead of the bladder.
> *Count five slowly—Relax. Repeat six times.*

POSTNATAL EXERCISE NO. 2 (*fourth day*)

Purpose

A. CORRECTION OF FAULTY POSTURE, PARTICULARLY LORDOSIS.
B. STANDING WITH GOOD POSTURE.
C. REPEAT ABDOMINAL AND PELVIC FLOOR EXERCISES.
D. WALKING WITH POISE AND GRACE.
E. HANDLING BABY.
F. PUSHING THE PRAM.

A. CORRECTION OF LORDOSIS

(*a*) Stand with heels 10·2 cm. (4 inches) from the wall, feet 22·9 cm. (9 inches) apart.
(*b*) Allow the body-weight to be transferred forwards on to the insteps and balls of the feet, not on the heels.
(*c*) Lean back against the wall, pressing the buttocks, then the small of the back and then the shoulders against the wall to straighten the back.

(*d*) **Relax the shoulders** and pull them backwards and downwards.

(*e*) **Hold the head high, chin pulled in.**

(*f*) **While pressing the small of the back against the wall** contract the lower abdomina muscles as in Exercise No. 1 B slowly.

Repeat five times. Relax.

(*g*) **Strengthen the pelvic floor muscles as in exercise No. 1 C** while maintaining this corrective posture.

Repeat five times. Relax.

(*The mothers are strongly recommended to practise the pelvic floor exercises four times daily at home. This can be done while standing at the sink or cooker.*)

B. STANDING WITH GOOD POSTURE
(*away from the wall*)

(*a*) **Feet are 22·9 cm. (9 inches) apart, toes flattened out and pointing straight forwards.**

(*b*) **Knees are gently straightened.**

(*c*) **Spine is erect but not stiff ; abdomen flat.**

(*d*) **The shoulders are relaxed and held back and down.**

(*e*) **The head is held high,** as primitive women do when carrying something on the head.

(*f*) **The chest is raised, arms hanging alongside thighs.**

C. *Repeat abdominal and pelvic floor exercises*

D. WALKING WITH POISE AND GRACE

(*a*) **Maintain good standing posture. Try to feel tall.**

(*b*) **Place heel then sole of foot on the ground,** lean slightly forwards propelling the weight of the body on to the tips of all the toes. The weight is borne mainly on the outer borders of the feet, the arches are drawn upwards. The movement should be smooth and graceful (avoid clamping the feet down in a solid mass).

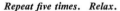

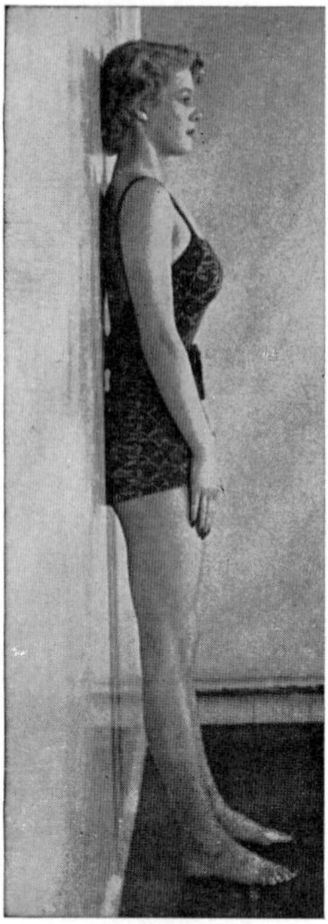

FIG. 496

CORRECT POSTURE.
Note straight spine.

E. HANDLING BABY

MAKING A LAP FOR BABY

For this procedure the nightdress should be lowered over the tights.

(*a*) **The women are requested to adopt the good sitting posture.**

(*b*) **Knees are held 15·2 cm. (6 inches) apart ; feet flat on floor,** but ready to go on tip toe instantly to adjust to baby's movements.

(*c*) **Midwife demonstrates how baby's head rests on her left thigh.**

TURNING BABY ON KNEE

With relaxed hands and arms baby is grasped by the body, gently lifted and rolled towards mother's body. To turn him on to his back again he is grasped and lifted in the same way and rolled towards mother's body. This is safer than rolling away from the body.

F. PUSHING THE PRAM

(*a*) **Good posture is maintained as in walking ;** the back ought to be straight and the tendency to bend forwards resisted.

(*b*) **Elbows are held close to the body.**

(*c*) **Arms and hands should be relaxed** and the handle grasped lightly, not clutched in a tense manner. The pram handle is kept close to the mother's body.

(*d*) **The shoulders are relaxed and held back and down, chest raised and ribs expanded sideways to facilitate deep breathing.** Mothers should be advised to take the pram away from heavy traffic (after shopping is completed).

POSTNATAL EXERCISE NO. 3 (*fifth day*)

Purpose
Handling baby ; using good body mechanics.

A. LIFTING BABY OUT OF COT.
B. HOW TO HOLD BABY WHILE WALKING OR SITTING.
C. LIFTING OBJECTS FROM FLOOR LEVEL.

A. **Bend knees rather than back when stooping over the cot.** Slip left hand under baby's shoulders until his head rests in the crook of the elbow. The arm supports his spine. Place right arm and hand over and under baby's buttocks. Straighten knees to resume the upright position.

B. **Practise the good walking and sitting positions while holding baby.**

C. LIFTING OBJECTS FROM FLOOR LEVEL

(*a*) **Stand with one foot slightly in front of the other.**
(*b*) **Bend both knees, placing most of the weight on the foot in front.**
(*c*) **Hold baby or object to be lifted close to the body.**
(*d*) **Maintain good postural position of spine and head.**
(*e*) **Stand up, straightening the knees and transferring the weight on to the back foot.**

(*Lifting a heavy object by stooping over it with flexed spine and straight knees puts very great strain on the back ; this is particularly undesirable because of the weakened state of the muscles of the abdomen, pelvic floor and back after childbirth.*)

PREPARING DRIED MILK FEEDS

Talk-Demonstration to Mothers

The need for cleanliness should be stressed, reasons given and the danger of infection by germs, causing baby to become seriously ill, explained.

1. HAND WASHING

This should be emphasized and carried out as part of the demonstration.

" **Hands that look clean may be covered with germs** which are so small they cannot be seen. Your hand must go into the carton to scoop up the powder and, if not clean, will infect the milk.

" **Wash your hands before preparing the feed,** also before feeding baby (*and always after changing the napkin, which is usually done just before feeding*)."

2. CLEAN UTENSILS

" **Everything used for making baby's food should be thoroughly washed** and kept, covered with a clean towel, in a cupboard free from dust and flies. A badly washed jug or dirty bottle brush will be a breeding ground for germs. Flies may infect the milk powder. Keep it in a glass jar with a screw top lid. The sugar jar should have a lid."

3. ACCURACY IN PREPARING FEEDS

" **Powdered milk, sugar and water must be measured carefully.** If given too much sugar, baby will become fat and flabby; too little will prevent adequate weight gain."

A few mothers have used the powder-scoop to measure the water: resulting in concentrated feeds having serious and in two cases fatal results.

Most dried milks have had sugar added to them except National Dried.

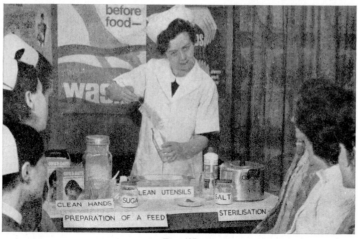

FIG. 497

PARENTCRAFT SISTER DEMONSTRATING TO EXPECTANT MOTHERS AND STUDENT MIDWIVES
PREPARATION OF BABY'S FEED.
(*Aberdeen Maternity Hospital.*)

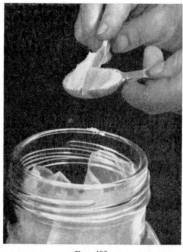

FIG. 498

Using knife edge to level scoop of dried milk
powder.
(*Aberdeen Maternity Hospital.*)

TO PREPARE ONE FEED
(*Demonstration*)

REQUIREMENTS

Carton of Dried Milk (half cream) with
scoop, jar of sugar if not in milk powder.

Kettle of water

Glass (*heat resisting*) measuring jug, 240
ml. (8 oz.).

Casserole containing pyrex feeding bottle
and teat in Milton, 15 ml./l. water.

Knife, 4 G. measure (teaspoon), bowl,
bottle brush, soapless detergent, coarse salt,
plastic measure for Milton.

PREPARATION

Wash hands; scald jug, bowl and bottle
brush with boiling water.

Allow kettle to cool for 10 minutes prior to
making feed. (*Boiling water separates out
the fat in the milk.*)

Method

1. Open pack or jar, remove lids from
casserole and sugar jar.

2. **Wash hands thoroughly.** Remove bottle and teat from Milton solution.

3. **Measure 90 ml. (3 oz.) boiled water,** pour into feeding bottle.

Measure 3 scoops powder (*level with edge of knife*), *put into jug.*

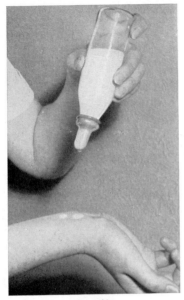

Fig. 499
Testing the heat of the milk on the sensitive inner aspect of wrist.

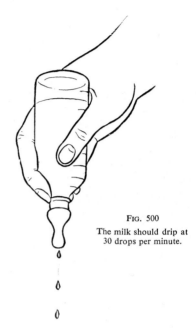

Fig. 500
The milk should drip at 30 drops per minute.

Measure 4 G. (one level teaspoonful) sugar, add to National Dried Milk.

(*Replace lids or close pack to avoid contamination by flies.*)

4. Add a little of the measured warm water in the bottle to powder in jug and mix to a smooth cream.

5. Add the remainder of the water, stirring constantly, to break down any lumps.

6. Pour into bottle and apply teat.

HOW TO GIVE THE FEED

1. The bottle is placed in a jug of hot water until the milk is about 37·2° to 37·7° C. (99° to 100° F.).

2. Test the heat of the milk by allowing it to drip on the sensitive inner aspect of the wrist milk should be at blood heat (gently warm).

Mothers must be told never to put the teats in their mouths, to test the heat of the milk: and only to touch the neck of the teat when putting it on to the bottle.

3. Test the rate of flow by holding the bottle upside down. The milk should drip at approximately 2 ml. (30 drops) per minute. If the hole is too small baby will take 15 or more minutes to get his feed and will swallow too much air and get colic. If the hole is too big baby will gulp his feed in less than five minutes.

(*Demonstrate how to enlarge a small hole with a darning needle heated by holding it in the flame of a match.*)

Feeding Position

Mothers should be warned against feeding baby in cot or pram with the bottle propped.

1. The mother sits in a low chair with one foot raised on a footstool, holding baby almost upright to avoid the risk of inhaling milk should choking occur.

2. A jug of hot water is within reach, a clock within view.

3. To keep baby's dress dry and sweet-smelling a bib (*not plastic*) **should be worn.**

4. It is advisable to hold the bottle like a pencil with the rim of the teat between the thumb and first finger. When the teat collapses, as it will when baby sucks the air out of the bottle, the fingers pinch the rim of the teat and allow air to enter. If the teat is removed from baby's mouth to do this he becomes annoyed.

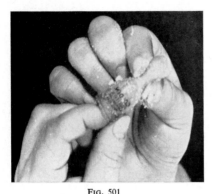

Fig. 501

Teat cleansed with coarse salt.
(*Aberdeen Maternity Hospital.*)

5. The bottle should be tilted at an angle to keep the neck of the bottle full of milk, thus avoiding undue sucking of air.

6. Wind should be broken half-way through the feed (see p. 512). If the stomach is distended with air baby may not wish to finish his feed. During this time the bottle should be shaken to prevent the fat from separating out, and then reheated. Wind is brought up again at the end of the feed, baby's bib being laid on mother's shoulder.

7. Rinse bottle and teat in cold water; turn teat inside out and rub between finger and thumb with coarse salt, rinse; clean bottle with brush and detergent, rinse and submerge in Milton 15 ml./l. water made up fresh daily. The bottle and teat must remain submerged in Milton between feeds.

N.B.—Mothers should be given the opportunity to test the heat of the milk on their wrists, count the drops, apply teats and hold the bottles in the manner recommended.

Advice should be given not to boil or add boiling water to orange juice; heat destroys vitamin C.

PLANNING THE DAY FOR MOTHER AND BABY

This talk is only a guide, for each midwife knows best what will suit the women in her own area. It is probably better to discuss the subject in general, as an hour-by-hour plan would not suit every woman, nor would it be remembered unless a typed copy was given to each mother.

The Talk as given

" Before you go home I would advise you to plan how you are going to manage your house-work and at the same time give baby the care he will need. Some mothers make a lot of unnecessary work and tire themselves out; others make no plan at all and get into a hopeless muddle.

" **Looking after baby will mean about three hours daily extra work,** especially if it is your first baby, because you will be slow until you become more expert in handling him. The main thing is that you start off by getting baby to fit in with your usual routine.

" **Babies are most accommodating;** they don't mind whether they are bathed in the morning or the evening, so long as you keep to one or the other. Feeding times can be put back or forwards half an hour, or even an hour, if they clash with family meals. Baby can be fed at 05.00; 09.00; 13.00; 17.00 hours instead of the usual 06.00; 10.00; 14.00; 18.00 hours. It is unnecessary and unwise to disorganize the household for baby."

TAKE THINGS EASILY

" **During the first month, you will tire readily** and will require some extra help with the heavy work, so do accept any offer of assistance you may get from relatives or friends. It is, however, better that you yourself should bath baby, a pleasant task at which you can sit down.

" **Encourage your husband to help with the heavier jobs,** such as turning mattresses, as this is not good for you: not for six to eight weeks should you lift heavy weights. Don't attempt to keep your house like a new pin if it means being on your feet from early morning until late at night. A home that is reasonably clean and tidy, well-cooked meals and a happy mother are better for everyone concerned than an immaculate house with a tired irritable mother."

HAVE A FLEXIBLE PLAN

" I am not going to set out a plan, hour by hour, from six in the morning until 22.00 hours at night. A hundred and one unexpected things may crop up in the course of the day, and some require your immediate attention; if life is a frantic race with the clock, you will soon be a nervous wreck. No rigid scheme will suit every household. **Mothers vary in their ability as housewives,** and some are stronger than others; babies differ in the amount of attention they demand; houses may be inconvenient, the rooms overcrowded.

" **By all means have a plan, but for baby's sake let it be a flexible one.**

" **Don't be too strict at first regarding feeding times,** for some babies object to being regimented by the clock. The restless wiry baby seems to need more food than the placid

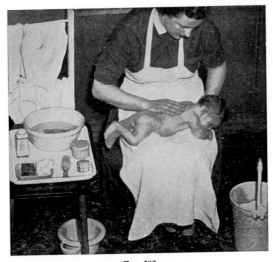

Fig. 502
Baby's morning toilet.
(*Bath given during evening.*)

sleepy one, and often likes to have it every three rather than every four hours. Let baby have some say regarding feeding times if he is the type who objects to the usual schedule.

" **The doctor at the child health clinic will advise you if any difficulty arises.**

" **Baby usually starts the day bright and early,** around 06.00 hours, but after you have fed him you can have another short sleep until it is time to prepare breakfast. When baby wakes up again, about 09.30 hours, give him his orange juice; then after face, hands and buttocks are washed and clean clothes put on, give the 10.00 hours feed and settle him for sleep in the pram out of doors.

" When you have finished baby's daily washing have a rest with your feet up while you take a nourishing drink. Housework and cooking usually occupy the remainder of the morning. If your husband and children do not come home at midday, be sure to have a proper meal yourself, as it is important that you keep up your strength and your supply of milk.

" Before the 14.00 hour feed allow baby to have at least five minutes on your lap kicking with his napkin off; chat to him, and he will learn to know the sound of your voice.

" These mothering times are essential for baby's happiness, and he enjoys the exercise, too. Finish your household jobs, and then have another rest with your feet up while you drink a cup of tea before you take baby out.

" The air in the parks or the suburbs does baby and you more good than the air in the crowded shopping centres, which is laden with dust and petrol fumes, so do get away from the traffic."

TAKE FATHER INTO CONSIDERATION

" Between 17.00 and 18.00 hours, depending on when father comes home, is a good time for baby's bath. You will find out, of course, whether father prefers to see baby being bathed or whether this should be done before he comes home. When fed and tucked into his warm cot baby will probably sleep until the 22.00 hour feed.

" Plan to have a quiet evening by the fire, reading, viewing television, or talking to your husband; bathing baby in the evening is one way of ensuring this. You should go to bed immediately after baby's last feed, and your husband will give you a beaker of cocoa, milk or Ovaltine to help to keep up your supply of breast milk. Relax and read if it is too early for you to go to sleep.

" Do try to arrange an outing with your husband at least once a week; it is good for you to get away from baby for a short time occasionally, and although you may be satisfied to stay at home, your husband will no doubt appreciate an outing with you.

" See that baby and father both get their fair share of your love and attention, but try to have a little leisure for yourself, or you will only become overtired and disgruntled. Remember, it is mainly the mother who makes the home a happy place. If baby, father and you are all thriving and contented, your plan is a success; you are a good wife and mother."

WHEN BABY CRIES

The Talk as given

" Many mistakes in baby care are made when trying to pacify a crying infant, so it is good that you should know some of the reasons why babies cry and how to deal with them. In moderation crying is good for babies; it expands their lungs, and the vigorous waving of arms and legs that accompanies crying is a splendid form of exercise.

" Crying is baby's language, and his only way of letting us know that something is annoying him. He may be uncomfortable, too hot, thirsty, hungry, or in pain, but even an experienced midwife cannot tell which of these is the cause during the first weeks of life. It doesn't take much to make tiny babies cry, so don't decide he is hungry or ill until you have investigated the other causes.

" A new baby may scream furiously as though in agony yet he may only be tired of lying on one side. Turn him over and give him a friendly pat and a word of comfort; he will very likely settle down and go to sleep again.

" You may expect your baby to have at least half a dozen spells of crying throughout the day, and occasionally at night. Always think of the simple things first before you conclude that he is in pain or ill. To a mother the cry of her infant makes such a tremendous appeal that she is apt to worry unnecessarily. Keep calm and investigate the situation.

"IS HIS NAPKIN WET ?

" It may be that his napkin is wet, but in my opinion babies are not disturbed by wet napkins if the cot is warm. Cold, wet napkins are uncomfortable, and if baby's buttocks are sore, they will hurt when he passes water or a motion.

"IS HE TOO WARM ?

" **Is his face red, and does his head look or feel moist ?** Is the bedroom stuffy ? Babies, like adults, sleep best in a well-ventilated room. Mothers often make the mistake of overclothing their babies, especially in summer. I saw a baby protesting bitterly about the heat one hot August afternoon ; he was swaddled in four layers of wool, yet his mother was wearing a cool cotton frock. By all means keep baby warm in winter, but allow the air to reach his skin in summer.

"IS HE UNCOMFORTABLE ?

" **Have you wrapped him up too tightly ?** Babies love to squirm and move their arms and legs when they want to, and it infuriates even tiny babies when they can't. I hope there isn't a belt on his nightgown ; they are quite unnecessary, and really out of date. If he is lying on the knot which you tied at the back or the side, he will certainly complain about it. It may be that the pure wool vest you knitted for him is driving him frantic ; many babies cannot tolerate wool next to their skins.

" **If baby continues to scream, you had better lift him.** Straighten his clothes, and make him comfortable ; **cuddle and soothe him before you lay him down again.** During the night, if he refuses to settle, give him a few ml. of boiled water ; he will be thirsty with crying, and more so if he is hot.

"IS HE HUNGRY ?

" **Water will not pacify a hungry baby, so you had better feed him.** With a first baby, the mother's milk supply may not be plentiful until the third or fourth week, so take nourishing drinks as well as three good meals a day.

" **You will never teach a baby to sleep all night by letting him cry for an hour or more,** and you have your husband to think of too ; he, as well as you, needs a good night's sleep. We used to condemn night feeds, but not now, although we only give them when necessary, and not routinely to all babies. When baby gets enough food during the day he usually sleeps all night.

" **If you have disturbed nights go to the child health clinic or consult the health visitor, who will be pleased to advise you.**

" **Persistent crying is more often due to some fault in the feeding routine rather than that the breast milk does not agree with baby.** He may be getting too much or too little food, take him to the child health clinic and this will be investigated.

" **No two babies are exactly alike in the amount of food they require ;** the thin restless infant often needs more food and more cuddling than the placid sleepy baby, so seek and take the advice of an expert.

" **Newborn babies do not cry because of bad temper.** Be patient, and don't expect too much of an infant who is only ten days old. Give him time to settle into a satisfactory sleeping and feeding routine."

PAIN OR ILLNESS

" **Wind may give rise to pain,** but you will avoid this by letting baby break wind after each feed.

" **Colic is rare in breast-fed babies.** With each piercing shriek baby will draw up his legs and will continue to cry even after you have picked him up. Lay him face downwards on your knee over a hot-water bottle with a little warm (not hot) water in it. Give him some warm water to drink.

" **A baby who is ill may whimper rather than cry** but you would notice that there was something wrong, such as **cough, cold, vomiting, diarrhœa, or feverishness.**"

GENERAL ADVICE

" **Try not to let crying become a habit ;** baby should not have to scream for the normal care all babies need.

" It is the placid, good-natured woman who makes the best mother; so make up your mind to keep calm. Mothers who are always in a state of anxiety about their babies seem to produce the same anxious state in their infants. **Don't get worked up over every whimper.**

" Babies may look very fragile, but they are not weaklings. This is when a patient, level-headed husband can be a tower of strength to a worried young mother, for sound common-sense can be applied to baby care as well as to other things.

" Baby's needs are simple.—Food, warmth, comfort and love, and when these are given satisfactorily baby will be as good as gold and brighten your home like a ray of sunshine."

SLEEP

TEACHING AIDS

A cot and bedding; a doll; sleeping garments.

Give demonstration of dressing baby for sleep; putting baby to bed.

The Talk as given

" It is easy to see what a soothing effect sleep has on babies, for no matter how cross they are when they fall asleep, they wake up good-natured and ready to smile again.

"At first baby will sleep 21 out of the 24 hours; he only stays awake long enough for napkin changing, feeding and bathing. Gradually he sleeps for shorter periods during the day, and at six months sleeps 18 out of the 24 hours.

" Baby feels drowsy after a feed, so you should settle him comfortably into the cot or pram then, and he will soon be fast asleep. The most important and the longest sleep is at night, and when baby is properly fed during the day, he is more likely to sleep all night."

A BED TO HIMSELF

" Baby should have a little bed of his own. If he sleeps with mother he breathes warm stale air, and there is always the danger that the heavy blankets or mother's arm might lie over his face. A basket may be suitable for the first three months, but baby very soon grows out of it and might topple it over in his attempts to sit up to see what is going on.

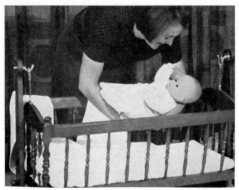

Fig. 503

Spine and head supported while laying baby in cot.

(*Aberdeen Maternity Hospital.*)

" **The mattress should be firm** and enveloped in a rubber cover. Pillows are not necessary: in fact, they are dangerous for young babies. If baby rolls over, and babies whose arms are wrapped in tightly are more likely to do this, he may burrow his face into a soft pillow with serious results.

" **Two light, wool, cotton or Acrilan cellular blankets will be needed,** and if a top sheet is not provided, the washable top cover may be folded in over the top of the blankets.

" **The cot should always be clean and sweet smelling.** Air it at feeding times; once a day you can strip and air it in the sunshine or fresh air.

" **A carry-cot** with adjustable straps is useful for travel during the first four months. In winter an extra lining blanket and mattress are needed for warmth if the carry-cot is used as a bassinet."

PUTTING BABY TO SLEEP

"**Always lay baby on his side in case he should be sick.** If lying on his back he might inhale into his lungs the milk he vomits and choke. A number of babies die each year because of this. Lay him on his right and left sides alternately so that both lungs will expand well.

" **Have baby's cot in your own bedroom during the first six months at least,** so that you can hear what is going on. For a number of years a separate room for baby was recommended, but in case he should vomit and choke, it is now considered safer to have baby near his mother. Don't worry about this, it is only a wise precaution. A baby alarm should be obtained if baby is not within hearing distance.

" **When baby is sleeping out of doors see that the back of the pram-hood faces into the wind,** and that in summer he is shaded from the rays of the mid-day sun. Choose a quiet spot, if you can. A cat net is necessary.

" **If babies are overtired they are very fretful,** and sometimes they scream, refuse food and cannot be pacified. When this happens you may think baby is ill, try cuddling and soothing him to sleep with a lullaby he knows.

"**As baby grows older he should go to sleep by himself,** so lay him down awake from the very beginning. This will save you time and trouble later on, and after a nursery rhyme or a story your child will go happily to sleep."

THE CARE OF BABY'S SKIN

The Talk as given

" **Baby's skin should be pink and smooth** like the petal of a rose, and as soft as silk. Because the texture is so fine, baby's skin is very easily irritated, therefore you should take every care to avoid this.

" **The time to begin is when you are planning baby's layette.** Choose vests with a mixture of silk or cotton and wool; they are much less irritating, but if the wool vests you have already knitted annoy baby, make a butter muslin slip to wear under them."

SKIN RASHES

" **The red blotches of a wool rash are so itchy and irritating that baby and you will have a few disturbed nights.** Should you bath him? Yes ! but let the water be slightly cooler than usual; pat him dry, gently, with a soft towel and apply a cooling substance such as calamine lotion.

"**A sweat rash is often troublesome,** especially in summer when baby is likely to be kept too hot. Tiny pin-point blisters that are hard, and make the skin feel rough, appear on the forehead and body. No wonder baby is cross. Bath him as usual to remove the perspiration, and dab on a very little baby talcum powder; keep him less warm and give extra water to drink."

SORE BUTTOCKS

" **Sore buttocks generally begin as a reddened area,** but with a little care they can usually be prevented. They are due to various causes, such as :

1. **Not washing baby's buttocks properly when they are soiled.**

" 2. **Leaving wet napkins on too long,** especially under plastic pants; the skin becoming soggy and then breaking.

" 3. **Using napkins that are too rough**; this happens when Turkish towelling is dried quickly, for example, near the fire. Napkins should, where possible, be dried out of doors.

" 4. **Washing the napkins with strong soap,** washing soda, bleaching powder or ' blue ' and not rinsing them properly. Napkins should be rinsed in three waters.

" **Sore buttocks sometimes occur during the first ten days of life,** when baby has loose stools because he is taking too much milk or is not digesting it properly. Copious oily applications combined with wearing plastic pants will make the skin soggy and encourage infection.

" **Prevention is the best treatment,** and that means the avoidance of the causes I have already mentioned. (The midwife should refer to page 501 for curative treatment.) "

SCURF

" **I'm sure you have all seen a baby with a dark greasy patch on the front of his head.** The scales from it fall on to the face, and the next thing you see is a red, sore area on baby's cheek. This may be the beginning of extensive skin trouble, so don't allow the scurf to form. Wash the softspot on baby's head every day, rinse off the soap thoroughly, and rub the hair briskly with a Turkish towel."

SENSITIVE SKINS

" **Some babies have extremely sensitive skins.**—I've seen little cheeks red and sore with rubbing on a harsh blanket or shawl. To avoid this, fold the cot sheet over the top of the blanket. **Tiny chins get sore, too, when dribbling or slavering.** Dry the chin gently, use a soothing face cream, change his bibs frequently, and tie a silk scarf around his neck.

" **Do dry baby's face thoroughly**; he objects, I know, but you must insist, or rough red patches will form on his cheeks and cold winds will make them raw and sore.

" **Crops of spots commonly appear during the first year which mothers often say are due to teething,** but are more likely to be the result of some new food baby isn't yet accustomed to. Always give new foods, such as eggs or fruit, in small quantities until you see what happens. **The treatment** is to dab on some cooling lotion and give him a few ml. of milk of magnesia.

" **Of course you mustn't expect all these skin conditions to affect your baby,** but it is wise to prevent them if you can. Aim at having the bloom of the fresh air and the tan of the sun on your baby's skin, and he won't have many skin blemishes. What is more, he is likely to be a healthy little lad."

THE NEW FATHER

This talk should be given to the mothers of first babies. So often the father's point of view is overlooked, and this leads to domestic disharmony.

The Talk as given

" Now that you are going home, have you given any thought as to how you are going to deal with that very important person : No, not His Majesty the baby—the new father. The average man has very little idea of what is expected of him, and it isn't easy being a father for the first time, so help him as much as you can.

" Don't make the mistake of being too possessive with your baby. True enough, you provide most of the care baby needs, but try to make your husband feel that he also is of importance. A baby should bind and not separate his parents. You have the advantage of having learned how to look after baby, but let your husband feel that baby is his as well as yours ; consult him, ask his opinion, bring him into the picture."

LET FATHER HANDLE BABY

"Allow your husband to share some of the pleasant little jobs for baby, but do try to let the first occasion be a happy one. Of course he is going to feel awkward and embarrassed too ; ignore this, and don't forget to give a word of encouragement.

"Use a little psychology. Do not hand a screaming infant to your hungry husband while you finish some item of housework ; it would be more tactful to get him to tuck baby into his cot, when drowsy after a feed, while you put the final touch to the evening meal. Be lavish in your praise, for success will encourage him to attempt the more complicated tasks.

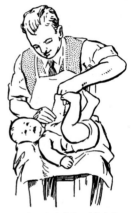

" There is no denying this is one of the dangerous corners in married life, and for your own happiness as well as your husband's you should try to negotiate it successfully. I wouldn't say a father would be actually jealous of his own child, but until now your husband has received all your love and attention; meals were ready on time, and a smiling wife greeted him at the end of the day. Now, the home is noisy and untidy, meals hastily prepared and often late, his wife harassed and irritable. The new father offers to help or maintains a friendly silence behind the newspaper, astonished that such a tiny scrap of humanity can have such a devastating effect on his home-life. Not until baby is old enough to give him a welcoming smile will he experience the real joy of fatherhood.

Note how baby's hand is being drawn through the sleeve.

" That is a gloomy picture, and I have purposely painted it like that as a warning, so that you will realize what can happen ; but you aren't going to let it be like that."

READJUST THE DAILY ROUTINE

" You may well be thinking, ' What about me, the mother, don't I get any consideration' : Of course you do. I know you need extra rest ; you may not be an experienced housewife, and the thought of the extra work you will have to do fills you with dismay. Fortunately, relatives and friends are often willing to lend a hand, and your husband should be encouraged to do so if extra domestic help is not available.

" It will be necessary to readjust your daily routine to allow for at least three hours' extra work. You will recall that I explained ' How to plan your day ' in a previous talk. You may have to lower temporarily your standards of housekeeping and do the essentials only until you feel stronger.

"Admittedly baby needs a lot of your attention, but he won't need as much as you are likely to lavish on him. Your second baby will get far less handling and will be a healthier, happier baby because of it.

" Make up your mind to make a success of motherhood by doing your best to keep your husband and children healthy and happy.

" Let your husband experience the joys as well as the responsibilities of fatherhood ; help him to adjust to this new home situation. Give him a fair share of your love and attention if you want him to be a home-loving, devoted husband and father. It is well worth making an effort to achieve this."

THE INFANT AFTER THE FIRST MONTH
SUN AND AIR-BATHS
TEACHING AIDS

Sun hat and suit.

The Talk as given

" You all know that baby must have fresh air ; that is why you buy a pram in which to take him to the park. Babies, like flowers, grow and flourish in fresh air and sunshine, so until the summer days are here catch every sunbeam.

" But there is little value in taking baby to the park for a short airing if he spends the remainder of the time in a room with closed windows.

" I have seen a pram out of doors in which it was impossible to see the baby. The hood was up and the front opening closed half-way by a waterproof protector. No fresh air could reach the baby at the bottom of that pram, so do not buy one that is too deep."

AIR-BATHS

" Besides having fresh air to breathe, baby will thrive better if you give him air-baths. This is one way of hardening baby so that he will not catch colds so readily. The baby who is always bundled up perspires so much that whenever the slightest breath of a cool breeze reaches him he gets another cold.

" Start air-baths when baby is 4 weeks old. Before his water-bath allow him to lie naked on your lap for five minutes. Don't chill him in a cold room or by having the window wide open. As time goes on take every opportunity to expose his arms and legs, and you will find he will develop a healthy tan even if there is no sunshine."

SUN-BATHING

" You may start sun-baths when baby is 3 months old. Go easily at first, for sun-tanning must be done slowly. Expose the legs only, for three minutes the first day. Increase the time by one minute each day, and expose a little more every day, until the whole body is getting the sun for 20 minutes. Then, when he is tanned all over he can remain in the sun for longer periods. Be sure to protect his head and the back of his neck with a suitable sun hat, especially from the hot mid-day sun.

" Whatever you do, don't attempt to tan your baby all in one day, especially at the seaside where the air is so much stronger. If you do, you will have a sick, sunburned child."

" You will soon see the results of sun and air-baths ; rosy cheeks will glow under a golden tan ; abundant energy, and a splendid appetite are signs of a healthy, thriving baby."

TREATMENT OF SUNBURN

" Sunburn is very painful, so baby will be as cross as can be ; he will be feverish—off his food—and he may vomit.

" Give him plenty of water to drink, but don't bath him. With the tips of your fingers, and using a feather-light touch, smear on plenty of cooling cream, and keep him out of the sun for a few days until he is better.

FROM KICKING TO WALKING
TEACHING AIDS

A play-pen with a blanket covered by a plastic or a rubber and a cotton sheet; examples of simple, safe playthings to be found in the home, such as—

A WOODEN SPOON: PLASTIC NAPKIN RING: REELS ON TAPE.

Stress the danger of toys with lead paint, sharp edges, and loose parts that may be swallowed.

The Talk as given

" Your baby at the moment is a helpless mite, yet at the end of a year he will be a sturdy little fellow, standing on his own two feet, and ready for walking. But before he can stand and walk, his bones must be strong and his muscles firm.

"A mother is apt to think that if her baby is properly fed and she gives him cod-liver oil and orange juice, and puts him out in the fresh air, she is doing all that is necessary. But that isn't enough, baby must get plenty of exercise. I have seen babies of 10 months whose legs were too weak and flabby to support the weight of their bodies. These babies had been bundled up in their prams for long periods, and their leg muscles were not developed because of lack of exercise.

" During the long summer days babies get a glorious opportunity to exercise. If you look into a pram and see a pair of active bare brown legs you will also see bright eyes and a beaming smile, for the baby who is given the chance to kick with perfect abandon amuses himself happily. In the winter, baby must, of course, be wrapped up to keep him warm, so he ought to get his exercise indoors.

" Stretching and squirming strengthen baby's back in readiness for sitting up. Kicking with freedom and vigour not only develops good leg muscles, it helps in the formation of straight bones and enables baby to strengthen those eager limbs of his in readiness for standing and walking."

EXERCISE DURING THE FIRST MONTHS

" Begin exercising baby as early as you like. At two weeks give him five minutes to kick when you change his napkin at feeding times. He will be hungry, so arms and legs will wave furiously. Then when you undress baby in the morning, and at bath-time in the evening, let him kick naked on your lap ; turn him over and stroke his back to encourage him to stretch.

" If you haven't got a play-pen lay baby on a clean napkin over a rubber and a cotton sheet, on the floor, the settee, or your own bed. (Don't leave him for a second, for it is surprising how a tiny baby can roll or wriggle to the edge of a wide bed in a matter of minutes.) Turn him over on his tummy, he will raise his head and arch his back. Let him roll about for 10 minutes.

"About the fourth month baby will start pushing his feet on your knee. Hold him around the body, taking the weight off his legs, and let him get the feel of his feet. His legs will grow stronger each week, and he will learn to control them. Encourage him to walk up your body, and he will gurgle with delight at this new game.

" Let baby have a few simple toys ; in the play-pen, a ball that he has to stretch to reach, four empty reels threaded on a tape, a red plastic napkin ring will please him as much as the expensive toys will. Rubber or woolly animals are more suitable for the pram. Out of doors there are so many things he loves to watch, and if you give him an occasional smile and a cheery word of greeting, baby will be perfectly content. Busy, active babies are healthy and happy."

STANDING AND WALKING

"A play-pen is a good investment for baby's health and happiness ; in it he gets more exercise than is possible in the pram. With safety he can roll about and get all the exercise he needs from about the fourth month. Play-pen babies rarely crawl ; their legs are so well developed that they stand and walk. During the ninth month, and sometimes before then, baby will pull himself on to his feet in his pen, and what fun it is ; he bumps down for the sheer delight of pulling himself up again.

" You needn't worry about early standing being the cause of bow-legs. It is the pale, fat, flabby baby who has had neither cod-liver oil nor exercise who gets bow-legs. You can depend on it that a baby will not attempt to stand until his legs are strong enough to bear his weight, but don't urge him to do so until he himself wants to. He may try to stand up in his pram, and I need hardly remind you how easily baby can fall out of it; so do use a set of safety harness after the seventh month, especially if his legs are strong.

" From the time baby stands it will be about two months before he walks by himself. To maintain his balance he keeps his feet wide apart, but very little will topple him over. Help him by removing bulky napkins. Clumsy, hard shoes are difficult to negotiate on polished floors, and after one or two nasty bumps baby loses confidence.

"A few babies walk before they are a year old, the majority are fifteen months."

SPOON AND CUP FEEDING

Much experience of baby feeding is necessary before the midwife is qualified to advise on this subject. The talk on weaning should probably be omitted until the need arises, when it could with greater advantage be given to individual mothers.

The Scottish report 1970 on infant feeding states that there is no need to give solids prior to 4 months.

TEACHING AIDS

Colourful baby-china : spoon and pusher : cod-liver oil : orange : tin of cereal baby food.

The Talk as given

" The first thing baby gets from a spoon is cod-liver oil, usually when he is three weeks old. It is given for sturdy growth. Start off cautiously with 0·3 ml. (five drops) and increase by 0·6 ml. (10 drops) a day until he is getting 4 ml. (one teaspoonful) daily. More than 4 ml. (one teaspoonful) would be harmful so keep to the exact dose. Babies having National Dried Milk only need 0·5 ml. (eight drops) daily. If you put 4 ml. (one teaspoonful) of cold cod-liver oil into baby's mouth it would surprise him, and he would probably spit it out ; it might even make him sick.

" Here is a good tip. Dip the spoon in warm water, don't make it hot ; put cod-liver oil on the warm, wet spoon and it will slip off easily into baby's mouth. It's a good idea to give the oil at bath time, when baby is undressed, to prevent staining his gown and the fishy smell that lingers.

" Orange juice may be started the next week, and breast-fed babies should have it as well as the bottle-fed ones. Start with 4 ml., (one teaspoonful) strain the juice and be sure to dilute it or it will make baby cough. Add 12 ml. (three teaspoonfuls) of lukewarm water and a few grains of sugar. Increase the orange juice by 4 ml. (one teaspoonful) every month until baby is having the juice of a whole orange. Give it by bottle if you like, but I'd suggest a plastic spoon, and when baby is five months old let him have it in his own little mug. Do not boil orange juice.

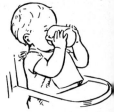

" Spoon-feeding should not be begun until baby is 12 weeks old, but baby experts have different opinions ; some begin later, others begin when baby weighs 7·7 kg. (15 lb.).

" Take the advice of the doctor who knows your baby ; he will tell you which foods baby should have ; I am just offering a few hints as to how you should prepare and give them."

CEREALS AND EGG YOLK

" Cereals are now being introduced during the fourth month, so baby can have 4 ml. of cereal baby food. After cooking mix it to a creamy consistency with whatever milk he is having. He will try to suck it at first and will spill most of it but he will soon learn. Gradually increase by 4 ml. every two weeks until he is getting 30 ml.

" Egg yolk is excellent for babies because it contains iron and other invaluable substances. Start with 4 ml. of lightly boiled egg—no more or you may upset him. Offer it as a great treat, let him see the yellow colour, and don't force it on him like medicine. As you already know, a speck of salt will improve the flavour. Give egg every other day before the 10.00 hours feed if you like. Baby should be 8 months old before he gets half an egg, and 15 months before he has a whole egg.

" Baby has to get accustomed to many different kinds of food, to the taste and feel of more solid things such as milk pudding and sieved vegetables. But if we are too late in introducing them baby may have become so attached to sucking milk that he refuses anything else. Tinned baby foods are convenient.

" At 3 months baby may have some strained vegetable soup. If it is thick dilute it and if greasy, be sure to skim it because fatty foods tend to upset babies. The foods mentioned are in addition to the milk he is having from the breast or bottle."

" Some infants get very annoyed when offered solid food before having the breast or bottle ; this is probably because they are thirsty and want a drink first. Try it at the end of the feed. Others resent solid food either before or after. A baby may object to any change in the routine he knows and enjoys, so humour him a little.

"At 4 months you could give sieved vegetable. Begin with cooked lettuce, as it is so easily digested, but you can use any fresh green vegetable that has been boiled until tender and rubbed through a fine sieve. 4 G. (one teaspoonful) will be enough to begin with. If he refuses it, try again in a week or two.

" The Mouli grinder and sieve is useful for fruit, vegetables, fish and meat.

" Putting a little egg yolk on the tip of the spoon with the vegetable might help, for it is quite a good plan to introduce a new food along with one he already knows."

LIVER IS GOOD FOR BABIES

" One very special food for babies is calf's or lamb's liver which helps baby to form rich red blood. Cut a small slice, 0·8 cm. (one-third of an inch) thick, put it between two saucers with 4 ml. (one teaspoonful) of warm water, and steam it for 20 minutes over a saucepan that is boiling briskly. Liver should be thoroughly cooked. Rub it through a fine sieve, and give 4 G. (one teaspoonful) with the sieved vegetable. Increase the amount until at 6 months he is having 15 G. (one tablespoonful).

WEANING

" Weaning proper is started at 8 months. Don't hurry over it, take about four weeks; it is better for baby and you that way. Baby is now accustomed to so many different foods that it is just a question of getting him to give up sucking and to use a cup and spoon instead. Continue with dried or evaporated milk.

" THE FIRST WEEK

" He will have one meal without sucking, usually the midday meal. Serve minced chicken, fish, liver or meat with 15 G. (one tablespoonful) of vegetable and potato. Give a small helping of pudding or stewed fruit and a drink of milk from his cup.

" THE SECOND WEEK

" He may have breakfast in addition to the midday meal: porridge; cereal; half an egg ; whole-wheat bread and butter.

" THE THIRD WEEK

" He will have supper at about 17.00 hours, as well as the other two meals: cereal; baby food. He will probably wish to have a drink of milk at 22.00 hours until he is about a year old.

"AT ONE YEAR

" Baby should be having 600 ml. (1 pint of milk) every day. Always remember it is the body-building foods as well as fruit and vegetables with their minerals and vitamins that baby needs. Starchy foods make fat, flabby babies, but a baby with strong straight bones and firm muscles is far healthier in every way.

" Don't worry if your baby is slow in drinking from a cup, giving up the bottle or in feeding himself; some babies develop at a slower rate without being actually backward.

"Allow him to feed himself as soon as he wants to even if he makes a mess. Some feed themselves at 12 months, others at 16 months. If he refuses to eat the foods you serve, don't fuss or show any anxiety or you will have more and more trouble.

" The mother who can keep calm at meal times will usually manage to get her infant to eat the foods that build bonny babies."

TRAINING BABY TO KEEP DRY

The Talk as given

" Ideas regarding the training of babies to keep dry have changed in recent years ; the modern method being to start potting at the ninth month.

" Babies take longer to gain control when potting is started early ; an investigation carried out on a large number of babies proved this quite conclusively.

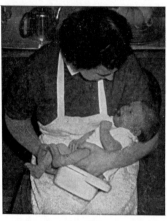

FIG. 504

" Catching what comes."

(*Real training starts at the eighth or ninth month.*)

" You may hold baby out from the second week, if you like, so long as you realize that you are not training him. Catch what comes, and be satisfied, but if you think you are teaching him to hold his water until you pot him again, you are going to be bitterly disappointed.

" Baby is too young to know what you are trying to teach him. After all, the sensation of water in the bladder is a very delicate one, and if after seven months he is no further ahead, you are going to get discouraged, and slack off in your efforts at the very time when you should be starting to train him.

" We all know the type of mother who is determined to have the perfectly trained baby, dry at all costs. She is thinking more of her own reputation as a good manager than of what is best for baby. Poor lamb, he is potted before and after feeds, before he goes out and when he comes in, before he goes to sleep and when he wakes up.

" No wonder he hates the pot and rebelliously refuses to use it on many occasions as soon as he is old enough to register his objection. He is shamed and blamed, scolded and spanked, and all this fuss gets him so worked up that he can't relax and do what is wanted. The happy baby becomes stubborn and bad tempered, and later develops into a defiant or sulky toddler."

WHEN TO START TRAINING

" START TRAINING BABY AT NINE MONTHS

" Study his habits ; note when he usually passes water and make your efforts coincide with ' his times,' which will most likely be every two or three hours.

"Always hold him out in the same place, so that he will learn where you want him to do it.

" Use a special word and he will soon know what it means.

" Show him the water when he has passed it, and again use the special word. It is at this point that baby is really beginning to learn bladder control.

" Don't hold him out for longer than three or four minutes. Praise his success with a word or two ; ignore failure. Be careful not to overpraise, or his feelings will be hurt on the days when he gets no praise. Keep steadily on, week after week, with persistent regularity, cheerful and hopeful.

" There will be periods of success and many setbacks; eventually, at about 15 months, he will tell you when he has passed water, and, not until about 18 months, will he tell you he wants to do it. Baby learns first that he has done it, later he learns that he is going to do it.

" Leave off the napkin when he can go for two hours. When busy playing, he may ignore the need until it is too late; remind him, for the memory of a child is short. Overlook occasional lapses.

"Active or highly strung children take longer than the placid type, and boys are rather slower than girls. It does, however, take longer to gain bladder control at night. Few children are dry all night at two years, and most are nearly three before they can do without napkins."

" Bowel training starts at the same time as bladder training, although baby may have had success with the pot prior to that time. He will be quite well trained at 12 or 15 months.

" It is the patient mother who plods steadily on, never expecting too much of a mere infant, who has the greatest success; the strict disciplinarian who makes such a ' to do ' about a perfectly natural function takes far longer to train her baby and may make him feel unloved. It is most important for a child to feel that he himself is loved although his behaviour may not be approved of.

" If at 3½ years he is still wetting, much encouragement is required; he needs all the help you can give him. Patience and perseverance are indeed excellent qualities in a mother."

TEETHING

The Talk as given

" There is always great rejoicing in the home when baby cuts his first tooth. The event is often anticipated for weeks and sometimes months, because from about the fourth month baby has been dribbling or slavering. But there is no connection at all between teething and dribbling, except that they occur at the same time. To digest starchy foods such as oat-flour or Farex, baby is now producing saliva, and it dribbles down his chin until he learns to swallow it.

" Day after day mother looks at his gums, and although it always seems as if a tooth is just ready to come through, nothing happens. Then without any warning two tiny teeth are seen peeping through the lower gum; baby has cut his first teeth and never even made a whimper. That is what usually happens; it is the double ones that are apt to upset baby and cause disturbed nights; they come through during the second year."

TIMES OF CUTTING TEETH

" The first two teeth may appear during the sixth month, but don't worry if your baby has no teeth even at 9 months as long as he is a sturdy infant; babies grow and develop at different rates. You will be attending your doctor or the child health clinic, and they will advise you what to do if teething is slow.

" If you would like to know when baby gets his teeth, I'll tell you an easy way to remember

" He should have six teeth less than his age in months.

AT 12 MONTHS BABY HAS	6	TEETH	
AT 18 ,,	,,	12	,,
AT 24 ,,	,,	18	,,

" By the time he is 2½ years old the 20 baby teeth will be cut."

CARE DURING TEETHING

" In cold weather see that baby has a cosy vest that fastens well up in front, for when his dress is sopping wet with saliva he is more likely to catch cold. Soft muslin bibs (four layers) are very satisfactory, but do not use a plastic bib : they have been known to blow over baby's nose and mouth with disastrous results.

" If baby is at the crawling stage his hands will get dirty, and as he is sucking his fingers a great deal at this time, wash them often. There is nothing to beat soap and water to prevent infection; have clean floors, clean clothes, clean toys.

" Baby's resistance to germs is lowered when he is upset with teething, and a cold may develop into bronchitis. Cotton play trousers with shoulder straps worn over a knitted dress or suit can be easily washed. They keep baby clean and warm.

" Give him something to bite on. Bone teething rings are usually recommended, but as a rule baby prefers something a little softer, a rubber toy or his own fingers.

" You will find baby prefers crusts rather than rusks, which may be so crisp that they irritate his tender gums. Don't give him too many, or you will upset his stomach; one after meals is sufficient.

" Use a plastic spoon with a rounded edge when feeding him, the sharp edge of a metal spoon will hurt his gums and make him cry."

TEETHING TROUBLES

" It is true some babies are upset, but we must not blame teething for every illness that occurs during the two years of teething time. If his gums are hot and painful he will be restless and cross. Give him frequent sips of cool water; it soothes his gums, and, if feverish, he needs the extra fluid. If he isn't hungry don't coax him to eat. Baby needs less food when he is feverish, and don't give any new foods or he may be upset.

" See that his bowels move every day; the extra water should help, but use a mild laxative, such as milk of magnesia, if necessary. If his water is dark in colour or has a strong smell, you will know he isn't getting enough to drink.

" Out of doors let him wear a helmet or hood, or tie a scarf round his ears if there is a cold blustering wind, for teething babies do get pain in their jaws.

"A teething baby has a very sensitive nervous system, so if he is having a bad day keep him quiet, give extra mothering and prevent the other children from trying to amuse him ; excitement only makes things worse. A warm bath and early to bed is good treatment.

" Some babies seem to have skin spots at teething time, but doctors think they are probably due to some food that baby hasn't become accustomed to. Moisten some bicarbonate of soda and dab it on to soothe the itching.

"All these things are not going to happen to any one infant, and the majority of babies cut their teeth with no trouble whatsoever, so don't let the teething bogey worry you unduly."

THE TODDLER AND THE NEW BABY

Some toddlers resent the intrusion of a new baby and may suffer intense jealousy if the parents do not show understanding. An endeavour should be made to avoid the psychological trauma which may ensue. Jealousy can be exhibited in various ways, such as temper tantrums, whining, bed-wetting and reversion to baby habits; these may not be manifest until months later.

It would be considerate if the toddler saw the new baby for the first time in a cot rather than in the mother's arms. Should domestic assistance be given by a relative or home-help, it might be discreet to allow her, rather than the mother, to attend to the new baby in the toddler's presence. Nor would it be advisable for the baby to be fed by the mother in the same room as the toddler. Allowing him to help with the bath and other matters will tend to make him feel that the baby belongs to him.

During this period the father usually devotes more time to the toddler who will revel in this. He should also be given a particularly coveted toy but should be spared hearing excessive adulation of the baby by visitors and ought not to see the gifts they bring.

If parents give the toddler extra attention and assure him of their love by a more than usual display of affection he will more readily accept and enjoy the new baby.

QUESTIONS FOR REVISION

What advice would you give in response to the mother's questions: What will I do if baby screams during the night ? How soon can I take baby out in the pram ? How will I know if baby is too hot ? How many hours should a baby sleep during 24 hours ? How will I know baby is crying too much ? If baby chokes when I am giving him his bottle what will I do ? Why should I not use a pillow ? Why are plastic bibs condemned ? My husband wants the baby to be circumcised. My mother says the baby is tongue-tied and thinks this should be cut. Are green motions serious ? How do I clean baby's nose and mouth? Should baby sleep in a separate room ?

C.M.B.(Scot.) paper, 1970.—Outline a programme for the education of the patient in preparation for labour and parenthood.

43

Suggestions on how to Teach Expectant Mothers

Preparation for childbirth and early parenthood is a practical subject which should be taught in a pleasant manner. If the teaching is ponderous or is mainly a dissertation on the generative organs the subject will fall into disrepute. In a limited series of talks where the need for instruction is immediate, the physiological approach should not be used except where it is necessary for a better understanding of some practical point.

THE TEACHER *(A Midwife)*

The teacher's knowledge and experience of obstetrics should be considerable, and to understand the difficulties under which women have to bring up their families she should be familiar with the community aspects of child bearing and rearing.

Additional experience with babies during the first year of life is an advantage in answering the questions mothers ask.

METHODS OF TEACHING

Preparing the Talk

Start preparing the talk in ample time ; read all the books available to you on the subject: draw on your own knowledge and experience. Jot down suitable facts under headings, each on a separate page ; check and re-check the facts, for all statements made must be correct and up to date, as well as practical. If in doubt consult an expert.

A clear plan should be made out and the subject-matter arranged in logical sequence rather than giving it as a jumble of unrelated facts. Search your brain for an exciting opening sentence. Set the matter aside for a few days and go back to it with a fresh outlook ; new ideas may come while the subject is simmering in your mind.

Write up the talk as fully as you wish, choosing words which depict what you mean to convey with vividness and exactitude. Again set the material aside, then read it over with a critical eye and select only the best of it, prune ruthlessly ; the improvement will be marked.

Polish it until the style is fluent yet lucid. Set it aside once more, then read it aloud and listen to the sound of the words, remembering that they are to be heard and not read. If you get someone to read it to you the faults in construction will be even more evident. Continue polishing and rearranging until it cannot be improved any further. By this time you are saturated with the subject-matter although you have not actually memorized it. " Time " it to the required length.

Arrange headings on filing cards, using red and blue ink to catch the eye. Think of these headings as islands between which you must swim ; you won't founder for you are buoyed up with a very comprehensive knowledge of the subject. Practise the delivery of one heading until it is mastered ; do the second one, then both together, and continue until the whole is ready for delivery in public. Then this apparently simple talk will, when given with effortless ease, belie all the hard work that has gone into its preparation.

PRESENTING THE SUBJECT

Arousing Interest

This is one of the essentials in teaching and as the expectant mother is intensely interested in mothercraft, teaching her is comparatively easy. To maintain that interest we must meet her needs by :

1. Telling her what she wants to know, *e.g.* " what happens during pregnancy and labour."

2. Showing her what she wants to see, *e.g.* " baby's model layette " and " how to bath baby."

We will, of course, teach her what we think she ought to know and this may entail giving two different subjects in one lesson in order that she may feel the class is worth while for her.

Holding Attention

To hold the attention of a group, the mind of each one must be kept active. The vitality of the teacher and her ability to paint vivid word pictures, the interest of the subject, the setting up of an attractive display, handing out typed recipes or instructions, passing round samples of fabrics and patterns, allowing the members of the group to participate in demonstration or discussion all help to maintain attention.

LEARNING SHOULD BE AN ENJOYABLE EXPERIENCE

The subject should be presented in such a way as to depict baby-care as a happy experience rather than a difficult responsible job ; " enjoy your baby " being the perfect motif. A little kindly humour will help to make the talks sparkle and the midwife should try to create a bright, friendly atmosphere.

In order that the expectant mothers of less than average intelligence will understand what is being taught, the language used ought to be within the range of their comprehension. The lay equivalent of medical terms should be given, *e.g.* (*fetus in utero*) – baby before he is born ; (*protein*) = body building food ; (*carbohydrates*) = starches.

Learning is a Slow Process

Most people have to be told or shown what to do at least three times before they really learn ; repetition is therefore very necessary, but it should not be too obvious (see p. 744 for an example of this).

Explanations should be made wherever possible, for unless people understand, they do not learn ; they may look without seeing, and hear without comprehending. The " reason why " should be stated in order to be convincing, particularly when something contrary to common practice is being recommended, *e.g.* babies' nightgowns without waist-bands. The reasons given may so impress the mother that she remembers what she is told, *e.g.* why cold water ought to be put into baby's bath before the hot water.

Every statement made should be crystal clear.

This may necessitate making a definite even dogmatic pronouncement, a measure usually advisable when instructing the novice. Having given what you consider is the best method, don't confuse the issue by making alternative suggestions. Do not clutter the talk with unnecessary words ; each sentence should carry the lesson a stage further on.

The Expectant Mother's Point of View

The subject ought to be approached from the expectant mother's point of view, and the teacher should try to imagine the thoughts and feelings of the woman at this time. She is going through one of life's most enriching experiences, her emotions are keyed up, sentiment runs high so the teacher must not be too mundane or matter of fact. The midwife should endeavour to catch a gleam of the mother's joy in creation and appreciate her strong maternal instinct.

Notes of lectures given to student midwives on pregnancy or babies are not suitable; they frequently contain bald statements of a scientific nature that will not appeal to the mother-to-be. A more personal approach is necessary, and many facts should be clothed in words with a sentimental bias.

HOW TO GIVE THE TALK

Posters and equipment should be set out in readiness to start without delay and in order that the rhythm of the talk will not be interrupted.

OVERCOMING NERVOUSNESS

The thought of the ordeal will no doubt make you nervous even though you are sure of your subject and well rehearsed.

All good speakers experience some degree of stage-fright which is a state of nervous tension rather than fear ; a necessary stimulus to effective public speaking.

Think of the audience instead of yourself ; it is almost certain that they know much less about the subject than you do. They are eager to learn, you should be eager to teach them.

Tension is usually evident in the hands and face so relax both ; slow, deep breathing helps to induce calmness.

Use a confident tone to bolster your own morale ; a thin tremulous voice will make you even more nervous and will distress the audience so much on your behalf that they will be unable to concentrate on what you are saying.

PLATFORM DEPORTMENT
An Attractive Appearance

It is the duty of a speaker to look her best as a compliment to the audience, and clothes with simple lines and clear contrasting colours show up well from a distance. A midwife ought to wear uniform if possible as a symbol of her competence to speak on the subject. An immaculate uniform appeals to the audience; it is becoming to the wearer and this gives her additional confidence; for demonstrating baby-care procedures it is most suitable.

Entering the Room

Have a smile in your heart if not on your lips and maintain a degree of poise and composure.

A chairman will not be necessary for an informal talk to a group of mothers who know you, but if being introduced by a chairman she will precede you when entering the room and show you to the seat on the right of " the chair."

All eyes will be on you and the slightest sign of nervousness will be noted, so resist the impulse to fiddle with your hair or uniform. Let your hands lie idly on your lap though you may feel tempted to clutch your notes.

Look over the audience with a friendly eye but give no visible sign of recognizing anyone you know.

OPENING THE TALK

When called on, rise gracefully and on no account must you speak until you are on your feet and facing the audience. With your gaze embrace the group, wait for silence and begin, turning slightly towards the chairman as you address her as " Madam Chairman."

Do not fix your eyes on any one individual, neither should you stare straight ahead into space as you concentrate intently on what you are saying. Looking at the floor gives the speaker a most pathetic demeanour and riveting the eyes on the ceiling, as though imploring help, will only rouse pity in the minds of the audience. If you gaze out of the window the group will do likewise and you will no longer hold their attention.

Avoid the trivial subterfuge of telling an amusing anecdote to get on good terms with the audience ; a friendly manner, a talk well prepared and delivered will do all that is necessary. The telling of stories to stress a point is an excellent teaching device but stories, humorous or otherwise, should arise out of and not be superimposed upon the subject-matter.

GRACEFUL STANCE AND APPROPRIATE GESTURES

Stand gracefully with the weight of the body poised lightly on the balls of the feet ; heels should be about 20 cm. (8 inches) apart, toes of the right foot being 10·2 cm. (4 inches) in front of the left to give a solid stance that allows free movement of knee, hip and shoulder joints without loss of balance, for your whole body is brought into play when speaking expressively. Hands ought to be cupped together lightly at waist level and shoulders held well back to give ample breathing capacity.

On no account lean on chair or table, an ungraceful even ugly attitude ; stand well away from both in case you are tempted to lean on either of them.

Make appropriate gestures, only when the urge to do so is spontaneous, in order to emphasize a point ; they should appear to be so natural that the audience is not aware that gestures are being made. Arms should be curved, wrists relaxed.

Avoid mannerisms, they distract and irritate the audience. Try to create an atmosphere of tranquillity by maintaining poise and making only the movements that are absolutely necessary. Do not pace the platform, fiddle with buttons, toy with the chalk, trifle with the duster, jingle coins or keys. These mannerisms are intensely annoying to an attentive audience ; they also develop into habits that are very difficult to eradicate.

MAKING CONTACT

This term is used to designate the mental and psychological link that a good teacher creates between the audience and herself and is one of the most vital factors in teaching.

Contact is made by the teacher when she looks at and talks to the audience as individuals in whom she is interested and to whom she is eager to pass on her ideas. Her gaze is directed towards the whole group yet every member feels that she is being looked at ; the spoken word is heard by each individual as though meant for her personally.

EXAMPLES OF HOW TO MAKE CONTACT

When demonstrating " baby's layette " the midwife's eyes ought to be on the audience so that her personality is projected towards them ; she should only glance at the garment she is displaying.

When demonstrating " baby's bath " she must frequently look at and address the group if only to say " watch carefully what I'm going to do now " or " I'll do that over again " or to explain a point. If the midwife's whole attention is concentrated on what she is doing with her hands no contact is made, and only an intense interest in the subject will hold the attention of the group.

When using teaching aids such as posters, blackboard or flannelgraphs they ought to be given only a fleeting glance.

Failing to Make Contact

No contact is made when a lecturer is so engrossed in her subject or indifferent to the educational needs of her audience that she appears to be quite oblivious of their presence.

Under no circumstances should a talk on a simple subject like baby-care be read. Listening to any lecture being read is dull and boring in the extreme because this breaks the vital contact so necessary between speaker and audience. When the eyes are glued to the reading desk there is no opportunity for the personality to bring the spoken word to life.

In painting vivid word-pictures the physical, mental, and emotional faculties must all be brought into play ; in fact a good speaker requires some of the attributes of the actor.

Teaching Aids

Every available aid should be used to amplify verbal teaching, but it should be realized that no matter how unique these are in conception or artistic in execution they are only of value if they simplify the lesson or make it more interesting and enjoyable.

POSTERS

They should be arresting in colour and design, conveying the message at a glance. Advice given should be positive, good rather than bad methods being depicted. Printing should be legible at a distance, captions short and pithy.

Many commercial posters are so colourful and pleasing that they introduce a note of vitality as well as having educational worth.

FLANNELGRAPHS

These supply a variation of poster and blackboard, but are somewhat limited in their usefulness. **Printed headings can be presented quickly ;** gaily coloured felt cut-outs are excellent to depict the generative organs and fetus *in utero* : cut-outs from glossy magazines make a colourful display of fruits and vegetables.

THE BLACKBOARD

This well-tried device is a most valuable teaching aid, too often used only to jot down words or on which to scribble a poorly conceived diagram. It is worth while going to the trouble of achieving proficiency in its use.

START WITH AN EMPTY BLACKBOARD

There is great educational value in teaching step by step while building up a drawing or setting out headings. The necessary action breaks the monotony of talk.

Coloured dust-free chalk should be used with vigour and gay abandon to give emphasis, variety and beauty. Study from a distance the colours that show up well in close proximity to each other, such as red and yellow, green and white. Blue can rarely be seen beyond the front row.

Do not hold the chalk like a pencil. Use half a stick, one end in the palm, the point projecting 1·25 cm. beyond the tips of the thumb and first two fingers.

Apply sufficient pressure to make a bold decisive line.

HOW TO DRAW

As an aid to drawing look at the object for six times as long as it will take to draw it, noting the proportions of length to breadth, the ratio of the size of one part to another, *e.g.* cervix to corpus, the convexity of curves and other details. Thus the visual image is transmitted to the brain which then guides the hand.

Practise drawing heavy bold lines, vertical, horizontal and semi-circular, right across the blackboard with a wide sweep of the arm, using shoulder and elbow rather than wrist. Continue until convincing lines can be executed under perfect control. Wavy thin lines are not readily visible and convey the impression that the teacher is lacking in resolution.

Printing is legible, but round writing is done more quickly. Practise writing rows of words 10, 5, 2·5, 1·25 cm. in size. From the back of the room it will be evident that medium size is the most legible.

A CLEAR PLAN

Decide how to arrange blackboard headings and sub-headings for each lesson. Avoid too much detail.

The outline should be intelligible, because of its orderly arrangement, to anyone who was not present at the lesson. It also provides an excellent means for recapitulation at the completion of a lecture.

Duplicate the foundation drawing rather than cluttering it with detail to such an extent that the structure or idea depicted is neither comprehensible nor recognizable.

LEARNING FROM THE BLACKBOARD

The blackboard is an aid to learning ; a means whereby understanding of the subject is enhanced, not merely a vehicle for the statement of facts.

The teacher is the link between audience and blackboard and the vital contact with the audience must be constantly maintained.

Teach the audience, not the blackboard.

While writing turn towards the audience as far as is possible.

Long silences while writing are wasteful and create an intangible barrier. Explain what you are drawing ; spell a difficult or new word, stop to explain a point.

Using the blackboard as an effective aid to learning requires teaching skill of a high order.

BULLETIN BOARD FOR EXPECTANT MOTHERS

A bulletin board is ideal for exhibiting printed matter or illustrations that will educate or interest expectant mothers.

The layout must be attractive to catch the eye. Bright, gaily coloured cut-outs from the cookery section of women's magazines. Booklets from baby food manufacturers are a source of attractive baby photographs ; pages from catalogues of baby equipment showing the latest in prams, baths, etc., are always appreciated.

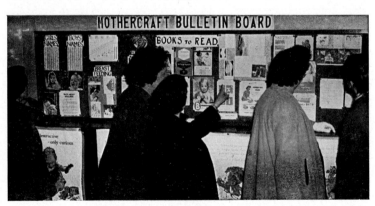

FIG. 505

Bulletin board placed in waiting or cloak room where small groups assemble.
Subject-matter changed weekly.
(*Simpson Memorial Maternity Pavilion, Edinburgh.*)

EDUCATIONAL EXHIBITS

Maternity benefits, immunization and **vaccination pamphlets.**

HEALTH EDUCATION

Foods that build bonny babies. Foods that prevent anæmia.

Keeping food clean, covered, cool. Good posture.

40

Mottoes and pictures relating to home and motherhood.

The Maternity Center Birth Atlas has been specially prepared for expectant mothers. *Illustrations from Midwifery textbooks are not suitable.*

FILMS AND FILM STRIPS

These are admirable to depict situations and procedures that are beyond the scope of presentation by the teacher, *e.g.* the birth of a baby. The teacher will make her own comments as the method shown may be at variance with those approved of by the teacher or her employing authority.

Films can be used to show the childbearing process as a whole and give expectant mothers insight into the facilities available for their welfare.

Their great disadvantage is that the viewers are passive observers rather than active participants and do not benefit from the personal relationship that should exist between the teacher and her audience.

RADIO AND TELEVISION BROADCASTS

These are of value in presenting another point of view to those who have basic knowledge and experience of the subject. They are apt to be talks or demonstrations given by experts on the subject rather than well-planned lessons by experienced teachers.

BABY CLOTHES AND EQUIPMENT

These are absolutely essential for teaching baby-care and can be displayed for their attractive, decorative value, and to create the atmosphere that appeals to mothers even although not utilized in the lesson being taught.

Some manufacturers will supply garments and equipment, patterns of materials and catalogues on request.

Baby equipment is discussed under the appropriate demonstrations.

THE DEMONSTRATION

Set up an attractive display ; hang model baby garments on the walls; buy or borrow the type of articles used in the home (not hospital equipment); see that everything is in perfect condition. You need hardly ask a busy mother to prepare things nicely for her baby if you don't do so when demonstrating.

Towels and baby's layette ought to be freshly laundered or pressed and arranged in the order in which they are to be used. Check each item so that nothing is missing.

Rehearse the procedure and know exactly what you will say when you are doing a certain thing. When undertaking a comprehensive demonstration such as bathing baby, it is a good idea to have an assistant to carry out the procedure while the teacher explains what is being done. In that case a complete rehearsal must be arranged beforehand.

Analyse each movement made before demonstrating such manœuvres as turning baby on the knee, *e.g.* show how to grasp baby's body and in which direction to turn him. These details are appreciated by the learner.

It is advisable to use a doll for bathing and dressing, because then you can be as slow as you wish without any danger of chilling: a crying baby distracts the audience.

When bathing a doll without the use of water, it is absolutely imperative that the face cloth be dipped into imaginary water and wrung out realistically, the non-existent soap rinsed off and the doll dried properly, otherwise the illusion is broken and the demonstration ruined.

Select the opening statement with discernment

While standing make a few remarks on the purpose or some other aspect of the demonstration. It may be worth while discussing the equipment, giving advantages and prices.

Speak slowly and deliberately, letting each sentence convey some particular point. **Repeat** any important part of the procedure.

Explain why you do a certain thing in a particular way, or the audience may think it is only a whim of yours. Draw attention to apparently trivial points, for they have neither the knowledge nor the experience of the teacher, *e.g.* the gentle drying of baby's fingers to avoid injury to the nail folds.

Look at the audience as often as you can to maintain contact.

Omit unnecessary detail, and do not make the mistake of the inexperienced teacher who tries to tell her students all that she knows on the subject; **teach a little at a time but teach it well.**

Short silent periods are invaluable to allow the mothers to concentrate on what you are doing; if you chatter the whole time, they become confused and cannot mentally absorb all that you are saying, nor differentiate between the significant and the insignificant.

Emphasize what they should, rather than what they should not, do. Use the words " don't " and " never" sparingly.

To bring the lesson to a close rise, if seated, and face the audience. Do not waver and then stop in an indecisive manner; work up to a climax by slowing the rate of speech and increasing intensity of feeling. Have the final sentence memorized, make it arresting or appealing.

Any remarks about leaflets or equipment can be made afterwards.

A woman less than 24 weeks pregnant may demonstrate again any procedure, under the guidance of the teacher.

Hints on Public Speaking

The following elementary facts on public speaking are intended to give the midwife confidence in speaking formally to larger groups and informally to smaller groups of expectant mothers.

Speech is concerned with breath control, voice production and diction. Beautiful audible speech can be acquired with training and practice. Voice is part of the personality and the mode of delivery must be in harmony with this.

BREATH CONTROL

The passage of a steady stream of air through the larynx is essential for the production of vocal sound. Fairly deep breaths should be taken in, through the nose and mouth, with no apparent effort; the shoulders not being raised during the process.

The expiration of air is controlled by the diaphragm and not by a tightening of the muscles of the throat, the vocalized breath being allowed to flow gently and evenly out of the mouth.

To be audible the voice must have carrying power and this requires sufficient breath. If the audience have to make an effort to hear they cannot absorb what is being said.

To amplify the volume of sound breathe more deeply but under control.

If not regulated properly the extravagantly used breath gives a gasping toneless quality to the spoken word and necessitates frequent inhalations: the sound produced lacks carrying power.

PRACTICE

Inhale a full breath and let it flow out steadily while you say " one, two . . . one, two . . ." for 20 to 30 seconds. Do not continue speaking after the breath is finished or the sound will be toneless. Increase the time taken to expel the breath as an exercise only; no attempt is made while speaking in public to breathe excessively deeply, but expiration must be steady and under control.

THE PRODUCTION OF TONE

Tone is produced in the larynx, but it emanates from the mind. The tone of voice expresses what is being felt emotionally, or can be made to simulate this as is done in acting. Facial expression also influences tone, *e.g.* it is not possible to speak in a pleasant tone of voice while frowning, or conversely to speak crossly with a smile on the face.

Variations in tone give interest and liveliness to the performance. Mental boredom will be evident in the tone of voice and it may be necessary to " pep-up " oneself in order to speak convincingly.

To produce a round musical tone the oral cavity must be resonant, and this is achieved by depressing the lower jaw as in yawning. The back of the tongue should be relaxed and must not block the passage of vocalized breath which should be directed forwards and on to the hard palate.

No tightening or squeezing of the throat muscles should take place, and the lips and mouth ought not to be forced beyond their normal limits in shaping words.

Much of the beauty and musical tone of the spoken word is dependent on the proper enunciation of the vowel sounds. In shaping these the cavity of the mouth may have to be round, ovoid or flattened, and many of the most exquisite words in the English language have the " oh " or " ah " vowel sounds, which permit the maximum of resonance in the oral cavity. Tones are also modified and beautified by the emotion of the speaker and her ability to interpret this in sound. An artistic quality can be given to words and conveyed by the tone of voice.

PRACTISE SAYING

" Lovely lilacs bloom in the valley."

Allow the mind to dwell on the mental image conjured up by these words, and try to interpret and convey it in colourful sound. Suffuse the vowel sounds with a warm glow ; allow the tongue to linger for a second on the consonant " L." Concentrate on tone and smooth flowing breath.

FOR COMPARISON REPEAT THE FOLLOWING LINES

" **Dirty British coaster with a salt-caked smoke stack** " Speak the words briskly, no beauty of tone is required ; accentuate the consonants and use a jerky rhythm to denote the chugging of a ship.

The volume of tone should be regulated according to the size of the room. The conversational tone suited to an informal small group would not project the voice to a large audience in a lecture theatre

Modulation is the passing from one tone to another in order to clothe the words with meaning and beauty and to give interest, variety and expression to speech. Speaking in a monotone, no matter how lovely the tone may be, is liable to act as a soporific.

Pitch is the level at which sound is produced on the vocal register, and may be high, middle or low. It is regulated by tightening or loosening the vocal cords. For a high note they are tightened ; for a low note the vocal cords are relaxed and a pleasing musical sound with good carrying power is produced. The middle pitch is most commonly used. When a high pitch is used the tone is thin and squeaky as in depicting excitement or agitation and is not pleasant to listen to. **A change of pitch is used to indicate a new idea or subject.**

Speakers sometimes make the mistake of raising pitch and shouting in response to complaints from members of the audience at the back of the hall that they cannot hear. This is quite wrong ; the speaker ought to lower pitch, articulate more precisely, relax the lower jaw, breathe deeply and increase the volume of air expelled.

Shouting tightens the throat muscles and interferes with voice production in the larynx.

Inflection is the gliding up and down of pitch on a syllable or individual word as an aid to clarifying the idea being expressed, *e.g.* when asking a question a rising inflection is used. Speaking on one pitch is most monotonous to listen to.

ARTICULATION

Articulation is concerned with the clear enunciation of vowel sounds and the precision with which consonants are delivered. Slovenly articulation of the consonants " T," " B," and " P " is a common cause of mumbling, and the consequent inaudibility of speech.

Words should be articulated by the lips, the teeth, the tip of the tongue, and when doing so, the voice is brought well forwards to facilitate its carrying power.

PRACTISE THE FOLLOWING

" Bat-pat " ; " Tip-top " ; " Pip-pop " ; " Bab-tab " ; also the sentence. " The lips, the teeth, the tip of the tongue." Exaggerate chipping off the consonants neatly like coins from the mint.

Avoid the hissing of sibilants.

This may occur when a word ends and the next one begins with the letter " S."

PRACTISE THE FOLLOWING

" Luscious strawberries " ; " Sing a song of sixpence " ; " English roses " ; " Irish shamrocks "; " Scottish thistles." " The hissing of sibilants is especially unpleasing."

Use the point of the tongue and speak well forward in the mouth, permitting the tongue to sound the letter " S " for the minimal length of time.

RATE

It is imperative when speaking in public, that the words are spoken slowly enough to be heard and understood. If a stream of words, indistinguishable one from another, is poured out, the audience will grasp only a minute part of their meaning. Even if the words are clearly articulated the rate at which new ideas are being presented is more rapid than the rate at which they can be absorbed. The necessary mental effort is so great that members of the audience allow their attention to wander.

Emphasis on some special point may be made by slowing the rate to an impressive degree, as in giving warning of impending danger or in working up to a climax. Unimportant points can be described rapidly but enunciation must be crisp to ensure clarity.

The pause is one of the most telling devices in public speaking; being not only effective, but almost dramatic in intensity. The audience listens more intently to hear what follows the pause or concentrates on what has just been said.

Multiple pauses are the refuge of the badly prepared speaker ; dull and boring.

As an aid to speaking more slowly, think in words, and not in sentences as is usually done during conversation. Give each word its full value, articulating the first and last letters meticulously (if they should be sounded) as well as the body of the word. Speak deliberately and make an effort to enunciate the words distinctly without actually disjointing them.

The Choice and Use of Words

Words are used to convey meaning and portray ideas, but they convey feeling also ; they should, therefore, be selected with care and discrimination. Vivid word-pictures may be used to recreate a scene or give vitality to an incident. Words may sound beautiful in themselves, or they may be loved by the hearer because of their association, *e.g.* " home " is more attractive than " hostel "; " a field of golden corn " than " a street littered with rubbish." These facts should be kept in mind when choosing words.

The meaning of words can be enhanced by the manner in which they are spoken, and the midwife can increase the effectiveness of her talk or demonstration in this way. *When saying,* " Rub the hair briskly with a Turkish towel," speak tersely to suggest the action ; use a fairly high pitch and sound consonants crisply. *When saying,* " Cuddle your baby," linger on the vowels, use a round musical tone, low pitch, slow rate ; above all " feel " in your mind what you are trying to express with your voice.

The fluent speaker has a deep and wide knowledge of her subject on which she can draw and a large and varied vocabulary from which she can select the appropriate word without hesitation. The reading of good prose is of inestimable value, experience in public speaking is, of course, beneficial, but adequate preparation of the talk is absolutely essential. Sheer garrulousness should not be emulated.

Some Common Faults in Public Speaking

Inadequate emotional power is often due to inhibition in expressing emotion. Forget yourself and think of the audience. Try to visualize the situation and to feel more acutely; use facial expression to suit the emotion.

Lack of emphasis may be due to insecurity regarding the subject-matter or in facing an audience. Volume should be amplified. Thorough preparation is essential.

Shrill or unmusical tone may be due to tightening the throat muscles or rigid lower jaw and lack of resonance.

Absence of variety occurs when the full range of tone, pitch and rate are not utilized.

Indistinct speech is due to rigidity of the lower jaw and immobility of the lips.

Slurred speech is due to flabbiness of the tip of the tongue: it should be used with precision.

Inaudibility may be due to insufficient volume or to dropping of the voice at the end of a sentence; the flow of breath must be sustained to the last letter of the final word in the sentence. Deeper inspiration and more frequent breaths are needed.

The persistent use of a word such as " now " prior to stating a new idea or saying quickly " Is that clear: " or " Do you see: " without waiting for a reply becomes a habit. This was said over forty times in one talk. (*There is no need to ask, except in rare instances. The good teacher anticipates the perplexities of her students and explains difficult points in various ways in order that all will understand.*)

Appendix I

Carcinoma of Cervix and Breast

Carcinoma of the cervix occurs usually in women over 25 who have borne children. Infected cervical erosions and lacerations are believed (*but this has not been proved*) to predispose to the disease in women who are susceptible to carcinoma.

CERVICAL CYTOLOGY
Early cancer of the cervix is detected by cytology (study of cell formation).

All epithelia desquamate their surface cells, and malignant epithelia do so more rapidly. The Papanicolaou cervical smear provides a means of detecting such malignant cells before any cancerous lesion of the cervix is clinically manifest; Ayres wooden spatula is used to scrape off surface cells from the region of the internal os. Should suspicious cells be found a cone biopsy is taken.

A cervical cytology service where a diligent search is made at gynæcological, prenatal, postnatal and infertility clinics, provides a means of accelerating the detection of early cancer of the cervix, which will result in a higher survival rate.

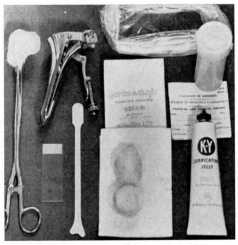

FIG. 506

Requirements for Papanicolaou cervical smear.

Sponge holder.	Glass slide.	3 wool balls.
Vaginal speculum.	Dispos-a-glove.	Laboratory form
Ayres spatula.	Tube of lubricant.	Bag for discard.

Container for slide with alcohol and ether.

(*Aberdeen Maternity Hospital.*)

SIGNS AND SYMPTOMS

Intermittent vaginal bleeding during pregnancy, not associated with abortion, moles or antepartum hæmorrhage, and a watery discharge should give rise to suspicion. On questioning the woman a history of metrorrhagia (bleeding between menstrual periods) prior to pregnancy may be elicited, but the bleeding may occur for the first time during pregnancy.

783

THE USUAL SEQUENCE IS

Vaginal discharge which is at first serous; bleeding, and later, pain and foul-smelling discharge.

No time should be lost. The patient is referred to her doctor, who will, in cases of suspected carcinoma, arrange for expert investigation. (*Late symptoms such as foul-smelling discharge and pain, are not usually seen by midwives in the course of their work, as in such cases the women do not become pregnant.*)

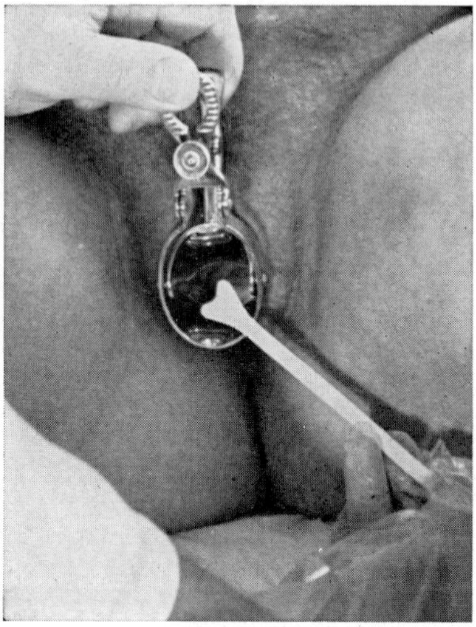

Early cancer is curable.

TREATMENT

1. In early pregnancy a radical hysterectomy (Wertheim) is performed followed by radiotherapy.

2. When diagnosed late in pregnancy, vaginal delivery is not permitted. After Cæsarean section, hysterectomy is performed because of the danger of sepsis and metastases via the placental site. Radical hysterectomy is performed, if operable; if not, subtotal hysterectomy and radiotherapy are employed.

Radiotherapy is being used more frequently, either alone or in conjunction with radical surgery, in the treatment of invasive cervical cancer.

FIG. 507
Using Ayres spatula to take Papanicolaou smear.
(*Aberdeen Maternity Hospital.*)

CARCINOMA OF THE BODY OF THE UTERUS

This is not found in association with pregnancy and tends to occur in women at the time of and following the menopause. Should the midwife's advice be asked about irregular or free bleeding at this period of life, the woman must be advised to see her doctor without delay.

CARCINOMA OF THE BREAST

This serious condition is occasionally diagnosed during pregnancy or the puerperium. Any lump during pregnancy, or which during the puerperium persists for longer than one month, should be investigated. The lump is painless, and not usually movable; there may be dimpling of the nipple. In some cases the area surrounding the nipple has the appearance of orange peel (*peau d'orange*).

Periodic screening by clinical examination of the breasts will detect cancer at an earlier date than formerly. Mammography and thermography as isolated screening procedures, although useful in certain cases, can be misleading.

The treatment is mastectomy and radiotherapy.

Immediate investigation should be advocated by the midwife if her advice is asked for by a woman of any age regarding a lump in the breast. The woman should be told that it may be a simple tumour which, if dealt with promptly, will be prevented from becoming serious.

QUESTIONS FOR REVISION

Explain how a Papanicolaou cervical smear is taken. What advice would you give a woman who complained of: (a) bleeding at the time of the menopause; (b) a lump in the breast.

C.M.B.(Eng.) paper. 50 word question.—Discuss the present arrangements for detecting early cancer of the cervix.

Appendix II

QUESTIONS FOR REVISION

THE QUESTIONS GIVEN BELOW ARE ASSOCIATED WITH
OR NAMED AFTER SOME NOTABLE PERSON.

To assess the percentage gained allow 2 marks for each correct answer.

	Name	See Page
1. The effect on which ultrasonic fetal pulse detection is based		665
2. Apparatus for abdominal decompression		796
3. Micro apparatus for testing pH of the blood		544
4. Wire saw decapitator		650
5. Pulmonary acid aspiration syndrome		635
6. Substance of the umbilical cord		39
7. Visible retraction ring		233
8. Suture applied for incompetent cervix in cases of habitual abortion		143
9. Placenta born fetal surface first		320
10. Scheme for scoring retraction in respiratory distress		542
11. Paralysis of arm due to injury of brachial plexus		590
12. Method of delivering " breech " shoulders by rotation and traction		370
13. Method of delivering aftercoming head of breech baby by carrying the body upwards until airway is clear		366
14. Test for Rhesus antibodies in the baby		575
15. The fetal stethoscope		118
16. Cervical smear taken to detect early carcinoma of cervix		783
17. Method of determining the degree of cephalo-pelvic disproportion by vaginal examination		122
18. Conservative method of treating unavoidable antepartum hæmorrhage		217
19. A reaction of the supine newborn when the supported head is allowed to drop a few cm.		524
20. Who introduced chloroform ?		251
21. Radiological sign of fetal death		654
22. Infant laryngoscope		557
23. Who first applied the use of ultrasonography to obstetrics?		663
24. The father of antenatal care		82
25. Valve used in cases of hydrocephaly		594
26. Post-coital test in cases of infertility		686
27. Intrauterine contraceptive device		472
28. Portable oxygen analyser		539

	Name	See Page
29. Alternative term for the mongol	*Down's*	603
30. Vacuum extractor applied to fetal head to aid its expulsion	*Malmstrom*	629
31. Scoring to evaluate condition of newborn . . .	*Apgar*	311
32. Blood test for phenylalanine (phenylketonuria) . .	*Guthrie*	799
33. Cerebral vein sometimes torn due to excessive or rapid head compression	*Galen* intra ventricle	584
34. Straight midwifery forceps		626
35. Method of placental extraction	*Caudal CT*	328
36. Bacteriological transport medium		565
37. Fetal scalp blood sampling		414
38. Neonate resuscitator with mask and hand bulb . .		682
39. Ducts opening in the urethra	*Skenes*	12
40. Test for congenital dislocation of hip . . .		601
41. Transverse abdominal incision for cæsarean section .	*Pfannenstiel*	639
42. Method of delivering aftercoming head of breech by jaw flexion and shoulder traction	*M SV*	372
43. Method of abdominal palpation, facing patient's head and grasping fetal head with right hand . .		115
44. The fetal skull perforator		649
45. Cricoid pressure		635
46. Semi-prone left lateral position.		424
47. Intravenous syringe pump		610
48. Test for number of fetal red cells in maternal blood (Rh-)		579
49. Blood clot observation test		666
50. Needle through which catheter is introduced for epidural anæsthesia		636

Short Examination Questions

CENTRAL MIDWIVES BOARD (N. IRELAND)

Write short notes on:

1. Hydramnios.   2. Atelectasis.   3. True conjugate.   4. Anencephaly.

1. Stillbirth.   2. Anuria.   3. Placenta prævia.   4. Hydatidiform mole.   5. Moulding.

1. Abnormal lochia.	2. Thrombo-phlebitis.
3. Engorgement of the breasts.	4. Postnatal exercises.

1. Cephalhæmatoma.   2. Spina bifida.   3. Prolapsed cord.   4. Foramen ovale.

1. Corpus luteum.   2. Moulding.   3. Episiotomy.   4. Proteinuria.

Write short notes on:

Induction of labour	Trichomonas vaginitis	Post-maturity
Pethilorfan.	Hydatidiform mole.	Engorged breasts.
Maternal mortality.	Anencephaly.	Unstable lie.
Moulding.	Caput succedaneum.	Third degree perineal tear.

Write short notes on:

Œsophageal atresia.	Cerebral hæmorrhage.	Hyaline membrane disease.
Hypoglycæmia.	Duodenal atresia.	Severe chilling due to cold.
Glycosuria in pregnancy.	Acetone in the urine, in labour.	Recognition of prolapsed cord.

Write short notes on:

Vitamin " K ".	Tube feeding.	Exchange transfusion.
Gastric lavage.	Oxygen.	Baby of diabetic mother.
An incubator.	Digoxin.	Hydrocephalus.

Write short notes on:

German measles in pregnancy.	Cervical cytology in pregnancy.	Cerebral hæmorrhage.
Heartburn in pregnancy.	Vaginal thrush in pregnancy.	Œsophageal atresia.
Anal atresia.	Congenital dislocation of the hip.	

Write short notes on:

Hæmoglobin.	Syntometrine.	Quickening.	Engagement of the fetal head.
Lochia.	Postnatal exercises.	Trial labour.	Cephalhæmatoma.
Club foot.	Cleft palate.	Cervical cytology.	Pulmonary embolus.

Write briefly on four of the following:

Urinary tract infection in pregnancy.	Syntometrine.	Postnatal exercises.
Engagement of the fetal head.	Cephalhæmatoma.	

Write short notes on four of the following:

The brim of the pelvis.	The liquor amnii.	Phenylketonuria.
Perinatal mortality.	Diagnosis of labour.	Recognition of fetal distress.

Write short notes on the following:

A complete tear.	Hæmoglobin.	Lochia.
Retention of urine.	Quickening.	

Write notes on the following:

Polyhydramnios.	Proteinuria.	" Free head " in a primigravida at term.
Oxytocic drugs.	Burns-Marshall manœuvre.	Amniocentesis.
Hydatidiform mole.	Trial labour.	Small for dates baby.

CENTRAL MIDWIVES BOARD (ENGLAND)

Write a short account of the following:

The outlet of the bony pelvis.	Breast changes in pregnancy.
Engagement of the fetal head.	Episiotomy.
Dangers of prematurity.	The dangers of the fifth and subsequent pregnancies.

Write short notes on:

Fetal Distress.	Hæmorrhagic disease of the newborn.	Lanugo.
Phenylketonuria.	Congenital dislocation of the hips.	Caput succedaneum.
Moulding.	Hydramnios.	

Write short notes on:

The use of pethidine in labour.	The detection of fetal distress.	Glycosuria in pregnancy.
Engorgement of the breasts.	Engagement of the fetal head.	Puerperal pyrexia.
Bleeding from the umbilical cord.	Varicose veins in pregnancy.	Postmaturity.
Vomiting in late pregnancy.	Heartburn in pregnancy.	
Auscultation of the fetal heart.	Engagement of the fetal head.	Œdema in pregnancy.
Blood tests in pregnancy.	Care of the umbilical cord.	Maternal distress.
The use of either Ergometrine or Syntometrine.		

Write brief notes on:

Placental insufficiency.
Suppression of lactation.
Fetal distress.
Puerperal psychosis.

Clothing in pregnancy.
Anæmia in pregnancy.
Entonox.
Rhesus incompatibility.

Weight gain in pregnancy.
Morning sickness.

Write brief notes on:

Varicose veins.
Diet in labour.
Indications for obtaining a catheter specimen of urine.

Vitamins in pregnancy.
Demand feeding.

The use of Syntometrine.
Congenital dislocation of the hip.
" After pains."

Write short notes on:

Congenital dislocation of the hip.
Deep transverse arrest.
Retained Placenta.
Polyhydramnios.

Moulding of the fetal head.
Gastro-enteritis in the newborn infant.
Involution of the uterus.
Treatment of the umbilical cord after delivery.

Ophthalmia neonatorum.
Prematurity.
Thrombophlebitis.

Write short notes on:

Treatment of asphyxia pallida.
Blood tests in pregnancy.
Infection of the stump of the umbilical cord.
Causes of a baby failing to gain weight in the first week of life.

Accidental hæmorrhage.
Third degree tear of the perineum.
Prodromal (warning) symptoms of eclampsia.

Rubella in pregnancy.
Postpartum hæmorrhage.

Write brief notes on:

Suppression of lactation.
Weight gain in pregnancy.
Antepartum hæmorrhage.

Lower uterine segment.
Perinatal mortality.
Transverse lie.

Ovulation.
Missed abortion.

Define the following:

Hæmolytic disease of the newborn.
Involution of the uterus.

Hæmorrhagic disease of the newborn.
Inversion of the uterus.

Transverse lie.
Deep transverse arrest.

Write definition of:

Pre-eclamptic toxæmia.
Engagement of the fetal head.

Puerperal pyrexia
Hæmolytic disease of the newborn.

Antepartum hæmorrhage.
A stillbirth.

Write short answers to each part of the question.

Describe the umbilical cord.
Give the average diameters of the normal
female pelvic brim.

What hormones are produced by the ovaries ?
What do you understand by the brim of the pelvis ?

Write not more than 100 words on each of the following:

Syntometrine.   Melæna neonatorum.   Pethidine.   Corpus luteum.   Cephalhæmatoma.
The causes of neonatal jaundice.   Neonatal cold syndrome.   Colostrum.

Write brief answers to these questions.

What do you mean by involution of the uterus ?
What are the causes of vaginal discharge in pregnancy ?

What are the signs of fetal distress ?
What is meant by a " dysmature baby " ?

Write notes on:

What are the anatomical relations of the vagina ?
What are the diameters of the fetal skull and why is the vertex the most favourable presentation ?

What are the functions of the placenta ?

Write briefly about:

What do you understand by polarity of the uterus ?
The differentiation between a caput succedaneum and a cephalhæmatoma.
Explain the reasons for taking blood samples in pregnancy.
The reasons why pregnant women frequently become " out of breath ".

The lower uterine segment.

Write short notes on:

    What are now the main causes of maternal mortality in England and Wales ?

    What blood samples should be taken after the delivery of the first baby of a Rhesus negative woman ?

    How would you recognize deep vein thrombosis during pregnancy ?

CENTRAL MIDWIVES BOARD (SCOTLAND)

Write short answers to each part of this question.

    Which hormone forms the basis of pregnancy diagnosis tests and what instructions would you give to a patient asked to collect urine for such a test ?

    Why is sugar often found in the urine of pregnant women ?

    What tissues are divided in a medio-lateral episiotomy ?

    What is an " incompetent cervix " ?   What history would lead you to suspect this condition ?

Write short notes on:

    Cephalhæmatoma.   Ophthalmia neonatorum.   Physiological jaundice.

         Quickening.   Binovular twins.   True knot in the umbilical cord.

         Meconium.   Anencephaly.   Colostrum.   Hydramnios.

Write short notes on the following:

         Weight gain in pregnancy.   Induction of labour.   Cephalhæmatoma.

  Battledore placenta.   Hydrops Fetalis.   Suppression of lactation.   Fetal distress.

Write notes on:

         Maternal distress in labour.   Hæmolytic disease in the newborn.

         Diagonal conjugate.   The significance of varicosities.

         Megaloblastic anæmia.   Inversion of the uterus.

                 Retained placenta.

Write notes on:

    Anuria.   Cephalhæmatoma.   Pigmentation in pregnancy.   Anencephaly.

Write notes on:

    Mid-stream specimen of urine.   Cervical cytology.   Pregnancy tests.

         The care of the umbilical cord.   Induction of labour.

Write notes on:

  Battledore placenta.   Uniovular twins.   Hydramnios.   Melæna neonatorum.

  Œsophageal atresia.   Uterine souffle.   Incompetent cervix.   Lochial discharges.

Define the following terms:

  Hydramnios   Placenta succenturiata.   Placenta accreta.   Incomplete abortion.

     Diagonal conjugate.   Perinatal mortality.   Extra-uterine gestation.

         Hydatidiform Mole.   Engagement of fetal head.

Write short notes on the following:

    Quickening.   Missed abortion.   Exchange transfusion in the newborn.

    Velamentous insertion of the cord.   Third degree tear.   Lochia.

    Pigmentation in pregnancy.   Sagittal suture.

  What is Apgar scoring ?   Define inevitable abortion.   What is meant by " attitude " of the fetus ?

  Enumerate the possible dangers to the infant following a breech delivery.   Define disproportion.

Write notes on:

    How may œdema be recognised in pregnancy ?   What is kernicterus and what are its causes ?

    What is neonatal hypothermia (cold injury) ?   Give the indications for episiotomy.

    Define presentation.   Name the bones which form the pelvis.

    Define a third degree tear (complete tear).   Give the positive (absolute) signs of pregnancy.

    What conditions may cause discharge during pregnancy ?   Give the definition of a stillbirth.

Write short notes on:

Œsophageal atresia. Brandt-Andrews manœuvre. Quickening.
Perinatal mortality. Umbilical cord. Episiotomy.
Uterine souffle. Trichomonas vaginitis. Neonatal hypothermia.

Write notes on:

How would you recognise Down's syndrome ? Define the term "position of the fetus".
What is a placenta succenturiata ? Describe the anterior fontanelle.
Differentiate between caput succedaneum and cephalhæmatoma.

Write short notes on:

Abruptio placentae. The lie of the fetus. Suppression of lactation. Cervical cytology.
The Guthrie test (Phenylketonuria). Blood pressure in pregnancy.

Define:

The vertex. The puerperium. Second stage of labour. Placenta velamentosa. Meconium.
Stillbirth. Internal rotation. Engagement of the head. Antepartum hæmorrhage.
Spalding's sign. Second stage of labour. Hydatidiform mole. Exomphalos.
C.M.B. Rule B. 11(h) (regarding frequency of antenatal visits).

Define the following:

Moulding of the fetal head. Neonatal mortality. Adoption order.
" At risk " register. Cord presentation. Ectopic pregnancy.
Meconium. Vasa prævia. Episiotomy. Show.

What is the Central Midwives Board for Scotland? Give the Rules of the Board relating to:

Intention to Practise (Rule B.4). Name and address (Rule B.5). Antenatal visits (Rule B.11(h)).
Second stage of labour (Rule B.13(b)). Baby's temperature (Rule B.16).

Define the following terms:

Mento-vertical diameter. Involution of the uterus. Restitution.
Retraction ring. Incompetent cervix.

Glossary

OF TERMS AND OBSTETRICAL CONDITIONS

ACARDIAC. Without a heart. An imperfectly formed fetus, sometimes consisting of the lower half of the trunk and lower extremities only, an acardiac acephalic (*without a head*) monster. It is one of monozygotic twins which has been deprived of its proper share of placental blood by the other well-developed twin. The one heart supplies both fetuses with blood, the cord from the healthy fetus bifurcating and entering the umbilicus of the imperfect fetus.

ACID-BASE BALANCE. The degree of acidity or alkalinity of the blood is governed by the amount of acid or bicarbonate present in the blood. This is reflected in the pH which rises in alkalæmia and falls in acidæmia.

Changes in the acid-base balance of fetal and neonatal blood are measured by the Astrup Micro-Equipment, *e.g.* when fetal distress or respiratory distress syndrome is present. This is essential prior to undertaking chemical correction by the administration of fructose and sodium bicarbonate.

ACCOUCHEMENT. Parturition, childbirth.

ACCOUCHEUSE. A female obstetrician, a midwife.

ACIDOSIS, METABOLIC. This condition is more serious than respiratory acidosis. The hypoxic cells produce lactic acid and a base deficit occurs. In respiratory distress syndrome there is combined respiratory and metabolic acidosis.

ACIDOSIS, RESPIRATORY. When the fetus is unable to excrete carbon dioxide, carbonic acid is produced in the blood so the pH falls (see pH).

ADNEXA. Appendages or adjacent parts; *e.g.* of the uterus.
The term " tenderness in the adnexa " is sometimes used when, on vaginal examination, tenderness is elicited on palpating the Fallopian tubes, ovaries or parametrium.

ANTE-. Prefix, meaning " before " or " in front of," *e.g.* antenatal, before birth; anteflexion of uterus, a uterus which bends forwards.

ARTIFICIAL INSEMINATION. A method of impregnation by means other than that of sexual intercourse; semen being introduced into the cervical canal by the use of a syringe and intra-uterine cannula. Donor semen may be used when the husband is sterile and the woman potentially fertile, but in such a case both husband and wife must sign an affidavit, indicating that they are fully aware of what is being done and that donor semen is being employed. The legal, moral and ethical objections to this procedure limit its practice.

ATRESIA. Closure or absence of a usual opening or canal; *e.g.* œsophageal atresia.

AUTOSOME. The chromosomes not concerned with sex determination are known as autosomes. The human cell has 22 pairs of autosomes and one pair of sex chromosomes.

AXIS-TRACTION. Used when pulling on the fetal head in the direction of the axis of the pelvic canal. For this purpose midwifery forceps are used, with a special axis-traction handle which permits alteration in the direction of pull, according to whether the head is in high or mid-cavity.

BAPTISM OF INFANTS. **This religious rite signifies entry into the Church** and is generally accompanied by name-giving. The ritual consists in the " pouring on " (*the baby's head*) of water at the same time saying: " I baptize thee in the name of the Father and of the Son and of the Holy Ghost."

A midwife may in an emergency be required to baptize a newborn infant whose condition is poor and who is likely to die. This is especially necessary when the family belong to the Roman Catholic church. Every effort should be made in such circumstances to summon the priest in time to perform the ceremony, but if this is not possible an adult Roman Catholic, in preference to a Protestant, should baptize a Roman Catholic baby. The fact that it is not essential to give the baby a name should be kept in mind. In hospital, during the night and in the absence of relatives a mother may be very upset if wakened and requested to state the baby's Christian name. She would no doubt suspect the reason why.

BI- *or* BIS-. **Prefix, meaning " two " ;** *e.g.* bi-manual, two hands, as in bi-manual examination of the pelvic organs, bi-manual compression of uterus ; bi-polar, two poles or extremities, as in bi-polar version ; bis-acromial diameter, the measurement between the two acromion processes.

BIFID. **Cleft, divided in two ;** *e.g.* spina-bifida.

BILIRUBIN. The orange pigment of bile. This gives the yellow tint to the skin and conjunctiva in cases of jaundice. The serum bilirubin test is carried out on the blood of babies suffering from icterus neonatorum.

BIOLOGY. **The science of life and of living things ;** *e.g.* biological pregnancy tests are those carried out by using animals such as the mouse, or toad as test animals.

BIOPSY. **Examination of tissue from the living body ;** *e.g.* from the cervix in cases of suspected carcinoma ; from the endometrium in cases of sterility.

BOHN'S NODULES. **Small white nodules,** having no significance, seen on the centre of the palate of the newborn. They may be present during the first few days of life and disappear spontaneously. Sometimes they are mistaken for thrush, which does not appear till after the fourth day.

BREAST-PUMP. **An appliance with glass funnel and rubber bulb,** used to extract milk from the lactating breast by suction ; it is worked either by hand or electricity.

CARDINAL LIGAMENTS. **The transverse cervical ligaments of the uterus (Mackenrodt's ligaments).**

CAUL. **A cap. This is the part of the amnion which covers the child's face when it is born with the amnion intact.**

-CELE. **Suffix, meaning a " tumour,"** usually one containing fluid ; *e.g.* cystocele, a protrusion of the bladder into the vagina ; meningocele, a tumour containing cerebro-spinal fluid.

CENTRAL VENOUS PRESSURE. **This is the pressure in the right cardiac atrium.** Measuring the central venous pressure is of value, when blood is being given rapidly by intravenous transfusion, as a guide (*a*) to avoid over-loading the heart, (*b*) in assessing the amount of blood required to restore the patient's blood volume to a value within the normal range, *i.e.* 5 to 12 cm. of water.

A radio opaque intra-cath is inserted through an arm or neck vein and passed into the superior vena cava. It is connected to the drip transfusion at a 3 way stop cock to which the venous manometer tubing is also attached. The strip of self adhesive tape with cm. scale is placed behind the manometer tubing; both being suspended from the pole of the I.V. stand.

41

The patient is positioned so that the level of her right atrium will correspond to zero on the manometer scale. By changing the stop-cock setting the infusion fluid will enter, and rise in, the manometer tubing. When a level of approximately 20 cm. has been reached the fluid in the manometer tubing is now connected through the stop-cock to the intra-cath. The level slowly falls and when it stabilizes the level is read from the cm. scale behind the manometer tubing which registers the measurement of the central venous pressure. A pressure of 10 cm. is usually aimed at.

CIRCUMCISION. **Excision of part of the prepuce or foreskin,** to allow it to be drawn back over the glans for the purpose of adequate cleansing of the part. This procedure is no longer recommended as a routine measure. Circumcision is a religious rite among Jewish people, being performed by the Mohel on the eighth day, if the health of the child permits.

CLIMACTERIC. **The change of life or menopause**

COLPOS. **The vagina;** *e.g.* colporrhaphy, suturing of the vagina; hæmatocolpos, collection of blood in the vagina, due to imperforate hymen or atresia of the vagina.

CRANIOTABES. **A condition characterized by thinning of the bones of the vault of the skull,** due to the failure of ossification. This is most common in premature babies, due to rapid growth and an insufficient supply of Vitamin D and calcium to meet the greater need. It is also an early sign of rickets. On applying pressure along the suture lines, the thin bone can be dented.

CYESIS. **Pregnancy;** *e.g.* pseudocyesis, a phantom or false pregnancy.

CYTOLOGY. **The study of tissue cells.** From desquamated fetal cells found in amniotic fluid, obtained by abdominal amniocentesis, the sex and maturity of the fetus can be determined. Chromosomal abnormalities, *e.g.* trisomy 21, as in Down's syndrome, can be detected. Cervical epithelial cells obtained by Papanicolaou smear are examined for the recognition of early cancer of the cervix.

DECIDUAL CAST. **The decidua, triangular in shape, when it is shed intact from the uterus, as occurs in some cases of tubal pregnancy.** The decidua is, however, usually passed in shreds.

DOLICHOCEPHALY. **A head which is long from front to back.** This is believed by some authorities to be a cause of face presentation; others consider dolichocephaly to be due to the moulding resultant from the extended head.

DOMICILIARY MIDWIFERY. **The delivery of women in their own homes** (either by doctors or midwives).

DUHRSSEN'S INCISIONS. **Incisions of the cervix, occasionally made in cases of extremely slow dilatation of the os,** to facilitate delivery of the child. Three incisions are usually made when the os is 6–7 cm. dilated.

ECTOMY. **Suffix, meaning " cutting out,"** *e.g.* hysterectomy, removal of the uterus.

ECTOPIA VESICÆ. **A congenital defect in which the bladder is exposed abdominally** and urine oozes from it. The treatment is transplantation of the ureters into the rectum.

ELECTROLYTE. **A substance which in solution is capable of conducting an electric current and is decomposed by it,** *e.g.* sodium, chloride, potassium, bicarbonate.

ENDO-. **Prefix, meaning " within " or " lining ";** *e.g.* endometrium, membrane lining the uterus.

EPISPADIAS. **A congenital malformation, in which the urethra opens in the upper surface of the penis.** Plastic repair is usually carried out. (*See also* Hypospadias).

EPITHELIOMA. A cancerous growth of epithelial tissue; *e.g.* squamous epithelioma of the cervix; chorionepithelioma, a malignant tumour derived from chorionic elements, commonly found in the uterine epithelium, and usually following hydatidiform mole.

ERYTHROBLASTOSIS FETALIS. A condition in which there are immature erythrocytes in the blood-stream of the newborn. This is the body's response to excessive destruction of red cells by hæmolysis, *e.g.* due to Rh incompatibility.

EUTOCIA. Easy, natural labour and delivery.

EX-. Prefix, meaning " out of "; *e.g.* exogenous source of puerperal sepsis, organisms introduced from " without " into the vagina; exomphalos, protrusion of the intestines out of the umbilicus (or omphalos).

EXTRA-UTERINE PREGNANCY. A pregnancy occurring outside the uterus; *e.g.* tubal, abdominal. (*See also* Ectopic gestation, p. 149.)

FECUNDATION. Impregnation or conception. (*See also* Superfecundation.)

FETATION. Impregnation or conception. (*See also* Superfetation.)

FONTANELLE. A little fountain. The membranous space at the junction of two or more sutures in the fetal skull. It was so named because, in days prior to the discovery of the circulation of blood, the pulsation felt suggested the bubbling of a small fountain.

GALACTAGOGUE. An agent or substance which stimulates the production of milk.

GAMMA GLOBULIN. Plasma proteins are divided into 4 main groups: albumin and the alpha, beta and gamma globulins. It is in the gamma globulin fraction that man carries his antibodies.

GANGLION. A semi-independent nervous centre from which nerves radiate; *e.g.* the paracervical ganglion, a sheath of nerves, situated behind and on either side of the cervix, also known as Frankenhäuser's plexus.

GENE. The genetic molecule or unit present in the chromosomes of the ovum and spermatozoon, which transmits the inherited factors or characteristics of the parents.

GENITALIA. The organs of generation; the external and internal genital organs.

GENOTYPE. The type characteristic of the species. This term is used when investigating paternal blood in cases of Rh incompatibility when the father's genotype may be Rh positive homozygous or Rh positive heterozygous.

GESTATION. Pregnancy; *e.g.* ectopic gestation.

GONAD. A reproductive gland; *e.g.* the ovary in the female, the testis in the male.

GONADOTROPHIC. The term used to describe a substance which stimulates the gonads; *e.g.* the follicle-stimulating hormone and the luteinizing hormone of the anterior pituitary gland.

GRAM-NEGATIVE. The term applied to bacteria which do not retain the stain when acted upon by Gram's iodine solution. The gonococcus is Gram-negative.

GRAVID. Pregnant; *e.g.* retroverted gravid uterus.

GRAVIDARUM. Meaning " of pregnant women "; *e.g.* hyperemesis gravidarum.

HÆM-. Prefix, meaning " blood "; *e.g.* hæmaturia, blood in the urine   hæmolysis, breaking-down of red blood cells.

HÆMATOCRIT. Expresses the percentage volume of red corpuscles in uncoagulated whole blood. It is used as a screening test for anæmia and in following the course of water and electrolyte disorders. Normal 50 to 60 per cent.

HERMAPHRODITISM. A condition in which the generative organs of both sexes are present. True hermaphroditism is exceedingly rare in human beings and pseudo-

41A

hermaphroditism is more commonly of the male type. The penis is small, the testes are present but undescended, and the scrotum being divided into two halves resembles the labia majora.

In the female type the clitoris is enlarged and resembles the penis, the labia may be adherent and contain the ovaries, thereby giving the appearance of male genitalia. The midwife must always examine the external genital organs carefully, prior to stating the sex, and in cases of doubt must obtain medical advice before making any pronouncement or filling up forms.

HERPES GESTATIONIS. **A skin disease affecting pregnant women and characterized by the appearance of papules, vesicles and pustules** which may extend over the whole body. The patient suffers from itching and burning which may cause insomnia. This rare condition is considered to be toxic in origin and may recur in subsequent pregnancies.

HETEROZYGOUS. **Having an inherited characteristic in which the zygotes are composed of diverse elements.** The term is applied in cases of Rh incompatibility, to describe the genotype of an Rh positive father. The positive heterozygous man has inherited an Rh negative gene from one of his parents and an Rh positive gene from the other. The genes in his spermatozoa may therefore be either negative or positive. If negative, the fetus will also be negative, and consequently there will be no incompatibility with the Rh negative mother. If positive, the fetus will also be positive, and there may be incompatibility with the Rh negative mother.

HEYN'S APPARATUS FOR ABDOMINAL DECOMPRESSION. **This apparatus, a fibre-glass dome, is placed over the abdomen, and is used to reduce the pain of labour.**

Negative pressure is produced by withdrawing the air from the dome. The abdominal wall rises about 15 cm. 6 inches) within the dome and by removing the pressure of the tense abdominal wall during contractions markedly reduces pain. **The apparatus is utilized when labour is established** and removed when the os is fully dilated. About 50 per cent of the women require pethidine, 100 mg.

HIRSUTES. **An abnormal growth of hair,** the term usually being applied to a female with the male distribution of hair.

HOME HELP SERVICES. **Each local authority is required to make provision for a home help service.** Social workers or health visitors usually make the necessary arrangements and a charge can be made for the service, which is available for illness, the ailing elderly, maternity cases and the welfare of young children. The home help attends for a number of hours during week days or as directed by the local authority.

HOMOZYGOUS. **Having an inherited characteristic in which the zygotes are composed of the same type of elements.** The term is applied in cases of Rh incompatibility to describe the genotype of an Rh positive father. The positive homozygous man has inherited an Rh positive gene from each of his parents. The genes in his spermatozoa will all be positive, the fetus will also be positive and there may be incompatibility with the Rh negative mother.

HUHNER'S POST-COITAL TEST. **This test is carried out in cases of infertility, to assess the number and activity of the spermatozoa.** The woman reports for examination within a few hours after coitus, and the seminal fluid in the posterior fornix is examined microscopically. The spermatozoa in this fluid and in the cervical canal are scrutinized.

HYDRO-. **Prefix, meaning " water ";** *e.g.* hydrocephaly, water in the ventricles of the brain ; hydræmia, a watery condition of the blood such as occurs normally during pregnancy.

HYDRORRHŒA GRAVIDARUM. **A condition in which, during the later months of pregnancy, there is a discharge from the uterus of clear fluid which may persist intermittently.** The fluid may be liquor amnii which escapes, owing to the rupture of the amniotic sac, at a high level. It may also be due to inflammation of the decidual glands, and in such cases there is pain in the lower abdomen.

HYPO-. **Prefix, meaning " under ";** *e.g.* hypotonic uterus, one which has poor tone

HYPOSPADIAS. A congenital malformation, in which the urethra opens in the under surface of the penis; in severe cases the opening is in the perineum. Plastic repair is usually carried out.

HYPOVOLÆMIA. Low or decreased blood volume.

ICHTHYOSIS (congenital). **A skin disease in which scales or plaques of smooth, dry, horny skin peel off,** the whole body being involved. Numerous fissures run between the plaques. The normal skin folds are obliterated and ectropion (eversion) of the eyelids is present. Such severe cases are fatal. Recovery may take place in mild forms of the disease which sometimes occur after birth.

IMMUNOGLOBULIN. A serum protein that is produced in response to an antigen and reacts specifically to it.

IMPACTION. **Tight wedging; jamming of one object inside another;** *e.g.* impaction of breech, face or shoulder (*presentation*) in the pelvic canal.

IMPETIGO HERPETIFORMIS GRAVIDARUM. **A dangerous form of impetigo, affecting pregnant women.** Pustules appear on the trunk and thighs; the temperature is raised; vomiting, delirium and grave prostration ensue. Injections of blood-serum from a normal pregnant woman have been given with varying degrees of success. The mortality rate is high, but, fortunately, the disease is rare.

INDICATING POINT. **The denominator or part of the presentation that indicates the position of the fetus** in relation to the six areas of the mother's pelvis.

INIENCEPHALY. **A fetus with a protrusion of the brain in the occipital region.**

INTER-. **Prefix, meaning " between ";** *e.g.* intertuberischial diameter, the distance between the inner borders of the ischial tuberosities.

INTRA-. **Prefix, meaning " within ";** *e.g.* intracranial hæmorrhage, bleeding within the skull; intrapartum eclampsia when the condition occurs during labour.

INTRA-LIGAMENTOUS PREGNANCY. **This occurs when the Fallopian tube ruptures and the fetus continues to develop within the folds of the broad ligament.**

ISO-IMMUNIZATION. **This has been defined as the process whereby antibodies are formed in an individual in response to the injection of an antigen from another individual of the same species,** *e.g.* Rhesus negative mother immunized by the antigens in the red cells of her Rh positive fetus or by the antigens in the red cells in a transfusion of Rh positive blood (inadvertently) given to her.

KLUGE'S SIGN OF PREGNANCY. **Varicosities of the veins in the region of the vaginal orifice.**

KLUMPKE'S PARALYSIS. **The forearm and hand are affected, due to injury of the lower part of the brachial plexus.** It is less common than Erb's paralysis in which the upper part of the brachial plexus is injured and the upper arm affected.

KORSAKOFF'S SYNDROME. (*A syndrome is a collection of symptoms.*) **This consists of the mental changes seen in cases of polyneuritis,** characterized by confusion, delirium and loss of memory. Symptoms similar to those of Korsakoff's syndrome are seen in serious cases of hyperemesis gravidarum.

KYPHOTIC PELVIS. When there is kyphosis (*angular curvature of the spine*) in the lumbar region, the misdirected body-weight causes a narrowing of the pelvis from side to side, particularly at the outlet. The deformity of hump-back is obvious in such a case. Cæsarean section is indicated.

LYSIS. A breaking down; *e.g.* hæmolysis, breaking down of red blood cells. This may occur in the fetal blood, due to Rh incompatibility.

MAL-. Prefix, meaning " bad "; *e.g.* malpresentation, such as breech, face, brow, shoulder; malposition, such as right and left occipito-posterior, right and left mento-posterior; malformation, such as cleft lip.

MATERNAL MORBIDITY RATE. This is the percentage of women whose postpartum temperature is raised to a level notifiable in Scotland as puerperal pyrexia or puerperal sepsis—It also includes any condition which impairs health or endangers life, and is always higher in hospitals to which unbooked obstetrical emergencies or booked complicated cases are admitted.

MENARCHE. The initial onset of menstruation.

MICRO-. Prefix, meaning " small "; *e.g.* microcephaly, a very small head; microcytic hypochromic anæmia, in which the red blood cells are small.

MISCARRIAGE. The word is synonymous with the word " abortion." Patients prefer the term " miscarriage " and use it to describe a spontaneous abortion : they associate the word " abortion " with criminal induction.

MICROGNATHIA. Because the mandible is poorly developed the lower jaw and chin recede. The baby should not lie on his back as the tongue may fall backwards and block the larynx.

MULTIGRAVIDA. Multi, meaning " more than one "; gravida, meaning " pregnant." A woman who has been pregnant more than once is a multigravida.

MULTIPARA. Multi, meaning " more than one "; parere, meaning " to bear." A woman who has borne more than one child is a multipara. A primigravida, having borne no child, is designated as para 0, a woman pregnant for the second time as para 1.

NATES. The buttocks. The natal cleft, the furrow between the buttocks.

NEO-. Prefix, meaning " new "; *e.g.* neonatal, the newborn; neoplasm, a new growth, a term usually applied to one that is malignant.

NULLIPARA. A woman who has not given birth to a child.

-OMA. Suffix, meaning " tumour "; *e.g.* carcinoma, tumour of malignant origin; fibroma, tumour of fibrous and muscle tissue.

-ORRHAPHY. Suffix, meaning " suturing of "; *e.g.* perineorrhaphy, suturing of perineum; trachelorrhaphy, suturing of cervix.

-OTOMY. Suffix, meaning " incision of " or " cutting into "; *e.g.* hysterotomy, cutting into the uterus.

PARA-. Prefix, meaning " alongside of " or " near "; *e.g.* parametrium, the connective tissue surrounding the uterus; parametritis, inflammation of the parametrium; paracervical nerve block.

PATHIC. Meaning " pertaining to disease "; *e.g.* pathogenic or disease-producing organisms; neonatal pathology, science of disease of the newborn.

PCO_2. This symbol denotes the pressure of carbon dioxide in the blood; normal being approx. 40 mm. Hg. In cases of respiratory acidosis the PCO_2 is raised.

PO$_2$ is the symbol for the pressure of oxygen in the blood, normal being approx. 100 mm. Hg in arterial blood. Levels below 70 mm. denote serious oxygen lack.

pH. **This is the symbol for expressing acidity or alkalinity.** The normal pH of the blood is 7·35 to 7·4. When the fetus is hypoxic the increased acid produced raises the acidity of the blood and the pH falls. When below 7·3 the fetus is at risk and its condition vigilantly monitored: if 7·20 or below, immediate delivery is essential; 6·9 could be fatal.

PHENYLKETONURIA. The Guthrie test for phenylalanine in the blood is the most efficient method available, 1-10,000 are positive; one drop of blood obtained by heel prick is dripped on to filter paper and dried, the test being done not before the 6th day of life and not after 14 days. Early dietary therapy prevents mental retardation.

PLACENTA MEMBRANACEA. **A thin layer of placental tissue, covering the whole of the amniotic sac** instead of being confined to one area. The condition is very rare.

POLY-. **Prefix, meaning " much " or " many ";** polyhydramnios, excessive liquor amnii; polydactyly, having supernumerary fingers or toes.

PRE-. **Prefix, meaning " before ";** *e.g.* prenatal, before birth; premonitory sign, a forewarning.

PREVIABLE BABY. **One of less than 28 weeks' gestation** and 1,134 G. (2½ lb.) in weight.

PRIMIGRAVIDA. **Gravida, meaning " pregnant."** A woman pregnant for the first time.

PRIMIPARA. **Parere, meaning " to bear."** A woman giving birth to a child for the first time. During pregnancy she is para 0. The author saw a patient, pregnant for the thirteenth time (*a case of habitual abortion*) give birth to her first baby. She was a primipara although a multigravida.

PRONE POSITION. **Lying face downwards;** *e.g.* semi-prone position as used in eclampsia.

PROSTAGLANDINS. **The prostaglandins, mainly group E,** have been used with success to induce labour at term. Intravenous infusion is usual as the oral route gives rise to vomiting. The substance which is derived from semen, is now being produced in a chemical synthetic form which will no doubt be available when trials are completed and approved. Prostaglandins are also being tried for inducing missed and other abortions.

PTYALISM. **Excessive salivation.** A slight increase in salivation may occur during pregnancy, and in rare cases the excessive flow amounts to 1,000 ml. per day. The woman does not swallow the saliva, because of nausea, and with loss of appetite, impaired digestion and dehydration her nutrition suffers. Sleep is interfered with. The treatment is to give fluids, intravenously if necessary, also sedatives and astringent mouthwashes. The condition is rare and usually occurs during the first half of pregnancy, sometimes being associated with hyperemesis gravidarum.

PUBIOTOMY. **An operation previously performed in cases of contracted pelvis, now superseded by Cæsarean section.** One transverse ramus of the os pubis is divided with a Gigli saw to enlarge the pelvic brim. The baby is then born *per vaginam.*

PYO-. **Prefix, meaning " pus ";** *e.g.* pyosalpinx, pus in the Fallopian tube; pyonephrosis, pus in the kidney.

RADIO-ACTIVE FIBRINOGEN UPTAKE TEST. This is a technique used to detect early deep vein thrombosis in patients "at risk" i.e. age over 30, history of varicose veins or thrombosis. Radio-active fibrinogen is injected I.V. within 8 hours after delivery. It becomes incorporated in the thrombus and can be detected by an external scintillation counter.

RECTO-VAGINAL FISTULA. This is an artificial opening between the rectum and vagina which occurs most commonly when a sutured third degree perineal tear does not heal properly. It may be suspected by the midwife when fæces are seen on the perineal pad, usually on the third or fourth day postpartum. A gynæcologist will repair the fistula.

RETRO-. Prefix, meaning " behind " ; *e.g.* retroplacental clot, a clot lying behind the placenta, occurring in severe abruptio placentæ; retroversion, backward displacement (*of uterus*).

RINGER'S LACTATE SOLUTION. Dextrose anhydrous 25·0 G.; sod. lactate 1·2 ml.; sod. chlor. 3·0 G.; Pot. chlor. 0·2 G.; calcium chlor. 0·1 G.; water to 500 ml. administered I.V. in prolonged labour and in hæmorrhage until blood is available.

SIBLING. One of a group of children of the same parents.

SPONTANEOUS EVOLUTION. A process by which the fetus may be expelled in cases of shoulder presentation. This can only occur with a large pelvis and a small fetus, and mainly when it is premature or macerated. One arm and shoulder are forced down on to the pelvic floor and are stemmed under the pubic arch. The body, breech and limbs, in that order, are driven past the shoulder. The head is born last.

SPONTANEOUS EXPULSION. This process begins in a manner similar to spontaneous evolution, but is even more rare. The shoulder presents and the body becomes doubled up and driven through the pelvis in that attitude until the breech and legs escape; the shoulders and head are born last.

SPURIOUS PREGNANCY. An imaginary or phantom pregnancy. (*See under* Pseudocyesis, p. 74).

STRIDOR (congenital). This is characterized by a crowing inspiration. In the absence of cyanosis or other pathological sign, the condition may be due to a poorly developed larynx, small glottis or large epiglottis. The pædiatrician will diagnose the cause.

SUPERFECUNDATION. The fertilization of two ova during one intermenstrual period, at different acts of coitus, will result in dizygotic twins. There is no way of proving that superfecundation has occurred.

SUPERFETATION. The fertilization of two ova during different intermenstrual periods (*the first three months of pregnancy*). This is a very rare occurrence. The fact that one twin weighs 1,361 to 1,814 G. (3 to 4 lb.) more than the other is not diagnostic of superfetation. A fetus papyraceous is sometimes wrongly attributed to superfetation.

TERATOGEN. An agent, *i.e.* drug, organism, believed to cause congenital abnormalities, *e.g.* Thalidomide, rubella.

TRIMESTER. A period of three months. The nine months of pregnancy can be divided into three trimesters (*a*) The first, (*b*) second or mid, and (*c*) the third.

TRISOMY. A chromosome additional to the normal complement = 47 instead of 46. In Down's syndrome the extra chromosome is commonly Trisomy 21.

VAGITUS UTERINUS. The crying of the fetus *in utero*. If air is introduced into the fetal sac, or if gases develop and the fetus inspires these, it may emit sound during their expiration. Cases have been reported by reliable observers, in which the baby has been born alive a number of hours after " cries " had been heard. It is a rare phenomenon.

INDEX

Printed by T. & A. CONSTABLE LTD., Edinburgh